FLUIDS AND ELECTROLYTES
WITH CLINICAL APPLICATIONS

Online Services

Delmar Online
To access a wide variety of Delmar products
and services on the World Wide Web, point your
browser to:
       http://www.DelmarNursing.com
       or email: info@delmar.com

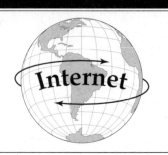

A service of **I**(**T**)**P**®

FLUIDS AND ELECTROLYTES
WITH CLINICAL APPLICATIONS

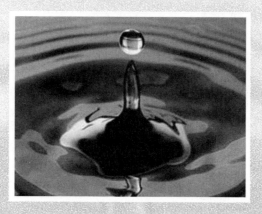

A Programmed Approach

Sixth Edition

Joyce LeFever Kee, RN, MS
Associate Professor Emerita
College of Health and Nursing Science
University of Delaware
Newark, Delaware

Betty J. Paulanka, RN, EdD
Dean and Professor
College of Health and Nursing Science
University of Delaware
Newark, Delaware

Delmar Publishers
an International Thomson Publishing company

Albany • Bonn • Boston • Cincinnati • Detroit • London • Madrid
Melbourne • Mexico City • New York • Pacific Grove • Paris • San Francisco
Singapore • Tokyo • Toronto • Washington

Notice to the Reader

Publisher does not warrant or guarantee any of the products described herein or perform any independent analysis in connection with any of the product information contained herein. Publisher does not assume, and expressly disclaims, any obligation to obtain and include information other than that provided to it by the manufacturer.

The reader is expressly warned to consider and adopt all safety precautions that might be indicated by the activities herein and to avoid all potential hazards. By following the instructions contained herein, the reader willingly assumes all risks in connection with such instructions.

The publisher makes no representation or warranties of any kind, including but not limited to, the warranties of fitness for particular purpose or merchantability, nor are any such representations implied with respect to the material set forth herein, and the publisher takes no responsibility with respect to such material. The publisher shall not be liable for any special, consequential, or exemplary damages resulting, in whole or part, from the readers' use of, or reliance upon, this material.

Cover Design: Scott Keidong's Image Enterprises

Delmar Staff

Publisher: William Brottmiller
Acquisitions Editor: Cathy L. Esperti
Developmental Editor: Patricia A. Gaworecki
Project Editor: Patricia Gillivan
Production Coordinator: Barbara A. Bullock
Art and Design Coordinator: Timothy J. Conners
Editorial Assistant: Darcy M. Scelsi

COPYRIGHT © 2000
By Delmar Publishers Inc.

an International Thomson Publishing company I(T)P®

The ITP logo is a trademark under license.
Printed in the United States of America

For more information, contact:

Delmar Publishers
3 Columbia Circle, Box 15015
Albany, New York 12212–5015
International Thomson Publishing Europe
Berkshire House 168–173
High Holborn
London, WC1V 7AA
England
Thomas Nelson Australia
102 Dodds Street
South Melbourne, 3205
Victoria, Australia
Nelson Canada
1120 Birchmount Road
Scarborough, Ontario
Canada, M1K 5G4

International Thomson Editores
Campos Eliseos 385, Piso 7
Col Polanco
11560 Mexico D F Mexico
International Thomson Publishing GmbH
Königswinterer Strasse 418
53227 Bonn
Germany
International Thomson Publishing Asia
60 Albert Street
#15–01 Albert Complex
Singapore 189969
International Thomson Publishing—Japan
Hirakawa-cho Kyowa Building, 3F
2–2–1 Hirakawa-cho
Chiyoda-ku, Tokyo 102
Japan

1 2 3 4 5 6 7 8 9 10 XXX 05 04 03 02 01 00 99

Library of Congress Cataloging-in-Publication Data
Kee, Joyce LeFever.
   Fluids and electrolytes with clinical applications: a programmed
approach / Joyce LeFever Kee, Betty J. Paulanka. — 6th ed.
      p.   cm.
   Includes bibliographical references and index.
   ISBN 0-7668-0332-5
   1. Body fluid disorders—Programmed instruction. 2. Water—electrolyte imbalances—Programmed instruction.
3. Body fluid disorders—Nursing—Programmed instruction. 4. Water—electrolyte imbalances—Nursing—
Programmed instruction. I. Paulanka, Betty J. II. Title.
      [DNLM: 1. Water-Electrolyte Imbalance—nursing programmed instruction. WY 18.2K26f 2000]
   RC630.K43 2000
   616.3'992'0077—dc21
   DNLM/DLC
   for Library of Congress   98-37022
                                                     CIP

Dedication

To
My Children—Eric, Katherine, and Wanda

Joyce LeFever Kee

To
My Children—Christie and Elaine

Betty J. Paulanka

Contents

UNIT II   FLUIDS AND THEIR INFLUENCE ON THE BODY / 30

UNIT VI   CLINICAL SITUATIONS: FLUID, ELECTROLYTE, AND ACID-BASE IMBALANCES / 338

Preface

Nurses and health professionals are involved continually in the assessment of fluid and electrolyte imbalance. Medical advances and new treatment modalities have increased the importance of a strong background in the physiologic concepts associated with these imbalances. Additionally, the expanded role of nurses in the community requires them to function more autonomously in assisting clients to control fluid and electrolyte imbalances. Every seriously or chronically ill person is likely to develop one or more of these imbalances, and the very young and the very old are especially vulnerable to changes in fluid and electrolyte balance. Even those who are only moderately ill are at high risk for these imbalances. Multiple health providers are responsible for maintaining homeostasis of fluid and electrolyte balance when caring for clients. After completing this book, the participant should understand more fully the effects of fluid, electrolyte, and acid-base balance and imbalance on the body as they occur in many clinical health problems.

New to This Edition

The sixth edition of this programmed text, *Fluids and Electrolytes with Clinical Applications,* has been completely revised to meet the current assessment, management, and clinical interventions recommended for fluid, electrolyte, and acid-base imbalances and related clinical health problems. The chapters include objectives, introduction, pathophysiology, etiology, clinical manifestations, clinical management, clinical applications, clinical considerations, case studies, and nursing diagnoses with clinical interventions, appropriate rationale, and evaluations. This new edition also includes:

- ▶ The reorganization of content into 6 units and 26 chapters helps set the foundation from simple to more complex fluid and electrolyte concepts.
- ▶ The design has been changed to make it more user friendly.
- ▶ Increased emphasis on evaluation and outcome for each chapter.
- ▶ The electrolytes sodium and chloride are presented as one chapter because of their close physiological relationship.
- ▶ Extensive revisions have been made for the chapters related to life-span issues in *Fluid Problems of Infants and Children* and *Fluid Problems of the Aging.*
- ▶ New summary charts, *Clinical Considerations,* for fluids and electrolytes, are included as quick reference sources for pertinent information related to the imbalance.
- ▶ A new chapter, *Chronic Diseases with Fluid and Electrolyte Imbalances,* contains the three common yet complex chronic health problems, congestive heart failure (CHF), diabetic ketoacidosis, and chronic obstructive pulmonary disease (COPD). This helps students learn how to apply multiple fluid and electrolyte concepts in complex situations.
- ▶ There are over 150 diagrams and tables. Many new tables and figures have been added for quick reference to pertinent information.
- ▶ There are five new appendices: (A) Clinical Pathways, (B) Summary of Acid-Base Imbalances, (C) Clinical Problems Associated with Fluid Imbalances, (D) Clinical Problems Associated with Electrolyte Imbalances, (E) Clinical Assessment Tool: Fluid, Electrolyte, and Acid-Base Imbalances, and (F) Foods Rich in Potassium, Sodium, Calcium, Magnesium, Chloride, and Phosphorus.

The content of this book has been geared to three levels of learning among the health professions. First, it is intended for beginning students who have had some background in the biological sciences or who have completed an anatomy and physiology course. Second, it is for students who have a sufficient background in the biological sciences, chemistry, and physics but who need to learn about intravenous therapy and specific clinical health problems that cause fluid and electrolyte imbalances. Many of these students might wish to review the entire text to reinforce their previous knowledge and/or practice their skills in handling clinical nursing assessments and interventions. Finally, this book is intended to aid graduate nurses who wish to review and improve their knowledge of fluid and electrolyte changes in order to assess their clients' needs and enhance the quality of client care. Summary charts have been included as quick reference sources for the working professionals.

What Is a Programmed Approach?

The programmed approach is a self-instructional method of learning that helps the instructor to use class time more efficiently, and enables students to work at their own pace while learning the principles, concepts, and applications of fluids and electrolytes.

Throughout, an asterisk (*) on an answer line indicates a multiple-word answer. The meanings for the following symbols are: ↑ increased, ↓ decreased, > greater than, < less than. A dagger (†) in tables indicates the most common signs and symptoms. A glossary covers words and terms used throughout the text. It should be useful to the student who has minimal preparation in the biological sciences.

Joyce LeFever Kee, RN, MS
Betty J. Paulanka, RN, EdD

Acknowledgments

For the sixth edition, we wish to extend our deepest appreciation to Ellen Boyda, Lisa Plowfield, Margaret R. Poppiti, Larry Purnell, Patricia H. Tagye, Gail Wade, Olga Ward, Julie Waterhouse, and Erlinda Wheeler for their contributions and assistance.

We especially wish to thank Don Passidomo, head librarian at the V.A. Medical Center, Wilmington, Delaware, for his valuable assistance and service and for the literature search on fluids and electrolytes.

We also offer our thanks to our editors Cathy L. Esperti and Patty Gaworecki at Delmar Publishers for their helpful suggestions and assistance with this revision.

Joyce LeFever Kee
Betty J. Paulanka

Contributors and Consultants

Ellen B. Boyda, RN, MS, CRNP
Family Nurse Practitioner
Pulmonary Clinical Nurse Specialist
Independent Practice
Boothywyn, PA
Unit 4 and 4 Chapters:
Acid-Base Balance

Linda Laskowski-Jones, RN, MS, CS, CCRN
Trauma Clinical Specialist
Trauma Service
Christiana Care Health Systems
Wilmington, Delaware
Trauma and Shock

Lisa Plowfield, RN, PhD
Assistant Professor
College of Health and Nursing Sciences
University of Delaware
Newark, Delaware
Increased Intracranial Pressure

Margaret R. Poppiti, RN, MS, CNN
Dialysis Center
V.A. Medical Center
Wilmington, Delaware
Renal Failure

Larry Purnell, RN, PhD
Associate Professor
College of Health and Nursing Sciences
University of Delaware
Newark, Delaware
Burns and Burn Shock

Patricia H. Tagye, RN
RCG Mainline Acute Dialysis Unit
Lankenau Hospital
Wynnwood, Pennsylvania
Hemodialysis and Peritoneal Dialysis

Gail H. Wade, RN, MS
Assistant Professor
College of Health and Nursing Sciences
University of Delaware
Newark, Delaware
Fluid Problems of Infants and Children

Olga Ward, RN
Parenteral Therapist
Christiana Care Health System
Wilmington, Delaware
Intravenous Therapy

Julie Waterhouse, RN, MS
Associate Professor
College of Health and Nursing Sciences
University of Delaware
Newark, Delaware
Clinical Oncology

Erlinda Wheeler, RN, PhD
Assistant Professor
College of Health and Nursing Sciences
University of Delaware
Newark, Delaware
Gastrointestinal Surgery

Reviewers

Sandra Cawley Baird, EdD, RN, CNS
Director, Professor
School of Nursing
University of Northern Colorado

Susanna Cunningham, BSN, MA, PhD
Associate Professor
University of Washington

Carol Della Ratta, RN, MS, CCRN
Clinical Assistant Professor
State University of New York at Stony Brook

David Derrico, RN, MSN
Assistant Clinical Professor
University of Florida

Deena B. Hollingsworth, RN, MSN
Assistant Professor
Marymount University

Helpful Suggestions from the Authors

To the Student

Many students believe that the subject of fluids and electrolytes is very difficult to comprehend. This programmed book provides you with important data on fluids and electrolytes from various points of view. If you apply this material to clinical problems and previous and present experiences, it is not so difficult to understand and retain.

By taking easy steps provided in this book, you can proceed through the chapters more quickly than you might expect. This book is written using a self-instruction format that allows you to proceed at your own speed. Each step is a learning process. A better quality of learning occurs when you either complete a chapter at a time or spend a minimum of two hours at one sitting. Never end the study period without at least completing all questions related to a single topic.

It is helpful to begin each study session with the final questions from the previous material; this enables you to check your retention of material that was presented previously. The case study reviews in each chapter give immediate reinforcement of the data learned. The assessment factors, diagnoses, and interventions should be useful when applying fluid, electrolyte, and acid-base concepts in various clinical settings. The six appendices act as a quick reference for obtaining data related to health problems of fluid and electrolyte imbalances. The clinical assessment tool is useful for determining fluid, electrolyte, and acid-base balance and imbalance. A glossary is included to assist you with words and terms used throughout the text.

Study each diagram and table before proceeding to the questions. If you make mistakes in the program, you need not be concerned so long as you rectify the mistakes. This learning modality and the content in this book should increase your knowledge and understanding of fluids and electrolytes. This model of learning can be a great asset for applying this knowledge to your clinical practicum experiences.

To the Instructor

Class time is frequently spent on reviewing material or presenting new material that can easily be given through programmed (learning) instruction. This method of instruction enables the teacher to minimize the time spent in lecture on fluids and electrolytes, thus devoting more time to clinical discussions and seminar format to enhance the students' understanding of fluid and electrolyte imbalance by active class participation.

You may find it helpful to cover the material in this book by one of three ways: (1) assigning the students a chapter at a time; (2) assigning a unit for the students to complete by a certain date; or (3) assigning the students a given length of time to complete the entire text and having them present material using their clinical experience.

Joyce LeFever Kee
Betty J. Paulanka

BODY FLUID AND ITS FUNCTION

OBJECTIVES

Upon completion of this unit, the reader should be able to:

- Compare the percentage of water found in the body of the average adult, newborn infant, and embryo.
- Identify the three compartments (spaces) where water is distributed in the body.
- Identify the two classifications of body fluid and their percentages.
- Describe five functions of body fluids.
- Define homeostasis in terms of its role in maintaining body fluid equilibrium.
- Describe how the body loses and maintains body fluid.
- Define the following homeostatic mechanisms: osmotic pressure, oncotic pressure, semipermeable membranes, selectively permeable membranes, osmol, and osmolality.
- Describe the effects of the above homeostatic mechanisms on the movement of body fluid.
- Describe four measurable pressures that determine the flow of fluid between the vessels and tissues in terms of their effects on the exchange of fluid.
- Describe the concept of a pressure gradient.
- Explain the significance in colloid osmotic (oncotic) and hydrostatic pressure gradients.
- Discuss the body's regulators of fluid balance.

(continued on next page)

OBJECTIVES (Continued)

● **Describe isotonic (iso-osmolar), hypotonic (hypo-osmolar), and hypertonic (hyperosmolar) solutions in terms of their effects on body cells.**

● **Discuss the relationship between milligrams and milliequivalents and the significance of this relationship in the body.**

● **Describe the effects of selected fluid changes on the observable symptoms of clients in your clinical area.**

▶ INTRODUCTION

The human body is a complex machine that contains hundreds of bones and the most sophisticated interaction of systems of any structure on earth. Yet, the substance that is basic to the very existence of the body is the simplest substance known—water. In fact, it makes up almost two-thirds of an adult's body weight.

The body is not static; it is alive, and solid particles within its framework are able to move into and out of cells and systems, and even into and out of the body, only because there is water.

The basis of all fluids is water, and as long as the quantity and composition of body fluids are within the normal range, we just take it for granted and enjoy being healthy. But if the water content of the body for some reason departs from this range, the whole delicate balance of body systems is disrupted, and disease can find an easy target.

An asterisk (*) on an answer line indicates a multiple-word answer. The meanings for the following symbols are: ↑ increased, ↓ decreased, > greater than, < less than.

Body Fluid, Its Function and Movement

CHAPTER

1

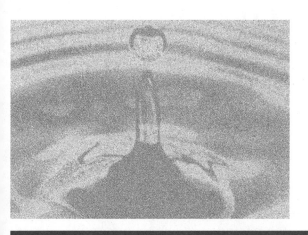

▶ INTRODUCTION

The greatest single constituent of the body is water. Body water movement and distribution are influenced by fluid intake, fluid pressures, and osmolality of the body fluid.

In this chapter, distribution of body fluids, fluid compartments, functions of body fluid, intake and output for homeostasis, definitions, fluid pressures, regulators of body fluid, and osmolality of body fluid and solutions are discussed. Also included are a case study review, assessment factors, diagnoses, interventions, and evaluation/outcome process.

1

The greatest single constituent of the body is water, which represents about 60% of the total body weight in the average adult, 45–55% of the older adult, 70–80% of a newborn infant, and 97% of the early human embryo.

Label the following drawings with the proper percentage of water to body weight.

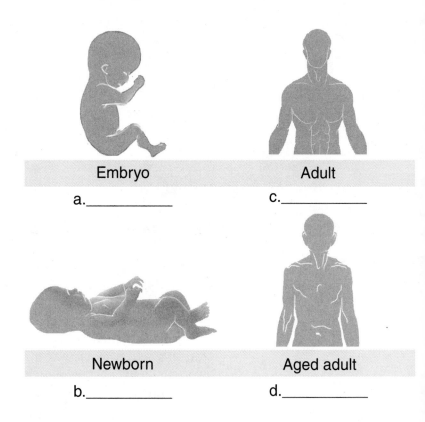

Embryo

a._____

Adult

c._____

Newborn

b._____

Aged adult

d._____

1   a. 97%; b. 77%; c. 60%; d. 54%

2

Which has the highest percentage of water in relation to body weight (adult, newborn infant, embryo, aged adult)? _____ Which has the lowest?_____

2   embryo; adult

3

Infants have a larger body surface area in relation to their weight, so extra water may act as a cushion against injury.

4

person weighing 125 pounds (lean)

5

a. cell; b. tissue space; c. blood vessel

3

Speculate why the early human embryo and the infant have a higher proportion of water to body weight than the adult.

*_____

_____

4

Because body fat is essentially free of water, the leaner the individual, the greater the proportion of water in total body weight.

　Who has more water as body weight, a person weighing 225 pounds or a person weighing 125 pounds? _____

▶ FLUID COMPARTMENTS

5

Body water is distributed among three types of "compartments": cells, blood vessels, and tissue spaces between blood vessels and cells that are separated by membranes.

　Label the three compartments where body water (fluid) is found.

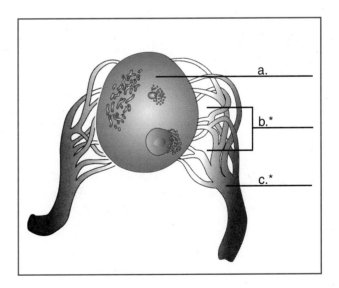

a. _____

b.* _____

c.* _____

6

The term for the water (fluid) in each type of "compartment" is as follows:

　　1. In the cell—*intracellular* fluid or *cellular* fluid

　　2. In the blood vessels—*intravascular* fluid

3. In tissue spaces between blood vessels and cells—
   interstitial fluid

Label the diagram with the proper terms for body water in each of the three compartments.

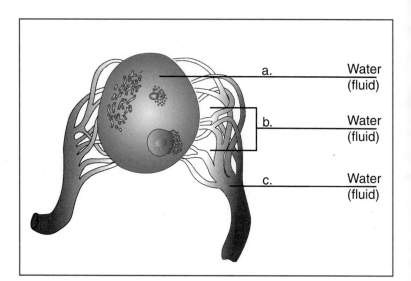

a. _____ Water (fluid)

b. _____ Water (fluid)

c. _____ Water (fluid)

6   a. intracellular; b. interstitial; c. intravascular

7

Fluid within the cell is classified as intracellular fluid, whereas intravascular fluid and interstitial fluid are classified as extracellular fluid.

The area within the cell is called the _____ space, whereas the tissue spaces between blood vessels and cells and the area within blood vessels are known as the _____ space.

7   intracellular; extracellular

8

Approximately two-thirds of the body fluid is contained in the intracellular compartment.

We have already said that the total body weight in the adult body is _____ % water; therefore, intracellular fluid must represent _____ % of the total body weight, and extracellular fluid represents _____ % of the total body weight.

8   60; 40; 20

9

If one-fourth of the extracellular fluid is intravascular fluid, then three-fourths of extracellular fluid is *_____ .

9   interstitial fluid

10

Therefore, extracellular fluid represents _____ % of the total body weight. Interstitial fluid represents _____ % of total body weight and intravascular fluid represents _____ % of total body weight.

10 20; 15; 5

▶ FUNCTIONS OF BODY WATER

The body is unable to maintain a healthy state without water. Five main functions of body water are listed in Table 1-1.

Table 1-1

Functions of Body Water

- Transportation of nutrients, electrolytes, and oxygen to the cells
- Excretion of waste products
- Regulation of body temperature
- Lubrication of joints and membranes
- Medium for food digestion

11

Name three of the five main functions of body water:

a. _____

b. _____

c. _____

11 Select three from the five functions listed in Table 1-1.

▶ INTAKE AND OUTPUT FOR HOMEOSTASIS

12

We already have learned that the percentage of body fluid varies with age and percentage of body fat. Then the proportion of intracellular and extracellular fluid in a person with more body fat would be (greater/lesser) _____ in proportion to body weight.

12 lesser

13

Homeostasis is a term used to describe the state of equilibrium of the internal environment. In relation to body fluids, homeostasis is the process of maintaining equilibrium or stability in relation to the physical and chemical properties of body fluid.

Explain the relationship of homeostasis to body fluid.

* _____

_____

14

The body normally maintains a state of equilibrium between the amount of water taken in and the amount of water lost. When body water is insufficient and the kidneys are functioning normally, urine volume diminishes and the individual becomes thirsty. Therefore, the client drinks more water to correct the fluid (excess/deficit) _____.

15

When we drink an excessive amount of water, our urinary output increases.

   a. If you did not drink any fluids or if the body loses excessive water, the urinary volume should (increase/decrease)

   _____ .

   b. If there were an excess of water in the body, the urinary volume would adapt by (increasing/decreasing)

   _____ .

16

The three normal sources of body water intake are * _____

_____

Refer to Figure 1-1.

17

The four avenues for daily water loss are * _____

_____ .

Refer to Figure 1-1.

18

If your water intake amounted to 2500 mL for the day and your water output was 2500 mL, your body has maintained a state of _____ of body fluid.

---

13 maintains equilibrium to the physical and chemical properties of body fluid

14 deficit

15 a. decrease; b. increasing

16 liquid, food, and oxidation of food

17 lungs, skin, urine, and feces

18 equilibrium or homeostasis

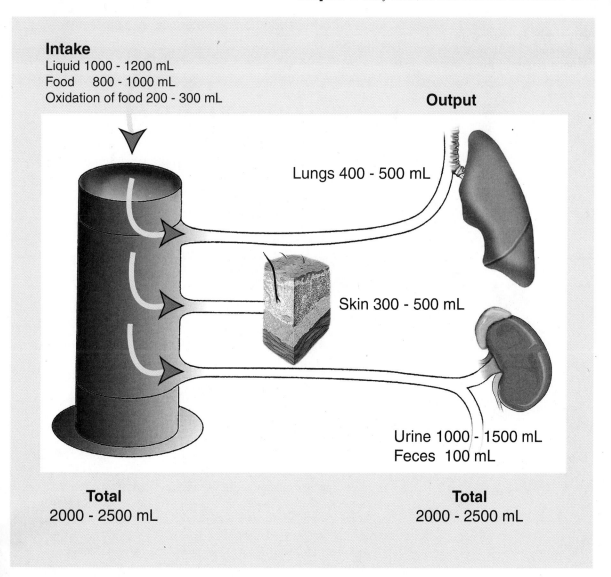

Intake
Liquid 1000 - 1200 mL
Food   800 - 1000 mL
Oxidation of food 200 - 300 mL

Output

Lungs 400 - 500 mL

Skin 300 - 500 mL

Urine 1000 - 1500 mL
Feces 100 mL

Total
2000 - 2500 mL

Total
2000 - 2500 mL

Figure 1-1 Normal pattern of water intake and loss.

---

19 When the summer atmospheric temperature is high, water loss via skin and lungs increases.

19
The rate of water loss and gain is different in summer and winter. Describe why you think this occurs. *_____

_____

20
Evaporation of water from the skin, as we perspire, is a protective mechanism against overheating the body.

20 It acts as a cooling system, keeping the body at a normal temperature.

Explain how evaporation of water acts as a protective mechanism. *_____

_____

▶ DEFINITIONS RELATED TO BODY FLUIDS

Definitions related to fluid movement are defined in Table 1-2. Questions that follow explain the physiologic terms that affect body fluid movement.

Table 1-2

Definitions Related to Fluid Functions and Movement

Membrane	A layer of tissue separating spaces or covering a surface or organ
Permeability	A capability of a substance, molecule, or ion to diffuse through a membrane
Semipermeable membrane	An artificial membrane such as cellophane membrane
Selectively permeable membrane	Permeability of the human membranes
Solvent	A liquid with a substance in solution
Solute	A substance dissolved in a solution
Osmosis	The passage of a solvent through a membrane from a solution of lesser solute concentration to one of greater solute concentration. *Note:* Osmosis may be expressed in terms of water concentration instead of solute concentration. Water molecules pass from an area of higher water concentration (fewer solutes) to an area of lower water concentration (more solutes).
Diffusion	The movement of molecules such as gas from an area of higher concentration to an area of lesser concentration. Large molecules move less rapidly than small molecules.
Osmol	A unit of osmotic pressure. The osmotic effects are expressed in terms of osmolality. A *milliosmol (mOsm)* is 1/1000th of an osmol and will determine the osmotic activity.
Osmolality	Osmotic pull exerted by all particles per unit of water, expressed as osmols or milliosmols per kilogram of water
Osmolarity	Osmotic pull exerted by all particles per unit of solution, expressed as osmols or milliosmols per liter of solution
Ion	A particle carrying a positive or negative charge
Plasma	Contains blood minus the blood cells (composed mainly of water)
Serum	Consists of plasma minus fibrogen (obtained after coagulation of blood)
Tonicity	The effect of fluid on cellular volume

21

21 movement of molecules/solutes; faster than an area of higher concentration; an area of lower concentration

Diffusion is the movement of molecules/solutes across a selectively permeable membrane along its own pathway, irrespective of all other molecules. Large molecules move *less* rapidly than small molecules. Molecules move faster from an area of higher concentration to an area of lower concentration.

Diffusion is the *_____ across a selectively permeable membrane. Small molecules move (faster than/slower than) *_____ large molecules.

Molecules/solutes tend to move faster from *_____ _____ to *_____ .

22

22 insensible; Heat and activity cause sufficient sweat gland activity. With comfortable temperature, normal loss occurs through insensible perspiration; thus water diffuses via skin and evaporates quickly.

Body water loss by diffusion through the skin that is immeasurable and independent of sweat gland activity is called *insensible perspiration.*

When sweat gland activity occurs and water appears on the skin, this is called *sensible perspiration.*

In a relatively comfortable temperature would insensible perspiration or sensible perspiration occur? _____

Why? *_____

_____

23

23 immeasurable water loss via skin; water on the skin due to sweat gland activity

Define the following terms:

Insensible perspiration *_____

Sensible perspiration *_____

24

24 decreased

The volume of body water is primarily regulated by the kidneys. When water loss increases, e.g., through perspiration or diarrhea, the urine output is (increased/decreased) _____ .

25

25 a liquid with a substance in solution; a substance dissolved in solution

Explain the difference between a solvent and a solute.

Solvent *_____

Solute *_____

26

In an effort to establish equilibrium, water in the body moves from a lesser solute concentration (fewer solute particles per

26 selectively permeable or human

unit of solvent) to a greater solute concentration (more solute particles per unit of solvent) through a *_____ membrane.

27

Osmotic pressure is the pressure or force that develops when two solutions of different strengths or concentrations are separated by a selectively permeable membrane.

To establish osmotic equilibrium, water moves from the (lesser/greater) _____ solute concentration to the (lesser/greater) _____ solute concentration.

The force that draws water across a selectively permeable membrane is called *_____ .

27 lesser; greater; osmotic pressure

▶ FLUID PRESSURES (STARLING'S LAW)

28

Extracellular fluid (ECF) shifts between the intravascular space (blood vessels) and the interstitial space (tissues) to maintain a fluid balance within the ECF compartment.

Four fluid pressures regulate the flow of fluid between the intravascular and interstitial spaces in order to maintain fluid homeostasis or equilibrium.

ECF flows back and forth between the _____ space and the _____ space to maintain _____ .

28 intravascular; interstitial; homeostasis or equilibrium

29

E. H. Starling states that equilibrium exists at the capillary membrane when the fluid leaving circulation and the amount of fluid returning to circulation are exactly equal.

There are four measurable pressures that determine the flow of fluid between the intravascular and interstitial spaces. These are the colloid osmotic (oncotic) pressures and the hydrostatic pressures that are in both the vessels and the tissue spaces.

According to Starling, equilibrium exists at the *_____ .

29 capillary membrane

30

Three new terms to define:

Colloid: a nondiffusible substance; a solute suspended in solution

Hydrostatic: pressure exerted by a stationary liquid
Oncotic pressure: osmotic pressure of a colloid (protein) in body fluid
Osmotic pressure is defined as *_____

_____

_____ .

31
The measurable pressures influencing body fluid flow within the ECF compartment that are present in both the blood vessels and tissue fluid are *_____ and *_____ .

32
The colloid osmotic pressure and the hydrostatic pressure of the blood and tissues influence the movement of fluid through the _____ membrane.

33
Do you know the meanings of the arterioles and venules? If not:
Arterioles: minute arteries that lead into a capillary bed
Venules: minute veins that lead from the capillary bed
Which is larger, the arteriole or the artery? _____ The venule or the vein? _____

34
Fluid exchange occurs only across the walls of capillaries and not across the walls of arterioles or venules. Therefore, fluid moves into the interstitial space at the arteriolar end of the capillary and out of the interstitial space into the capillary at the *_____ of the capillary.

35
Fluid flows only when there is a difference in pressure at the two ends of the system. This difference in pressure between two points is known as the *pressure gradient.*
    If the pressure at one end was 32 mm Hg (millimeters of mercury) and at the other end was 26 mm Hg, the pressure gradient is *_____ .

---

30 the pressure that develops when two solutions of different strengths or concentrations are separated by a selectively permeable membrane OR the force that draws water (fluid) across a selectively permeable membrane

31 the hydrostatic pressure; the colloid osmotic pressure (oncotic pressure)

32 capillary

33 artery; vein

34 venular end

35 6 mm Hg

36

The plasma in the capillaries has hydrostatic pressure and colloid osmotic pressure. The tissue fluids have hydrostatic pressure and colloid osmotic pressure.

The difference in pressure between the plasma colloid osmotic pressure and the tissue colloid osmotic pressure is known as the *_____.

The difference in pressure between the plasma hydrostatic pressure and the tissue hydrostatic pressure is known as the *_____.

It is this difference in pressure that makes the fluid flow between and among compartments.

37

The plasma colloid osmotic pressure is 28 mm Hg and the tissue colloid osmotic pressure is 4 mm Hg. Refer to Figure 1-2.

The colloid osmotic pressure gradient would be *_____ .

36 colloid osmotic pressure gradient; hydrostatic pressure gradient

37 24 mm Hg

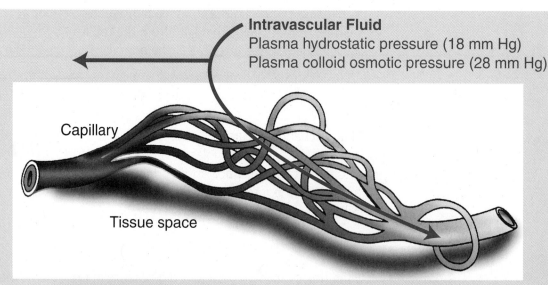

Intravascular Fluid
Plasma hydrostatic pressure (18 mm Hg)
Plasma colloid osmotic pressure (28 mm Hg)

Capillary

Tissue space

Interstitial Fluid
Tissue hydrostatic pressure (-6 mm Hg)
Tissue colloid osmotic pressure (4 mm Hg)

Figure 1-2 Pressures in the intravascular and interstitial fluids.

38 24 mm Hg

39 equal or same pressure

40 The plasma hydrostatic pressure is higher than the tissue pressure. Plasma osmotic pressure is higher than tissue pressure.

41 is; Fluid stays in the tissues, causing accumulation and tissue swelling. insufficient

42 Starling; Plasma and tissue colloid osmotic and hydrostatic pressures regulate the flow of blood constituents between the interstitial and intravascular compartments.

38

The hydrostatic fluid pressure is 18 mm Hg in the capillary, and the hydrostatic tissue pressure is −6 mm Hg; therefore, the hydrostatic pressure gradient is *_____ . Refer to Figure 1-2.

39

The hydrostatic pressure gradient across the capillary membrane (24 mm Hg) is equal to the colloid osmotic pressure gradient across the membrane (24 mm Hg). Thus, the two pressures are

_____ .

40

The plasma hydrostatic pressure gradient tends to move fluid out of the capillary. Why? *_____ Refer to Figure 1-2 if reply is unknown.

The colloid osmotic pressure gradient tends to move fluid into the capillary. Why? *_____

41

The balance between the two forces keeps the blood volume constant for circulation. In this way fluid does not accumulate in the intravascular or the interstitial compartments.

Without the colloid osmotic forces, fluid (is/is not) _____ lost from circulation. Explain. *_____

_____

The blood volume is (sufficient/insufficient) _____ to maintain circulation.

42

Name the man who formulated the Law of Capillaries.
_____ Define this law in your own words. *_____
_____ .

▶ REGULATORS OF FLUID BALANCE

43

Thirst, electrolytes, protein and albumin, hormones, lymphatics, skin, and kidneys are the major regulators that maintain body fluid balance. Thirst alerts the person that there is a fluid loss, thus stimulating the person to increase his or her oral intake.

43 prone to fluid loss (deficit) and dehydration

The thirst mechanism in the medulla may not respond effectively to fluid deficit in the older adult and young child. Therefore, these groups of individuals are * _____ .

44
When there is a body fluid deficit, what mechanism alerts the person that there is a fluid need? _____

44 thirst or thirst mechanism

A discussion regarding regulators of fluid balance follows Table 1-3. Study the actions of these substances or regulators.

45
The electrolyte sodium promotes the (retention/excretion) _____ of body water.

45 retention

46
Protein and albumin help in promoting the (retention/excretion) _____ of body fluid (water). A decrease in protein can (increase/decrease) _____ the colloid osmotic pressure.
    Another name for colloid osmotic pressure is * _____ .

46 retention; decrease; oncotic pressure

47
The two major hormones that influence fluid balance are _____ and _____ .

47 ADH (antidiuretic hormone); aldosterone

48
The antidiuretic hormone, or ADH, increases the permeability of the cells of the kidney tubules to water, thus allowing more water to be reabsorbed. With a decrease in the production of ADH, what would occur? * _____

_____

48 an increased excretion of water from the kidney tubules

49
The posterior pituitary gland is influenced by the solute (sodium, protein, glucose) concentration of the plasma. If there is an increase in the amount of solute in the plasma, the posterior pituitary gland releases the hormone, ADH, which holds water in the body.
Explain how. * _____
    For what reason should there be more water? * _____

_____

49 It absorbs water from the kidney tubules; to dilute the solute

Table 1-3

Regulators of Fluid Balance

Regulators	Actions
Thirst	An indicator of fluid need.
Electrolytes and Nonelectrolytes Sodium	Sodium promotes water retention. With a water deficit, less sodium is excreted via kidneys; thus more water is retained.
Protein, albumin	Protein and albumin promote body fluid retention. These nondiffusible substances increase the colloid osmotic (oncotic) pressure in favor of fluid retention.
Hormones and Enzymes Antidiuretic hormone (ADH)	ADH is produced by the hypothalamus and stored in the posterior pituitary gland (neurohypophysis). ADH is secreted when there is an ECF volume deficit or an increased osmolality (increased solutes). ADH promotes water reabsorption from the distal tubules of the kidneys.
Aldosterone	Aldosterone is secreted from the adrenal cortex. It promotes sodium, chloride, and water reabsorption from the renal tubules.
Renin	Decreased renal blood flow increases the release of renin, an enzyme, from the juxtaglomerular cells of the kidneys. Renin promotes peripheral vasoconstriction and the release of aldosterone (sodium and water retention).
Body Tissues and Organs Lymphatics	Plasma protein that shifts to the tissue spaces cannot be reabsorbed into the blood vessels. Thus, the lymphatic system promotes the return of water and protein from the interstitial spaces to the vascular spaces.
Skin	Skin excretes approximately 300–500 mL of water daily through normal perspiration.
Lungs	Lungs excrete approximately 400–500 mL of water daily through normal breathing.
Kidneys	The kidneys excrete 1000–1500 mL of body water daily. The amount of water excretion may vary according to the balance between fluid intake and fluid loss.

50 ADH; a. ADH would not be released; b. More water would be excreted from the body.

51 It becomes diluted.; reduces

52 by drinking water or other liquids when thirsty

53 sodium; loss

54 extracellular fluid (ECF) or vascular spaces

55 ADH and aldosterone

56 decreased renal blood flow; It promotes aldosterone secretion.

50

A small increase of solute concentration in the plasma above the normal amount is sufficient to stimulate the posterior pituitary gland to release _____ .

Name two things that occur when there is less solute concentration in the plasma.

a. * _____

b. * _____

51

When you drink a lot of fluids, what happens to the solute concentration of your plasma? * _____

The posterior pituitary then (releases/reduces) _____ ADH.

52

When the solute concentration increases, the thirst mechanism is stimulated and the individual ingests water.

Based on the above statement how can homeostasis be maintained? * _____

_____

53

Aldosterone promotes (water/sodium) _____ retention.

An increase in aldosterone release can be due to fluid volume (loss/excess) _____ and stress.

54

Sodium retention stimulates water retention in the * _____

_____

55

An ECF deficit causes the release of two (2) hormones called * _____ .

56

Increased renin (enzyme) secretion is a response to * _____

_____ .

How does renin affect fluid balance? * _____

_____

57 to promote the return of ECF and protein from the interstitial to the vascular spaces

58 loss; 300–500 (normal perspiration)

59 increase; lungs; 400–500

60 fluid balance or homeostasis; 1000–1500

61 urea and glucose

57

The response of the lymphatic system to the maintenance of fluid balance is *_____

_____ .

58

If a person is febrile (increased body temperature) or there is an increase in humidity, diaphoresis may occur. This causes a fluid (loss/gain) _____ .

  Normally the amount of fluid lost through daily perspiration is _____ mL.

59

Overbreathing or hyperventilation can (increase/decrease) _____ fluid loss through the _____ . The lungs normally cause a daily fluid loss of _____ mL.

60

Kidneys conserve or excrete body water to maintain *_____ .

  The amount of urine excreted per day is approximately _____ mL.

❱ OSMOLALITY

61

Osmolality is determined by the number of dissolved particles (sodium, urea, and glucose) per kilogram of water. Sodium is the largest contributor of particles to osmolality. The other two major particle groups that contribute to osmolality are *_____

_____ .

  These dissolved particles exert an osmotic pull or pressure.

62

An *osmol* is a unit of osmotic pressure. The osmotic effects are expressed in terms of osmolality. A *milliosmol* (mOsm) is 1/1000th of an osmol and will determine the osmotic activity. Refer to Table 1-2 for definitions of osmol and osmolality. The basic unit used to express the force exerted by the concentration of solute or dissolved particles is a(n) _____ .

The osmotic effect of a solute concentration in water is expressed as _____ , a property that depends on the number of osmols or milliosmols contained in a solution.

62 osmol; osmolality

63

Osmolality of fluid may be determined in serum and intravenous solutions. In serum, sodium, urea, and glucose are the most plentiful solutes and are the major contributors of serum osmolality. Sodium is most abundant in (extracellular/intracellular) _____ fluid and is available with most laboratory test results.

63 extracellular

64

The normal serum osmolality range is 280–295 mOsm/kg (milliosmols per kilogram). The serum osmolality may be estimated by doubling the serum sodium level. For example, if the serum sodium is 142 mEq/L, the serum osmolality would be _____ mOsm/kg.

This provides a "rough estimate" of the serum osmolality.

Why is the serum sodium level used as an indicator of serum osmolality? _____

64 284; Sodium is the most abundant solute/particle in the ECF.

65

Another formula that may be used to determine the serum osmolality is

$$2 \times \text{serum sodium} + \frac{\text{BUN}}{3} + \frac{\text{glucose}}{18} = \text{serum osmolality}$$

The two formulas that may be used to determine serum osmolality are

a. * _____

b. * _____

65 a. 2 × serum sodium level = serum osmolality;
b. 2 × serum sodium + $\frac{\text{BUN}}{3}$ + $\frac{\text{glucose}}{18}$ = serum osmolality

66

Which of the two formulas (see question 65) would be the most accurate indicator of serum osmolality?

* _____

66 the formula that contains sodium, BUN, and glucose

67 289.5

68 iso-osmolality

69 1. c; 2. b; 3. a; 4. c; 5. a

70 hypertonicity;
hyperosmolality

67

Determine the serum osmolality from the following laboratory test results: serum sodium, 140 mEq/L; BUN, 12 mg/dL; serum glucose, 99 mg/dL.

Complete the following formula:

$$2 \times 140 + \frac{12}{3} + \frac{99}{18} = \underline{\hspace{2cm}} \text{ mOsm/kg}$$

68

A serum osmolality of 288 mOsm/kg would be (hypo/iso/hyper) _____ osmolality.

69

Match the serum osmolality concentrations on the left with the type of osmolality:

_____ 1. 299 mOsm/kg   a. Hypo-osmolality
_____ 2. 292 mOsm/kg   b. Iso-osmolality
_____ 3. 274 mOsm/kg   c. Hyperosmolality
_____ 4. 305 mOsm/kg
_____ 5. 269 mOsm/kg

70

The terms *osmolality* and *tonicity* have been used inter-changeably; though similar, they are different. Osmolality is the concentration of body fluids and tonicity is the effect of fluid on cellular volume. Increased osmolality (hyperosmolality) can result from impermeant solutes such as sodium and from permeant solutes such as urea (blood urea nitrogen). Hypertonicity results from an increase of impermeant solutes such as sodium but *not* of permeant solutes such as urea (BUN).

A high sodium level can cause (hypertonicity/hyperosmolality) _____ . High BUN and sodium levels can cause (hypertonicity/hyperosmolality/both) _____ .

71

The osmolality of an intravenous solution can be hypo-osmolar or hypotonic, iso-osmolar or isotonic, and hyperosmolar or hypertonic. The osmolality of the intravenous (IV) solution is determined by the average serum osmolality, which is 290 mOsm/L. The normal range for the osmolality of a solution is +50 mOsm or −50 mOsm of 290 mOsm.

Early literature refers to the concentration of solutions as hypotonic, isotonic, and hypertonic. These terms are still in use; however, since the solute concentration is determined by the number of osmols or milliosmols in solution, hypo-osmolar, iso-osmolar, and hyperosmolar are the suggested terms.

The average osmolality of IV solution is 240 to _____ mOsm/L.

71 340

72

Plasma (from vascular fluid) is considered to be a(n) (hypo-osmolar/iso-osmolar/hyperosmolar) _____ fluid.

The osmolality of solutions is compared to *_____ .

72 iso-osmolar; plasma osmolality or serum osmolality

73

Match the types of solutions on the left with their solute concentrations:

_____ 1. Iso-osmolar   a. Higher solute concentration than plasma

_____ 2. Hypo-osmolar   b. Same solute concentration as plasma

_____ 3. Hyperosmolar   c. Lower solute concentration than plasma

73 1. b; 2. c; 3. a

74

An IV solution having less than 240 mOsm is considered _____ , and a solution having more than 340 mOsm is considered _____ .

74 hypotonic (hypo-osmolar); hypertonic (hyperosmolar)

75

The following is a list of milliosmol values of IV fluids (solution). Classify them as iso-osmolar, hypo-osmolar, or hyperosmolar.

Milliosmol Values (mOsm)	Type of Osmolality
220	_____
75	_____
350	_____
310	_____
560	_____

75 hypo-osmolar; hypo-osmolar; hyperosmolar; iso-osmolar; hyperosmolar

76

Extracellular hyperosmolar fluid has a greater osmotic pressure than the cell; thus, intracellular water moves out of the cells and into the extracellular hyperosmolar (hypertonic) fluid by the process of _____ .

When cells lose water, what happens to their form and size? *_____ Cellular (hydration/dehydration) _____ results.

77

A liter of 5% dextrose in water (D_5W) is 250 mOsm, and a liter of 0.9% sodium chloride or normal saline is 310 mOsm, having somewhat the same osmotic pressure as _____ .

These solutions are (isotonic/hypotonic/hypertonic) _____ .

78

The sum of 5% dextrose in normal saline equals _____ mOsm. This solution is a(n) _____ solution.

79

Dextrose in normal saline is eventually metabolized leaving the solution as_____ .

▶ MILLIGRAMS VS MILLIEQUIVALENTS

80

In studying serum chemistry alterations and concentrations, one is concerned with how much the ions or chemical particles weigh. The weight of ions and chemical particles is measured in milligrams percent (mg%), which is the same as mg/100 mL or mg/dL. The number of electrically charged ions is measured in milliequivalents per liter (1000 mL), or mEq/L.

The term *milliequivalent* involves the chemical activity of elements, whereas milliosmol involves the _____ activity of the solution.

How do milligrams and milliequivalents differ? *_____

---

76 osmosis; Cells shrink and become smaller in size.; dehydration

77 plasma; isotonic (Dextrose is metabolized so hypotonic eventually occurs.)

78 560; hypertonic

79 isotonic

80 osmotic; Milligrams: the weight of ions.; *Milliequivalents:* the chemical activity of ions.

81 weight

82 15 girls and 15 boys; Otherwise, you would have an unequal number of boys and girls, for not every child weighs exactly 100 pounds.

83 milliequivalents

81

Milliequivalents provide a better method of measuring the concentration of ions in the serum than milligrams.

Milligrams measure the _____ of ions and give no information concerning the number of ions or the electrical charges of the ions.

82

The following is a simple analogy to compare milligrams and milliequivalents.

If you were having a party and wanted to invite equal numbers of boys and girls, which would be more accurate—inviting 1500 pounds of girls and 1500 pounds of boys or inviting 15 girls and 15 boys? * _____ .
Why? * _____

_____ .

83

From the example in question 82, which would be more accurate in determining the serum chemistry of chemical particles or ions in the body—milliequivalents or milligrams?

_____ .

You will find both measurements used in this book and in your clinical settings for determining changes in our serum chemistry. However, when referring to ions, milliequivalents will be used in this book.

▶ CLINICAL APPLICATIONS

84

There are several diseases that affect the plasma colloid osmotic pressure due to the loss of serum protein.

Memorize these five important definitions:
Protein: a nitrogenous compound, essential to all living organisms
Plasma protein: relates to albumin, globulin, and fibrinogen
Serum protein: relates to albumin and globulin
Serum albumin: a simple protein; constitutes about 50% of the blood protein
Serum globulin: a group of simple protein

Clients with diagnoses of kidney and liver diseases or malnutrition lose serum protein. What are the two groups of simple proteins found in the serum?

* _____

84 albumin and globulin

85

The main function of serum albumin is to maintain the colloid osmotic pressure of blood.

Without colloid osmotic pressure, what would happen to the fluid in the tissues? *_____

_____

85 Fluid would accumulate in the tissues (interstitial spaces) and swelling would occur. This is known as edema.

86

Identify three possible responsibilities you think are important when caring for clients with diseases that cause abnormal serum albumin and serum globulin levels.

    a. *_____
    b. *_____
    c. *_____

86 Possible answers include: a. Report abnormal serum laboratory findings immediately.; b. Observe and report physical findings of swelling or edema.; c. Keep an accurate record of fluid intake and output.

87

Edema, or swelling, occurs when there is fluid retention. Dehydration occurs with excess fluid removal or loss.

If the osmolality of intravascular fluid is greater than the osmolality of intracellular fluid, the cells would (lose/gain) _____ water.

(Edema/dehydration) _____ would occur to the cells.

87 lose; dehydration

88

With any vein obstruction, there is an increased venous hydrostatic pressure. This in turn inhibits the fluid moving out of the tissues, causing the tissues to *_____

_____ .

88 retain/accumulate fluid and swell (edema)

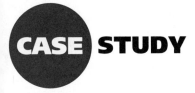

CASE STUDY REVIEW

Mr. Kendall had been vomiting for several days. His urine output decreased. He was given 1 liter of 5% dextrose in water and then 1 liter of 5% dextrose in normal saline (0.9% NaCl).

1. In his adult stage, Mr. Kendall's body water represents _____ % of his total body weight. What percentage of his total body weight is in the intracellular compartment? _____ % What percent of water is in the extracellular compartment? _____ %

1. 60; 40; 20

2. Explain why Mr. Kendall's urine output is decreased. * _____
_____

2. Mr. Kendall is losing body fluid from vomiting and a lack of fluid intake.

3. The three primary sources for water intake are * _____
_____ .

The four primary mechanisms for daily water loss (output) are * _____
_____

3. liquid, food, and oxidation of food; lungs, skin, urine, and feces

4. Vomiting caused Mr. Kendall to lose body fluids and caused a decrease in urine output. The solute concentration was increased. As a result of an increased solute concentration, the posterior pituitary gland will release (more/less) _____ ADH.

4. more

5. Define osmolality and osmolarity.
Osmolality * _____
Osmolarity * _____

5. osmols or milliosmols per kilogram of water; osmols or milliosmols per liter of solution

6. Mr. Kendall received 1 liter of 5% dextrose in water, which has a similar osmolality as plasma. A solution with osmolality similar to that of plasma is considered to be (isotonic/hypotonic/hypertonic) _____ .

6. isotonic

7. The second liter he received was 5% dextrose in normal saline. This solution is a(n) _____ solution.

7. hypertonic

8. The osmolality of plasma is _____ mOsm. A solution with less than 240 mOsm is considered _____ .

8. 290; hypotonic

9. One-half of normal saline (0.45% NaCl) solution has 155 mOsm/L. What is this type of solution? _____ .

9. hypotonic

Mr. Kendall developed edema of the lower extremities. Laboratory results documented a lower than normal serum protein.

10. Starling's Law of Capillaries

11. a. difference in pressure between two points in a fluid; b. diffusible substances; c. nondiffusible substances; d. simple protein

12. tissues

13. protein and albumin

14. a. capillaries; surrounding tissues (interstitial spaces); b. tissues; capillary

15. edema

16. Fluid accumulates in the tissue, causing swelling (edema).

10. Factors regulating the movement of body constituents between the interstitial and intravascular compartments are stated by *_____ .

11. Define the following four terms.
    a. *Pressure gradient* *_____
    b. *Crystalloids* *_____
    c. *Colloids* *_____
    d. *Albumin* *_____

12. Pressure gradients are responsible for the exchange of fluid between the capillaries and the _____ .

13. The amount of colloid osmotic pressure that develops depends on the concentration of nondiffusible substances such as *_____ .

14. The direction of the movement of fluid depends on the results of the opposing forces.
    a. The hydrostatic pressure is greater than the colloid osmotic pressure at the arterial end of the capillary; thus the fluid moves out of the _____ and into the *_____ .
    b. The osmotic pressure is greater than the hydrostatic pressure at the venous end of the capillary; thus the fluid moves out of the _____ and reenters the _____ .

15. Mr. Kendall's decrease in serum protein could account for his (edema/dehydration) _____ .

16. Mr. Kendall has a venous obstruction due to varicosities. This causes an increase in venous hydrostatic pressure, preventing fluid from moving out of tissues and into the circulation. Explain what happens to the fluid. *_____
_____

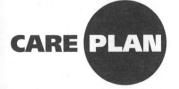

Client Management: Fluid Volume Deficit and Fluid Volume Excess

Assessment Factors

▶ Assess the intake and output status of the client. Fluid intake and urine output are normally in proportion to each other.

▶ Recognize that infants and thin people have a higher proportion of body water than adults, older adults, and people with increased body fat.

▶ Assess excess fluid loss from the skin and lungs. Diaphoresis (excess sweating) and tachypnea (rapid breathing) cause excess body water loss through the skin and lungs.

▶ Obtain baseline vital signs. Baseline vital signs are used for comparison with future vital signs.

▶ Assess for fluid balance by checking the client's serum osmolality with the laboratory test results. The serum sodium, BUN, and glucose results are used in calculating the serum osmolality status of clients. If only the serum sodium value is available, double the sodium level for a rough estimate of the serum osmolality. A serum osmolality >295 mOsm/kg can indicate hemoconcentration due to fluid loss. A serum osmolality <280 mOsm/kg can indicate hemodilution due to fluid excess.

Diagnosis

Fluid volume deficit and fluid volume excess related to body fluid imbalance.

Interventions and Rationale

1. Monitor vital signs. Report abnormal vital signs or significant changes from baseline measurements.

2. Monitor intake and output. Report urine output of less than 600 mL/day and less than 25 mL/hr.

3. Check the daily osmolality of IV solutions. Know that IV solutions with osmolality between 240 and 340 mOsm/L are isotonic and are similar to plasma. Remember that a solution of 5% dextrose in water is 250 mOsm and a normal saline solution (0.9% sodium chloride) is 310 mOsm; both are isotonic solutions. Continuous use of hypotonic (0.45% sodium chloride) and hypertonic [10% dextrose in water ($D_{10}W$)] IV solutions may cause a fluid imbalance. However, remember that dextrose is metabolized rapidly; with D_5W, the solution eventually becomes hypotonic. D_5/NSS (normal saline solution) is hypertonic but becomes isotonic after dextrose is metabolized. With the continuous use of dextrose in normal saline solutions, hyperosmolality occurs.

4. Monitor the fluid status of the client: check laboratory studies to determine the serum osmolality. Serum sodium, BUN, and glucose levels should be used to assess the serum osmolality.

5. Monitor the serum albumin and serum protein levels of clients with malnutrition, liver disease such as cirrhosis of the liver, and kidney disease. Low serum albumin and serum protein levels decrease the colloid osmotic (oncotic) pressure; thus fluid remains in the tissue spaces (edema). While diuretics are helpful in decreasing edema, they can also markedly decrease the circulating fluid volume.

Evaluation/Outcome

1. Maintain intake and output approximately equal to one another.

2. Determine that the serum osmolality level has remained within normal range.

3. Evaluate the types of intravenous solutions prescribed daily to ensure that these solutions are within a normotonicity.

UNIT II

FLUIDS AND THEIR INFLUENCE ON THE BODY

OBJECTIVES

Upon completion of this unit, the reader should be able to:

- Describe the physiologic factors leading to extracellular fluid volume deficits, extracellular fluid volume excess, and intracellular fluid volume excess.

- State the difference between a hyperosmolar fluid deficit and an iso-osmolar fluid deficit.

- Compare the extracellular fluid volume shift in hypovolemia with the extracellular fluid volume shift in hypervolemia.

- Identify assessments associated with dehydration, edema, and water intoxication.

- Develop selected diagnoses appropriate for clients with clinical manifestations of extracellular fluid volume deficits and excess and intracellular fluid volume excess.

- Identify selected interventions to alleviate the symptoms of dehydration, edema, and water intoxication.

- Identify selected outcomes appropriate to the management of dehydration, edema, and water intoxication.

▶ INTRODUCTION

Many disease entities have some degree of fluid and electrolyte imbalance. Much of the imbalance is the result of fluid loss, fluid excess, and/or fluid volume shift. Four major fluid imbalances—extracellular fluid volume deficit (ECFVD), extracellular fluid volume excess (ECFVE), extracellular fluid volume shift (ECFVS), and intracellular fluid volume excess (ICFVE)—are discussed in four separate chapters with regard to pathophysiology, etiology, clinical manifestations (signs and symptoms), clinical applications, clinical management, and clinical consideration. Assessment factors, diagnoses, interventions, and evaluations are listed for ECFVD, ECFVE, and ICFVE. Case reviews related to clients with fluid imbalances are presented.

The health care provider computes and orders fluid replacement; however, the nurse should understand reasons for various types of fluid imbalances and should assess physical changes that may occur before and during clinical management. Refer to Chapter 1 for background information related to body fluids and its concentration and function. If there is previous knowledge of body fluids and its concentration, then proceed to Chapter 2.

An asterisk (*) on an answer line indicates a multiple-word answer. The meanings for the following symbols are: ↑ increased, ↓ decreased, > greater than, and < less than.

Extracellular Fluid Volume Deficit (ECFVD)

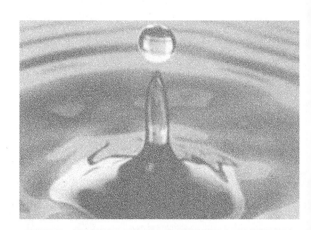

▌ INTRODUCTION

Extracellular fluid volume deficit (ECFVD) is a loss of body fluid from the interstitial (tissue) and intravascular (vascular-vessel) spaces. With a severe ECF loss and an increase in serum osmolality (more solutes than water), there is an intracellular (cellular-cells) fluid loss. If the loss of water and loss of solutes are equal, then intracellular fluid loss is unlikely to occur.

Dehydration means a lack of water. Dehydration may occur due to ECF loss. It may also result from a decrease in fluid intake.

1
Extracellular fluid loss results primarily from the loss of body fluid in the _____ and _____ spaces.

2
Severe loss of ECF, causing an increase in osmolality, results in _____ fluid loss.

3
Severe loss of ECF (may/may not) _____ cause fluid loss from the cells.

4
Dehydration is another name used to describe *_____ .
　　Dehydration may be due to *_____

PATHOPHYSIOLOGY

5
The concentration of body fluids or plasma/serum osmolality is determined by the number of particles or solutes in relation to the volume of body water (refer to Chapter 1 for a description of osmolality).
　　The normal range of plasma/serum osmolality is *_____
_____ .

6
If the serum osmolality is less than 280 mOsm/kg, there are (more/less) _____ solutes/particles in proportion to the volume of body water. This body fluid is described as (hypo-osmolar/iso-osmolar/hyperosmolar) _____ .

7
If the serum osmolality is greater than 295 mOsm/kg, there are (more/less) _____ solutes in proportion to body water; the fluid imbalance is known as _____ .

Answer Column:

1　interstitial and intravascular

2　intracellular or cellular

3　may not

4　loss of body water; ECF loss

5　280–295 mOsm/kg (milliosmols per kilogram)

6　less; hypo-osmolar or hypotonic

7　more; hyperosmolar or hypertonic

8

A loss of the electrolyte sodium is usually accompanied by a simultaneous fluid loss. With a loss of sodium, ECF is usually decreased or moves from the ECF to the ICF compartment.

When fluid and sodium are lost in equal amounts, the type of fluid deficit that usually occurs is (iso-osmolar/hyperosmolar) _____ .

9

When the amount of water lost is in excess of the amount of sodium lost, the serum sodium level is (elevated/decreased) _____ .

This type of fluid deficit is called (hypo-osmolar/iso-osmolar/hyperosmolar) _____ fluid volume deficit.

10

Plasma/serum osmolality increases with the retention of sodium or the loss of water. This causes water to be drawn from the cells. With the elevation of serum sodium, the ECF becomes (hyperosmolar/hypo-osmolar) _____ , which results in a(an) (increase/decrease) _____ in plasma/serum osmolality. This change in serum osmolality causes a withdrawal of fluid from the _____ compartment.

11

Hyperosmolar ECF causes intracellular (dehydration/hydration) _____ .

Explain. *_____

12

With an iso-osmolar fluid volume loss, the loss of water and solute is (equal/varied) _____ . The plasma/serum osmolality is (increased/decreased/unchanged) _____ .

13

An iso-osmolar fluid volume loss is not classified as dehydration, although dehydration could occur with this type of fluid loss.

A hyperosmolar fluid volume loss is referred to as _____ . Explain.

*_____

8   iso-osmolar or isotonic

9   elevated; hyperosmolar

10 hyperosmolar; increase; cell or intracellular

11 dehydration; The hyperosmolar ECF will pull ICF from the cells by osmosis.

12 equal; unchanged

13 dehydration; Moderate to severe fluid volume losses can cause symptoms of dehydration.

14

Compensatory mechanisms such as an increased heart rate and blood pressure attempt to maintain the fluid volume necessary for vital organs to receive adequate perfusion.

When more than one-third of the body fluid is lost, what might occur? *_____

_____

14 vascular collapse or shock or inadequate organ perfusion

▶ ETIOLOGY

The causes of hyperosmolar and iso-osmolar fluid volume deficits differ. Both types of fluid volume deficits may be caused by vomiting and diarrhea; however, in most cases, the severity of vomiting and diarrhea indicates the type of ECFVD. Table 2-1 discusses the types and causes with rationale for ECFVD. Study the table carefully and refer to it as needed.

15

Usually with severe vomiting and diarrhea, the loss of water is greater than the loss of sodium. This type of fluid loss causes
*_____ .

15 hyperosmolar fluid volume deficit

16

With "equal" proportional loss of fluid and solutes due to mild or moderate vomiting or diarrhea, what type of fluid volume deficit might occur? _____

With severe body fluid and solute loss due to severe vomiting and/or diarrhea, what type of fluid volume deficit might occur?

_____

16 iso-osmolar; hyperosmolar

17

Match the type of ECFVD with its possible cause.
a. IFVD (iso-osmolar fluid volume deficit)
b. HFVD (hyperosmolar fluid volume deficit)
_____ 1. Hemorrhage
_____ 2. Diabetic ketoacidosis
_____ 3. Increased salt and protein intake
_____ 4. Burns
_____ 5. GI suctioning
_____ 6. Inadequate fluid intake
_____ 7. Profuse diaphoresis and/or fever

17 1. a; 2. b; 3. b; 4. a; 5. a; 6. b; 7. a

Table 2-1

Causes of Extracellular Fluid Volume Deficits

Types and Causes	Rationale
Hyperosmolar Fluid Volume Deficit	
Inadequate fluid intake	A decrease in water intake results in an increase in the numbers of solutes in body fluid. The body fluid becomes hyperosmolar.
Increased solute intake (salt, sugar, protein)	An increase in solute intake increases the solute concentration in body fluid; the body fluids can become hyperosmolar with a normal or decreased fluid intake.
Severe vomiting and diarrhea	Cause a loss of body water greater than the loss of solutes such as electrolytes, resulting in hyperosmolar body fluid.
Diabetes ketoacidosis	An increase in glucose and ketone bodies can result in body fluids becoming more hyperosmolar, thus causing diuresis. The resulting fluid loss is greater than the solute loss (sugar and ketones).
Sweating	Water loss is usually greater than sodium loss.
Iso-osmolar Fluid Volume Deficit	
Vomiting and diarrhea	Usually result in fluid losses that are in proportion to electrolyte (sodium, potassium, chloride, bicarbonate) losses.
Gastrointestinal (GI) fistula or draining abscess and GI suctioning	The GI tract is rich in electrolytes. With a loss of GI secretions, fluid and electrolytes are lost in somewhat equal proportions.
Fever, environmental temperature, and profuse diaphoresis	Result in fluid and sodium losses via the skin. With profuse sweating, the sodium is usually lost in proportions equal to water losses. Depending upon the severity of the sweating and fever, symptoms of mild, moderate, or marked fluid loss may be observed.
Hemorrhage	Excess blood loss is fluid and solute loss from the vascular fluid. If hemorrhage occurs rapidly, fluid shifts to compensate for blood losses can be inadequate.
Burns	Burns cause body fluid with solutes to shift from the vascular fluid to the burned site and surrounding interstitial space (tissues). This may result in inadequate circulating fluid volume.
Ascites	Fluid and solutes (protein, electrolytes, etc.) shift to the peritoneal space, causing ascites (third-space fluid). A decrease in circulating fluid volume may result.
Intestinal obstruction	Fluid accumulates at the intestinal obstruction site (third-space fluid), thus decreasing the vascular fluid volume.

18

Indicate which situations are representative of iso-osmolar or hyperosmolar fluid volume deficits.

    a. Iso-osmolar

    b. Hyperosmolar

      _____ 1. There is a proportional loss of both body fluids and solutes.

      _____ 2. The loss of body fluids is greater than the loss of solutes.

      _____ 3. A serum osmolality of 282 mOsm/kg occurring with ECFVD may indicate which type of fluid loss?

      _____ 4. A serum osmolality of 305 mOsm/kg occurring with ECFVD may indicate which type of fluid loss?

18 1. a; 2. b; 3. a; 4. b

▶ CLINICAL MANIFESTATIONS

The clinical manifestations (signs and symptoms) of ECFVD are listed in Table 2-2. The table describes the degrees of ECF loss, percentage of body weight loss, symptoms, and body water deficit by liter for a man weighing 150 pounds.

Study this table carefully; be able to name the degrees of dehydration, their symptoms, the percentage of body weight loss, and an estimation of body fluid loss in liters. Hopefully, you will be able to recognize and identify degrees of dehydration that can occur to your clients during your clinical experience. Refer back to this table as you find necessary.

19

Thirst is a symptom that occurs with mild, marked, and severe fluid loss. Lack of water intake is usually the contributing cause of mild dehydration.

How can mild dehydration be corrected? *_____

_____

19 by increasing water (fluid) intake

20

With mild dehydration, the percentage of body weight loss is _____ %, which is equivalent to _____ liter(s) of body fluid loss.

20 2; 1–2

Table 2-2

Degrees of Dehydration

Degrees of Dehydration	Percentage of Body Weight Loss (%)	Symptoms	Body Water Deficit by Liter
Mild dehydration	2	1. Thirst	1–2
Marked dehydration	5	1. Marked thirst 2. Dry mucous membranes 3. Dryness and wrinkling of skin—poor skin turgor 4. Hand veins: slow filling with hand lowered 5. Temperature— low-grade elevation, e.g., 99°F (37.2°C) 6. Tachycardia (pulse greater than 100) as blood volume drops 7. Respiration >28 8. Systolic BP 10–15 mm Hg ↓ in standing position 9. Urine volume <25 mL/h 10. Specific gravity >1.030 11. Body weight loss 12. Hct ↑, Hgb ↑, BUN ↑ 13. Acid-base equilibrium toward greater acidity	3–5
Severe dehydration	8	1. Same symptoms as marked dehydration, plus: 2. Flushed skin 3. Systolic BP <60 mm Hg 4. Behavioral changes, e.g., restlessness, irritability, disorientation, and delirium	5–10
Fatal dehydration	22–30 total body water loss can prove fatal	1. Anuria 2. Coma leading to death	

Abbreviations: BP, blood pressure; Hct, hematocrit; Hgb, hemoglobin; BUN, blood urea nitrogen.

21

In the elderly, the thirst mechanism in the medulla does not alert the older person that there is a water deficit. Therefore, the older person may become *_____ without experiencing the symptom of thirst.

22

Common symptoms of marked ECF loss include decreased skin turgor, dry mucous membranes, increased pulse rate, weight loss, and decreased urine output.

What percentage of weight loss is associated with marked dehydration? _____ This weight loss is equivalent to _____ liter(s) of body water loss.

23

The percentage of body weight loss is a guide for *_____
_____ therapy.

24

With marked and severe body fluid loss, the hematocrit, hemoglobin, and blood urea nitrogen (BUN) may be (increased/decreased) _____ . Why? *_____
_____

25

The red blood cell count, hemoglobin, hematocrit, and plasma/serum protein may be elevated as a result of hemoconcentration (increased blood cells and decreased vascular fluid).

Hemoconcentration occurs with dehydration. Why? *_____
_____

26

With marked dehydration, increased urine concentration usually results. The specific gravity (SG) may be (increased/decreased) _____ , such as SG (<1.008/>1.025) _____ . The urine output is (increased/decreased) _____ .

---

21 dehydrated or mildly dehydrated

22 5%; 3–5

23 replacement fluid or intravenous (IV) fluid

24 increased; because of the increased number of solutes such as BUN and red blood cells or hemoconcentration

25 With body fluid loss, red blood cell count is increased, along with other solutes.

26 increased; >1.025; decreased

27

Indicate which symptoms are associated with *severe* dehydration.

( ) a. Bradycardia
( ) b. Tachycardia as blood volume drops
( ) c. Temperature 99.6°F
( ) d. Urine volume is increased
( ) e. Specific gravity of urine of 1.030 and higher
( ) f. Skin flushed
( ) g. Irritability
( ) h. Restlessness and disorientation
( ) i. Specific gravity of urine lower than 1.020
( ) j. Marked thirst

What percentage of fluid loss is associated with severe dehydration? _____

27 b, c, e, f, g, h, j; 8%

▶ CLINICAL APPLICATIONS

28

During early dehydration, the serum osmolality may not show any significant changes. As dehydration continues, fluid is lost in greater quantities from the extracellular than from the intracellular fluid space. This results in an ECF (excess/deficit) _____ .

28 deficit

29

When dehydration is severe, the serum osmolality increases, causing water to leave the cells.

A severe ECF deficit can lead to an ICF (excess/deficit) _____ .

29 deficit

30

When there is a marked or severe fluid volume loss, hypovolemia occurs. Hypovolemia may be a new term to you. The prefix *hypo* indicates _____ . Volemia comes from the Latin word *volumen,* meaning "volume."

Hypovolemia is a diminished volume of circulating blood or vascular fluid. It is frequently referred to as a decrease in blood volume.

30 loss, less, deficit, or diminished

31

The health professional can make a quick assessment of dehydration, or hypovolemia, by checking the peripheral veins in the hand. First hold the hand above heart level for a short time and then lower the hand below heart level. The peripheral veins in the hand below heart level should be engorged within 5–10 seconds with a normal blood volume and circulating blood flow.

If the peripheral veins do not engorge in 10 seconds, this may be indicative of _____

_____ .

32

Body weight is an important tool for assessing fluid imbalance. Two and two-tenths (2.2) pounds of body weight loss or gain is equivalent to 1 liter of water loss or gain.

Intake and output give the approximate amount of body fluid intake and output. What provides the more accurate assessment of fluid balance (body weight, intake and output balance)?
* _____

33

Vital signs provide another tool for assessing hypovolemia, or loss of body fluid. With fluid loss due to dehydration, what physiologic symptoms occur with the following vital measurements?
Temperature * _____
Pulse * _____
Respirations * _____
Blood pressure * _____
Urine volume * _____

▶ CLINICAL MANAGEMENT

In replacing body water loss, the total fluid deficit is estimated according to the percentage of body weight loss. The health care professional computes the fluid replacement for his or her client. The following is only an example. Many health care professionals use this method for replacement of fluid loss.

Mr. Smith, who was admitted to the hospital, had a weight loss of 10 pounds due to dehydration. His weight had originally

---

31 dehydration or hypovolemia (low blood volume)

32 body weight

33 temperature: low-grade elevation; pulse: tachycardia (rate over 100); respirations: increased; systolic blood pressure: <10–15 mm Hg (standing position); urine volume: decreased or small amount and highly concentrated; (Kidney damage can occur if the systolic blood pressure is less than 60 for several hours.)

been 154 pounds, or 70 kg (kilograms). To determine the percentage of body weight loss, divide the weight loss by the original weight; therefore, 10 ÷ 154 = 0.06, or 6%. To determine the total fluid loss, multiply the percentage of body weight loss by kilograms of body weight; therefore, 0.06 × 70 kg = 4.2 liters.

34
Clinically, Mr. Smith has (mild/marked/severe) dehydration.
_____

35
To determine the percentage of body weight loss, one *_____
_____
To determine the total fluid loss, one *_____
_____

36
One-third of body water deficit is from ECF (extracellular fluid), and two-thirds of body water deficit is from ICF (intracellular fluid) (Chapter 1). To determine replacement therapy for the first day, you would multiply:
(a) $\frac{1}{3}$ × 4.2 L = 1.4 L (ECF replacement)
Replacement fluid needed for ECF is _____ liter(s), or
_____ mL.
(b) $\frac{2}{3}$ × 4.2 L = 2.8 L (ICF replacement)
Replacement fluid needed for ICF is _____ liter(s), or
_____ mL.
(c) 2.5 L, or 2500 mL, is added to replace the current day's losses (constant daily amount)
The total fluid replacement for the first day is _____ liter(s), or _____ mL (sum of ECF and ICF and current day's losses).

37
One-third of the water deficit is from the *_____ , and two-thirds of the water deficit is from the *_____ .

38
The sodium (Na) deficit is the amount contained in the ECF loss of 1.4 liters. Sodium is the main cation of (ECF/ICF) _____ .

34 marked

35 divides the weight loss by the original weight; multiplies the percentage of body weight loss by kilograms of body weight

36 a. 1.4; 1400; b. 2.8; 2800; c. 6.7; 6700

37 extracellular fluid; intracellular (cellular) fluid

38 ECF

Normally there is a loss of sodium when there is a loss of ECF. However, the serum sodium level may be elevated if the fluid loss is greater than the sodium loss.

39

The potassium (K) deficit is the amount contained in the ICF loss of 2.8 liters. Potassium is the main cation of (ECF/ICF)

_____ .

Usually when there is cellular fluid loss, there is potassium loss. However, the serum potassium level may be elevated when potassium leaves the cells and accumulates in the ECF. When diuresis occurs, the serum potassium (elevates/decreases)

_____ .

39 ICF; decreases

40

In severe dehydration, cellular breakdown usually occurs and acid metabolites such as lactic acid are released from the cells; thus, metabolic acidosis results. The serum CO_2 and the arterial bicarbonate (HCO_3) levels are decreased. Why do you think this happens? *_____

_____

Bicarbonate is usually added to a liter or two of IV fluids to neutralize the body's acidotic state. Constant use of saline (NaCl) is not indicated. Explain why. *_____

_____

40 Because of acidosis, the body bicarbonate is decreased.; Chloride would combine with the hydrogen ion and increase acidosis.

41

As potassium is being restored to the cells (when there is a potassium deficit), fluid flows into the cells with potassium replacement. Cellular fluid is then (decreased/increased)

_____ ; thus, the cells become (hydrated/dehydrated)

_____ .

Refer to table 2-3 for suggested solution replacement needed to correct dehydration.

41 increased; hydrated

42

When potassium is being administered intravenously, explain your assessment concerns and the appropriate rationale related to the client's urinary output? *_____

_____

42 Eighty to 90% of potassium is excreted via kidneys. Poor urinary output leads to potassium excess, so urine output should be 250 mL per 8 hours.

Table 2-3

Suggested Solution Replacement for ECF Deficit

1. Lactated Ringer's, 1500 mL, to replace ECF losses (varies according to the serum potassium and calcium levels).
2. Normal saline solution (0.9% NaCl solution), 500 mL.
3. Five percent dextrose in water (D_5W), 4700 mL, to replace the water deficit and increase urine output.
4. Potassium chloride, 40–80 mEq, may be divided into 3 liters to replace potassium loss. The serum potassium level must be closely monitored.
5. Bicarbonate as needed if an acidotic state exists.

43 replace fluid volume and assess degree of dehydration

43

In correcting dehydration, two goals are to * _____

_____ .

44

Select all true statements.

Lactated Ringer's solution is helpful in treating ECFVD because:
( ) a. It resembles the electrolytic structure of normal blood serum.
( ) b. It replaces the extracellular fluid volume.
( ) c. It replaces all of the electrolyte loss.
( ) d. It replaces potassium loss.

M/6 sodium lactate is helpful in treating dehydration because:
( ) a. It replaces the sodium loss.
( ) b. It aids in decreasing the CO_2 combining power of the plasma.
( ) c. It aids in increasing the CO_2 combining power of the plasma.
( ) d. It is helpful in the correction of metabolic acidosis.
( ) e. It is helpful in the correction of metabolic alkalosis.

Dextrose 5% in water is helpful in treating dehydration because:
( ) a. It replaces water deficit.
( ) b. It aids in increasing urine output.
( ) c. It aids in decreasing urine output.
( ) d. It replaces the sodium deficit.

44 a, b; a, c, d; a, b

45

Mild dehydration is frequently treated with dextrose, water, and small amounts of electrolytes.

Dextrose 5% in water (D_5W) is frequently given first followed by a solution of low electrolyte content such as *_____

_____.

(These solutions could be given in reverse, according to the client's condition and health care professional's choice.)

When administering D_5W, dextrose is metabolized quickly, leaving _____ .

45 lactated Ringer's solution or $D_5/\frac{1}{2}$ NSS (5% dextrose in 0.45% normal saline solution); water

● **Clinical Considerations**

1. Thirst is an early symptom of ECFVD, or dehydration. Encourage fluid intake.

2. The serum osmolality is one method to detect dehydration. A serum osmolality of >300 mOsm/kg indicates dehydration.

3. Decreased skin turgor, dry mucous membranes, an increased pulse rate, a systolic blood pressure (while standing) <10–15 mm Hg of the regular BP, and/or decreased urine output are some signs and symptoms of dehydration.

4. A quick assessment of hypovolemia or dehydration can be accomplished by checking the peripheral veins in the hand. First hold the hand above heart level for 10 seconds and then lower the hand below the heart level. The peripheral veins in the hand below the heart level become engorged within 5–10 seconds with a normal blood volume.

5. Lactated Ringer's and 5% dextrose in $\frac{1}{3}$ or $\frac{1}{2}$ normal saline are solutions that are helpful for treating ECFVD.

CASE STUDY REVIEW

Mr. Cooper, age 55, has been vomiting persistently for 3 days. On admission, he weighed 153 pounds. His original weight was 165 pounds (75 kg). The nurse assessed his fluid state and noted that his mucous membranes and skin were dry. His temperature was 99.4°F (37.5°C), pulse 112, respirations 32, blood pressure 110/88, and urine output in 8 hours 125 mL with a specific gravity of 1.036. Electrolyte findings were serum K, 3.5 mEq/L; Na, 154 mEq/L; and Cl, 102 mEq/L. His hematocrit and BUN were elevated.

1. Name the type of Mr. Cooper's dehydration (fluid volume loss). *_____ Explain the rationale for your selection.

   *_____

   _____

1. hyperosmolar dehydration; Serum sodium is elevated with the fluid loss.

2. Another name for dehydration is *_____

   _____ .

2. extracellular fluid volume deficit, or hypovolemia

3. The nurse assesses Mr. Cooper's body fluid state. Name four of his symptoms and laboratory findings that are suggestive of the fluid imbalance (dehydration).

   a. *_____

   b. *_____

   c. *_____

   d. *_____

3. a. dry mucous membrane and dry skin; b. vital signs—temperature slightly elevated, tachycardia, respiration increased, systolic blood pressure ↓; c. elevated sodium level; d. Hct and BUN increased; Others— weight loss, urinary output ↓

4. Determine the percentage of Mr. Cooper's body weight loss.

   *_____

   _____

4. $12 \div 165 = 0.07 \times 100 = 7\%$

5. Clinically, Mr. Cooper has (mild/marked/severe) _____ dehydration.

5. marked dehydration

6. Mr. Cooper's total fluid loss is *_____ . (Work space is provided.)

6. $75 \text{ kg} \times 0.07 = 5.25 \text{ L loss}$

7. a. Calculate the replacement fluid needed for ECF loss.

   *_____

   b. Calculate the replacement fluid needed for ICF loss.

   *_____

   c. Calculate the replacement fluid needed for current day's losses. *_____

   (constant daily amount)

7. a. $\frac{1}{3} \times 5.25 \text{ L} = 1.75 \text{ L or}$ 1750 mL

   b. $\frac{2}{3} \times 5.25 \text{ L} = 3.5 \text{ L or}$ 3500 mL

   c. 2.5 L or 2500 mL

8. What two laboratory results were indicative of dehydration other than the electrolytes? *_____

8. elevated Hct and BUN

9. Hypernatremia frequently results from *_____ .

9. water depletion

10. decreased; With dehydration, K leaves cells.

11. decreased; With hydration, K moves from the ECF back into cells; thus, serum K is lowered.

12. lactated Ringer's

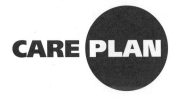

10. Mr. Cooper's serum potassium level of 3.5 mEq/L is considered low average. Do you think his cellular potassium is (increased/decreased) _____ ? Explain your rationale.

    _____

    _____

11. If Mr. Cooper is hydrated without potassium added, the nurse should expect his serum potassium to be (increased/decreased) _____

    Why? * _____

    _____

12. What intravenous solution resembles the electrolyte concentration of plasma? * _____

Client Management: Extracellular Fluid Volume Deficit (ECFVD)

Assessment Factors

▸ Complete a client history identifying factors that may cause a fluid volume deficit (ECFVD), such as vomiting, diarrhea, limited fluid intake, diabetes mellitus or insipidus, large draining wound, or diuretic therapy.

▸ Assess the skin for poor skin turgor by pinching the skin (pinched skin that remains pinched or returns slowly to its normal skin surface is indicative of poor skin turgor), dry mucous membranes, and/or dry cracked lips or tongue.

▸ Check vital signs: pulse rate, respiration, and blood pressure. When the blood volume decreases, the heart compensates for the fluid loss by increasing the heart rate. When the fluid volume continues to decrease, the systolic blood pressure begins to fall. Check the blood pressure, first, while the client is sitting and, then, while the client is standing (a fall of 10–15 mm Hg in systolic pressure may indicate marked dehydration). A narrow pulse pressure of less than 20 mm Hg can indicate severe hypovolemia.

▸ Check the urine output for volume and concentration. A decrease in urine output may be due to a lack of fluid intake or excess body fluid loss.

▸ Monitor weight gain/loss to assist in accurate fluid replacement.

▶ Assess hand and/or neck vein filling. A decrease in venous filling (in the vessels of the hand) when the hand is below the heart level and in the jugular vein when the client is in a low Fowler's position may suggest a fluid volume deficit.

▶ Check laboratory findings such as BUN, hematocrit, and hemoglobin. Record and report abnormal findings.

Diagnosis 1

Fluid volume deficit: dehydration related to inadequate fluid intake, vomiting, diarrhea, hemorrhage, or third-space fluid loss (burns or ascites).

Interventions and Rationale

1. Monitor vital signs every 4 hours depending upon the severity of the fluid loss. Compare the vital signs to the client's baseline vital signs. Check the blood pressure in lying, sitting, and standing positions.

2. Provide fluid intake hourly using fluids client prefers and those indicated by electrolyte deficits. If intravenous (IV) method is used for fluid replacement, monitor IV flow rate. Guard against overhydration and infiltration of the IV fluids.

3. Monitor skin turgor, mucous membranes, and lips and tongue for changes: improvement or deterioration.

4. Routinely check body weight. Remember 2.2 pounds (1 kg) loss is equivalent to 1 liter (1000 mL) of fluid loss.

Diagnosis 2

Impaired tissue integrity related to a fluid deficit.

Interventions and Rationale

1. Utilize preventive measures to preserve skin and mucous membrane integrity. The client's position should be changed on a regular schedule.

2. Apply lotion to increase circulation to the bony prominences.

3. Check skin turgor. Note skin color and temperature.

Diagnosis 3

Altered oral mucous membranes related to dehydration.

Interventions and Rationale

1. Provide oral hygiene several times a day. Inspect mouth for sores, lesions, or bleeding. Avoid use of drying agents such as lemon and glycerine swabs or certain mouth washes. Use half-strength hydrogen peroxide (H_2O_2) to remove dry debris from the mouth.

2. Apply water-soluble lubricant to the lips to prevent cracking and promote healing.

3. Promote adequate fluid replacement.

4. Avoid irritants (foods, fluids, temperature, etc).

Diagnosis 4

Altered tissue perfusion, renal, related to decreased renal blood flow and poor urine output secondary to ECFVD, or hypovolemia.

Interventions and Rationale

1. Monitor urinary output. Report if urine output is less than 30 mL/h or 250 mL/8 h. Absence of urine output for 5–12 hours may indicate renal insufficiency due to decreased renal blood perfusion.

2. Note presence of pain on urination.

3. Monitor; report abnormal laboratory findings such as elevated BUN and elevated serum creatinine. Measure the specific gravity of urine every shift.

4. Weigh client daily, at the same time in the morning.

Evaluation/Outcome

1. Evaluate that the cause of extracellular fluid volume deficit (ECFVD) has been controlled or eliminated.

2. Evaluate the effects of clinical management for ECFVD. The fluid deficit is lessened.

3. Remain free of signs and symptoms of dehydration; skin turgor improved, moist mucous membranes, vital signs within normal range, and body weight increased.

4. Urine output is within normal range (600–1500 mL/24 h).

5. Determine if the serum electrolytes are within normal range.

6. Determine support measures for the client and family.

CHAPTER 3

Extracellular Fluid Volume Excess (ECFVE)

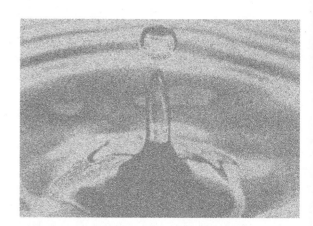

▌ INTRODUCTION

Extracellular fluid volume excess (ECFVE) is increased fluid in the interstitial (tissues) and intravascular (vascular or vessel) spaces. Usually it relates to the excess fluid in tissues of the extremities (peripheral edema) or lung tissues (pulmonary edema).

ANSWER COLUMN

1 excess fluid volume in circulating blood volume

2 hypervolemia, overhydration, and edema

3 interstitial spaces of the ECF compartment or in serous cavities

4 hemodilution; decreased

1

Hypervolemia and *overhydration* are interchangeable terms for ECFVE and edema.

Hypervolemia means *_____ .

Hypervolemia and overhydration contribute to fluid excess in tissue spaces, or edema.

Fluid overload is another term for overhydration and hypervolemia.

2

Edema is the abnormal retention of fluid in the interstitial spaces of the ECF compartment or in serous cavities. Frequently, edema results from sodium retention in the body, causing a retention of water and an increase in extracellular fluid volume. Three terms used for extracellular fluid volume excess are *_____

_____ .

3

Edema is the abnormal retention of fluid in the *_____

_____ .

▶ PATHOPHYSIOLOGY

4

When sodium and water are retained in the same proportion, the fluid is referred to as iso-osmolar fluid volume excess. Total body sodium is increased but concentration is unchanged because there is retention of sodium, chloride, and water. Usually the sodium level may be within the normal range. This is most likely due to (hemoconcentration/hemodilution) _____ .

If only free water is retained, the excess is referred to as hypo-osmolar (hypotonic) fluid volume excess. Serum sodium levels would be (increased/decreased) _____ due to the increase of free water.

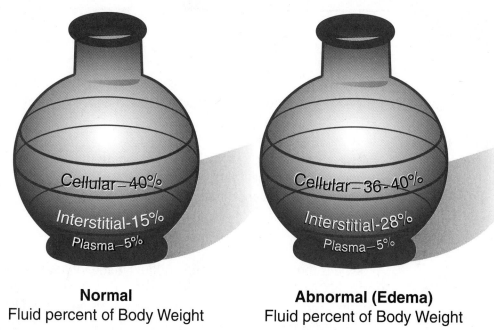

Normal
Fluid percent of Body Weight

Abnormal (Edema)
Fluid percent of Body Weight

Figure 3-1 Body fluid compartments and edema. Demonstrates the makeup of normal body fluid versus abnormal body fluid, such as with edema. As you recall from Chapter 1, 60% of the adult body weight is water; 40% of that is intracellular or cellular water, and 20% is extracellular water. Of the extracellular fluid, 15% is interstitial fluid and 5% is intravascular fluid or plasma. Note that with edema there is an increase of fluid in the interstitial space, which is between tissues and cells. The intracellular fluid may be decreased in extreme cases. (Adapted with permission, from H. Statland (1963). *Fluid and Electrolytes in Practice*, 3rd ed. Philadelphia, Pa: J. B. Lippincott Co., p. 177.)

5
Normally there is an exchange of fluid between the intravascular and interstitial spaces to maintain fluid balance in the ECF compartment.
　　The hydrostatic pressure in the arteries pushes fluid into the tissue spaces, and oncotic pressure in the arteries, which are made up of protein and albumin, holds fluid in the vessels. When there is fluid volume excess, the fluid pressure is greater than the oncotic pressure; therefore, (more/less) _____ fluid is pushed into the tissue spaces.

5　more

6
When standing for a period of time, excess fluid in the lower extremities can occur due to fluid overload, known as

(peripheral/pulmonary) _____ edema. The excess fluid that crosses the alveolar-capillary membrane of the lungs is known as (peripheral/pulmonary) _____ edema.

6   peripheral; pulmonary

7

Edema in the extremities (peripheral edema) occurs when there is a dysfunction of the heart, kidney, and/or liver. The fluid pressure in the vessels is increased and the fluid is pushed into the tissue spaces, primarily in the extremities.

   If the kidneys cannot excrete excess vascular fluid, what might happen? *_____

_____ .

7   peripheral edema, or fluid
       is pushed into the tissue
       spaces

8

Excess vascular fluid may lead to (peripheral edema/pulmonary edema/eventually both)*_____ .

8   peripheral and pulmonary
       edema (both)

▶ ETIOLOGY

   Edema is commonly associated with excess extracellular body fluid or excess fluid.

   Physiologic factors leading to edema may be caused by various clinical conditions such as congestive heart failure (CHF), kidney failure, cirrhosis of the liver, steroid excess, and allergic reaction. Table 3-1 lists the physiologic factors for edema, the rationale, and the clinical conditions associated with each physiologic factor.

9

Blood backed up in the venous system increases the capillary pressure, forcing more fluid into *_____

_____ .

   The clinical conditions in which edema may occur as a result of an increase of plasma hydrostatic pressure are:

   a. *_____
   b. *_____
   c. *_____
   d. *_____

9   the tissue spaces (inter-
       stitial spaces); a. CHF
       (congestive heart failure);
       b. kidney failure; c. venous
       obstruction; d. pressure on
       the veins, e.g., from casts or
       bandages

Table 3-1

Physiologic Factors Leading to Edema

Physiologic Factors		Rationale	Clinical Conditions
Plasma hydrostatic pressure in the capillaries	↑ Increased	Blood dammed in the venous system can cause "back" pressure in capillaries, thus raising capillary pressure. Increased capillary pressure will force more fluid into tissue areas, thus producing edema.	1. Congestive heart failure with increased venous pressure. 2. Kidney failure resulting in sodium and water retention. 3. Venous obstruction leading to varicose veins. 4. Pressure on veins because of swelling, constricting bandages, casts, tumor, pregnancy.
Plasma colloid osmotic pressure	↓ Decreased	Decreased plasma colloid osmotic pressure results from diminished plasma protein concentration. Decreased protein content may cause water to flow from plasma into tissue spaces, thus causing edema.	1. Malnutrition due to lack of protein in diet. 2. Chronic diarrhea resulting in loss of protein. 3. Burns leading to loss of fluid containing protein through denuded skin. 4. Kidney disease, particularly nephrosis. 5. Cirrhosis of liver resulting in decreased production of plasma protein. 6. Loss of plasma proteins through urine.
Capillary permeability	↑ Increased	Increased permeability of capillary membrane will allow plasma proteins to leak out of capillaries into interstitial space more rapidly than lymphatics can return them to circulation. Increased capillary permeability is predisposing factor to edema.	1. Bacterial inflammation causes increased porosity. 2. Allergic reactions. 3. Burns causing damage to capillaries. 4. Acute kidney disease, e.g., nephritis.

continues on the following page

Table 3-1

(Continued)

Physiologic Factors	Rationale	Clinical Conditions
Sodium retention	↑ I n c r e a s e d — Kidneys regulate level of sodium ions in extracellular fluid. Kidney function will depend on adequate blood flow. Inadequate blood flow, presence of excess aldosterone or glucocorticosteroids, and diseased kidneys are predisposing factors to edema since they cause sodium chloride and water retention.	1. Congestive heart failure causing inadequate circulation of blood. 2. Renal failure—inadequate circulation of blood through kidneys. 3. Increased production of adrenal cortical hormones—aldosterone, cortisone, and hydrocortisone—will cause retention of sodium. 4. Cirrhosis of liver. Diseased liver cannot destroy excess production of aldosterone. 5. Trauma resulting from fractures, burns, and surgery.
Lymphatic drainage	↓ D e c r e a s e d — Blockage of lymphatics will prevent return of proteins to circulation. Obstructed lymph flow is said to be high in protein content. With inadequate return of proteins to circulation, plasma colloid osmotic pressure will be decreased, thus causing edema.	1. Lymphatic obstruction, e.g., cancer of lymphatic system. 2. Surgical removal of lymph nodes. 3. Elephantiasis, which is parasitic invasion of lymph channels, resulting in fibrous tissue growing in nodes, obstructing lymph flow. 4. Obesity because of inadequate supporting structures for lymphatics in lower extremities. Muscles are considered the supporting structures.

10

A decrease in plasma protein results in a(n) (increase/decrease) _____ in the plasma colloid osmotic (oncotic) pressure. This causes water to move from the vessels into the *_____ .

Name at least four clinical conditions in which edema occurs as a result of decreased plasma/serum colloid osmotic (oncotic) pressure *_____

_____

10 decrease; tissue spaces malnutrition, burns, kidney disease, and liver disease (all clinical conditions due to loss or lack of protein intake)

11

An increase in the capillary membrane permeability will permit plasma proteins to escape from _____ , causing more water to move into * _____ .

Name at least three situations in which edema occurs as a result of increased capillary permeability. * _____

_____

12

The kidneys regulate the gain/loss of sodium, chloride, and water via the renin-angiotensin-aldosterone system. An inadequate blood flow, the presence of excess aldosterone, or diseased kidneys results in sodium (excretion/retention) _____ .

Name at least three clinical conditions that can cause sodium retention. _____

13

Obstruction of the lymph flow prevents the return of proteins to the circulation. The obstructed lymph fluid is high in _____ content.

A decrease in protein content in the plasma causes the water to move from * _____ into * _____ .

Name at least three clinical conditions that cause a decrease in lymphatic drainage. * _____

_____

14

Edema of the lungs, often called *pulmonary edema,* can occur in clients with limited cardiac or renal reserve. When the heart is not able to function adequately and the kidneys cannot excrete a sufficient amount of urine, the fluid backs up into the pulmonary circulatory system.

When the hydrostatic pressure of the blood in the pulmonary capillaries rises to equal or exceed the plasma colloid osmotic pressure, the water moves from vessels into the * _____ , leading to pulmonary edema.

---

11 capillaries; the tissue spaces (interstitial spaces); bacterial inflammation, allergic reactions, acute kidney disease (e.g., nephritis), and burns

12 retention; CHF (congestive heart failure), renal failure, adrenal cortical hormones (e.g., cortisone), cirrhosis of the liver, and trauma

13 protein; the intravascular space; the tissue spaces; cancer of the lymphatic system, removal of the lymph nodes, obesity, and elephantiasis

14 lung tissues

15

Giving excessive amounts of intravenous infusions to a person with pulmonary edema may cause the blood volume to increase. This increased blood volume is called _____ .

Intravenous infusions should be regulated so that the rate of flow is not in excess of the urinary _____ .

15 hypervolemia; output

▶ CLINICAL MANIFESTATIONS

There are numerous clinical manifestations of ECFVE as they relate to pulmonary edema and peripheral edema.

16

When the fluid volume excess (overhydration/hypervolemia) causes a "backup" of fluid that seeps into the lung tissue, *_____ results.

16 pulmonary edema

17

An early symptom of ECFVE is a constant, irritated cough. This is a sign of *_____

_____ .

17 overhydration or hypervolemia or fluid volume excess or early pulmonary edema

Table 3-2 lists the clinical signs and symptoms of ECFVE related to pulmonary and peripheral edema. Laboratory test results influenced by ECFVE are included. Rationale for each sign and symptom and potential abnormal laboratory results are listed.

18

One of the first clinical symptoms of ECFVE excess (hypervolemia or overhydration) is a *_____

_____ .

18 constant, irritating cough

19

Identify which of the following are signs and symptoms of pulmonary edema.

_____ a. Dyspnea
_____ b. Neck vein engorgement
_____ c. Hand vein engorgement
_____ d. Pitting edema in the extremities
_____ e. Tight, smooth, shiny skin over edematous site
_____ f. Moist rales in lung

19 a, b, c, f

Table 3-2

Clinical Manifestations of ECFVE—Hypervolemia, Overhydration, Edema

Signs and Symptoms	Rationale
Pulmonary Edema	
Constant, irritated cough	An irritated cough is frequently the first clinical symptom of hypervolemia. It is caused by fluid "backed up" into the lungs (fluid is in the alveoli).
Dyspnea (difficulty in breathing)	Breathing is labored and difficult due to fluid congestion in lungs.
Neck vein engorgement	Jugular vein remains engorged when the patient is in semi-Fowler's or sitting position.
Sublingual vein engorgement	Engorged veins under the tongue may indicate hypervolemia.
Hand vein engorgement	Peripheral veins in the hand remain engorged with hand elevated above heart level for 10 seconds.
Moist rales in lung	Lungs are congested with fluid. Moist rales in lung can be heard with the stethoscope.
Bounding pulse	A full, bounding pulse may be present with hypervolemia. The pulse rate may increase.
Cyanosis	Can be a late symptom of pulmonary edema as a result of impaired gas exchange caused by fluid in the alveolar space.
Peripheral Edema	
Pitting edema in extremities	Peripheral edema present in the morning may result from inadequate heart, liver, or kidney function. A positive test of pitting edema is a finger indentation on the edematous area.
Tight, smooth, shiny skin over edematous area	Excess fluid in the peripheral tissues may cause the skin to be tight, smooth, and shiny.
Pallor, cool skin at edematous area	Excess fluid causes a decrease in circulation. The skin becomes pale, shiny, and cool.
Puffy eyelids (periorbital edema)	Swollen eyelids occur with generalized edema.
Weight gain	A gain of 2.2 pounds is equivalent to a gain of 1 liter of body water.
Laboratory Tests	
Decreased serum osmolality	Excess fluid dilutes solute concentration; thus serum osmolality is below 280 mOsm/kg.
Decreased serum protein and albumin, BUN, Hgb, Hct	Serum protein, albumin, BUN, and Hgb and Hct levels can be decreased due to excess fluid volume (hemodilution).
Increased CVP (central venous pressure)	An increase in CVP measurement of more than 12–15 cm H_2O is indicative of hypervolemia, evidenced as an increase in the fluid pressure.

20

Pulmonary edema causes poor or inadequate ventilation.

20

In pulmonary edema, the alveoli (air sacs) are filled with fluid. Explain the effect this fluid has on ventilation throughout the lung tissue. *_____

_____

21

extracellular fluid volume excess or hypervolemia

21

When the jugular vein remains engorged after a person is put in a semi-Fowler's position (45° elevated), what type of fluid imbalance might this indicate? *_____

_____ .

22

hypervolemia or over-hydration; Hypervolemia is assessed with the hand above the heart level for vein engorgement and hypovolemia is assessed with the hand below the heart level for flat vein or no engorgement.

22

A quick assessment for hypervolemia, or overhydration, can be done by checking the peripheral veins in the hand. Instruct the client to hold a hand above the heart level. If the peripheral veins of the hand remain engorged after 10 seconds, this can be an indication of _____ .

   Explain how peripheral vein assessment for hypervolemia differs from peripheral vein assessment for hypovolemia.
*_____

_____ .

23

moist rales

23

The nurse can assess the lungs for evidence of hypervolemia by listening for *_____ with a stethoscope.

24

late

24

Cyanosis is a(n) (early/late) _____ symptom of pulmonary edema due to hypervolemia.

25

less

25

The influence of gravity has an effect on the distribution of fluid in the edematous person. In a lying position, there is a more equal distribution of edema, whereas in an upright position the edema is more prevalent in the lower extremities. This is called *dependent edema.*

   The eyelids of a person with generalized edema may be swollen in the morning, but by afternoon, with increased activity, the swelling is (more/less) _____ marked.

26 ankles and feet; eyes or sacrum and buttocks, or more equally distributed

27 dependent edema

28 Dependent edema should not be present after the client has been in a prone or supine position for the night. If edema is present in the morning, it is most likely due to cardiac, renal, or liver disease and can be called *nondependent edema* (to differentiate between edema due to gravity versus edema due to cardiac, renal, or liver dysfunction; it can also be called *refractory edema* when edema does not respond to diuretics).

29 1 (one)

30 hypervolemia; hypovolemia or dehydration

31 protein; It increases plasma colloid osmotic pressure and thus pulls fluid out of the tissues.

26
With clients who are up and about, the peripheral edema is frequently found in the (ankles and feet/sacrum and buttocks) *_____ . For those who are bedridden, edema fluid is most likely found in the *_____ .

27
The type of edema associated with gravity and the person's body position is called *_____ .

28
Explain why a nurse should assess for edema in the ankles and feet early in the morning.*_____

_____

_____ .

29
Another tool for assessing edema and hypervolemia is body weight.
 If the client has edema and has gained 2.2 pounds, this weight gain is equivalent to _____ liter(s) of water.

30
When hemoglobin and hematocrit measurements have been in a normal range and suddenly decrease, not due to hemorrhage or loss of blood supply, the change in fluid imbalance is (hypovolemia/hypervolemia) _____ .
 If the hemoglobin and hematocrit increase, the fluid imbalance might be indicative of _____ .

▶ CLINICAL APPLICATIONS

31
Many edematous persons are malnourished due to a loss of proteins or electrolytes. Unless contraindicated, the nurse should encourage the edematous client to eat foods high in _____ . Why? *_____

_____

32 The edema fluid is trapped in the interstitial space (tissue) and is not circulating, e.g., ascites and peripheral edema.

33 decubiti (bedsores); tissue breakdown or constant pressure on the edematous tissues

34 frequent change of body position (e.g., every 2 hr)

35 will not; Salt (sodium) has a water-retaining effect and without the sodium the water would not increase the edema. However, caution should be taken with giving excess amounts of water.

36 water

37 diuretics, digoxin (digitalis preparation), and diet (low sodium)

32

Edematous persons may suffer from decreased vascular volume. Explain why? *_____

33

The tissues of an edematous person are said to be more vulnerable to injury, resulting in tissue breakdown.

A bedfast person with edema of the sacrum and buttocks is apt to develop _____ due to *_____

_____ .

34

Identify a nursing intervention to prevent decubiti in the edematous person. *_____

▶ **CLINICAL MANAGEMENT**

35

When edema is present, salt and water intake often increases the fluid retention.

Water intake alone probably (will/will not) _____ increase the edema. Why? *_____

_____

36

Thiazide diuretics such as hydrochlorothiazine (HydroDiuril) and loop or high ceiling diuretics such as furosemide (Lasix) assist in decreasing fluid volume excess by promoting sodium and water excretion.

Decreasing fluid pressure in the vascular system assists fluid in flowing back from the tissue spaces into the vessels in order to be excreted.

Diuretics aid in the excretion of body sodium and _____ .

37

In cardiac insufficiency, the digitalis preparation digoxin may be needed to improve heart function and circulation.

The three D's are frequently prescribed for the clinical management of ECFVE. They are *_____ .

38

Increasing protein intake in a malnourished person should (increase/decrease) _____ the oncotic pressure in the vessels, thus pulling water out of the tissues.

38 increase

● Clinical Considerations

1. ECFVE, overhydration or hypervolemia, usually relates to excess fluid in tissues of the extremities (peripheral edema) or lungs (pulmonary edema).

2. Body water retention (edema) usually results from sodium retention. If only free water is retained, the excess is referred to as hypo-osmolar (hypotonic) fluid volume excess.

3. A constant, irritating cough is frequently the first clinical symptom of hypervolemia. It is caused by excess fluid "backed up" into the lungs.

4. For quick assessment of ECFVE, check for hand vein engorgement. If the peripheral veins in the hand remain engorged when the hand is elevated above the heart level for 10 seconds, ECFVE or hypervolemia is present.

5. Moist rales in the lung usually indicate that the lungs are congested with fluid.

6. Peripheral edema present in the morning may result from inadequate heart, liver, or kidney function. Peripheral edema in the evening may be due to fluid stasis, dependent edema. Peripheral edema should be assessed in the AM before the client gets out of bed.

7. A weight gain of 2.2 pounds is equivalent to the retention of 1 liter of body water.

8. Excess fluid dilutes solute concentration in the vascular space. A serum osmolality of <280 mOsm/kg indicates an ECFVE.

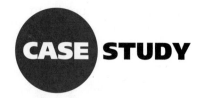

REVIEW

Mrs. Shea, age 72, was admitted to the hospital with complaints of shortness of breath, coughing, and swollen ankles and feet. Her blood pressure was 190/110, pulse 96, and respirations 28 and labored. Her hemoglobin and hematocrit were slightly low. She has a history of a "heart condition" and hypertension.

ANSWER COLUMN

1. extracellular fluid volume excess or edema; edema, hypervolemia, and overhydration

2. constant, irritating cough

3. increased hydrostatic pressure, decreased colloidal osmotic pressure, increased capillary permeability, increased sodium retention, and decreased lymphatic drainage
4. increased hydrostatic pressure and increased sodium retention

5. nondependent; inadequate heart, kidney, or liver function

6. extracellular fluid volume excess, or hypervolemia

7. pulmonary; observe the jugular veins for engorgement when Mrs. Shea is in semi-Fowler's position and assess chest sounds for moist rales
8. inadequate heart and kidney function

9. 2; 2000

---

1. The nurse assesses Mrs. Shea's physical state. Her shortness of breath, coughing, and swollen ankles and feet may be indicative of *_____ . Other names for extracellular fluid volume excess include _____ , _____ , and _____ .

2. An early symptom of extracellular fluid volume excess or hypervolemia is a *_____ _____ .

3. The five main physiologic factors that lead to edema are *_____ _____

4. The two physiologic factors that may have caused Mrs. Shea's edema are *_____ .

5. The nurse assesses Mrs. Shea's ankles and feet in the morning to differentiate between dependent and nondependent edema. If Mrs. Shea's ankles and feet remain swollen before she arises in the morning, the edema is described as _____ edema. The cause of this type of edema is *_____ .

6. The nurse assesses Mrs. Shea's peripheral veins. Her veins are still engorged after holding her hand above the heart level for 10 seconds. This can be indicative of *_____ _____ .

7. Mrs. Shea's shortness of breath or dyspnea and coughing may be due to _____ edema. Identify two assessment factors to assist the nurse in determining the type of edema present. *_____ _____

8. Identify two causes of pulmonary edema. *_____

9. Mrs. Shea gained 5 pounds in 2 days. This weight gain would be approximately _____ liter(s) of body water gain, which is equal to _____ mL of body water.

10. hypervolemia; dilution of red blood cells (RBCs) with a decrease in RBCs and an increase in water

11. decubiti; change body position, e.g., every 2 hours

12. anasarca

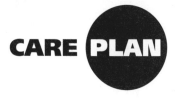

10. Mrs. Shea's hemoglobin and hematocrit have been normal. At present, they are decreased, which may indicate _____ . Why?*_____
_____

11. If Mrs. Shea developed generalized edema and was bedfast, what skin complication might result? _____
Identify a nursing intervention that can be taken to prevent this complication?*_____
_____

12. Identify the name for generalized edema. _____

Client Management: Extracellular Fluid Volume Excess (ECFVE)

Assessment Factors

▶ Complete a client history to identify health problems that may contribute to the development of ECFVE. Examples of such health problems may include a recurring heart problem such as CHF; kidney or liver disease; infection; or malnutrition. Ask if there has been a recent weight gain.

▶ Obtain a dietary history that emphasizes sodium, protein, and water intake.

▶ Assess vital signs. Obtain baseline data that can be compared with past and future vital signs. Assess for a bounding pulse.

▶ Assess for signs and symptoms of hypervolemia (overhydration) such as constant and irritated cough, difficulty in breathing, neck and hand vein engorgement, chest rales, and abnormal laboratory results such as a decreased hematocrit and hemoglobin level that had previously been normal. Serum sodium levels may or may not be elevated.

▶ Make a quick assessment of hypervolemia by checking the peripheral veins in the hand: first lowering the hand and then raising the hand above the heart level. Overhydration is present if the peripheral veins remain engorged after 10 seconds.

▶ Assess extremities for peripheral edema. Check for pitting edema in the lower extremities in the morning before the client arises. Nondependent edema or refractory edema may be due to cardiac, renal, or liver dysfunction. Dependent edema (edema caused by gravity) is usually not present in the morning.

▶ Assess urine output. Decreased urinary output may be a sign of body fluid retention and/or renal dysfunction.

▶ Assess pulmonary status. Observe for the presence of pulmonary congestion or changes in respiratory status.

Diagnosis 1

Fluid volume excess: edema related to body fluid overload secondary to heart, renal, or liver dysfunction.

Interventions and Rationale

1. Monitor vital signs. Report elevated blood pressure and bounding pulse.

2. Monitor weight daily. Check weight every morning before breakfast. A weight gain of 2.2 pounds (1 kg) is equivalent to 1 liter or quart of water (1000 mL). Usually edema does not occur unless there is 3 or more liters of excess body fluids. Restrict fluids as necessary. Teach the client to monitor intake, output, and weight.

3. Observe for the presence of edema daily. Check for pitting edema in the extremities every morning. Press one or two fingers on the edematous area, and if indentation is present for 15 seconds or more, the degree of pitting edema should be recorded according to the length of time it takes for the indentation to disappear (+1 to +4). Monitor all IV fluids carefully.

4. Monitor diet. Teach appropriate food selections. Instruct the client to avoid using excess salt on foods [salt (sodium) holds water and increases the edematous condition]. Teach the client to avoid over-the-counter drugs without first checking with a nurse or physician.

5. Encourage the client with a liver disorder such as cirrhosis of the liver to eat foods rich in protein. Protein increases the plasma/serum oncotic (colloid osmotic) pressure, thus pulling fluids from the tissue spaces and decreasing edema.

6. Encourage rest periods to support diuresis.

Diagnosis 2

Ineffective breathing patterns related to increased capillary permeability causing fluid overload in the lung tissue (pulmonary edema).

Interventions and Rationale

1. Monitor breathing patterns. Assess rate and depth of respiration. Check chest sounds and chest excursion. Note changes and location of adventitious sounds.
2. Observe for changes in skin color and nasal flaring. Note any coughing. Report any progression of symptoms to physician.
3. Use semi-Fowler's position for those with dyspnea or orthopnea.

Diagnosis 3

Impaired tissue integrity related to edematous tissues (peripheral edema).

Interventions and Rationale

1. Monitor client's mobility. Turn edematous clients frequently to prevent decubiti. Edematous persons are prone to tissue breakdown.
2. Identify and record changes in skin surfaces regarding color, temperature, and skin turgor.
3. Ambulate the client to improve circulation and enhance fluid reabsorption from the tissue spaces to the vascular space.
4. Monitor laboratory results pertinent to electrolyte status and fluid balance. Report changes.

Diagnosis 4

Altered tissue perfusion related to hypervolemia as manifested by peripheral (tissue) edema.

Interventions and Rationale

1. Monitor fluid intake. Water and sodium restrictions may be necessary.
2. Monitor urine output. Urine output should be >30 mL/h or >250 mL/8 h. Large amounts of urine output can indicate a decrease in urine retention.
3. Administer diuretics as ordered. Assess fluid balance.
4. Check serum electrolyte values while client is receiving diuretics. The more potent diuretics excrete not only sodium

but also the important electrolyte potassium. Encourage foods high in potassium; potassium supplements may be necessary. Urine output should be closely monitored when potassium is given.

Evaluation/Outcome

1. Evaluate that the cause of extracellular fluid volume excess (ECFVE) has been controlled or eliminated.

2. Evaluate the effects of clinical management for ECFVE. Pulmonary edema and/or peripheral edema are absent or decreased because of clinical management.

3. Remain free of signs and symptoms of overhydration/ hypervolemia. Dyspnea, neck vein engorgement, moist rales in the lungs, and peripheral edema are absent.

4. Urine output is increased; vital signs are normal.

5. Maintain a patent airway and the breath sounds are improved.

6. Determine that the serum electrolytes are within normal range.

7. Maintain a support system for client.

CHAPTER
4

Extracellular Fluid
Volume Shift (ECFVS)

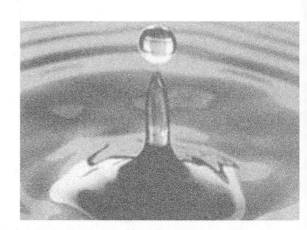

▌ INTRODUCTION

In the ECF compartment, fluid volume with electrolytes and protein shifts from the intravascular to the interstitial spaces. This fluid is referred to as *third-space fluid*. The fluid is nonfunctional and is considered to be physiologically useless. Later, third-space fluid shifts back from the interstitial space to the intravascular space.

1

Extracellular fluid is constantly shifting between the intravascular and interstitial spaces for the purpose of maintaining fluid balance.

When abnormal amounts of fluid shift into the tissue spaces and remain there, it is called *_____.

1　third-space fluid

▶ PATHOPHYSIOLOGY

Refer to the Pathophysiology section in Chapters 2 (ECFVD) and 3 (ECFVE).

2

Excess fluid in the tissue spaces, or third-space fluid, is nonfunctional and is considered *_____

_____ .

2　physiologically useless

▶ ETIOLOGY

3

Clinical causes could be as simple as a blister or sprain or as serious as massive injuries, burns, ascites, abdominal surgery, a perforated peptic ulcer, and intestinal obstruction.

When massive amounts of fluid shift to the tissues and remain there, what happens to the state of vascular fluids? *_____

_____

3　Hypovolemia, or fluid loss
　　from the vascular space. If
　　severe, shock can develop.

4

Minor causes of third-space fluid may be _____ and

_____ .

Identify three severe health problems that can cause third-space fluid. *_____

4　blisters; sprains; burns,
　　trauma (massive injuries),
　　and ascites (severe liver
　　disease) (also, abdominal
　　surgery, intestinal obstruc-
　　tion, or perforated ulcer)

5

Burns and abdominal surgery are common causes of third-space fluid. With these two conditions, there are two phases of fluid shift.

In the first phase fluid is shifting from the intravascular space to the interstitial space. With burns, fluid loss occurs at the surface of the burned area and surrounding tissues. Fluid from the vascular space "pours" into the burned site and remains for approximately 3–5 days.

In the second phase of fluid shift, fluid then shifts from the *_____ to the *_____ .

5 interstitial space (tissue and injured area); intravascular space

▶ CLINICAL MANIFESTATIONS

In a fluid shift due to tissue injury, it takes approximately 24–48 hours for the fluid to leave the blood vessels and accumulate in the injured tissue spaces. Edema may or may not be visible.

Table 4-1 presents the two phases of fluid volume shift and the causes, time occurrence, and possible resulting type of fluid imbalance.

6

When fluid shifts out of the vessels, changes in the vital signs occur that are similar to shocklike symptoms. These vital signs are similar to those of fluid volume deficit—marked dehydra-

Table 4-1

Fluid Volume Shift

Phase	Fluid Shift	Cause	Time Occurrence	Resulting Type of Fluid Imbalance
I	Intravascular (vessel) to the interstitial (tissue) spaces	*Minor:* blister, sprain *Major:* burns, abdominal surgery, intestinal obstruction, crushing wounds, severe infections	24–48 h	Hypovolemia
II	Interstitial to intravascular spaces		3–5 days	Hypervolemia

6 increased pulse rate; increased respiration; decreased systolic blood pressure (depends on the severity of fluid loss to the injured site)	tion. Indicate whether the following vital signs increase or decrease in such fluid shifts. * _____ Pulse rate * _____ Respiration * _____ Systolic blood pressure

7
Three to five days after an injury causing tissue destruction, fluid shifts from the injured site to * _____ .

7 blood vessels or intravascular space	

8
If the kidneys cannot excrete the excess fluid from the vascular space (blood vessels) that resulted from the fluid shift, what type of fluid imbalance might occur? _____
_____

8 hypervolemia or ECFVE	
9 constant, irritated cough, dyspnea, and moist chest rales (also hand and neck vein engorgement and full bounding pulse)	**9** Name three clinical signs and symptoms of hypervolemia. * _____ _____

▶ CLINICAL APPLICATIONS

Refer to the Clinical Applications sections of Chapters 2 (ECFVD) and 3 (ECFVE).

▶ CLINICAL MANAGEMENT

10
An assessment must be completed in order to determine the cause of the third-space fluid. In the case of burns when severe tissue destruction results, the fluid shift may be so severe that (hypervolemia/hypovolemia) _____ occurs.

10 hypovolemia	

11
During the first phase of a fluid shift to the burn tissue site, intravenous infusion in the amount of two to three times the urine output may be necessary to maintain the circulating fluid volume.

During the second phase of fluid shift, (more/less) _____ IV fluids would be needed. Why? * _____
_____

11 less; Large quantities of fluid shift back into the vascular space and too much intravenous fluid may cause a fluid overload.	

12 increases; Urine excretion increases, with sufficient kidney function, to prevent fluid overload.

12
During the second phase of the fluid shift, the urine output (increases/decreases) _____ .
Explain. *_____

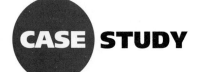

CASE STUDY

REVIEW

John Thomas had massive tissue injuries and was admitted to the hospital. His vital signs were blood pressure (BP) 98/54, pulse (P) 102, respiration (R) 32. Urine output was <30 mL/h.

ANSWER COLUMN

1. ECFVD or hypovolemia

1. John's vital signs could indicate what type of fluid imbalance? _____

2. third-space fluid

2. When an abnormal amount of fluid shifts into the injured tissue space and remains there, the fluid in that space is called *_____ .

3. massive tissue injury; With massive tissue injury, abnormal amounts of fluid shift to the injured site.

3. The cause for Mr. Thomas' fluid shift is *_____ .
Explain. *_____
_____

Clinical management for John Thomas included the administration of 4000 mL of 5% dextrose in 1/2 normal saline (0.45% NaCl) solution and 5% dextrose in water. Mr. Thomas' vital signs after a few days were BP 114/64, P 92, and R 30.

4. to correct fluid loss from vascular space to tissue space

4. Why was John given a large amount of intravenous fluids?
*_____

5. ECFVE or overhydration or hypervolemia; John is receiving large amounts of IV solutions and at the same time the fluid is shifting back into the vascular space from the injured tissue area.

Three days after John received daily large amounts of IV fluids, he developed a constant, irritated cough, mild dyspnea, and neck and hand vein engorgements.

5. What type of fluid imbalance is John exhibiting? _____
Explain? *_____
_____ .

6. Intravenous fluids administration should be greatly reduced or discontinued.
7. phase 1, fluid in the intravascular space shifts to the injured site, and phase 2, fluid shifts from the injured area to the vascular space

8. sprain and blister

6. What corrective measures for this imbalance should be taken?* _____

7. What are the two phases of ECFV shift?* _____

_____

8. Two examples of minor causes for third-space fluid are
* _____

_____ .

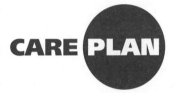

Client Management: Extracellular Fluid Volume Shift (ECFVS)

Assessment Factors

For extracellular fluid volume shift, refer to Chapters 2 (ECFVD, phase 1) and 3 (ECFVE, phase 2).

Diagnosis

For extracellular fluid volume shift, refer to Chapters 2 (ECFVD, phase 1) and 3 (ECFVE, phase 2).

Interventions and Rationale

For extracellular fluid volume shift, refer to Chapters 2 (ECFVD, phase 1) and 3 (ECFVE, phase 2).

Evaluation/Outcome

For extracellular fluid volume shift, refer to Chapters 2 (ECFVD, phase 1) and 3 (ECFVE, phase 2).

Intracellular Fluid Volume Excess (ICFVE)

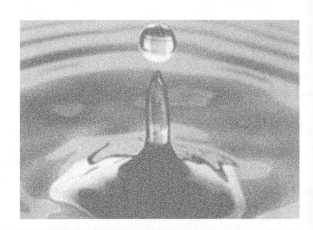

▶ INTRODUCTION

1

Intracellular fluid volume excess (ICFVE), also referred to as water intoxication, results from an excess of water or decrease in solutes in the intravascular system. With an ICFVE there is an excess of fluid in the intracellular compartment. Fluid in the blood vessels is (hypo-osmolar/iso-osmolar/hyperosmolar) _____ when there is an ICFVE.

1   hypo-osmolar

2

water intoxication;
decreased

2

Another name for ICFVE is *_____ . As a result of this fluid imbalance, the serum osmolality is (increased/decreased) _____ .

▶ PATHOPHYSIOLOGY

Hypo-osmolar fluid (decreased solute concentration in the circulating vascular fluid) moves by the process of osmosis from the areas of lesser solute concentration to the areas of greater concentration. The intracellular fluid (cells) is iso-osmolar, so the hypo-osmolar fluid from the vascular space moves into the cells, thus causing the cells to swell.

3 osmosis

3

Fluid shifts from the areas of lesser solute concentration to the areas of greater solute concentration due to the process of (diffusion/osmosis) _____ .

4 (intra)cellular fluid overload or cellular edema

4

Excess fluid that may accumulate in the cells can cause *_____ _____ .

5 cerebral edema or cellular fluid overload

5

In an ICFVE, the cerebral cells are usually the first cells involved in the fluid shift from the vascular to the cellular space.
    What might happen if there are large amounts of fluid shifting into the cerebral cells? *_____ _____ .

6 hypo-osmolar

6

An excess secretion of the antidiuretic hormone (ADH) causes fluid to be reabsorbed from the renal tubules. This can result in what type of vascular fluid? _____

7 sodium; water; extracellular fluid; intracellular fluid

7

Edema may result from an excess of _____ , whereas water intoxication results from an excess of _____ .
    With edema, there is excessive fluid in the *_____ compartment, whereas with water intoxication there is excess fluid in the *_____ compartment.

8

Water intoxication (is/is not) _____ the same as edema. Generally, edema is the accumulation of fluid in the interstitial spaces. With water intoxication, the excess hypo-osmolar fluid (increases/lowers) _____ serum osmolality.

As the result of the hypo-osmolar fluid in the vascular space, water moves into the cells, causing the cells to (shrink/swell) _____ .

8 is not; lowers; swell

▶ ETIOLOGY

Intracellular fluid volume excess is not as common as ECFVD and ECFVE, but if untreated, it can cause serious health problems.

Common causes of water intoxication are the intake of water-free solutes and the administration of hypo-osmolar intravenous fluids such as 0.45% sodium chloride ($\frac{1}{2}$ normal saline solution) and 5% dextrose in water (D_5W). Dextrose 5% in water is an iso-osmolar IV solution; however, the dextrose is metabolized quickly, leaving water or a hypo-osmolar solution.

9 ECFVD and ECFVE; intracellular fluid volume excess

9

The two most common types of fluid imbalance are * _____ _____ . The acronym ICFVE stands for * _____ .

10

There are four major conditions that may cause ICFVE:
  a. Excessive nonsolute water intake
  b. Solute deficit (electrolytes and protein)
  c. Increased secretion of antidiuretic hormone (ADH)
  d. Kidney dysfunction (inability to excrete excess water)

These conditions may cause an increase in (hypo-osmolar/hyperosmolar) _____ fluid in the vascular space (vessels).

10 hypo-osmolar

Table 5-1 lists four major conditions and laboratory tests to assess for ICFVE, their causes, and rationale. Study the table carefully and refer to it as needed.

11 excess nonsolute water intake, solute deficit or lack of electrolytes and protein, increased secretion of inappropriate ADH (SIADH), and kidney dysfunction or renal impairment

11

Name four major conditions that might cause water intoxication. * _____

Table 5-1

Causes of Intracellular Fluid Volume Excess: Water Intoxication

Conditions	Causes	Rationale
Excessive water intake	Excessive plain water intake	Water intake with few or no solutes dilutes the vascular fluid.
	Continuous use of IV hypo-osmolar solutions (0.45% saline, D$_5$W)	Overuse of hypo-osmolar solutions can cause hypo-osmolar vascular fluid. Dextrose is metabolized rapidly, leaving water.
	Psychogenic polydipsia	Compulsive drinking of plain water can result in water intoxication.
Solute deficit	Diet low in electrolytes and protein	Decrease in electrolytes and protein may cause hypo-osmolar vascular fluids.
	Irrigation of nasogastric tube with water (not saline)	GI tract is rich in electrolytes. Plain water can wash out the electrolytes.
	Plain water enema	Plain water can wash out the electrolytes.
Excess ADH secretion	Stress, surgery, drugs (narcotics, anesthesia), pain, and tumors (brain, lung)	Overproduction of ADH is known as secretion (syndrome) of inappropriate antidiuretic hormone (SIADH), which causes mass amounts of water reabsorption by the kidneys and results in hypo-osmolar fluids.
	Brain injury or tumor	Cerebral cell injury may increase ADH production, causing excessive water reabsorption.
Kidney dysfunction	Renal impairment	Kidney dysfunction can decrease water excretion.
Abnormal laboratory tests	Decreased serum sodium level and decreased serum osmolality	Because of hemodilution, the solutes in the vascular fluid are decreased in proportion to water.

12 dextrose is metabolized rapidly, leaving water solution. When D$_5$W is used continuously without other solutes, hypo-osmolar fluid results.

12

The iso-osmolar IV solution D$_5$W becomes a hypo-osmolar solution when * _____

_____

13

Overproduction of ADH or SIADH causes (more/less) _____ water reabsorption from the tubules of the kidneys.

    Two causes of excess secretion of ADH are * _____

_____ .

13 more; stress and surgery [also drugs (narcotics) and pain]

14

If the circulation through the kidneys is impaired and there is an excessive amount of plain water intake, the fluid imbalance most likely to occur is * _____ .

    Impairment of the renal circulation can occur due to arteriosclerosis. If the kidneys do not receive sufficient blood circulation, kidney (function/dysfunction) _____ can result.

14 water intoxication from water taken without solutes; dysfunction

15

If there is a water excess, the serum osmolality is most likely * _____ , and the serum sodium level is most likely _____ .

15 low or decreased or <280 mOsm/kg; decreased

▶ CLINICAL MANIFESTATIONS

    The clinical signs and symptoms and rationale of water intoxication or ICFVE are explained in Table 5-2. Study the table and be cognizant of the signs and symptoms. Refer to the table as necessary.

16

Identify four early symptoms of water intoxication. * _____

_____

16 headache, nausea and vomiting, excessive perspiration, and weight gain

17

Central nervous system symptoms are (least/most) _____ prominent with water intoxication. Explain why? * _____

_____

17 most; Hypo-osmolar body fluids pass into cerebral cells; swollen cerebral cells cause behavioral changes.

Table 5-2

Clinical Signs and Symptoms of Intracellular Fluid Volume Excess—Water Intoxication

Type of Symptoms	Signs and Symptoms	Rationale
Early	Headache Nausea and vomiting Excessive perspiration Acute weight gain	Cerebral cells absorb hypo-osmolar fluid more quickly than other cells.
Progressive Central nervous system (CNS)	Behavioral changes: progressive apprehension, irritability, disorientation, confusion Drowsiness, Incoordination Blurred vision Elevated intracranial pressure (ICP)	Hypo-osmolar body fluids usually pass into cerebral cells first. Swollen cerebral cells can cause behavioral changes and elevate ICP.
Vital signs (VS)	Blood pressure ↑ Bradycardia (slow pulse rate) Respiration ↑	VS are the opposite of shock. VS are similar to those in increased ICP.
Later (CNS)	Neuroexcitability (muscle twitching) Projectile vomiting Papilledema Delirium Convulsions, then coma	Severe CNS changes occur when water intoxication is not corrected.
Skin	Warm, moist, and flushed	

18 apprehension, irritability, disorientation, and confusion

18

Name three behavioral changes that occur with progressive symptoms of water intoxication.*_____

_____

19 increased

19

The intracranial pressure is (increased/decreased) _____ with water intoxication.

20

With progressive intracellular fluid volume excess, the vital sign measurements reflect:

20 a. increased; b. decreased, or bradycardia; c. increased

a. Blood pressure _____
b. Pulse rate * _____
c. Respiration _____

21
Name five later symptoms of water intoxication. * _____
_____
_____

21 muscle twitching, projectile vomiting, papilledema, delirium, and convulsions

22
The skin in the later stages of water intoxication is * _____
_____ .

22 warm, moist, and flushed

▶ **CLINICAL APPLICATIONS**

23
It is difficult for a person to drink himself into water intoxication unless the renal mechanisms for elimination fail or psychogenic polydipsia occurs.

If excessive water has been given and the kidneys are not functioning properly, what is most likely to occur? * _____
_____

23 water retention or water intoxication

24
The most common occurrence of water intoxication is seen in postoperative clients when oral and intravenous fluids have been forced without compensatory amounts of salt. In these situations, the amount of water taken in exceeds that which the kidneys can excrete.

A postoperative client receiving several liters of 5% dextrose in water (D_5W) with ice and sips of water PO (by mouth) can develop a fluid imbalance called * _____
_____ .

24 water intoxication or ICFVE (due to intake of copious amounts of hypo-osmolar fluids)

25
Also, after surgery, an overproduction of the antidiuretic hormone (ADH), known as the syndrome of inappropriate ADH secretions (SIADH), can occur due to trauma, anesthesia, pain,

and narcotics. Because of the overproduction of ADH, water excretion (increases/decreases) _____ , causing the urine volume to (rise/drop) _____ and the vascular (intravascular) fluid volume to (rise/drop) _____ .

25 decreases; drop; rise

▶ CLINICAL MANAGEMENT

The overall objective of clinical management for ICFVE is to reduce excess water in the body. Two ways to reduce water intoxication in the body are to reduce the water intake and promote water excretion.

26

In *less* severe cases of water intoxication, water restriction may be sufficient, or an extracellular replacement solution such as lactated Ringer's or normal saline solution may be given to increase the osmolality of the extracellular fluid.

The overall objective in the clinical management of water intoxication is *_____

_____ .

Name two ways in which this objective is accomplished.
*_____

26 to reduce excess water in the body; reduce water intake and promote water excretion

27

Concentrated saline (3% NaCl) may be given in severe cases of water intoxication to raise extracellular electrolyte concentration in hope of drawing water out of the (intracellular space/ interstitial space) *_____ and (increasing/decreasing) _____ urinary output.

27 intracellular space; increasing

28

However, administration of additional salt to a person who already has too much water can result in expansion of the interstitial fluid and blood volume and the development of (water intoxication/edema) _____.

An osmotic diuretic, e.g., mannitol, includes diuresis and a loss of retained fluid, especially from the cerebral cells.

28 edema

29 water restriction; extracellular replacement solution, e.g., lactated Ringer's or normal saline solution (0.9% NaCl); concentrated saline solution; and osmotic diuretics, e.g., mannitol or other diuretics

30 water restriction; extracellular replacement solution; intravenous concentrated saline solution; osmotic diuretics

31 diuresis and a loss of retained fluid, especially from cerebral cells

29

Identify three methods for promoting water excretion. *_____

_____

_____

_____

_____

30

For less severe cases of water intoxication, the clinical management includes *_____ and/or *_____

_____

 For more severe cases of water intoxication, identify two possible clinical management interventions.*_____

_____

and/or *_____

31

An osmotic diuretic induces *_____

_____ .

● Clinical Considerations

1. ICFVE is also known as water intoxication, excess water in the cells. It usually results from an excess of hypo-osmolar (hypotonic) vascular fluid. Water intoxication is not the same as edema. Edema usually results from sodium retention whereas water intoxication results from excess water.

2. In ICFVE, cerebral cells are usually the first cells involved in the fluid shift from the vascular to the cellular (cell) space. Large amounts of fluid shifting into the cerebral cells can result in cerebral edema.

3. Continuous administration of intravenous solutions that are hypotonic or the continuous use of 5% dextrose in water can result in ICFVE. In the latter case, dextrose is metabolized rapidly in the body; thus water remains. At least 1 or 2 liters of the dextrose solution should contain a percentage of a saline solution or be administered in combination with solutes such as lactated Ringer's.

4. Headache and nausea and vomiting are early signs and symptoms of ICFVE. As ICFVE progresses, behavioral changes such as irritability, disorientation, and confusion may occur. Drowsiness and blurred vision may result.

5. Changes in vital signs are similar to those of cerebral edema: increased blood pressure, decreased pulse rate, increased respiration.

6. A concentrated saline solution (3% NaCl) can be administered for severe ICFVE. It is given if the serum sodium is <115 mEq/L. Also it draws the water out of the swollen cells.

7. Water restriction is suggested for mild ICFVE.

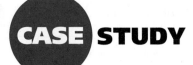

REVIEW

Ms. Cline, age 19, returned from having an appendectomy performed. She received 1 liter of 5% dextrose in water during the procedure and another liter postoperatively. She was allowed to have crushed ice and sips of water. That evening she became nauseated, and the third liter of 5% dextrose in water was added. The following day she received 2 more liters of 5% dextrose in water. Ms. Cline took several glasses of crushed ice. Her first day postoperatively she complained of a headache. Later she was drowsy, disoriented, and confused. Her blood pressure evidenced a slight increase, and a drop in her pulse rate was noted.

ANSWER COLUMN

1. water intoxication or intracellular fluid volume excess
2. water intoxication; With 5% dextrose in water, the dextrose is metabolized by the body, leaving water. The intravenous solution and crushed ice cause the plasma to become hypo-osmolar.
3. Headache. If your answer was nausea—possibly; however, early nausea is most likely the result of the surgery and anesthesia.
4. drowsiness, disorientation, and confusion

1. The nurse assessed Ms. Cline's fluid state. From the history and her symptoms, the nurse assessed a fluid imbalance was present indicative of * _____
   _____ .

2. Excessive amounts of 5% dextrose in water along with glasses of crushed ice without any other solute intake can cause * _____ .
   Explain why. * _____
   _____

3. Name Ms. Cline's early symptoms of intracellular fluid volume excess. * _____

4. As the fluid imbalance progressed, name three symptoms that indicated water intoxication or ICFVE. _____
   _____

5. increased intracranial pressure
6. yes; After surgery, there can be an increased secretion of ADH, due to trauma, anesthesia, pain, and narcotics. This increases water retention and, with the hypo-osmolar fluids she received, could increase the state of water intoxication.
7. concentrated saline solution, e.g., 3% saline, hyperosmolar solution to "pull" water out of the cells
8. Ms. Cline should have received intravenous fluids containing saline (solute) together with dextrose.

5. Her vital signs were similar to those of *._____ _____

6. Can an overproduction of ADH increase her water intoxication? _____ Explain how. *_____ _____

7. Name the type of intravenous solution to be administered to correct severe cases of water intoxication. *_____ _____

8. Identify how this fluid imbalance could have been prevented. *_____ _____

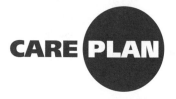

Client Management: Intracellular Fluid Volume Excess (ICFVE)

Assessment Factors

▶ Complete a history to identify possible causes of intracellular fluid volume excess (ICFVE) such as excessive administration of hypo-osmolar solutions [continuous use of D_5W without solutes (saline)], oral fluid without solutes, major surgical procedure that might cause SIADH, and kidney dysfunction in which urine output is decreased.

▶ Assess vital signs. Obtain baseline data that can be compared with past and future vital signs. Note if the systolic blood pressure increases even slightly, pulse rate decreases, and respirations increase. These signs are indicative of an accumulation of cerebral fluid (cerebral edema).

▶ Assess for behavioral changes, such as confusion, irritability, and disorientation. Headache is an early symptom of ICFVE. These symptoms can result when hypo-osmolar fluid in the vascular space shifts to the cells, increasing cellular fluid. Cerebral cells are usually the first cells affected.

▶ Assess for weight changes. With ICFVE or water intoxication, there is normally an acute weight gain. With peripheral edema, the weight gain occurs more slowly.

Diagnosis 1

Fluid volume excess: water intoxication related to excessive ingestion and infusion of hypo-osmolar fluids and solutions, major surgical procedure causing SIADH.

Interventions and Rationale

1. Monitor fluid replacement. Assess osmolality of fluid replacement and consult with the health care provider for appropriate replacement balance. Report if the client is receiving only 5% dextrose in water continuously. Dextrose is metabolized rapidly by the body, leaving water, a hypo-osmolar solution.

2. Offer fluids that contain solutes, such as broth and juices, to the postoperative client. Giving plain water and ice chips increases the hypo-osmolar state. Immediately postoperatively and for 24–48 hours, there may be an overproduction of ADH [SIADH, or secretion (syndrome) of inappropriate antidiuretic hormone], causing an increase in water reabsorption.

3. Monitor fluid balance. The urine output after surgery and trauma can be compromised. The SIADH is frequently seen following surgery and trauma, which causes more water to be reabsorbed from the kidney tubules and dilution of the vascular fluid. Urine output is decreased due to water reabsorption.

Diagnosis 2

Risk for injury related to cerebral edema secondary to ICFVE.

Interventions and Rationale

1. Monitor vital signs and observe for behavioral changes. Assess the client for progressive signs and symptoms of water intoxication such as headache, behavioral changes (irritability, drowsiness, confusion, disorientation, delirium), changes in the vital signs (increased blood pressure, decreased pulse, increased respiration), and warm, moist, flushed skin.

2. Protect the client from injury during periods of confusion and disorientation. Keep bed rails up, assist the client with ambulation, assist the client with meals, and frequently reorient to place and time.

3. Observe for signs of seizure activity. Convulsions usually occur with severe ICFVE.

Evaluation/Outcome

1. Evaluate that the cause of intracellular fluid volume excess (ICFVE) has been corrected or controlled.

2. Evaluate the effects of clinical management for ICFVE: hypotonic/hypo-osmolar solutions discontinued, solutes offered with fluids.

3. Remain free of signs and symptoms of ICFVE or water intoxication. Vital signs return to normal ranges. Headaches have been lessened or absent.

4. Responds clearly without confusion.

5. Maintain a support system for client.

ELECTROLYTES AND THEIR INFLUENCE ON THE BODY

OBJECTIVES

Upon completion of this unit, the reader should be able to:

- Describe the relationship of nonelectrolytes, electrolytes, and ions in body fluids.
- Name the principal cation and anion of the extracellular and intracellular fluids.
- Describe the physiologic functions of potassium, sodium, calcium, magnesium, phosphorus, and chloride.
- List the normal ranges of serum and urine potassium, sodium, calcium, magnesium, phosphorus, and chloride.
- Identify the various clinical causes (etiology) of potassium, sodium, calcium, magnesium, phosphorus, and chloride deficits or excesses.
- List the signs and symptoms of hypo-hyperkalemia, hypo-hypernatremia, hypo-hypercalcemia, hypo-hypermagnesemia, hypo-hyperphosphatemia, and hypo-hyperchloremia.
- Relate the electrolyte imbalances to drug action and interaction.
- Describe methods commonly utilized in electrolyte replacement therapy.
- Explain the assessment factors, diagnoses, and interventions to selected clinical situations (clinical applications).
- List foods that are rich in potassium, sodium, calcium, magnesium, phosphorus, and chloride.

▶ INTRODUCTION

Chemical compounds may react in one of two ways when placed in solution. In one way, their molecules may remain intact as in urea, dextrose, and creatinine in the body fluid. These molecules do not produce an electrical charge and are considered nonelectrolytes.

In the other reaction, the compound develops a tiny electrical charge when dissolved in water. The compound breaks up into separate particles known as ions; this process is referred to as ionization, and the compounds are known as electrolytes. Some electrolytes develop a positive charge (cations) when placed in water; others develop a negative charge (anions).

The chemical composition of seawater and human body fluid is very similar. The principal cations of seawater are sodium, potassium, magnesium, and calcium, and so it is with the body fluid. The seawater contains as principal anions chloride, phosphate, and sulfate, the same as body fluid.

In this unit six electrolytes [potassium, sodium, calcium, magnesium, phosphorus (phosphate), and chloride] are discussed in relation to human body needs (functions), pathophysiology, etiology, clinical manifestations, and clinical management. Normal serum and urine levels, drug-laboratory test interactions, and foods rich in these electrolytes are presented. Clinical applications, clinical considerations, and case studies are discussed using the nursing process format—assessment, diagnoses, interventions, and evaluations/outcome.

An asterisk (*) on an answer line indicates a multiple-word answer. The meanings for the following symbols are: ↑ increased, ↓ decreased, > greater than, < less than.

▶ ELECTROLYTES: CATION AND ANION

ANSWER COLUMN

1

Electrolytes are compounds that, when placed in solution, conduct an electric current.

Pure water does not conduct electricity, but if a pinch of salt, which contains sodium and chloride, is dropped into it, what do you think happens to the water? *_____

_____

2

Ions are dissociated particles of electrolytes that carry either a positive charge called a *cation* or a negative charge called an *anion*.

Dissociated particles of electrolytes are called _____ .
The particles that carry a positive charge are called _____ ,
and those that carry a negative charge are called _____ .

3

What is the difference between a cation and an anion? *_____

_____

Table U3-1 gives the principal cations and anions in human body fluid. Since we will be referring to these elements and their symbols throughout the program, take a few minutes now to memorize them. Be sure to note the + and − symbols.

4

Place a C in front of the cations and an A in front of anions.
_____ a. K   _____ e. Na
_____ b. Mg   _____ f. Ca
_____ c. Cl   _____ g. HPO_4
_____ d. HCO_3

1   Salt would produce an electrical charge. The water would conduct electricity.

2   ions; cations; anions

3   A cation carries a positive charge and an anion a negative charge.

4   a. C; b. C; c. A; d. A; e. C; f. C; g. A

Table U3-1

Cations and Anions

Cations		Anions	
Na^+	(Sodium)	Cl^-	(Chloride)
K^+	(Potassium)	HCO_3^-	(Bicarbonate)
Ca^{2+}	(Calcium)	HPO_4^{2-}	(Phosphate)
Mg^{2+}	(Magnesium)		

5 two positive charges

6 osmotic; *Milligrams*. The weight of ions.; *Milliequivalents*. The chemical activity of ions.

7 weight

8 15 girls and 15 boys; Otherwise, you would have an unequal number of boys and girls, for not every child weighs exactly 100 pounds.

9 milliequivalents

5

For electrical balance, the quantities of cations and anions in a solution, expressed in milliequivalents (mEq), always equal each other.

Electrolytes differ in their chemical activity, for sodium has one positive charge and calcium has * _____ .

6

In studying serum chemistry alterations and concentrations, one is concerned with how much the ions or chemical particles weigh. The weight of ions and chemical particles is measured in milligrams percent (mg%), which is the same as mg/100 mL or mg/dL. The number of electrically charged ions is measured in milliequivalents per liter (1000 mL), or mEq/L.

The term *milliequivalent* involves the chemical activity of elements, whereas milliosmol involves the _____ activity of the solution.

How do milligrams and milliequivalents differ? * _____

7

Milliequivalents provide a better method of measuring the concentration of ions in the serum than milligrams.

Milligrams measure the _____ of ions and give no information concerning the number of ions or the electrical charges of the ions.

8

The following is a simple analogy to compare milligrams and milliequivalents.

If you were having a party and wanted to invite equal numbers of boys and girls, which would be more accurate—inviting 1500 pounds of girls and 1500 pounds of boys or inviting 15 girls and 15 boys? * _____
Why? * _____

_____

9

From the example in question 7, which would be more accurate in determining the serum chemistry of chemical particles or ions in the body—milliequivalents or milligrams? _____

You will find both measurements used in this book and in your clinical settings for determining changes in our serum chemistry. However, when referring to ions, milliequivalents will be used in this book.

10
The term *milliequivalents* is used to express the number of ionic charges of each electrolyte on an equal basis. It measures the _____ activity of ions or elements.
  The total cations in milliequivalents must equal the total _____ in milliequivalents.

11
Milliequivalents consider electrolytes in terms of their *_____ rather than their weight.

12
Electrolytes have different weights but are considered during therapy in terms of their chemical activity, which is expressed as (milliequivalents/milligrams) _____ .

  Table U3-2 gives the weights and equivalences of five ions. Note how the weights of the named ions differ but the equivalences remain the same according to their ionic charge. You are not expected to memorize the weights of these ions.

13
Name a cation and an anion with the same equivalence but different weights. *_____
_____

10 chemical; anions

11 chemical activity

12 milliequivalents

13 sodium and chloride or potassium and chloride

Table U3-2

Electrolyte Equivalents

Ion	Weight (mg)	Equivalence (mEq)
Na^+	23	1
K^+	39	1
Cl^-	35	1
Ca^{++}	40	2
Mg^{++}	24	2

14

intracellular and extracellular; intravascular and interstitial

14

The electrolyte composition of fluid differs within the two main classes of body fluid.

The two main classes of body water are* _____ fluid. What are the two main compartments of extracellular fluid?

* _____

Table U3-3 gives the ion concentrations of the intravascular fluid (which is frequently referred to as plasma), interstitial fluid, and intracellular fluid. Take a few minutes to memorize the fluids and their greatest concentration of ions. Memorizing the numbers is not necessary. Refer back to the table when necessary.

15

sodium; potassium

15

According to Table U3-3, the cation that is most plentiful in the extracellular body fluid is _____ and the cation that is most plentiful in the intracellular body fluid is _____ .

16

sodium or Na, chloride or Cl, and bicarbonate or HCO_3; same as in intravascular fluid; potassium or K, magnesium or Mg, and phosphate or HPO_4

16

What are the three principal ions in intravascular fluid? * _____

_____

What are the three principal ions in interstitial fluid? * _____

_____

What are the three principal ions in intracellular fluid? * _____

_____

Figure U3-1 shows the various cations and anions in extracellular and intracellular fluids. Pay special attention to the principal cations and anions in these fluids. Refer to the figure when necessary.

17

sodium or Na; potassium or K

17

The principal cation in extracellular fluid is _____ .
The principal cation in intracellular fluid is _____ .

18

chloride or Cl; phosphate or HPO_4

18

The principal anion in extracellular fluid is _____ .
The principal anion in intracellular fluid is _____ .

Table U3-3

Electrolyte Composition of Body Fluid (mEq/L)

| Ions | Extracellular | | Intracellular |
	Intravascular or Plasma	Interstitial	
Na^+	142	145	10
K^+	5	4	141–150
Ca^{++}	5	3	2
Mg^{++}	2	1	27
Cl^-	104	116	1
HCO_3^-	27	30	10
HPO_4^{--}	2	2	100

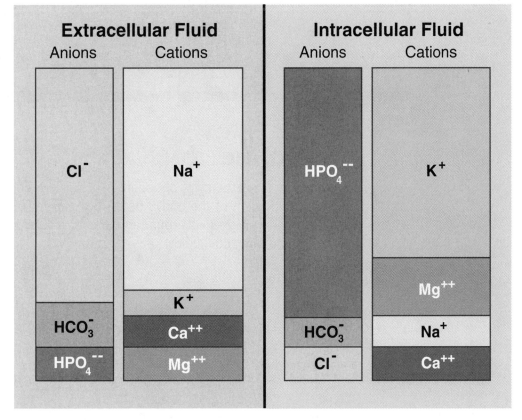

Figure U3-1 Anions and cations in body fluid.

CHAPTER
6

Potassium Imbalances

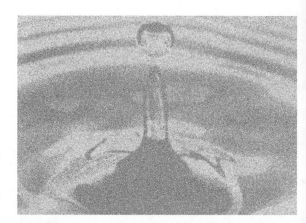

▌ INTRODUCTION

Potassium (K) is the most abundant cation in the body cells. Ninety-seven percent of the body's potassium is found in the intracellular fluid, and 2–3% is found in the extracellular fluid (intravascular and interstitial fluids).

ANSWER COLUMN

1
Although potassium is present in all body fluids, it is found predominantly in ̲i̲n̲t̲r̲a̲c̲e̲l̲l̲u̲l̲a̲r̲ fluid.
    What kind of ion is potassium? _̲C̲a̲t̲i̲o̲n̲_ .

1 intracellular; cation

    Figure 6-1 tells the effect of too much potassium or not enough in our body cells. Memorize the normal range of serum potassium. You may wonder why the range of serum potassium and not cell potassium is used to measure the potassium level, since the cells have the highest concentration of potassium. Serum potassium can be aspirated from the intravascular fluid but cannot be aspirated from potassium cells. When you are ready, go

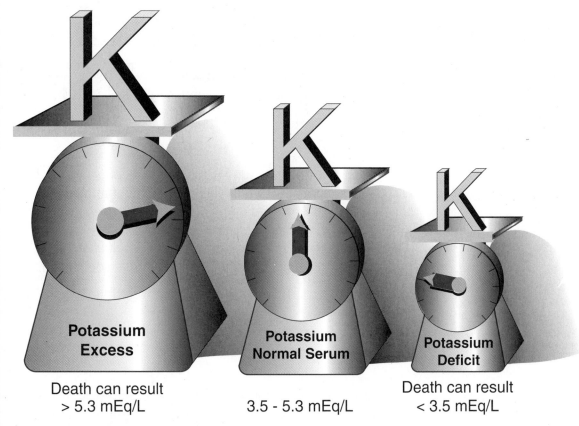

Potassium Excess	Potassium Normal Serum	Potassium Deficit
Death can result > 5.3 mEq/L	3.5 - 5.3 mEq/L	Death can result < 3.5 mEq/L

Figure 6-1 Potassium—balance and imbalance.

ahead to the frames following the figure and refer to the figure when necessary.

2

3.5-5.1

The normal serum potassium range is _____ mEq/L. The intracellular potassium level is 150 mEq/L, but the concentration cannot be determined.

The kidneys excrete 80–90% of the potassium lost from the body. If the kidneys fail to function, what might result? *_____

_____hyper kalemia_____

3

Either too much or too little potassium can cause a cardiac arrest. The heart needs potassium for conducting nerve impulses and contracting the heart muscle.

Why do you think too much potassium can cause a cardiac arrest? *___l_____

_____

Why do you think too little potassium can cause a cardiac arrest? *_____

_____

Note: If the answers are unknown, refer to the section on Functions and Pathophysiology and, particularly, question 11.

▶ FUNCTIONS

Table 6-1 gives the various functions of potassium according to body systems. Study the table and refer to it as needed.

4

Potassium is needed for transmission and conduction of
*_____ . Also potassium is needed for the contraction of
*_____ muscles.

5

Name two cellular activities of potassium. *_____

6

The average daily oral intake of potassium is 50–100 mEq/day. Within the first hour, potassium from oral absorption shifts into the cells. Renal excretion is slower in response to increased

---

2 3.5–5.3; excess potassium buildup, leading to death

3 Too much potassium causes irritability of the heart muscle, increasing and then decreasing the rate.; Too little potassium changes the conduction rate of nerve impulses and weakens the heart muscle, causing the heart to beat irregularly.

4 nerve impulses; skeletal and smooth muscle and the myocardium
5 enzyme action and glycogen deposits in liver, also regulates intracellular osmolality

---

Table 6-1

Potassium and Its Functions

Body Involvement	Function
Neuromuscular	Transmission and conduction of nerve impulses Contraction of skeletal and smooth muscles
Cardiac	Nerve conduction and contraction of the myocardium
Cellular	Enzyme action for cellular energy production Deposits glycogen in liver cells Regulates osmolality of intracellular (cellular) fluids

---

6 Potassium shifts into the cells after 1 hour of K ingestion. Renal excretion of potassium decreases the serum potassium level. (Renal excretion is a slower process.)

potassium level. It takes 4–6 hours for the kidneys to excrete potassium.

Identify two ways the body avoids excessive serum potassium levels after large oral potassium consumptions. * _____

_____

_____

7

Because potassium is not well stored in body cells, a daily potassium intake of 40–60 mEq is needed. Dietary potassium restriction does not necessarily cause a low serum potassium level unless the decreased potassium intake is prolonged or severely deficient.

The average daily oral potassium intake is _____ mEq. The daily potassium intake needed for body function is _____ mEq.

7 50–100; 40–60

8

Foods rich in potassium include fruits (fresh, dry, and juices), vegetables, meats, and nuts. Particularly rich sources include bananas, dry fruits, and orange juice. If a person's serum potassium level is slightly decreased (3.4 mEq/L), what would you suggest? * _____

_____

8 Consume bananas and other fruits as well as vegetables.

9

insulin and aldosterone

10

increases

11

hypokalemia; hyper-
kalemia; 1. c; 2. c; 3. b; 4. a; 5. a;
6. b

12

cardiac arrest

9

Potassium is continually moving between the intracellular fluid and the extracellular fluid, which is controlled by the sodium-potassium pump. Hormones increase the sodium-potassium pump activity. Insulin promotes cellular potassium uptake by shifting glucose and potassium into the cells. Aldosterone promotes potassium excretion and cellular potassium uptake.

The two hormones that can decrease the serum potassium level and increase the cellular potassium level are * _____

_____ .

10

Insulin (increases/decreases) _____ the sodium-potassium pump activity.

▶ PATHOPHYSIOLOGY

11

A serum potassium level below 3.5 mEq/L is known as (hypokalemia/hyperkalemia) _hypo_ , and a serum potassium level above 5.3 mEq/L is called _hyper_ .

Cardiac arrest may occur if the serum potassium level is less than 2.5 mEq/L or greater than 7.0 mEq/L. Too little potassium (<3.5 mEq/L) changes the conduction rate of nerve impulses to the heart, causing dysrhythmia. Also too much potassium (>5.3 mEq/L) can cause irritability of the heart muscle, increasing and then decreasing the heart rate.

Match the serum potassium levels on the left with the type of potassium imbalance or balance.

normal 1. 3.7 mEq/L	a. Hypokalemia
normal 2. 4.8 mEq/L	b. Hyperkalemia
hyper 3. 5.9 mEq/L	c. Normal
hypo 4. 2.7 mEq/L	
hypo 5. 3.1 mEq/L	
hyper 6. 6.8 mEq/L	

12

If the client's serum potassium level is less than 2.5 mEq/L, what might occur? * _____

13

The assimilative processes involved in the formation of new tissue (the synthesis of complex molecules from simple molecules) are referred to as *anabolism,* and the reactions concerned with tissue breakdown (the breakdown of complex molecules to simple molecules with a release of chemical energy) are referred to as *catabolism.*

When cellular activity is *anabolic* (state of building up), potassium enters the cells. When cellular activity is *catabolic* (state of breaking down), potassium leaves the cells.

Potassium enters the cells in _____ states and leaves the cells in _____ states.

13 anabolic; catabolic

14

Potassium may leave the cells under various conditions. When tissues are destroyed as a result of trauma, starvation, or wasting diseases, large amounts of potassium *_____ .

Potassium leaves the cells in _____ states.

14 leave the cells; catabolic

15

During exercise, when muscles contract, the cells lose potassium and absorb a nearly equal quantity of sodium from the extracellular fluid. After exercise, when the muscles are recovering from fatigue, potassium reenters the cells and most of the sodium goes back into the extracellular fluid.

During exercise which ion may be increased over usual levels in the extracellular fluid—the potassium ion or the sodium ion?

*_____

_____

15 The potassium ion. Of course it depends on how much exercise.

16

During exercise, potassium leaves the cells, causing muscular fatigue.

After exercise, potassium *_____ .

Potassium enters the cells in _____ states.

16 reenters the cells; anabolic

17

After releasing potassium from the cells, the muscles are soft.

The soft muscles are a result of (hyperkalemia/hypokalemia) _____ .

17 hypokalemia

18 trauma, exercise,
starvation, wasting disease

18

Name as many conditions as you can in which potassium might leave the cells. *_____

_____

19

In stress caused by a harmful condition or severe emotional strain, an excessive amount of potassium is lost through the kidneys. The potassium leaves the cells, depleting the cells' supply. From the adrenal gland one of the adrenal cortical hormones, aldosterone, is produced in abundance during stress. This hormone influences the kidneys to excrete potassium and to retain sodium, chloride, and water.

Frequently the cations K and Na have an opposing effect on each other in the extracellular fluid. When one is retained, the other is excreted.

Therefore, with an excessive production of aldosterone, what happens to the cations K and Na in the extracellular fluid?
*_____

19 Potassium will be excreted
and Na will be retained.

20

When kidney function is normal, the excess potassium will be slowly excreted by the kidneys. The range of potassium excreted daily by the kidneys is 20–120 mEq/L.

If potassium intake is decreased or if no potassium is taken orally or given intravenously, potassium is still excreted by the kidneys. Potassium is lost from the cells and the extracellular fluid (ECF) when potassium intake is diminished or absent. What type of potassium imbalance will occur? _____

20 hypokalemia

21

If the kidneys are injured or diseased and the urine output is markedly decreased, which of the following happen?

( ) a. The potassium concentration increases in the extracellular fluid.

( ) b. The potassium concentration increases in the intracellular fluid.

( ) c. The potassium is excreted through the skin.

21 a

▶ ETIOLOGY

The causes of hypokalemia and hyperkalemia are divided into two separate tables. Table 6-2 lists the etiology and rationale for hypokalemia and Table 6-3 gives the etiology and rationale for hyperkalemia. Study both tables carefully, noting the causes and reasons for these changes. Then proceed to the questions that follow. Refer to the tables as needed.

22 malnutrition and alcoholism (also reducing diets, anorexia nervosa)

23 40–60 mEq

24 The diuretics promote loss of water, sodium, and potassium

25 vomiting, diarrhea, and GI suctioning (also laxative abuse, bulimia)

26 deficit; Potassium is lost from the cells due to tissue injury with normal kidney function.

27 hypokalemia; Licorice has an aldosteronelike effect, thus promoting potassium excretion and sodium retention.

28 Insulin moves potassium into the cells along with glucose, and alkalosis promotes the exchange of potassium ions for hydrogen ions in the cells. Either can cause a low serum potassium level (hypokalemia).

22
Name two causes of hypokalemia related to dietary changes.
*_____

23
What is the daily potassium need for body function? _____

24
The major cause of a potassium deficit is potassium-wasting diuretics. Why? *_____

25
Gastrointestinal (GI) losses account for the second major cause of a potassium deficit. List three GI causes of hypokalemia.
*_____

26
Trauma and injury to tissues as a result of burns and surgery can cause a potassium (deficit/excess) _____ . Why? *_____

_____

27
Excessive ingestion of licorice can cause (hypokalemia/hyperkalemia) _____ .
    Why? *_____

_____

28
How do insulin and alkalotic states affect potassium balance?
*_____

_____

Table 6-2

Causes of Hypokalemia (Serum Potassium Deficit)

Etiology	Rationale
Dietary Changes Malnutrition, starvation, alcoholism, unbalanced reducing diets, anorexia nervosa, crash diets	Potassium is poorly conserved in the body. For a potassium deficit to occur, a prolonged, inadequate potassium intake must occur.
Gastrointestinal Losses Vomiting, diarrhea, gastric/intestinal suctioning, intestinal fistula, laxative abuse, bulimia, enemas	Potassium is plentiful in the GI tract. With the loss of GI secretions, large amounts of potassium ions are lost.
Renal Losses Diuretics, diuretic phase of acute renal failure, hemodialysis and peritoneal dialysis	The kidneys excrete 80–90% of the potassium lost. Diuretics are the major cause of hypokalemia, especially potassium-wasting diuretics [thiazides, loop (high-ceiling), osmotic]
Hormonal Influence Steroids, Cushing's syndrome, stress, excessive intake of licorice	Steroids, especially cortisone and aldosterone, promote potassium excretion and sodium retention. Stress increases the production of steroids in the body. In Cushing's syndrome, there is an excess production of adrenocortical hormones (corticol and aldosterone). Licorice contains glyceric acid, which has an aldosteronelike effect.
Cellular Damage Trauma, tissue injury, surgery, burns	Cellular and tissue damage cause potassium to be released in the intravascular fluid. More potassium is needed to repair injured tissue.
Redistribution of Potassium Insulin, alkalotic state	Insulin moves glucose and potassium into cells. Metabolic alkalosis promotes the movement of potassium into cells.

Table 6-3

Causes of Hyperkalemia (Serum Potassium Excess)

Etiology	Rationale
Excessive Potassium Intake	
Oral potassium supplements	A potassium consumption rate greater than the potassium excretion rate increases the serum potassium level.
IV potassium infusions	Adequate urinary output must be determined when giving a potassium supplement.
Decreased Renal Function	
Acute renal failure	Because potassium is generally excreted in the urine, anuria and oliguria
Chronic renal failure	cause a potassium buildup in the plasma.
Potassium-sparing diuretics	Potassium-sparing diuretics can cause an aldosterone deficiency, promoting potassium retention.
Altered Cellular Function	
Severe traumatic injury	Cellular injury increases potassium loss due to cell breakdown. Potassium excretion may be greater than cellular K reabsorption. Potassium can accumulate in the plasma.
Metabolic acidosis	In acidosis, the hydrogen ion moves into the cells and potassium moves out of the cells, increasing the serum potassium level.
Blood for transfusion that is 1–3 weeks old	As stored blood for transfusion ages, hemolysis (breakdown of red blood cells) occurs; potassium from the cells are released into the ECF.
Hormonal Deficiency	
Addison's disease	Reduced secretion of the adrenocortical hormones causes a retention of potassium and a loss of sodium.
Pseudohyperkalemia	
Hemolysis	With hemolysis, ruptured red blood cells release potassium into the ECF.
Tourniquet application Phlebotomy	A tourniquet that has been applied too tightly or rapidly drawing blood with a small needle lumen (<18 gauge) can cause a falsely elevated potassium level in the blood specimen.

29 *a. diarrhea, vomiting, gastric suction; b. starvation, anorexia nervosa, bulimia; c. diuretics—potassium wasting; d. burns; e. trauma or injury; f. surgery; Also: stress; increase of adrenal cortical hormones (steroids); metabolic alkalosis*

29

List six clinical conditions causing a potassium deficit:

a. _____

b. _____

c. _____

d. _____

e. _____

f. _____

30 The kidneys excrete 80–90% of excess potassium. With increased potassium ingestion and poor urine output, hyperkalemia can result.

30

The serum potassium level should be monitored for clients taking large doses of a potassium supplement. This is especially true when the daily urine output is diminished.

Why? *_____

_____

31

A client should not receive more than 10 mEq of IV potassium per hour that has been diluted in intravenous solution. Usually 20–40 mEq of potassium chloride is diluted in 1 liter of IV fluids.

Potassium in IV fluids administered at a rate faster than 20 mEq/L per hour for 24–72 hours can result in (hypokalemia/ hyperkalemia) _____ .

31 hyperkalemia

32 hemolysis or a tightly applied tourniquet to obtain blood sample; also, rapidly drawing blood through a small needle lumen

32

Pseudo-hyperkalemia may occur due to _____ or *_____

_____ .

33

Which of the following are causes of potassium excess (hyperkalemia)?

( ) a. Potassium-wasting diuretics
( ) b. Potassium-sparing diuretics
( ) c. Adrenal gland insufficiency
( ) d. Vomiting, diarrhea
( ) e. Multiple transfusions of old blood
( ) f. Metabolic acidosis with poor kidney function
( ) g. Renal shutdown

33 b, c, e, f, g

▶ CLINICAL MANIFESTATIONS

34

Although 98% of potassium is found in cells, focus is placed on the extracellular fluid, for it is more readily available for study. Intracellular levels are not clinically available.

The normal serum potassium level (in extracellular fluid) is _____ mEq/L.

34 3.5–5.3

Table 6-4 lists the signs and symptoms associated with hypokalemia and hyperkalemia. Clinical manifestations can be determined by the serum potassium level, electrocardiography (ECG/EKG), and signs and symptoms related to gastrointestinal, cardiac, renal, and neurologic abnormalities. The serum potassium level and the ECG play the most important role in determining the severity of the potassium imbalance.

Clients with hypokalemia and hyperkalemia can be found in many clinical settings. You may save a client's life by recognizing and reporting symptoms of potassium imbalance. If you are not familiar with these words, refer to the glossary.

Table 6-4

Clinical Manifestations of Potassium Imbalances

Body Involvement	Hypokalemia	Hyperkalemia
Gastrointestinal Abnormalities	*Anorexia Nausea *Vomiting Diarrhea †Abdominal distention †Decreased peristalsis or silent ileus	*Nausea *Diarrhea †Abdominal cramps
Cardiac Abnormalities	†Dysrhythmias †Vertigo Cardiac arrest when severe	Tachycardia, later †bradycardia, and finally cardiac arrest (severe)
ECG/EKG	†Flat or inverted T wave Depressed ST segment	†Peaked, narrow T wave Shortened QT interval Prolonged PR interval followed by disappearance of P wave. Prolonged QRS interval if level continues to rise
Renal Abnormalities	Polyuria	†Oliguria or anuria
Neuromuscular Abnormalities	†Malaise Drowsiness †Muscular weakness Confusion Mental depression Diminished deep tendon reflexes Respiratory paralysis	Weakness, numbness, or tingling sensation Muscle cramps
Laboratory Values Serum potassium	<3.5 mEq/L	>5.3 mEq/L

†Most commonly seen symptoms of hypo-hyperkalemia
*Commonly seen symptoms of hypo-hyperkalemia

35

Hypokalemia causes the muscle to become soft, like "half-filled water bottles," and weak. The abdomen becomes bloated due to smooth-muscle weakness and not due to flatus. The blood pressure goes down (hypotension) and dizziness occurs. Malaise or uneasiness occurs.

The heart beat is irregular, known as _____ . Eventually, if the irregularity of the heart beat is not corrected, bradycardia occurs and finally cardiac arrest.

36

A weak grip, an irregular pulse, and dizziness upon standing may be signs of _____ .

37

T wave changes on the ECG/EKG can indicate a potassium imbalance. Match the T wave changes on the left with the type of potassium imbalance.

_____ 1. Peaked T wave   a. Hypokalemia
_____ 2. Flat T wave   b. Hyperkalemia
_____ 3. Inverted T wave

38

Name the six most commonly seen symptoms of hypokalemia.
*_____

_____

39

With hyperkalemia, the heart beats very fast, which is known as *tachycardia,* and then it slows down (*bradycardia*). The heart goes into a block, with few or no impulses being transmitted, and finally cardiac arrest occurs.

You recall that the kidneys are responsible for excreting excessive amounts of potassium not needed by the body. If the kidneys excrete a small amount of urine, known as *oliguria,* or no urine, known as *anuria,* what can occur to the potassium level? *_____

What would you think happens to the heart rate? *_____

_____

---

35 dysrhythmia (arrhythmia)

36 hypokalemia

37 1. b; 2. a; 3. a

38 abdominal distention, decreased peristalsis or silent ileus, dizziness, dysrhythmia/arrhythmia, malaise, and muscular weakness

39 increase in potassium (hyperkalemia); increase (tachycardia) and later decrease (bradycardia)

40 abdominal cramps,
tachycardia and later
bradycardia, and oliguria
or anuria

41 cardiac arrest

40

Name the three most commonly seen symptoms of
hyperkalemia. *_____

_____

41

With prolonged hypokalemia, circulatory failure and eventual
heart failure can result. The electrocardiogram frequently shows
a flat or inverted T wave. With potassium excess, the
electrocardiogram shows a peaked T wave.

    Serum potassium levels below 2.5 mEq/L and above 7.0 mEq/L
are extremely dangerous and need immediate attention. Without
correction, what type of heart condition can occur? *_____

    Figures 6-2 and 6-3 note electrocardiographic changes found
with hypo-hyperkalemia. Students who have had a physiology
course and/or have a basic knowledge of electrocardiography,

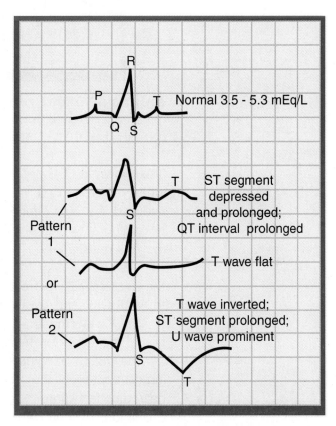

Figure 6-2 Electrocardiographic changes in serum potassium deficit.

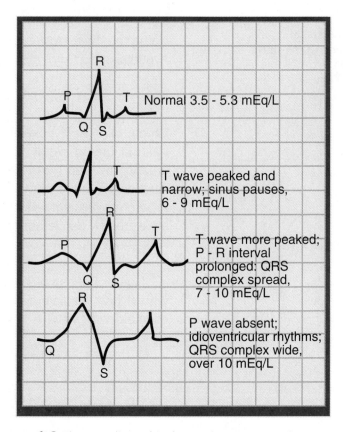

Figure 6-3 Electrocardiographic changes in serum potassium concentration. Changes that do occur are most marked in the precordial leads over the right side (V_1–V_4 position) of the heart.

also known as ECG or EKG, will find these diagrams most useful when monitoring clients. Students who do not have this basic knowledge should refer to a physiology text and/or text on electrocardiography. Students who do not need this information may move to question 49.

A brief review of the electrocardiogram. The ECG measures the electrical activity from various areas of the heart and records this as P, QRS, and T waves.

The *P wave* measures the electrical activity initiating contraction of the atrium or the atrial muscle.

The *QRS wave complex* measures the electrical activity initiating contraction of the ventricle, which is the thickest part of the heart muscle responsible for forcing blood from the heart into the circulation. A "heart attack," also known as myocardial infarction, frequently affects this part of the heart muscle.

The *T wave* is the electrical recovery of the ventricles.

Abnormal potassium levels affect the T wave of the electrocardiogram. Note the normal T wave structure in Figure 6-2 and compare the normal with the abnormal, with patterns 1 and 2. Study this figure and then proceed to the questions.

42

The two abnormal changes in the T wave that occur with hypokalemia are *_____ .

43

The ST segment is prolonged in both patterns in Figure 6-2. This change relates to a *_____ .

44

With a serum potassium *deficit* which of the following electrocardiographic changes may occur?

( ) a. Flat T wave
( ) b. Inverted T wave
( ) c. High-peaked T wave
( ) d. Depressed and prolonged ST segment

High peaked-T waves are an early electrocardiographic sign of hyperkalemia. Heart block can result from severe hyperkalemia, e.g., 8–10 mEq/L of serum potassium. Study Figure 6-3 carefully, noting especially the T waves, QRS complex, and P wave. If any of the words are unfamiliar, refer to a physiology text and/or a text on electrocardiography.

45

Name the abnormal change in the T wave occurring with hyperkalemia. *_____

46

A flat or inverted T wave on an electrocardiogram frequently indicates a _____ state, whereas a high-peaked T wave can indicate a _____ state.

47

Which of the following electrocardiographic changes can occur with a high serum potassium?

---

42 flat T wave and inverted T wave

43 potassium deficit

44 a, b, d

45 high-peaked T wave

46 hypokalemic; hyperkalemic

( ) a. Flat T wave
( ) b. Inverted T wave
( ) c. High-peaked T wave
( ) d. Depressed and prolonged ST segment
( ) e. QRS complex spread
( ) f. Prolonged P-R interval

47 c, e, f

48

Match the following ECG changes on the left with the electrolyte abnormalities on the right. Refer to Figures 6-2 and 6-3 as needed.

___1.

A. Hypokalemia

B. Hyperkalemia

___2.

___3.

48 1. b; 2. a; 3. a; 4. b

___4.

◗ CLINICAL MANAGEMENT

Clinical management of hypokalemia consists of oral supplements (tablets, capsules, liquid) and/or IV potassium diluted in an IV solution. To correct hyperkalemia, potassium intake is restricted and various drugs can be used to lower the serum potassium level. First, potassium replacement for hypokalemia is discussed and, then, drug modalities are presented for correcting hyperkalemia.

Potassium Replacement

Oral potassium supplements help to replace potassium losses due to potassium-wasting diuretics, inadequate nutritional intake, and disease entities that increase potassium losses. Table 6-5 contains examples of frequently ordered oral potassium supplements.

49

Name a drug that corrects serum potassium and serum chloride deficits. *_____

49 potassium chloride (liquid or tablet)

Table 6-5

Oral Potassium Supplements

Preparation	Drug
Liquid	Potassium chloride 10% = 20 mEq/15 mL; 20% = 40 mEq/15 mL
	Kay Ciel (potassium chloride)
	Kaochlor 10% (potassium chloride)
	Kaon Cl 20 (potassium chloride)
	Potassium Triplex (potassium acetate, bicarbonate, citrate)
Tablet/capsule	Potassium chloride (enteric-coated tablet)
	Kaon—plain (potassium gluconate)
	Kaon Cl (potassium chloride)
	Slow K (potassium chloride—8 mEq)
	Kaochlor (potassium chloride)
	K-Lyte—plain (potassium bicarbonate-effervescent tablet)
	K-Lyte/Cl (potassium chloride)

50 Potassium triplex and K-Lyte—plain (also Kaon—plain). The gluconate in Kaon is converted to bicarbonate. Kaon comes with or without Cl.

51 no; Because 80–90% of potassium is excreted from the body by the kidneys; hyperkalemia might result.

52 hyperkalemia; potassium accumulation in the ECF; also ECG changes

53 Cardiac arrest. Potassium concentration is extremely irritating to the myocardium (heart muscle); phlebitis (inflammation of the vein) and infiltration (tissue sloughing or necrosis)

50

Oral potassium may be extremely irritating to the gastric mucosa and should be diluted in at least 6–8 ounces of water or juice.

   Name two oral potassium supplements that contain bicarbonate. *_____

_____

51

There have been reports of deaths related to hyperkalemia caused by oral potassium supplements.

   Would oral potassium supplements be recommended for a person with poor kidney function? _____

Why? *_____

_____

52

Severe serum hyperkalemia may occur from administering an intravenous potassium solution too rapidly, thus not allowing enough time for the potassium to pass into the cells.

   The normal dose of intravenous potassium is 20–40 mEq in 1 liter of solution to run over 8 hours or no more than 10 mEq of KCl per hour. What might result from administering 40 mEq of potassium per hour? _____

   Why? *_____

53

Intravenous potassium is irritating to blood vessels (can cause phlebitis) and tissues (can cause sloughing and necrosis).

   Potassium should NEVER be given as a bolus (injected directly into the vein).

   What might happen if a bolus injection of potassium chloride (KCl) is given?

*_____

   The nurse should assess the infusion site when the client is receiving intravenous KCl for _____ and _____ .

54

For severe hypokalemia (<3.0 mEq/L) 40–60 mEq of KCl can be diluted in 1 liter of IV fluids, and no more than 20 mEq per hour should be given.

For a life-threatening hypokalemic situation (<2.6 mEq/L), 30–40 mEq of KCl can be diluted in 100–150 mL of D_5W and administered through a central venous line in 1 hour.

What is the recommended KCl dosage to be diluted in 1 liter of IV fluids? *_____

54 20–40 mEq/L

55

In hypokalemia, if the serum potassium level is 3.0–3.5 mEq/L, 100–200 mEq of KCl is needed to raise serum level 1 mEq/L. Remember, do not administer the KCl all at once; a high concentration is toxic to the heart muscle and irritating to the blood vessels.

If the serum potassium level is below 3.0 mEq/L, 200–400 mEq of KCl is needed to raise serum level 1 mEq/L.

If an individual has a serum potassium level of 2.7 mEq/L, how much KCl, administered, is needed to raise the serum level to 3.7 mEq/L? *_____

55 200–400 mEq

56

The daily potassium requirement is 40–60 mEq. A client with a serum potassium of 3.3 mEq/L must (increase/decrease) _____ daily potassium intake.

56 increase

Hyperkalemia Correction

In mild hyperkalemic conditions (5.4–5.6 mEq/L), correcting the cause of the potassium excess and restricting the potassium intake may correct the hyperkalemic state. Interventions to temporarily correct a moderate hyperkalemic state (6.0 mEq/L) include IV sodium bicarbonate infusion, insulin and glucose infusion, and IV calcium salt. Correcting the cause of the potassium excess is often successful in lowering the serum potassium level. In severe hyperkalemic conditions (>6.7 mEq/L), kayexalate and sorbitol are usually prescribed.

Table 6-6 describes various methods used to correct a potassium excess (hyperkalemia). Study the table carefully and refer to it as needed.

57

To correct mild hyperkalemia, restriction of potassium intake is suggested.

Table 6-6

Correction of Potassium Excess (Hyperkalemia)

Treatment Methods	Rationale
Potassium restriction	Restriction of potassium intake will slowly lower the serum level. For mild hyperkalemia (slightly elevated K levels), i.e., 5.4–5.6 mEq/L, potassium restriction is normally effective.
IV sodium bicarbonate ($NaHCO_3$)	By elevating the pH level, potassium moves back into the cells, thus lowering the serum level. This is a temporary treatment.
10% Calcium gluconate	Calcium decreases the irritability of the myocardium resulting from hyperkalemia. It is a temporary treatment and does not promote K loss. *Caution:* Administering calcium to a patient on digitalis can cause digitalis toxicity.
Insulin and glucose (10–50%)	The combination of insulin and glucose moves potassium back into the cells. It is a temporary treatment, effective for approximately 6 hours, and is not always as effective when repeated.
Kayexalate (sodium polystyrene) and sorbitol 70%	Kayexalate is used as a cation exchange for severe hyperkalemia and can be administered orally or rectally. Approximate dosages are as follows: *Orally:* Kayexalate—10–20 g 3 to 4 times daily Sorbitol 70%—20 mL with each dose *Rectally:* Kayexalate—30–50 g Sorbitol 70%—50 mL; mix with 100–150 mL water (Retention enema—20–30 minutes)

57 no; It is severe hyperkalemia, and this method is too slow.

Would you correct a hyperkalemia of 7.0 mEq/L by restricting potassium intake? _____

Why? *_____

58

For temporary correction of a moderate potassium excess, indicate which methods are most effective:

( ) a. Potassium restriction diet
( ) b. IV sodium bicarbonate
( ) c. 10% Calcium gluconate
( ) d. Insulin and glucose
( ) e. Kayexalate and sorbitol

58 b, c, d

59
If a client is taking digitalis and has a serum potassium of 7.4 mEq/L, is 10% calcium gluconate indicated for temporary correction of hyperkalemia? _____
   Explain. * _____

60
Drugs such as Kayexalate (sodium polystyrene sulfonate), a cation exchange resin, and sorbitol 70% are given for severe hyperkalemia. They cause a sodium-potassium ion exchange, and the potassium is excreted.
   What treatment is suggested for mild hyperkalemia?
*
_____
   What treatment is suggested for severe hyperkalemia?
* _____

Drugs and Their Effect on Potassium Balance

61
Diuretics are divided into two categories: potassium wasting and potassium sparing. Potassium-wasting diuretics excrete potassium and other electrolytes such as sodium and chloride in the urine. Potassium-sparing diuretics retain potassium but excrete sodium and chloride in the urine.
   Indicate the electrolytes that are lost when potassium-sparing diuretics are taken:
   ( ) a. Potassium
   ( ) b. Sodium
   ( ) c. Chloride

   Table 6-7 lists the trade and generic names of potassium-wasting and potassium-sparing diuretics and a combination of potassium-wasting and potassium-sparing diuretics. Study the types of diuretic in each category and refer to the table as needed.

62
Name the potassium imbalance that is most likely to occur in people taking a potassium-sparing diuretic, who have poor kidney function. * _____

---

59 no; Calcium administration enhances the action of digitalis, causing digitalis toxicity.

60 Restrict potassium intake.; Kayexalate and sorbitol— ion exchange

61 b, c

62 potassium excess (hyperkalemia)

Table 6-7

Potassium-Wasting and Potassium-Sparing Diuretics

Potassium-Wasting Diuretics	*Potassium-Sparing Diuretics*
Thiazides	Aldosterone antagonist
Chlorothiazide/Diuril	Spironolactone/Aldactone
Hydrochlorothiazide/Hydrodiuril	Triamterene/Dyrenium
Loop diuretics	Amiloride/Midamor
Furosemide/Lasix	
Ethacrynic acid/Edecrin	*Combination: K-Wasting*
Carbonic anhydrase inhibitors	*and K-Sparing Diuretics*
Acetazolamide/Diamox	Aldactazide
Osmotic diuretic	Spironazide
Mannitol	Dyazide
	Moduretic

63

Potassium-wasting diuretics can cause (hypokalemia/ hyperkalemia) _____ .

63 hypokalemia

64

Enter W for potassium-wasting, S for potassium-sparing, and C for a combination of potassium-wasting and potassium-sparing diuretics for the following drugs. Refer to Table 6-7 as needed:

( ) a. Chlorothiazide/Diuril
( ) b. Aldactazide
( ) c. Triamterene/Dyrenium
( ) d. Acetazolamide/Diamox
( ) e. Amiloride/Midamor
( ) f. Dyazide
( ) g. Spironolactone/Aldactone
( ) h. Hydrochlorothiazide/Hydrodiuril
( ) i. Furosemide/Lasix
( ) j. Ethacrynic acid/Edecrin
( ) k. Mannitol

64 a. W; b. C; c. S; d. W; e. W; f. C; g. S; h. W; i. W; j. W; k. S

Laxatives, corticosteroids, antibiotics, and potassium-wasting diuretics are the major drug groups that can cause a potassium deficit, or hypokalemia. The drug groups attributed to potassium excess, or hyperkalemia, are oral and intravenous potassium salts, central nervous system (CNS) agents, and potassium-sparing diuretics. Table 6-8 lists the drugs that affect potassium balance.

65

Enter KD for potassium deficit/hypokalemia and KE for potassium excess/hyperkalemia beside the drugs that can cause a potassium imbalance. Refer to Table 6-8 as needed:

_____ a. Laxatives
_____ b. Corticosteroids
_____ c. Barbiturates
_____ d. Narcotics
_____ e. Indomethacin/Indocin
_____ f. Licorice
_____ g. Antibiotics
_____ h. Levodopa
_____ i. Heparin
_____ j. Potassium chloride
_____ k. Succinylcholine/Anectine
_____ l. Terbutaline/Brethine

66

Digitalis is a drug that strengthens the heart muscle and slows down the heart beat. A serum potassium deficit, or hypokalemia, enhances the action of digitalis and causes the drug to become more potent. Digitalis toxicity or intoxication (slow and irregular pulse, nausea and vomiting, anorexia) can result from a low serum potassium level.

Thiazides and loop diuretics can cause (hypokalemia/hyperkalemia) _____ .

The nurse needs to be alert for what type of drug toxicity when a client is taking potassium-wasting diuretics and digitalis?
*_____

67

Common symptoms of digitalis toxicity are bradycardia (slow heart beat) and/or dysrhythmia (arrhythmia).

Can you name two other symptoms of digitalis toxicity?
a. *_____
b. _____

65 a. KD; b. KD; c. KE; d. KE; e. KE; f. KD; g. KD; h. KD; i. KE; j. KE; k. KE; l. KD

66 hypokalemia; digitalis toxicity

67 a. nausea and vomiting; b. anorexia

Table 6-8

Drugs Affecting Potassium Balance

Potassium Imbalance	Substances	Rationale
Hypokalemia (serum potassium deficit)	Laxatives Enemas (hyperosmolar)	Laxative abuse can cause potassium depletion.
	Corticosteroids 　Cortisone 　Prednisone	Ion exchange agent. Steroids promote potassium loss and sodium retention.
	Kayexalate	Exchange potassium ion for a sodium ion.
	Licorice	Licorice action is similar to aldosterone, promoting K loss and Na retention.
	Levodopa/L-dopa Lithium	Increases potassium loss via urine.
	Antibiotic I 　Amphotericin B 　Polymyxin B 　Tetracycline (outdated) 　Gentamicin 　Neomycin 　Amikacin 　Tobramycin 　Cisplatin	Toxic effect on renal tubules, thus decreasing potassium reabsorption.
	Antibiotic II 　Penicillin 　Ampicillin 　Carbenicillin 　Ticarcillin 　Nafcillin 　Piperacillin 　Azlocillin	Potassium excretion is enhanced by the presence of nonreabsorbable anions.
	Alpha-adrenergic blockers Insulin and glucose	These agents promote movement of potassium into cells, thus lowering the serum potassium level.
	Beta$_2$ agonists 　Terbutaline 　Albuterol 　Estrogen Potassium-wasting diuretics	See Table 6-7

continues on the following page

Table 6-8

(Continued)

Potassium Imbalance	Substances	Rationale
Hyperkalemia (serum potassium excess)	Potassium chloride (oral or IV) Potassium salt (no salt) K penicillin KPO_4 enema	Excess ingestion or infusion of these agents can cause a potassium excess.
	Indomethacin Captopril (Capoten) Heparin	Decrease renal excretion of potassium.
	CNS agents Barbiturates Sedatives Narcotics Heroin Amphetamines	These CNS agents are usually characterized by muscle necrosis and cellular shift of potassium from cells to serum.
	Nonsteroidal anti-inflammatory drugs (NSAIDS): ibuprofens Alpha agonists Beta blockers	Blocks cellular potassium uptake.
	Succinylcholine Cyclophosphamide	Loss of potassium from cells.
	Potassium-sparing diuretics	See Table 6-7.

68

A serum potassium excess (hyperkalemia) inhibits the action of digitalis. If a person has a serum potassium of 5.8 mEq/L, (more/less) _____ digitalis will be needed to obtain the appropriate digitalis dosage.

68 more

69

Quinidine is an antidysrhythmic drug used to correct irregular heart rates. Hypokalemia blocks the effects of quinidine; therefore more quinidine may be needed to produce therapeutic action. Hyperkalemia enhances the action of quinidine and can produce quinidine toxicity and myocardium depression.

　　Explain the effect of hypokalemia:

On digitalis * _____

On quinidine * _____

69 it enhances the action of digitalis; it decreases the action of quinidine

70

Cortisone causes excretion of potassium and retention of sodium. If a person takes digoxin (digitalis), hydrochlorothiazide/Hydrodiuril, and prednisone/cortisone daily, what type of severe electrolyte imbalance can result?
*_____

Explain the effect this imbalance has on digitalis. *_____
_____

70 hypokalemia or potassium deficit; Hypokalemia precipitates digitalis toxicity by enhancing the action of digoxin.

▶ CLINICAL APPLICATIONS

71

Approximately 2% of healthy adults develop hypokalemia. Twenty to 80% of persons taking potassium-wasting diuretics develop hypokalemia. Hypokalemia is present in about 20% of hospitalized clients, and hyperkalemia occurs in approximately 10% of hospitalized clients.

The most common potassium imbalance in hospitalized clients is (hypokalemia/hyperkalemia) _____ .

71 hypokalemia

72

Five percent of hospitalized clients with hypokalemia have a serum potassium level lower than 3.0 mEq/L. One to 2% of hospitalized clients having hyperkalemia have a serum potassium level greater than 6.0 mEq/L.

A client with a serum potassium level below 3.0 mEq/L requires approximately _____ mEq of potassium to raise the serum potassium level 1 mEq/L.

72 200–400

73

An example of a severe serum potassium deficit that is life threatening is a serum potassium level of _____ mEq/L. An example of a severe serum potassium excess that is life threatening is _____ mEq/L.

73 <2.5; >7.0

74

Eighty to 90% of potassium excretion is lost in the urine, and only a very small percentage is lost in the feces.

Which of the following promotes a greater loss of potassium?
( ) a. An individual taking a laxative
( ) b. An individual taking a diuretic

74 b

75

Hyperglycemia, an increased blood sugar, is a symptom of diabetes mellitus. Cells cannot utilize glucose; thus, catabolism (cellular breakdown) occurs, and potassium leaves the cells and is excreted by the kidneys. If the kidneys are not functioning adequately (<600 mL/day), potassium can accumulate and serum potassium excess can occur.

When cells do not receive their proper nutrition, what happens to the cells? *_____

_____

In hyperglycemia (hypokalemia/hyperkalemia) _____ occurs due to cellular breakdown and polyuria. If there is kidney shutdown, (hypokalemia/hyperkalemia) _____ occurs.

75 catabolism—cellular breakdown with loss of potassium; hypokalemia; hyperkalemia

76

Administering glucose and insulin to correct abnormal cellular metabolism in a diabetic client may lead to rapid transfer of potassium from the extracellular fluid to the cell. In this situation, the serum potassium rapidly (increases/decreases)

_____ .

76 decreases

77

When oliguria develops because of poor renal function, potassium is no longer excreted, which results in a high serum potassium level.

If there is poor renal function, do you think potassium should be administered? *_____
Why? *_____

77 no, NEVER with poor renal function; Hyperkalemia can be brought to a dangerous level.

78

Potassium therapy should not be administered to clients with untreated adrenal insufficiency and * _____ .

78 renal failure or poor renal function

79

In the cirrhotic client with degenerated liver cells, hypokalemia can precipitate hepatic coma or liver failure.

As a nurse caring for a client with cirrhosis you would alert the physician of any low serum K levels, and you should watch for symptoms of *_____ .

79 hypokalemia and hepatic coma

80 no; Magnesium deficit usually needs to be corrected first, which may automatically correct potassium deficit by making potassium that is given usable by the body.

80

The serum levels of magnesium, chloride, and protein should be checked when correcting hypokalemia. Low serum levels of Mg, Cl, and protein inhibit potassium utilization by the body.

If hypokalemia and hypomagnesemia (Mg deficit) are present, should a potassium deficit be corrected by giving potassium chloride? _____ Why? * _____

_____

● Clinical Considerations

1. Oral potassium should be taken with food and/or 8 ounces of fluid. Potassium is irritating to the gastric mucosa and can cause a gastric ulcer.

2. Mild hypokalemia, 3.4 mEq/L, can be avoided by eating foods rich in potassium, i.e., fresh/dry fruits, fruit juices, vegetables, meats, nuts.

3. IV potassium should be well diluted in IV solution. NEVER administer IV potassium as a bolus (IV push). It can cause cardiac arrest.

4. Normal dose for IV potassium is 20–40 mEq in 1 liter of IV fluids to run for 8 hours.

5. Infiltration of IV potassium salt in solution causes sloughing of the subcutaneous tissues. IV potassium is irritating to blood vessels, and with prolonged use, phlebitis might occur.

6. Potassium should NOT be administered if the urine output is <600mL/day. Eighty to 90% of potassium is excreted in the urine.

7. Potassium deficit can enhance the action of digoxin; digitalis toxicity could result.

8. Potassium-wasting diuretics, i.e., thiazides [hydrochlorothiazide (HydroDIURIL)], and loop/high ceiling [furosemide (Lasix)] cause potassium loss via kidneys. Steroids promote potassium loss and sodium retention.

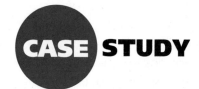

CASE STUDY

REVIEW

Mr. Johnson, 68 years old, has been vomiting and has had diarrhea for 2 days. He takes digoxin, 0.25 mg, and HydroDIURIL, 50 mg, daily. His serum potassium level is 3.2 mEq/L. He complains of being dizzy. The nurse assesses his physiologic status and notes that his muscles are weak and flabby, his abdomen is distended, and peristalsis is diminished.

1. hypokalemia

2. 3.5–5.3 mEq/L

3. yes; Hypokalemia will enhance the action of digoxin, causing digitalis toxicity.

4. loss

5. dizziness; muscles weak and flabby; distended abdomen; diminished peristalsis

6. hypokalemia

7. 40–60 mEq/L

8. hyperkalemia, which is toxic to heart muscle and can cause phlebitis (irritated blood vessel)

9. abdominal cramps, tachycardia and later bradycardia, and oliguria

10. Potassium chloride. Also potassium triplex, Kaon, or K-Lyte since the chloride level is normal.

11. causes loss of potassium

---

1. What was his potassium imbalance? _____

2. The "normal" range of potassium balance is * _____ .

3. Should the nurse have checked his pulse rate, since he was receiving digoxin? _____ Explain. * _____
   _____

4. Vomiting will cause a potassium (gain/loss) _____ .

5. Name the signs and symptoms of Mr. Johnson's potassium deficit. _____ , * _____ , * _____ , and
   * _____ .

Mr. Johnson's heart activity was monitored with an ECG. He received 1 liter of 5% dextrose in water with 40 mEq/L of KCl.

6. A flat T wave would be indicative of _____ .

7. The daily potassium requirement is * _____ .

8. A concentration of KCI in IV fluids higher than 40 mEq/L can cause * _____
   _____ .

9. List at least three common symptoms found with hyperkalemia. * _____
   _____

A week after his acute illness, his serum potassium was 3.7 mEq/L and his serum chloride was in the "normal" range. The health care provider ordered Mr. Johnson to take an oral potassium supplement with his daily digoxin and HydroDIURIL (hydrochlorothiazide). For Mr. Johnson's arthritis, prednisone 4 times a week was ordered.

10. Name an oral potassium supplement that can be prescribed.
    * _____
    _____

11. Explain the effect of cortisone on potassium in the body.
    * _____ .

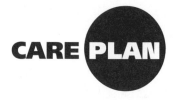

12. Aldactone or Dyrenium

12. If a potassium supplement was not prescribed, name a potassium-sparing diuretic that can be taken in conjunction with hydrochlorothiazide. _____

Client Management

Hypokalemia

Assessment Factors

▶ Obtain a history observing for a clinical health problem that may cause hypokalemia, i.e., vomiting, diarrhea, fad-reducing diet, potassium-wasting diuretics.

▶ Assess for signs and symptoms of hypokalemia, i.e., dizziness, dysrhythmia, soft muscles, abdominal distention, and decreased peristalsis or paralytic ileus.

▶ Check the serum potassium level that can be used as a baseline for comparison of future serum potassium levels. A serum potassium level below 3.5 mEq/L indicates hypokalemia. A serum potassium level below 2.5 mEq/L may cause cardiac arrest.

▶ Check the ECG/EKG strips for changes in the T wave (flat or inverted) that may indicate hypokalemia.

▶ Assess the urine output for 24 hours. Excess urine excretion increases the amount of potassium being excreted.

▶ Assess for signs and symptoms of digitalis toxicity (i.e., nausea, vomiting, anorexia, bradycardia, dysrhythmias) when a client is receiving a potassium-wasting diuretic and/or steroids with a digitalis preparation. Hypokalemia enhances the action of digitalis product.

Diagnosis 1

Risk for injury: vessels, tissues, or gastric mucosa related to phlebitis from concentrated potassium solution, infiltration of potassium solution into subcutaneous tissues, or ingestion of concentrated oral potassium irritating and damaging to the gastric mucosa.

Interventions and Rationale

1. Dilute oral potassium supplements in at least 8 ounces of water or juice. Concentrated potassium is irritating to the gastric mucosa.

2. Check infusion site for phlebitis or infiltration when KCl is given intravenously. Potassium is irritating to blood vessels and subcutaneous tissue. NEVER administer potassium intravenously as a bolus or IV push.

3. Monitor serum potassium levels. A serum potassium level less than 3.5 mEq/L can cause neuromuscular dysfunction and injury to tissues.

4. Monitor the ECG for changes that indicate hypokalemia such as a flat or inverted T wave. Report changes immediately.

Diagnosis 2

Altered nutrition: less than body requirements, related to insufficient intake of foods rich in potassium or potassium losses (gastric suctioning).

Interventions and Rationale

1. Instruct clients to eat foods rich in potassium when hypokalemia is present or when they are taking potassium-wasting diuretics and steroids. Examples of such foods are fresh fruits, fruit juices, dry fruits, vegetables, meats, nuts, cocoa, and cola.

2. Monitor the serum potassium level of clients receiving potassium-wasting diuretics and steroids (cortisone preparations).

3. Irrigate GI tube with normal saline solution to prevent electrolyte loss. Gastrointestinal fluid loss from GI suctioning, vomiting, and diarrhea should be measured.

4. Recognize other drugs and substances (i.e., glucose, insulin, laxatives, lithium carbonate, salicylates, tetracycline, and licorice) that decrease serum potassium levels.

5. Monitor serum magnesium, chloride, and protein when hypokalemia is present. Attempts to correct the potassium deficit may not be effective when hypomagnesemia, hypochloremia, and hypoproteinemia are also present.

Hyperkalemia
Assessment Factors

▶ Obtain a history of clinical health problems or procedures that may cause hyperkalemia (i.e., renal insufficiency or failure, administration of large doses of intravenous potassium or rapid administration of potassium, and Addison's disease).

▶ Assess for signs and symptoms of hyperkalemia [i.e., cardiac dysrhythmia (tachycardia and later bradycardia), decreased urine output, abdominal cramps].

▶ Check the ECG/EKG strips for changes in the T wave (peaked) that may indicate hyperkalemia.

▶ Check the serum potassium level, which can be used as a baseline for comparison of future serum potassium levels. A serum potassium level greater than 5.3 mEq/L is indicative of hyperkalemia. A serum potassium level greater than 7.0 mEq/L can be a factor in causing cardiac arrest.

▶ Assess urine output for 24 hours. A decrease in urine output of less than 600 mL/day can indicate an inadequate fluid intake, decreased cardiac output, or renal insufficiency.

▶ Check the age of whole blood before administering it to a client with hyperkalemia. Blood, for transfusion, that is 10 or more days old has an elevated serum potassium level due to the hemolysis of aging blood cells.

Diagnosis 1

Risk for decreased cardiac output: related to dysrhythmia secondary to hyperkalemia.

Interventions and Rationale

1. Monitor vital signs. Report presence of tachycardia or bradycardia.

2. Monitor ECG strips. Report presence of peaked T wave, wide QRS complex, and prolonged P-R interval.

3. Monitor serum potassium levels. Report precipitous decrease or increase in serum potassium level.

Diagnosis 2

Altered urinary elimination: related to renal dysfunction, cardiac insufficiency.

Interventions and Rationale

1. Monitor daily urine output. Urine output that is less than 600 mL per day should be reported.

2. Monitor urine output for clients receiving potassium supplements (orally or intravenously). If urine output is poor while

the client is receiving potassium supplements, the serum potassium level will be increased.

3. Regulate the flow rate of intravenous fluid with potassium so that no more than 10 mEq/L of KCl is administered per hour. Rapidly administered KCl can cause hyperkalemia.

4. Monitor medical treatments for hyperkalemia. Know which corrective treatments are used for mild, moderate, and severe hyperkalemia.

5. Note if the client is on digitalis when calcium gluconate is ordered for temporary correction of hyperkalemia. Hypercalcemia enhances the action of digitalis, causing digitalis toxicity.

6. Administer Kayexalate and sorbitol orally or rectally, according to the amount prescribed by the physician. The serum potassium should be checked frequently during treatment to prevent hypokalemia resulting from overcorrection of hyperkalemia.

7. Administer fresh blood (blood transfusion) to clients with hyperkalemia. The serum potassium level of fresh blood is 3.5–5.5 mEq/L. With blood that is 3 weeks old, the serum potassium level can be as high as 25 mEq/L.

Evaluation/Outcome

1. Evaluate that the cause of potassium imbalance has been corrected.

2. Evaluate the effect of therapeutic regimen in correcting potassium imbalance. The serum potassium levels are within normal range.

3. Remain free of clinical signs and symptoms of hypokalemia or hyperkalemia. Client's ECG, vital signs, and muscular tone are or return to a normal pattern.

4. Diet includes foods rich in potassium while taking drugs that promote potassium loss.

5. Urine output is adequate ($>$600 mL/day or $1\frac{1}{2}$ pints of urine per day).

6. Document compliance with the prescribed drug therapy and medical and dietary regimens.

7. Client and family recognize risk factors related to hypokalemia.

8. Maintain a support system, i.e., health professionals, family members, friends.

9. Schedule follow-up appointments.

CHAPTER

7

Sodium and Chloride Imbalances

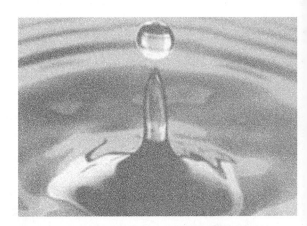

▶ INTRODUCTION

Sodium (Na) and chloride (Cl) are the principal cations and anions in the extracellular fluid (ECF). Sodium and chloride levels in the body are regulated by the kidneys and are influenced by the hormone aldosterone. Sodium is mainly responsible for water retention, which influences the serum osmolality level.

1 extracellular or
    intravascular

2 anion; extracellular fluid

3 sodium loss

4 extracellular fluid

5 135–146

6 more

1

Sodium is the main cation found in _____ fluid.

2

Chloride is a(n) (anion/cation) _____ .
    The chloride ion frequently appears in combination with the sodium ion. Which fluid has the greatest concentration of chloride—intracellular or extracellular? *_____

3

Sodium loss from the skin is negligible under normal conditions. Environmental conditions related to temperature and humidity, fever, and/or muscular exercise can influence the loss of sodium.
    If an individual runs a race and the atmospheric temperature is 100, what do you think happens to the sodium in his or her body? *_____

4

The normal concentration of sodium in the extracellular fluid is 135–146 mEq/L.
    The normal concentration of sodium in perspiration is 50–100 mEq, which is less than the concentration found in the
*_____ .

5

Perspiration is regarded as a by-product of temperature regulation. Therefore, when the body's sodium level is elevated, perspiration is not a means of regulating sodium excretion. Bones contain as much as 800–1000 mEq of sodium, but only a portion of the sodium is available for exchange with sodium in other parts of the body.
    The normal concentration of sodium in the extracellular fluid is _____ mEq/L.

6

Bones contain (more/less) _____ sodium than extracellular fluid.

7

Thirst often leads to the replacement of water, but not of sodium.

One (can/cannot) _____ replace sodium by drinking lots of water.

7   cannot

8

Ocean water is about three times as salty as our body fluid—far too salty for our body organs, i.e., stomach and intestines.

Ocean water is a (hypo-osmolar/hyperosmolar) _____ fluid. Therefore, in cases of ocean water ingestion, the water is drawn from the body fluid into the stomach and intestines by the process of (osmosis/diffusion) _____ .

8   hyperosmolar; osmosis

9

An elevated serum sodium is known as sodium excess or *hypernatremia* and a decreased serum sodium is known as sodium deficit or *hyponatremia.*

Hypernatremia is also known as *_____ . Hyponatremia is also known as *_____ .

9   sodium excess; sodium
     deficit

10

One of the main functions of sodium is to influence the distribution of water in the body. Water accompanies sodium.

A name for a sodium excess is _____ .

A name for a sodium deficit is _____ .

A function of sodium is to influence the distribution of

*_____ .

10 hypernatremia; hypona-
     tremia; body water (water
     accompanies sodium)

11

The normal serum chloride (Cl) range is 95–108 mEq/L. The chloride concentration in the intracellular fluid is 1 mEq/L.

A serum chloride level less than 95 mEq/L is called (hypochloremia/hyperchloremia) _____ .

A serum chloride level greater than 108 mEq/L is called (hypochloremia/hyperchloremia) _____ .

11 hypochloremia;
     hyperchloremia

▶ FUNCTIONS

Sodium action is influenced by the kidneys, the posterior pituitary gland, and the adrenal glands. The kidneys have an im-

Table 7-1

Influences Affecting Serum Sodium

Organ Kidneys	Kidneys are regulators that maintain homeostasis through excretion or absorption of water and sodium from the renal tubules according to excess or deficit of serum sodium.
Glands 1. Posterior hypophysis or posterior pituitary gland	The antidiuretic hormone (ADH), secreted by the pituitary gland, favors water absorption from the distal tubules of the kidneys and thus limits sodium excretion.
2. Adrenal cortex of the adrenal glands	Adrenal cortical hormones, e.g., cortisone and aldosterone, secreted by the adrenal cortex, favor sodium absorption from the renal tubules. These steroids stimulate the kidneys to absorb sodium and excrete potassium.

portant role in maintaining homeostasis of body sodium. The hypothalamus produces ADH (antidiuretic hormone) and the posterior hypophysis (posterior pituitary gland) stores and secretes ADH. This hormone facilitates the absorption of large quantities of water from the kidneys. The adrenal glands are composed of two sections, the cortex and the medulla, each secreting its own hormones. The hormones from the adrenal cortex are frequently referred to as steroids. Table 7-1 explains how one organ and two glands influence serum sodium. Study this table carefully. Refer to a physiology text for any further clarification.

12

12 kidneys

The chief regulation of sodium occurs within the _____ .

13

13 They stimulate the kidneys to absorb sodium and excrete potassium.

Explain the effect of cortisone and aldosterone on the regulation of sodium and potassium. *_____

_____

Table 7-2 explains the functions of sodium. The two most important functions of sodium are water balance and neuromuscular activity. Study Table 7-2 carefully and refer to the table as needed.

Table 7-2

Sodium and Its Functions

Body Involvement	Functions
Neuromuscular	Transmission and conduction of nerve impulses (sodium pump— see Cellular).
Body fluids	Largely responsible for the osmolality of vascular fluids. Doubling Na level gives the approximate serum osmolality. Regulation of body fluid (increased sodium levels cause water retention).
Cellular	Sodium pump action. Sodium shifts into cells as potassium shifts out of the cells, repeatedly, to maintain water balance and neuromuscular activity. When Na shifts into the cell, depolarization occurs (cell activity); and when Na shifts out of the cell, K shifts back into the cell, and repolarization occurs. Enzyme activity.
Acid-base levels	Assist with the regulation of acid-base balance. Sodium combines readily with chloride (Cl) or bicarbonate (HCO_3) to regulate the acid-base balance.

14 potassium, magnesium, or calcium

15 sodium; doubling the serum sodium level

16 Sodium shifts in as potassium shifts out of the cells, stimulating depolarization and cell activity. K shifts in and Na shifts out for repolarization (cell rest).; water balance and neuromuscular activity

17 chloride and bicarbonate

14
An important function of sodium is neuromuscular activity. Name another electrolyte responsible for neuromuscular activity.

_____

15
The concentration or osmolality of vascular fluids is determined by which electrolyte? _____
   A rough estimate of the serum osmolality can be obtained by
* _____ .

16
Explain the action of the sodium pump. * _____

_____

Name two purposes for the sodium pump. * _____

_____

17
What are the two anions that combine with sodium to help regulate acid-base balance? * _____

18

Sodium in increased quantities is contained within the following body secretions: saliva, gastric secretions, bile, pancreatic juice, and intestinal secretions.

Indicate which of the following body secretions contain large quantities of sodium:

( ) a. Saliva
( ) b. Thyroid secretions
( ) c. Gastric secretions
( ) d. Bile
( ) e. Parathyroid secretions
( ) f. Pancreatic juice
( ) g. Intestinal secretions

18 a, c, d, f, g

Table 7-3 lists the four functions of the chloride ion. Study the table and refer to it as needed.

19

Chloride, like sodium, influences the serum osmolality.

What two ions are usually increased when the serum osmolality is elevated? *_____

19 sodium and chloride

Table 7-3

Chloride and Its Functions

Body Involvement	Functions
Osmolality (tonicity) of ECF	Chloride, like sodium, changes the serum osmolality. When serum osmolality is increased, >295 mOsm/kg, there are more sodium and chloride ions in proportion to the water. A decreased serum osmolality, <280 mOsm/kg, results in less sodium and chloride ions, and a lower serum osmolality.
Body water balance	When sodium is retained, chloride is frequently retained, causing an increase in water retention.
Acid-base balance	The kidneys excrete the anion chloride or bicarbonate, and sodium reabsorbs either chloride or bicarbonate to maintain the acid-base balance.
Acidity of gastric juice	Chloride combines with the hydrogen ion in the stomach to form hydrochloric acid (HCl).

20

20 a. increases; b. increases; c. is reabsorbed

When there is a body water deficit, what occurs to the:
a. Serum sodium and serum chloride levels? _____
b. Serum osmolality? _____
c. Body water? _____

21

For every sodium ion absorbed from the renal tubules, a chloride or bicarbonate ion is also absorbed; thus the proportion of sodium and chloride lost can differ.

21 kidneys

The organs responsible for electrolyte homeostasis by the excretion and absorption of ions are the _____ .

22

If metabolic alkalosis is present, the kidneys excrete the bicarbonate ion and sodium is reabsorbed with the (bicarbonate/chloride) _____ ions.

22 chloride; chloride; bicarbonate

If metabolic acidosis is present, the kidneys excrete (bicarbonate/chloride) _____ ion, and the sodium is reabsorbed with which ion? _____

▶ PATHOPHYSIOLOGY

23

The pathophysiologic effects of hyponatremia are evidenced in the membranes of the central nervous system (CNS), the neuromuscular tissues, and the smooth muscles of the gastrointestinal (GI) tract.

The cells of the CNS are more sensitive to a decreased serum sodium level than other cells. The cardiac muscle is usually not affected by changes in the serum sodium level.

Hyponatremia has an effect on the membranes of:

23 a. central nervous system; b. neuromuscular tissues; c. smooth muscles of the GI tract

a. * _____
b. * _____
c. * _____

24

Hyponatremia can occur when the kidneys are unable to excrete enough urine. Reduced urine excretion increases the amount of body water, which in turn dilutes the serum sodium concentration.

The type of electrolyte imbalance that can result when the body fluid volume is increased is known as (hyponatremia/hypernatremia) _____ .

24 hyponatremia

25

When the serum sodium level is increased, sodium passes more freely across the cell membranes, accelerating the rate of depolarization. This can cause (decreased/increased) _____ cellular activity (irritability). As the hypernatremic state intensifies, less sodium passes across the cell membrane, ultimately resulting in (more/less) _____ cellular activity.

25 increased; less

26 Increases. The serum osmolality is the concentration of solutes in the plasma.

26

An increased serum sodium level (hypernatremia) (increases/decreases) _____ the serum osmolality.

▶ ETIOLOGY

The general causes of hyponatremia and hypochloremia are GI losses, altered cellular function, renal losses, electrolyte-free fluids, and hormonal influences. Table 7-4 lists the various causes and gives the rationale concerning the sodium and chloride loss. Study this table carefully and refer to it as needed.

27

The hemodilution of body fluids that can cause hyponatremia and hypochloremia includes which of the following symptoms:

( ) a. Drinking excessive amounts of plain water
( ) b. Increased adrenocortical hormone
( ) c. SIADH
( ) d. Gastric suction
( ) e. Hypervolemic state due to CHF
( ) f. Increased environmental temperature

27 a, c, e

28 decrease; The high concentrations of sodium and chloride in the GI tract are reduced.

28

Vomiting and diarrhea can (increase/decrease) _____ the serum sodium and chloride levels. Explain * _____

_____

Table 7-4

Causes of Hyponatremia and Hypochloremia
(Serum Sodium and Chloride Deficit)

Etiology	Rationale
Dietary Changes Low-sodium diet Excessive plain water intake "Fad" diets/fasting Anorexia nervosa Prolonged use of IV D$_5$W	A low-sodium intake over several months can lead to hyponatremia. Drinking large quantities of plain water dilutes the ECF. Administration of continuous IV D$_5$W dilutes the ECF and can cause water intoxication. Gastric juice is composed of the acid hydrogen chloride (HCl).
Gastrointestinal Losses Vomiting, diarrhea GI suctioning Tap-water enemas GI surgery Bulimia	Sodium and chloride are in high concentration in the gastric and intestinal mucosas. Sodium and chloride losses occur with vomiting, diarrhea, GI suctioning, and GI surgery.
Loss of potassium	Loss of potassium is accompanied by loss of chloride.
Renal Losses Salt-wasting kidney disease Diuretics	In advanced renal disorders, the tubules do not respond to ADH; therefore, there is a loss of sodium, chloride, and water. The extensive use of diuretics or excessively potent diuretics can decrease the serum sodium and chloride levels.

continues on the following page

---

29 sweating, increased environmental temperature and humidity, fever, and muscular exercise

29

Name four conditions that cause an increased sodium and chloride loss through the skin. *_____

_____

30 deficit; Excess or continuous ADH secretion (SIADH) causes water to be reabsorbed from the kidney, thus diluting ECF.

30

Wound drainage, bleeding, and vomiting postoperatively can cause a sodium and chloride (deficit/retention)_____ .

   SIADH may occur following surgery. Explain how it causes a sodium and chloride deficit. *_____

_____

Table 7-4

(Continued)

Etiology	Rationale
Hormonal Influences Antidiuretic hormone (ADH), syndrome of inappropriate ADH (SIADH)	ADH promotes water reabsorption from the distal renal tubules. Surgical pain, increased use of narcotics, and head trauma, cause more water to be reabsorbed, thus diluting the ECF.
Decreased adrenocortical hormone: Addison's disease	Decreased adrenocortical hormone production related to decreased adrenal gland activity (Addison's disease) causes sodium loss and potassium retention.
Altered Cellular Function Hypervolemic state: CHF, cirrhosis	In hypervolemic states due to CHF, cirrhosis, and nephrosis, the ECF is increased, thus diluting the serum sodium and chloride levels.
Burns	Great quantities of sodium and chloride are lost from burn wounds and from oozing burn surface areas.
Skin	Large amounts of sodium and chloride are lost from the skin due to increased environmental temperature, fever, and large skin wounds.
Acid-Base Imbalance Metabolic alkalosis	An increase in the concentration of bicarbonate ions is associated with a decrease in the concentration of chloride ions.

31 decreased; metabolic alkalosis

32 hyponatremia; Gastric and intestinal secretions are lost through the gastric tube/suction.

31

Increased bicarbonate ion concentration (HCO_3) is associated with a(n) (increased/decreased) _____ chloride ion concentration.

　　What type of acid-base imbalance results? *_____

32

The use of gastric suction for the purpose of drainage can cause (hypernatremia/hyponatremia) _____ . Why? *_____

33 insufficiency; loss

34 water, sodium, and chloride loss; due to oozing at the burn surface

35 hypernatremia; hyperchloremia; Water loss is greater than sodium and chloride loss (hypovolemic with hypernatremic/ hyperchloremic effect).

36 a, b, d, f, g

37 retention; Reduced glomerular filtration. Sodium retention usually causes an increase in body fluid and may give a false indication that the serum sodium level is normal or low.

38 overproduction; retention

33

Addison's disease occurs when there is an adrenocortical hormone (insufficiency/overproduction) _____ .

In Addison's disease, there is a sodium (loss/gain) _____ .

34

Clients recovering from burn injuries experience numerous fluid shifts as the body attempts to compensate for the trauma to its tissues. Burns promote increased *_____. Why? *_____

Table 7-5 lists the various causes and gives the rationale concerning sodium excess.

35

Severe vomiting and diarrhea can cause (hyponatremia/ hypernatremia) and (hypochloremia/hyperchloremia) _____ . Why? *_____

_____

36

Which of the following situations can cause an increased serum sodium and chloride level:

( ) a. Excessive use of table salt.
( ) b. Continuous use of canned vegetables and soups
( ) c. Increased water intake
( ) d. Use of intravenous 3% saline solutions
( ) e. Use of diuretics
( ) f. Large doses or prolonged uses of oral cortisone therapy
( ) g. Severe vomiting

37

Congestive heart failure (CHF) or obstruction of the arterial blood supply to the kidney can cause sodium and chloride (excretion/retention) _____ . Why? *_____

_____

38

Cushing's syndrome occurs when there is an adrenocortical hormone (insufficiency/overproduction) _____ .

In Cushing's syndrome, there is a sodium and chloride _____ .

Table 7-5

Causes of Hypernatremia and Hyperchloremia
(Serum Sodium and Chloride Excess)

Etiology	Rationale
Dietary Changes Increased sodium intake Decreased water intake Administration of 3% saline solutions	Inadequate fluid intake and increased use of table salt, canned vegetables, and soups can increase the serum sodium and chloride levels. Administration of concentrated 3% saline solutions can cause hypernatremia and hyperchloremia.
GI Disorders Vomiting (severe) Diarrhea	With severe vomiting, water loss can be greater than sodium loss, causing a dangerously high serum sodium level. This is particularly true in babies who have diarrhea. Their loss of water can be greater than their loss of sodium.
Decreased renal function	Reduced glomerular filtration causes an excess of sodium in the body.
Environmental Changes Increased temperature and humidity Water loss	Increased environmental and body temperatures may cause profuse perspiration. Water loss can be greater than sodium and chloride losses.
Hormonal Influence Increased adrenocortical hormone production: oral or IV cortisone	Excess adrenocortical hormone can cause a sodium and chloride excess in the body whether it is due to cortisone ingestion or hyperfunction of the adrenal gland (Cushing's syndrome).
Altered Cellular Function CHF, renal diseases	Usually with CHF and renal disease, the body's sodium and chloride are greatly increased. If water retention is greatly enhanced, pseudohyponatremia may result.
Trauma: head injury	Chloride ions are frequently retained with the sodium.
Acid-base imbalance: metabolic acidosis	Increased chloride (Cl) ion concentration is associated with a decreased bicarbonate ion concentration.

39

39 decreased; metabolic
   acidosis

An increased chloride level is associated with a(n)
(increased/decreased) _____ bicarbonate (HCO_3) level.
What type of acid-base imbalance occurs? *_____

▶ CLINICAL MANIFESTATIONS

The severity of the clinical manifestations of hypo-hypernatremia
varies with the onset and extent of sodium deficit or excess. Mild
hypernatremia is normally asymptomatic, and early nonspecific
symptoms such as nausea and vomiting may be overlooked. Table
7-6 gives the signs and symptoms associated with hypo-hypernatremia. Memorize the common symptoms, which are marked with
an asterisk. Study this table carefully. Refer to the glossary for any
unknown words. Refer back to this table as needed to complete
the frames on hypo-hypernatremia.

Table 7-6

Clinical Manifestations of Sodium Imbalances

Body Involvement	Hyponatremia	Hypernatremia
Gastrointestinal Abnormalities	*Nausea, vomiting, diarrhea, abdominal cramps	*Nausea, vomiting, anorexia *Rough, dry tongue
Cardiac Abnormalities	Tachycardia, hypotension	*Tachycardia, possible hypertension
Central Nervous System (CNS)	*Headaches, apprehension, lethargy, confusion, depression, seizures	*Restlessness, agitation, stupor, elevated body temperature
Neuromuscular Abnormalities	*Muscular weakness	Muscular twitching, tremor, hyperreflexia
Integumentary Changes	Dry skin, pale, dry mucous membrane	*Flushed, dry skin, dry, sticky membrane
Laboratory Values Serum sodium	<135 mEq/L	>146 mEq/L
Urine sodium		<40 mEq/L
Specific gravity	<1.008	>1.025
Serum osmolality	<280 mOsm/kg	>295 mOsm/kg

Note: *Most common clinical manifestations of hyponatremia and hypernatremia.

40

40 135; above 146

In hyponatremia, the serum sodium level is below
_____ mEq/L. What is the serum value in hypernatremia?
*_____ mEq/L

41

41 hyponatremia

Headaches, lethargy, depression, and muscular weakness
are clinical manifestations of (hyponatremia/hypernatremia)
_____ .

42

Which of the following signs and symptoms indicate
hypernatremia?
( ) a. Rough, dry tongue
( ) b. Tachycardia
( ) c. Apprehension, confusion
( ) d. Flushed, dry skin
( ) e. Restlessness, agitation
( ) f. Elevated body temperature

42 a, b, d, e, f

43 hyponatremia (also
indicates ECF dilution
caused by a sodium deficit
or excess water retention);
hypernatremia

43

A serum osmolality below 280 mOsm/L can indicate
(hyponatremia/hypernatremia) _____ , while a serum
osmolality above 295 mOsm/L can indicate _____ .

44

Hypochloremia neuromuscular abnormalities are similar to the
symptoms of tetany. Tetany symptoms are evidenced as
(hypo/hyper) _____ excitability of the nerves and muscles.

44 hyper; tremors; twitching

Examples of these symptoms are _____ and _____ .

45

With hyperchloremic neuromuscular abnormalities, there is a
decrease in nerve and muscle activity. Two examples of these

45 weakness and lethargy

symptoms are *_____ .

46

In hypochloremia, the respiratory symptom is similar to
metabolic alkalosis.

46 a; The lungs conserve carbon dioxide ($CO_2 + H_2O = H_2CO_3$) or carbonic acid to increase acid and restore the pH.

Indicate which type of breathing occurs with a chloride deficit.

( ) a. Slow, shallow breathing
( ) b. Deep, rapid, vigorous breathing

Explain why. *_____

_____

47

In hyperchloremia, the respiratory symptom is similar to metabolic acidosis.

Indicate which type of breathing occurs with a chloride excess.

( ) a. Slow, shallow breathing
( ) b. Deep, rapid, vigorous breathing

47 b; The lungs blow off carbon dioxide to prevent the formation of H_2CO_3— carbonic acid.

Do you know why? *_____

_____

Table 7-7 lists the clinical manifestations of hypochloremia and hyperchloremia according to the body areas affected. Hypochloremic symptoms are similar to metabolic alkalosis, and hyperchloremic symptoms are similar to metabolic acidosis. Study the table carefully and refer to it as needed.

Table 7-7

Clinical Manifestations of Chloride Imbalances

Body Involvement	Hypochloremia	Hyperchloremia
Neuromuscular Abnormalities	Hyperexcitability of the nerves and muscles (tremors, twitching)	Weakness Lethargy Unconsciousness (later)
Respiratory Abnormalities	Slow and shallow breathing	Deep, rapid, vigorous breathing
Cardiac Abnormalities	↓ Blood pressure with severe Cl and ECF losses	
Laboratory Values Milliequivalent per liter	<95 mEq/L	>108 mEq/L

▶ CLINICAL MANAGEMENT

Sodium Correction

48

The majority of Americans consume 3–5 g of sodium per day (some consume 8–15 g daily). Daily sodium requirements are 2–4 g. A teaspoon of salt has 2.3 g of sodium.

When sodium intake increases, what happens to the water intake and to the body fluids? *_____

48 Sodium holds water. Extracellular fluid (ECF) is increased.

49

To restore the sodium balance due to a sodium deficit, either normal saline solution (0.9% NaCl) or a 3% salt solution is recommended. Several health professionals suggest that the serum sodium fall below 130 mEq/L before giving saline and ≤115 mEq/L before giving a concentrated salt solution, i.e., 3% saline.

Remember, a rapid infusion of concentrated salt solutions can result in pulmonary edema. Explain why. *_____

_____

49 Sodium retains fluid. A high concentration of sodium pulls intracellular fluid from cells, thus overexpanding the vascular compartment. Fluid collects in the lungs.

50

Excessive intravenous administration of dextrose and water can cause sodium dilution. Dextrose is metabolized, leaving free water. Copious amounts of plain water can cause sodium

_____ .

Explain how sodium can be diluted. *_____

_____

50 dilution; Following the utilization of dextrose, the remaining water dilutes the sodium and other electrolytes.

Drugs and Their Effect on Sodium Balance

Diuretics, certain antipsychotics, antineoplastics, and barbiturates can cause a sodium deficit. Corticosteroids and the ingestion and infusion of sodium are the major causes of a sodium excess. Table 7-8 lists the drugs that affect sodium balance.

51

Enter SD for sodium deficit/hyponatremia and SE for sodium excess/hypernatremia beside drugs that affect sodium balance. Refer to Table 7-8 as needed.

Table 7-8

Drugs Affecting Sodium Balance

Sodium Imbalance	Drugs	Rationale
Hyponatremia (serum sodium deficit)	Diuretics	Diuretics, either K wasting or K sparing, cause sodium excretion.
	Lithium	Lithium promotes urinary sodium loss.
	Antineoplastics/Anticancer 　Vincristine 　Cyclophosphamide 　Cisplatin Antipsychotics 　Amitryptyline (Elavil) 　Thioridazine (Mellaril) 　Thiothixene (Navane) 　Tranylcypromine (Parnate) Antidiabetics 　Chlorpropamide (Diabenase) 　Tolbutamide (Orinase) CNS depressants 　Morphine 　Barbiturates 　Ibuprofens (Motrin) 　Nicotine 　Clonidine (Catapres)	Anticancer drugs, antipsychotics, and antidiabetics stimulate ADH release and cause hemodilution and decrease sodium level.

continues on the following page

_____ a. Lithium

_____ b. Cortisone

_____ c. Diuretics

_____ d. Sodium penicillin

_____ e. Antipsychotic agents

_____ f. Ibuprofen/Motrin

_____ g. Amphoterin B

_____ h. Lactulose

_____ i. Barbiturates

_____ j. Cyclophosphamide/Cytoxan

_____ k. Tolbutamide/Orinase

51 a. SD ; b. SE; c. SD; d. SE; e. SD;
f. SD; g. SE; h. SE; i. SD; j. SD;
k. SD

Table 7-8

(Continued)

Sodium Imbalance	Drugs	Rationale
Hypernatremia (serum sodium excess)	Corticosteroids Cortisone Prednisone	Steroids promote sodium retention and potassium excretion.
	Hypertonic saline Sodium salicylate Sodium phosphate Sodium bicarbonate Cough medicines	Administration of sodium salts in excess.
	Antibiotics Azlocillin Na Penicillin Na	Many of the antibiotics contain the sodium salt, which increases drug absorption.
	Mezlocillin Na Carbenicillin Ticarcillin disodium	Ion exchange.
	Cholestyramine Amphotericin B Demeclocycline Propoxyphene (Darvon)	These miscellaneous drugs promote urinary water loss without sodium.
	Lactulose	Water loss in excess of sodium via GI tract.

---

52 Steroids promote sodium retention (sodium-retaining effect).

52
Clients who are receiving steroids, such as cortisone and prednisone, should be cautioned in the use of excess salt. Explain * _____

53
Hyponatremia enhances the action of quinidine and hypernatremia reduces or decreases the action of quinidine.
  With a serum sodium of 156 mEq/L would the action of quinidine be (increased/decreased)? _____

53 decreased

54
Cough medicines, most antibiotics, and sulfonamides can (increase/decrease) _____ the serum sodium level.

54 increase

▶ CLINICAL APPLICATIONS

55

55 Hyponatremia thus results from hemodilution. May be receiving a low-sodium diet and taking a diuretic.

You have a cardiac client who has edema and his serum sodium concentration is reduced. Why do you think this occurs?
*_____

_____

56

56 yes; A low urine sodium indicates sodium retention in the body, especially with symptoms of overhydration. A low serum sodium level can be misleading. Hyponatremia can also occur with a fluid volume excess (hypervolemia), by causing the sodium to be diluted.

A 24-hour urine sodium test is helpful for determining sodium retention or loss within the body. A normal range for a 24-hour urine sodium is 40–220 mEq/L.

A client's 24-hour urine sodium is 32 mEq/L, the serum sodium level is 133 mEq/L, and the client has symptoms of heart failure. Do you think the client is retaining sodium?
_____ . Explain. *_____

_____

57

A normal urine chloride level in 24 hours is 150–250 mEq/L. The amount of chloride excreted depends on the amount of salt intake, body fluid imbalance, and acid-base imbalance.

With a body fluid deficit, the serum chloride and sodium levels are increased due to hemoconcentration. In this situation do you expect the urine chloride level to be (increased/decreased)? _____

57 decreased

58

If your client is vomiting following a surgical intervention and is receiving dextrose and water intravenously, one may expect a sodium and chloride (excess/deficit) _____ if the vomiting persists.

A client experiencing severe vomiting without water replacement is at high risk for a sodium (excess/deficit) _____ . Why? *_____

_____

58 deficit; excess; The loss of water is greater than the loss of sodium in severe vomiting.

59

59 retention; Poor circulation reduces the glomerular filtration; therefore, Na and Cl are retained.

In congestive heart failure, there is sodium and chloride (retention/excretion) _____ . Why? *_____

_____

60

If a feeble or debilitated client receives numerous tap-water enemas for the purpose of cleaning the bowel, the enemas can cause a sodium and chloride _____ .

60 loss (deficit)

61

Diarrhea can cause either a sodium deficit or a sodium excess. Babies having diarrhea can lose more _____ than the . sodium; therefore, a sodium _____ can result.

61 water; excess

62

Hypochloremia usually indicates alkalosis (hypochloremic alkalosis) due to increased levels of bicarbonate.

Persistent vomiting and gastric suction cause a loss of hydrogen and chloride ions. A loss in hydrogen and chloride results in *_____ .

62 hypochloremic alkalosis

63

A potassium deficit cannot be fully corrected until a chloride deficit is corrected.

With vomiting, what type of potassium supplement (Kaon/ K-Lyte/potassium chloride) _____ is needed to replace the potassium and chloride deficits.

Explain. *_____

63 potassium chloride; Both chloride and potassium are lost due to vomiting.

● Clinical Considerations

1. Serum osmolality of body fluids (ECF) can be estimated by *doubling the serum sodium level.* For a more accurate serum osmolality level, use the formula

$$2 \times serum\ Na + \frac{BUN}{3} + \frac{glucose}{18} = serum\ osmolality\ (mOsm/kg)$$

The normal serum osmolality range is 280–295 mOsm/kg.

2. Sodium causes water retention.

3. One teaspoon of salt is equivalent to 2.3 g of sodium. The daily sodium requirement is 2–4 g. Most Americans consume 3–5 g of sodium per day, and some consume 8–15 g daily.

4. Vomiting causes sodium and chloride losses, and diarrhea causes sodium, chloride, and bicarbonate losses.

5. A 3% saline solution should be given when there is a severe serum sodium deficit, e.g., <115 mEq/L. When administering a 3% saline solution, check for signs and symptoms of pulmonary edema.

6. A serum potassium cannot be fully corrected until the chloride deficit is corrected.

7. Sodium and potassium have opposite effects on cellular activity. The sodium pump effect causes sodium to shift into the cells resulting in depolarization. When sodium shifts out of the cells, potassium shifts into cells and repolarization occurs. The sodium pump action is continuously repeated.

8. Continuous use of a saline solution causes a calcium loss.

9. Steroids promote sodium retention and, thus, water retention. Cough medicine, sulfonamides, and some antibiotics containing sodium can increase the serum sodium level.

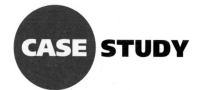

CASE STUDY **REVIEW**

Mrs. Unger has a high temperature and diaphoresis. She has been nauseated and has taken only ginger ale for the last several days. Her serum sodium is 129 mEq/L.

ANSWER COLUMN

1. sodium deficit or hyponatremia

2. 135–146 mEq/L

3. fever; diaphoresis; ginger ale intake for several days (lack of food)

4. abdominal cramps; muscular weakness; headaches; nausea and vomiting

1. What type of sodium imbalance does Mrs. Unger have?
   *_____
   _____

2. Give the "normal" serum sodium range. *_____

3. Give some of the reasons for Mrs. Unger's imbalance.
   a. *_____
   b. *_____

4. Name some of the clinical signs and symptoms the nurse might observe.
   a. *_____
   b. *_____
   c. *_____
   d. *_____

5. **a.** 1.010 or below

6. Yes. She could have a loss of potassium from lack of food and due to illness. Arrhythmia may be a sign of hypokalemia

7. flushed skin; elevated body temperature; rough, dry tongue; tachycardia

8. It reduces or decreases quinidine's action.

9. They increase the hypernatremic state. Cortisone causes sodium, chloride, and water retention, and certain antibiotics increase sodium levels.
10. During cell catabolism, potassium leaves the cells and sodium enters the cells.

5. When testing Mrs. Unger's urine, what would you expect the specific gravity level to be?
   (   ) a. 1.010 or below
   (   ) b. 1.015
   (   ) c. 1.020 or above

Mrs. Unger was given 3% sodium chloride solution. Her serum sodium level rose to 152 mEq/L. She was given quinidine for her irregular pulse rate.

6. Do you think her serum potassium should have been evaluated? _____ Why?* _____
   _____

7. Name some of the clinical signs and symptoms the nurse observes with hypernatremia.
   a. * _____
   b. * _____
   c. * _____

8. Explain the effect of hypernatremia on quinidine. _____
   _____

9. If Mrs. Unger were to receive cortisone and antibiotic, penicillin G Na, what would this do to her hypernatremic state?
   * _____
   _____

10. Sodium is most plentiful in the extracellular compartment. Explain why sodium might enter the cells. * _____
    _____

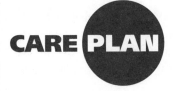

Client Management: Sodium and Chloride

Hyponatremia and Hypochloremia

Assessment Factors

▶ Obtain a history of high-risk factors for decreased serum sodium and chloride levels, i.e., GI loss from vomiting, diarrhea, or GI suctioning; eating disorders such as anorexia nervosa and bulimia; SIADH as a result of surgery; hypervolemic state resulting in hemodilution; use of potent diuretics with a low-sodium diet; or continuous use of D_5W.

▶ Assess for signs and symptoms of hyponatremia, i.e., headache, nausea, vomiting, lethargy, confusion, tachycardia, and/or muscular weakness.

▶ Obtain serum sodium and chloride levels that can be used as baseline values for comparison. A serum sodium level less than 135 mEq/L would indicate hyponatremia. A sodium level less than 125 mEq/L should be reported immediately to the health care provider. A serum chloride level below 95 mEq/L is indicative of hypochloremia.

▶ Check other electrolytes, such as potassium and chloride, when serum sodium levels are not within normal range.

▶ Check the serum osmolality level and urine specific gravity. A serum osmolality level of less than 280 mOsm/kg indicates hyponatremia. A specific gravity below 1.010 can indicate hyponatremia.

Diagnosis 1

Altered health maintenance: related to vomiting, diarrhea, gastric suction, SIADH resulting from surgery, potent diuretics.

Interventions and Rationale

1. Monitor the serum sodium and chloride levels. Sodium replacement with chloride may be needed if the serum sodium deficit is due to GI losses. Hypervolemic conditions such as CHF can indicate a pseudo-hyponatremia.

2. Keep an accurate intake and output record. Excess water intake can cause hyponatremia and hypochloremia due to hemodilution.

3. Observe changes in vital signs, especially the pulse rate. If hyponatremia is due to hypovolemia (loss of fluid and sodium), shocklike symptoms such as tachycardia can occur. Frequently, hyponatremia is due to hemodilution from an excess fluid volume.

4. Check for signs and symptoms of water intoxication, i.e., headaches and behavioral changes, when hyponatremia is due to SIADH.

5. Restrict water when hyponatremia is due to hypervolemia (excess fluid volume).

6. Monitor serum CO_2 or arterial HCO_3. An increased serum CO_2, >32 mEq/L, and/or increased arterial HCO_3, >28 mEq/L, can

indicate metabolic alkalosis and hypochloremia (hypo-chloremic alkalosis).

7. Observe for respiratory difficulties, i.e., slow, shallow breathing due to hypochloremic alkalosis.

Hypernatremia and Hyperchloremia

Assessment Factors

▶ Obtain a history of high-risk factors for increased serum sodium and chloride levels, i.e., increased sodium intake, decreased water intake, administration of concentrated saline solutions, renal diseases, and increased adrenocortical hormone production.

▶ Assess for signs and symptoms of hypernatremia, i.e., nausea, vomiting, tachycardia, elevated blood pressure, flushed-dry skin, dry-sticky membrane, restlessness, and elevated body temperature. Obtain serum sodium and chloride values. Serum sodium levels greater than 146 mEq/L indicate hypernatremia. A serum chloride level greater than 108 mEq/L is indicative of hyperchloremia.

▶ Check the serum osmolality level and urine specific gravity. A serum osmolality level greater than 295 mOsm/kg can indicate hypernatremia. A specific gravity above 1.025 can indicate hypernatremia.

Diagnosis 1

Altered nutrition: more than body requirements, related to excess intake of foods rich in sodium.

Interventions and Rationale

1. Instruct the client with hypernatremia to avoid foods rich in salt, i.e., canned foods, lunch meats, ham, pork, pickles, potato chips, and pretzels.

2. Identify drugs that have a sodium-retaining effect on the body, i.e., cortisone preparations, cough medicines, and certain laxatives containing sodium.

3. Monitor the serum sodium level. Check for chest rales and for edema in the lower extremities.

4. Monitor the serum sodium levels daily or as ordered. A serum sodium level above 146 mEq/L can indicate hypernatremia. A serum sodium level above 160 mEq/L should be reported im-

mediately to the health care provider. Report serum chloride level greater than 108 mEq/L.

5. Monitor serum CO_2 or arterial HCO_3. A decreased serum CO_2 level, <22 mEq/L, and/or decreased arterial HCO_3, <24 mEq/L, can indicate metabolic acidosis and hyperchloremia.

6. Observe for respiratory difficulties, i.e., deep, rapid, vigorous breathing due to hyperchloremia and an acidotic state (metabolic acidosis).

7. Check the serum osmolality level and the urine specific gravity. A serum osmolality level exceeding 295 mOsm/kg can indicate hypernatremia. Sodium is primarily responsible for the serum osmolality value.

8. Check the urine sodium level. A decreased urine sodium, <40 mEq/L, frequently indicates sodium retention in the body, even though the serum sodium level may be within normal range (caused by hemodilution). Also check for rales in the lung and for pitting edema from sodium and fluid retention.

9. Check for signs and symptoms of pulmonary edema when the client is receiving several liters of normal saline (0.9% NaCl) or 3% saline. Sodium holds water in the blood vessels, and when administering a concentrated saline solution, overhydration can occur. Symptoms include dyspnea, cough, chest rales, and neck and hand vein engorgement.

10. Keep an accurate intake and output record. A decrease in urine output could indicate hypervolemia due to sodium excess.

Diagnosis 2

Impaired Tissue Integrity: related to peripheral edema secondary to sodium and water excess.

Interventions and Rationale

1. Provide skin care to the body, especially the edematous areas.
2. Change the client's positions frequently to maintain skin integrity.
3. Promote increased mobility.
4. Use lotions as needed to keep skin moist.

Evaluation/Outcome

1. Evaluate that the cause of sodium and chloride imbalances has been corrected or controlled.

2. Evaluate the effect of the therapeutic regimen in correcting sodium and chloride imbalances. Serum sodium and chloride levels should be periodically checked.

3. Remain free of signs and symptoms of hyponatremia and hypernatremia.

4. Check that fluid imbalances are not contributing to sodium and chloride imbalances. The client is not dehydrated or overhydrated.

5. Urine output is adequate (>600 mL/day).

6. Maintain a support system, i.e., health professionals, family members, friends.

CHAPTER
8

Calcium Imbalances

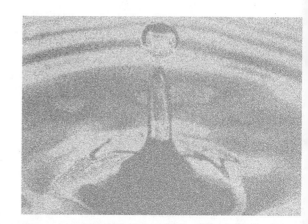

▶ INTRODUCTION

Calcium (Ca) is an electrolyte that can be found in both the extracellular and intracellular fluids; it is in somewhat of a greater concentration in the extracellular fluid. Approximately 55% of serum calcium is bound to protein and 45% is free, ionized calcium. It is the free calcium that is physiologically active.

1

Calcium is a(n) (anion/cation) _____ found in the
(extracellular/intracellular/both) _____ body fluids.
    Which body fluid has the greater calcium concentration?
*_____

1 cation; both; extracellular
    fluid

2

Calcium is a durable chemical substance of the body that is the
last element to find its place in the adult body composition and
the last element to leave after death.
    The element that preserves the bony remains of dead
creatures and is responsible for the x-ray photograph of bones

2 calcium

is _____ .

3

The normal range of the serum (plasma) calcium concentration
level in the blood is 4.5–5.5 mEq/L, or 9–11 mg/dL. Approximately 99% of the body's calcium is in teeth and bones; the
remaining 1% is in the extracellular and intracellular fluids.
    Most of the body's calcium is in the _____ and

3 teeth and bones

_____ .

4

About one-half of the body's serum calcium is bound to plasma
proteins and the other half is free, ionized calcium that serves as
a catalyst to stimulate a physiologic cellular response. Do you
think the calcium that is bound to protein can cause a cellular

4 No. For calcium to cause a
    physiologic response, it
    must be free, ionized
    calcium.; 4.5–5.5; 9–11

response? _____
    The serum calcium level is _____ mEq/L
_____ mg/dL.

5

When calcium becomes unbound from the plasma protein, the
calcium is free, active calcium. This free calcium (can/cannot)

5 can

_____ cause a physiologic cellular response.

6

Today's blood analyzers allow the ionized calcium (iCa) level to be measured. The normal serum ionized calcium level is 2.2–2.5 mEq/L, or 4.25–5.25 mg/dL.

Certain changes in the blood composition can either increase or decrease the serum iCa level. During acidosis, decreased pH, calcium is released from the serum proteins, which (increases/decreases) _____ the serum iCa level.

With alkalosis, there is an increased pH level that (increases/decreases) _____ the calcium bound to protein. This results in a(n) (increase/decrease) _____ in the amount of free serum calcium, and thus, the serum iCa level is (increased/decreased) _____ .

7

The normal serum calcium (Ca) range is _____ mEq/L, or _____ mg/dL.

The normal ionized calcium (iCa) range is _____ mEq/L, or _____ mg/dL.

▶ FUNCTIONS

8

Vitamin D is an element that is needed for calcium absorption from the gastrointestinal tract. The anion phosphorus (P) inhibits calcium absorption. Thus, the actions of these two ions on the body have an opposite physiologic effect. When the serum calcium level is increased, the serum phosphorus level (increases/decreases) _____ . However, both calcium and phosphorus are stored in the bone and are excreted by the kidneys.

9

The parathyroid glands, which are four small oval-shaped glands located on the posterior thyroid gland, regulate the serum level of calcium. These glands secrete the parathyroid hormone (PTH), which is responsible for the homeostatic regulation of the calcium ion in the body fluids.

When the serum calcium level is low, the parathyroid gland secretes more parathyroid hormone. Explain what happens when the serum calcium level is high. *_____

_____

---

6 increases; increases; decrease; decreased

7 4.5–5.5; 9–11; 2.2–2.5; 4.25–5.25

8 decreases

9 It inhibits or limits the secretion of the parathyroid hormone (PTH).

10

Calcitonin from the thyroid gland increases calcium return to the bone, thus decreasing the serum calcium level. Figure 8-1 diagrams the sequence of PTH and calcitonin which are secreted from the thyroid and parathyroid glands, and their effects on bone and serum Ca levels.

The parathyroid hormone (PTH) can (increase/decrease) _____ the serum calcium level by promoting calcium release from the bone as needed.

Indicate which of the hormones listed on the left increase or decrease the serum calcium levels.

_____ 1. Calcitonin   a. Increase
_____ 2. PTH   b. Decrease

10 increase; 1. b; 2. a

11

The regulation of serum calcium is maintained by the negative-feedback system. A low serum calcium stimulates the parathyroid gland to *_____ . What do you think happens when there is a high serum calcium? *_____
_____

11 secrete parathyroid hormone (PTH); It inhibits the secretion of parathyroid hormone (PTH) from the parathyroid gland.

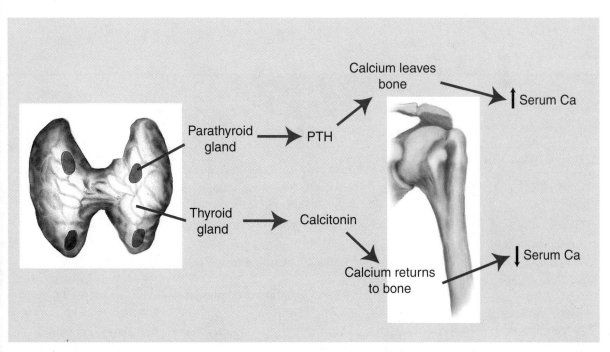

Figure 8-1 Functions of PTH and calcitonin.

12

A low serum calcium level tells the parathyroid gland to secrete more parathyroid hormone (PTH). The parathyroid hormone increases serum calcium by mobilizing calcium from the bone, increasing renal absorption of calcium and promoting calcium absorption from the intestine in the presence of vitamin D.

PTH increases serum calcium by which of the following mechanisms:

( ) a. Mobilizing calcium from the bone
( ) b. Decreasing renal absorption of calcium
( ) c. Increasing renal absorption of calcium
( ) d. Promoting calcium absorption from the intestine with vitamin D

Table 8-1 explains the functions of calcium. Calcium is needed for neuromuscular activity, contraction of the myocardium, normal cellular permeability, coagulation of blood, and bone and teeth formation. Study the table carefully, and refer to it as needed.

13

Name five functions of calcium in the body. Refer to Table 8-1 as needed.

12 a, c, d

Table 8-1

Calcium and Its Functions

Body Involvement	Functions
Neuromuscular	Normal nerve and muscle activity. Calcium causes transmission of nerve impulses and contraction of skeletal muscles.
Cardiac	Contraction of heart muscle (myocardium).
Cellular and Blood	Maintenance of normal cellular permeability. ↑ calcium decreases cellular permeability and ↓ calcium increases cellular permeability. Coagulation of blood. Calcium promotes blood clotting by converting prothrombin into thrombin.
Bones and Teeth	Formation of bone and teeth. Calcium and phosphorus make bones and teeth strong and durable.

13 a. normal nerve and muscle activity; b. contraction of myocardium; c. maintenance of normal cellular permeability; d. coagulation of blood; e. formation of bone and teeth

a. * _____
b. * _____
c. * _____
d. * _____
e. * _____

14
A high serum concentration of calcium (increases/decreases) _____ the permeability of membranes, whereas a low serum concentration of calcium (increases/decreases) _____ the permeability of membranes.

14 decreases; increases

15
A calcium deficit causes neuromuscular excitability (tetany symptoms). How does calcium promote blood clotting?
* _____

Explain how tetany occurs. * _____

15 Calcium converts prothrombin into thrombin.; A calcium deficit causes neuromuscular excitability.

▶ PATHOPHYSIOLOGY

16
A decrease in the serum calcium level is known as *hypocalcemia*. What do you think an increase in the serum calcium level is called? _____
The normal serum calcium level is * _____ .

16 hypercalcemia; 4.5–5.5 mEq/L, or 9–11 mg/dL

17
A serum calcium level less than 4.5 mEq/L is (hypocalcemia/hypercalcemia/normal) _____ .
A serum calcium level greater than 5.5 mEq/L is known as (hypocalcemia/hypercalcemia/normal) _____ .

17 hypocalcemia; hypercalcemia

18
Match the serum calcium levels on the left with the type of calcium imbalance or balance.
_____ 1. 5.0 m Eq/L   a. Hypocalcemia
_____ 2. 6.5 mEq/L   b. Hypercalcemia
_____ 3. 5.8 mEq/L   c. Normal
_____ 4. 4.2 mEq/L
_____ 5. 8.2 mg/dL
_____ 6. 9.6 mg/dL

18 1. c; 2. b; 3. b; 4. a; 5. a; 6. c; 7. b

_____ 7. 11.8 mg/dL

19

When the parathyroid hormone (PTH) level is low, calcium release from the bones is (increased/inhibited) _____ .

What type of calcium imbalance can occur? _____

20

Tissues most affected by hypocalcemia include peripheral nerves, skeletal and smooth muscles, and the cardiac muscle.

A prolonged serum calcium deficit leads to osteoporosis, and a marked serum calcium deficit impairs the clotting time (clot formation).

Neuromuscular excitability of the skeletal, smooth, and cardiac muscles can result from (hypocalcemia/hypercalcemia) _____ .

A decrease in blood coagulation resulting in bleeding may be due to a serum calcium (deficit/excess) _____ .

21

There is a correlation between calcium and magnesium levels. Usually, when there is a magnesium deficit, there is an accompanying calcium deficit.

Hypomagnesemia (serum magnesium deficit) causes a decrease in PTH secretion. A PTH deficiency causes (hypocalcemia/hypercalcemia) _____ .

22

With a magnesium deficit, PTH secretions (increase/decrease) _____ .

As a result of the PTH secretion, what happens to the serum calcium level? _____

23

Hypercalcemia is frequently the result of calcium loss from the bones. Hypophosphatemia (serum phosphorus deficit) promotes calcium retention.

As a result of hypercalcemia, cellular permeability is _____ . (Refer to Table 8-1 as needed.)

24

Increased calcium enhances hydrochloric acid, gastrin, and pancreatic enzyme release. Hypercalcemia decreases GI

peristalsis; thus gastrointestinal motility is (increased/decreased)
_____ .

24 decreased

25

Hypercalcemia can decrease the activity of the smooth muscles in the GI system as well as the cardiac muscle activity. Dysrhythmias, heart block, and ECG/EKG changes are likely to occur from hypercalcemia.

Indicate the effects of a calcium deficit (CD) or calcium excess (CE) for the following physiologic changes:

_____ a. Impaired clotting time
_____ b. Decreased GI peristalsis
_____ c. Increased capillary permeability
_____ d. Neuromuscular excitability of skeletal, smooth, and cardiac muscles
_____ e. Decreased cardiac muscle activity
_____ f. Decreased capillary permeability

25 a. CD; b. CE; c. CD; d. CD; e. CE; f. CE

▶ ETIOLOGY

The causes of hypocalcemia and hypercalemia are presented in two separate tables. Table 8-2 lists the etiology and rationale for hypocalcemia and Table 8-3 gives the etiology and rationale for hypercalcemia. Proceed to the questions and refer to the tables as needed.

26

Name three causes of hypocalcemia related dietary changes.

*_____

_____

26 lack of calcium intake, inadequate vitamin D intake, and lack of protein in the diet

27

What effect does vitamin D insufficiency have on calcium?

*_____

_____

27 Vitamin D must be present for calcium absorption.

28

What effect does an inadequate protein diet have on calcium?

*_____

_____

28 It inhibits the body's utilization of calcium.

Table 8-2

Causes of Hypocalcemia (Serum Calcium Deficit)

Etiology	Rationale
Dietary Changes Lack of calcium intake, inadequate vitamin D, and/or lack of protein in diet	A calcium (Ca) deficit resulting from lack of Ca intake is rare. Vitamin D must be present for calcium absorption from GI tract. Inadequate protein intake inhibits the body's utilization of calcium.
Chronic diarrhea	Chronic diarrhea interferes with adequate calcium absorption.
Renal Dysfunction Renal failure	Renal failure causes phosphorus and calcium retention. Lack of PTH decreases renal calcium absorption.
Hormonal and Electrolyte Influence Decreased parathyroid hormone (PTH) Increased serum phosphorus (phosphate) Increased serum magnesium Severe decreased magnesium Increased calcitonin	With hypoparathyroidism, there is less PTH secreted. Secondary hypoparathyroidism may be caused by sepsis, burns, surgery, or pancreatitis. Overuse of phosphate laxatives can decrease calcium retention. Magnesium imbalances inhibit PTH secretion.
Calcium Binders or Chelators Citrated blood transfusions Alkalosis Increased serum albumin level	Rapid administration of citrated blood binds with calcium, inhibiting ionized (free) Ca. Alkalosis increases calcium protein binding. With an increase in serum albumin, more calcium is bound and less calcium is free and active.

29 deficit; Less parathyroid hormone (PTH) is secreted.

29
Hypoparathyroidism can cause a calcium (deficit/excess) _____ . How? *_____

30
Which of the following are the effects of an insufficient PTH level?

Table 8-3

Causes of Hypercalcemia (Serum Calcium Excess)

Etiology	Rationale
Dietary Changes: Increased Calcium Salts (supplements)	Excessive use of calcium supplements, calcium salts, and antacids can increase the serum calcium level.
Renal Impairment, Diuretics: Thiazides	Kidney dysfunction and use of thiazide diuretics decrease the excretion of calcium.
Cellular Destruction Bone Immobility	A malignant bone tumor, a fracture, and/or a prolonged immobilization can cause loss of calcium from the bone. Some malignancies cause an ectopic PTH production. Increased immobility promotes calcium loss from the bone.
Hormonal and Drug Influence Increased PTH Decreased serum phosphorus Steroid therapy Thiazide diuretics	Hyperparathyroidism increases the production of PTH and increased PTH, then promotes the release of calcium from the bone. A decreased phosphorus level can increase the serum calcium level to the extent that the kidneys are unable to excrete excess calcium. Thiazides increase the action of PTH on kidneys, promoting calcium reabsorption. Steroids such as cortisone mobilize calcium absorption from the bone.

( ) a. Calcium release from the bone is inhibited.
( ) b. Less calcium is absorbed from the kidney tubules.
( ) c. Calcium release from the bone is promoted.
( ) d. Calcium absorption from the kidneys is promoted.

30 b, c

31

Calcium and phosphorus, which are found in many foods, are regulated by the parathyroid gland and absorbed together. The serum values of calcium and phosphate (ionized phosphorus) are opposites. With hyperphosphatemia, (hypocalcemia/hypercalcemia) _____ is more likely to occur.

31 hypocalcemia

32

What effect does prolonged immobilization have on calcium?
* _____

_____

32 It increases the serum calcium level by releasing Ca from the bones.

33

Hypercalcemia occurs because of increased amounts of calcium being released from the bone due to which of the following conditions: Refer to Table 8-3 as needed.

( ) a. Fractures
( ) b. Immobilization
( ) c. Decreased parathyroid hormone (PTH) secretion
( ) d. Bone cancer
( ) e. Malignancies promoting PTH production

33 a, b, d, e

34

Multiple fractures cause the release of calcium into the intravascular fluid, thus (increasing/decreasing) _____ the serum calcium level.

34 increasing

35

Loop or high-ceiling diuretics (furosemide) decrease the serum calcium level. Thiazide diuretics such as HydroDiuril (increase/decrease) _____ the serum calcium level.

Hypercalcemia (increases/decreases) _____ cellular permeability.

35 increase; decreases

36

Hypercalcemia occurs in 25–50% of malignancies occurring in the lung, breast, ovaries, prostate, and bladder. These cancers can cause bone destruction due to metastasis or (increased/decreased) _____ ectopic PTH secretion.

36 increased

37

Prolonged steroid therapy can cause increased serum calcium levels. Explain. *_____

_____

37 Prolonged use of steroids mobilizes calcium release from the bone.

▶ CLINICAL MANIFESTATIONS

38

Clinical manifestations of hypocalcemia and hypercalcemia are determined by the signs and symptoms of calcium imbalance, ECG/EKG changes, and the serum calcium level.

The normal serum calcium range is _____ mEq/L, or _____ mg/dL. Levels less than _____ mEq/L indicate hypocalcemia and those greater than _____ mEq/L indicate hypercalcemia.

38 4.5–5.5; 9–11; 4.5; 5.5

39

A commonly seen clinical manifestation of hypocalcemia is tetany. A calcium deficit causes neuromuscular excitability. With hypocalcemia, the amount of circulating free, ionized calcium is (increased/decreased) _____ .

39 decreased

Table 8-4 lists the clinical manifestations of hypocalcemia and hypercalcemia according to the body areas that are affected. The serum calcium level and the specific ECG changes determine the severity of the calcium imbalance. Study the table and refer to it as needed.

40

Tetany symptoms are due to a decrease in free, (ionized/nonionized) _____ circulating calcium. Symptoms of tetany include which of the following:

_____ a. Twitching around the mouth
_____ b. Tingling and numbness of the extremities
_____ c. Carpopedal spasms
_____ d. Laryngeal spasm
_____ e. Spasmodic contractions
_____ f. Muscular hypertrophy

40 ionized; a, b, c, d, e

41 absent; With metabolic acidosis, more calcium is freed from protein-binding sites. When the acidotic state is corrected, calcium will bind again with albumin/protein and the tetany symptoms can occur.

41

Tetany symptoms are (present/absent) _____ when the client with hypocalcemia is in an acidotic state (metabolic acidosis). Explain your response. *_____

_____

42

Two tests, Chvostek and Trousseau, may be used to test for severe hypocalcemia and presence of tetany. Figure 8-2 describes the technique for checking for positive Chvostek and Trousseau signs.

A positive test for Chvostek and/or Trousseau indicates a calcium (deficit/excess) _____ .

42 deficit

Table 8-4

Clinical Manifestations of Calcium Imbalances

Body Involvement	Hypocalcemia	Hypercalcemia

CNS and Muscular Abnormalities	Anxiety, irritability
	Tetany
	    Twitching around mouth
	    Tingling and numbness of fingers
	    Carpopedal spasm
	    Spasmodic contractions
	    Laryngeal spasm
	    Convulsions
	Abdominal cramps
	Muscle cramps
		Depression/apathy
		Muscles are flabby

Chvostek's Sign	Positive	
Trousseau's Sign	Positive	
Cardiac Abnormalities	Weak cardiac contractions	Signs of heart block Cardiac arrest in systole
ECG/EKG	Lengthened ST segment Prolonged QT interval	Decreased or diminished ST segment Shortened QT interval
Blood Abnormalities	Blood does not clot normally, reduction of prothrombin.	
Skeletal Abnormalities	Fractures occur if deficit persists.	Pathologic fractures Deep pain over bony areas Thinning of bones apparent
Renal Abnormalities		Flank pain Calcium stones formed in the kidney
Laboratory Values Serum Ca Ionized serum Ca Serum Ca Ionized serum Ca	 <4.5 mEq/L <2.2 mEq/L <9.0 mg/dL <4.25 mg/dL	 >5.5 mEq/L >2.5 mEq/L >11.0 mg/dL >5.25 mg/dL

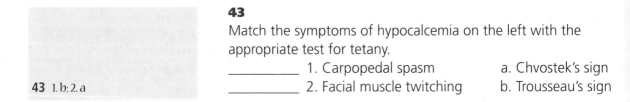

43

Match the symptoms of hypocalcemia on the left with the appropriate test for tetany.

_____ 1. Carpopedal spasm   a. Chvostek's sign

_____ 2. Facial muscle twitching   b. Trousseau's sign

43 1. b; 2. a

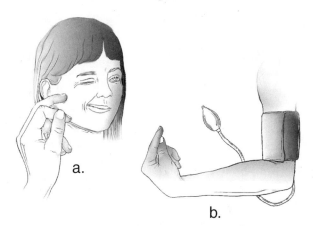

Figure 8-2 A. Chvostek's sign: The face is tapped over the facial nerve (2 cm anterior to the earlobe). B. Trousseau's sign: Inflate a blood pressure cuff (20–30 mm Hg) on the upper arm to constrict circulation. A positive Trousseau is evidenced as the occurrence of a carpopedal spasm of the fingers and hands within 1–5 minutes.

44

With hypercalcemia, kidney stones (calcium) may occur. This may result when calcium leaves the bones due to immobilization, bone tumors, or increased PTH associated with a secondary malignancy. Increased PTH promotes *_____ .

44 calcium release from the bone

45

For the following clinical manifestations, indicate which is the result of a calcium deficit (CD) or a calcium excess (CE).

_____ a. Muscles are flabby
_____ b. Tetany symptoms
_____ c. Muscle cramps
_____ d. Positive Chvostek's sign
_____ e. Deep pain over bony areas
_____ f. Kidney stones
_____ g. Blood does NOT clot normally

45 a. CE; b. CD; c. CD; d. CD; e. CE; f. CE; g. CD

Figures 8-3A and B note the electrocardiographic changes found with hypocalcemia and hypercalcemia. The normal ECG/EKG tracing is found on pages 107 and 108. The ECG changes that may occur with hypocalcemia are shown in Figure 8-3A.

The ECG changes that may occur with hypercalcemia are shown in Figure 8-3B.

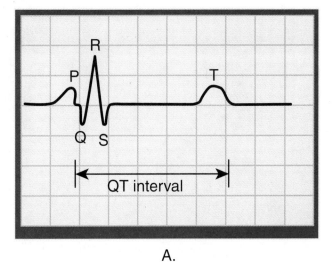

A.

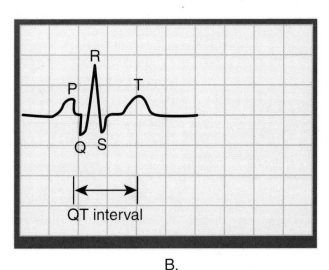

B.

Figure 8-3 A. Lengthened ST segment; prolonged QT interval.
B. Decreased ST segment; shortened QT interval.

46
The hypocalcemia effect on the ECG causes the ST segment to
be _____ and the QT interval to be _____ .

46 lengthened; prolonged

47
The hypercalcemia effect on the ECG causes the ST segment to
be _____ and the QT interval to be _____ .

47 decreased; shortened

▶ CLINICAL MANAGEMENT

Clinical management of hypocalcemia consists of oral supplements and intravenous calcium diluted in 5% dextrose in water (D_5W). Calcium should not be diluted in normal saline solution (0.9% NaCl) since the sodium encourages calcium loss.

The goal of management for hypercalcemia is to correct the underlying cause of the serum calcium excess. Drugs such as calcitonin or IV saline solution administered rapidly and followed by a loop diuretic can be used to promote urinary excretion of calcium.

Calcium Replacement

48

Identify food products high in calcium that can be used to prevent or correct the body's calcium deficit. *_____

49

Normally, calcium is not required for IV therapy since there is a tremendous reservoir in the bone. However, the body needs vitamin D for the utilization of dietary calcium.

What other essential composition of the diet is needed for calcium utilization? _____

Table 8-5 lists the oral and intravenous preparations of calcium salts and their dosages and drug form. The drugs are listed in alphabetic order. The drug dosage is given in milligrams per gram and indicates the elemental calcium amount within that gram. Study the table carefully and refer to it as needed.

50

Asymptomatic hypocalcemia is normally corrected with oral calcium gluconate, calcium lactate, and calcium carbonate. Calcium carbonate can cause GI upset due to carbon dioxide (CO_2) formation. For better calcium absorption, a calcium supplement containing vitamin D should be given 30 minutes before meals.

Why should the calcium supplement contain vitamin D?
*_____

48 milk and milk products with vitamin D

49 protein

50 Vitamin D is needed for calcium absorption from the intestine.

Table 8-5

Calcium Preparations

Calcium Name	Drug Form	Drug Dose
Orals		
Calcium carbonate	650–1500-mg tablets	400 mg/g*
Calcium citrate	950-mg tablet	211 mg/g*
Calcium lactate	325–650-mg tablets	130 mg/g*
Calcium gluconate	500–1000-mg tablets	90 mg/g*
Intravenous		
Calcium chloride	10 mL size	272 mg/g*; 13.5 mEq
Calcium gluceptate	5 mL size	90 mg/g*; 4.5 mEq
Calcium gluconate	10 mL size	90 mg/g*; 4.5 mEq

*Elemental calcium is 1 gram (1 g).

51

Acute hypocalcemia with tetany symptoms needs immediate correction. Intravenous 10% calcium chloride or 10% calcium gluconate is given slowly, 1–3 mL/min, to avoid hypotension, bradycardia, and other dysrhythmias.

Calcium chloride provides more ionized calcium than calcium gluconate; however, it is more irritating to the subcutaneous tissue, and if calcium chloride infiltrates, sloughing of the tissue results.

For intravenous administration calcium salts should be diluted in which of the following solution(s):

( ) a. Normal saline (0.9% NaCl)
( ) b. Five percent dextrose in water

51 b

52

The suggested rate of IV flow for a calcium solution is
*_____ . If the rate of IV flow is too rapid, what might occur? *_____

52 1–3 mL/min; cardiac
dysrhythmias
(bradycardia), hypotension

Table 8-6 gives the suggested clinical management for hypocalcemia.

> ### Table 8-6
>
> ### Suggested Clinical Management for Hypocalcemia
>
> | Calcium Deficit | Suggested Clinical Management |
> | --- | --- |
> | Mild | Oral calcium salts with vitamin D, take twice a day.
 10% IV calcium gluconate (10 mL) in D$_5$W solution. Administer slowly, 1–3 mL/min. |
> | Moderate | 10% IV calcium gluconate (10–20 mL) in D$_5$W solution. Administer slowly, 1–3 mL/min. |
> | Severe | 10% IV calcium gluconate (100 mL) in 1 liter of D$_5$W. Administer over 4 hours. |

53 dilute 100 mL of 10% IV calcium gluconate in D$_5$W and administer over 4 hours.

54 does not (elevated calcium level enhances the action of digoxin)

55 decreases; a decrease in the T wave

53

For moderate hypocalcemia, 10–20 mL of 10% IV calcium gluconate is diluted in 5% dextrose and water (D$_5$W). The solution is administered at a rate of 1–3 mL/min.

For severe hypocalcemia, the suggested clinical management is to * _____ .

54

Care should be taken when administering calcium to a client who is taking digoxin daily (digitalis preparation). An elevated serum calcium level enhances the action of digoxin; thus digitalis toxicity can result.

A decreased calcium level (does/does not) _____ cause digitalis toxicity.

55

Intravenous calcium salts may be used to counteract the effect of a potassium excess on the heart muscle (myocardium). IV calcium (increases/decreases) _____ the effect of hyperkalemia?

What type of ECG improvement should the nurse observe when using calcium supplements to correct hyperkalemia? * _____

Hypercalcemia Correction

56

Immediate correction of a moderate and severe serum calcium excess is essential. An intravenous normal saline solution is given

56 It promotes urinary calcium excretion.

rapidly with furosemide (Lasix) to prevent a fluid overload. Explain how this increases the calcium loss. *_____

_____

57
Which diuretic promotes urinary calcium excretion?
_____ a. Hydrochlorothiazide (HydroDiuril)
_____ b. Furosemide (Lasix)

57 b

58
Other drugs that can decrease the serum calcium level are:
  a. Calcitonin, a thyroid hormone that inhibits the effects of PTH on the bone and increases urinary calcium excretion
  b. Glucocorticoids (Cortisone), which compete with vitamin D, thus decreasing the intestinal absorption of calcium
  c. Intravenous phosphates, which promote calcium excretion
  d. Mithracin (plicamycin), which inhibits the action of PTH
  The four drugs that may be used to treat hypercalcemia are

58 furosemide, calcitonin, cortisone, and IV phosphate; also plicamycin

*_____

_____ .

59
The antitumor antibiotic plicamycin (Mithracin) inhibits the action of PTH on osteoclasts in bone. The result of this drug action is a(n) (increase/decrease) _____ in the serum calcium level.

59 decrease

60
Malignancies are a common cause of hypercalcemia. A metastatic bone lesion can destroy the bone, which releases calcium into the circulation, thus (increasing/decreasing) _____ serum calcium level.
  Some cancers promote the secretion of the parathyroid hormone (PTH) and may be referred to as tumor-secreting (ectopic) PTH production. The most common types of cancer that can cause hypercalcemia are lung, breast, ovary, prostate, leukemia, and gastrointestinal cancers.
  Parathyroid hormone (increases/decreases) _____ the release of calcium from the _____ .

60 increasing; increases; bone

Drugs and Their Effect on Calcium Balance

Phosphate preparations, corticosteroids, loop diuretics, aspirin, anticonvulsants, magnesium sulfate, and plicamycin are some of the groups of drugs that can lower the serum calcium level. Excess calcium salt ingestion and infusion and thiazide and chlorthalidone diuretics are drugs that can increase the serum calcium level. Table 8-7 lists drugs that affect calcium balance.

61

Enter CD for calcium deficit/hypocalcemia and CE for calcium excess/hypercalcemia opposite the following drugs. Refer to the table as needed.

_____ a. Magnesium sulfate
_____ b. Aspirin
_____ c. Anticonvulsants
_____ d. Calcium sulfates
_____ e. Thiazide diuretics
_____ f. Corticosteroids
_____ g. Loop diuretics
_____ h. Vitamin D
_____ i. Aminoglycosides

61 a. CD; b. CD; c. CD; d. CE; e. CE; f. CD; g. CD; h. CE; i. CD

62

Mithracin, an antineoplastic antibiotic, is used to treat hypercalcemia. This agent lowers the serum calcium level.

Steroids and mithracin (increase/decrease) _____ the serum calcium level.

62 decrease

63

Hypercalcemia can cause cardiac dysrhythmias. An elevated serum calcium enhances the effect of digitalis and can cause digitalis toxicity.

Give three signs and symptoms of digitalis toxicity. *_____
_____

63 bradycardia (slow heart rate) with or without dysrhythmias, nausea and vomiting, and anorexia

64

During a hypercalcemic state the dose of digitalis preparations, e.g., digoxin, should be (increased/decreased)? _____

64 decreased

Table 8-7

Drugs Affecting Calcium Balance

Calcium Imbalance	Drugs	Rationale
Hypocalcemia (serum calcium deficit)	Magnesium sulfate Propylthiouracil/Propacil Colchicine Plicamycin/Mithracin Neomycin Excessive sodium citrate	These agents inhibit parathyroid hormone/PTH secretion and decrease the serum calcium level.

	Acetazolamide
	Aspirin
	Anticonvulsants
	Glutethimide/Doriden
	Estrogens
	Aminoglycosides
	   Gentamicin
	   Amikacin
	   Tobramycin
		These agents can alter the vitamin D metabolism that is needed for calcium absorption.

	Phosphate preparations:
	Oral, enema, and intravenous
	   Sodium phosphate
	   Potassium phosphate
		Phosphates can increase the serum phosphorus level and decrease the serum calcium level.

	Corticosteroids
	   Cortisone
	   Prednisone
		Steroids decrease calcium mobilization and inhibit the absorption of calcium.

	Loop diuretics Furosemide/Lasix	Loop diuretics reduce calcium absorption from the renal tubules.
Hypercalcemia (serum calcium excess)	Calcium salts Vitamin D	Excess ingestion of calcium and vitamin D and infusion of calcium can increase the serum Ca level.
	IV lipids	Lipids can increase the calcium level.

	Kayexalate, androgens
	Diuretics
	   Thiazides
	   Chlorthalidone/Hygroten
		These agents can induce hypercalcemia.

65

Steroids such as cortisone tend to decrease calcium mobilization and inhibit the absorption of calcium.

Steroids (increase/decrease) _____ the serum calcium level.

66

A loop (high-ceiling) diuretic affects the renal tubules by reducing the absorption of calcium and increasing calcium excretion. Give the name of a loop diuretic. _____

Name two other electrolytes that are excreted by loop diuretics. *_____

▶ CLINICAL APPLICATIONS

67

For body utilization, calcium must be in the ionized form. In body fluids, calcium is found in both ionized and nonionized (bound to plasma proteins) forms.

In an alkalotic state (body fluids are more alkaline), large amounts of the calcium become protein bound and cannot be utilized. When the body fluids are more acid (acidotic state), calcium is more likely to be (ionized/nonionized)? _____ .

68

Calcium acts on the central nervous system (CNS).

Let us say you are caring for a debilitated client who becomes severely agitated. You notice the client's hands trembling and mouth twitching. These symptoms may indicate a calcium (excess/deficit) _____ .

69

Lack of calcium causes neuromuscular irritability. Explain.
*_____
_____

What does hypocalcemia do to blood clotting? *_____
_____

70

Prolonged vomiting leads to alkalosis due to the loss of hydrogen and chloride ions from the stomach.

---

65 decrease

66 Furosemide/Lasix; potassium and sodium

67 ionized (hence calcium can be utilized)

68 deficit

69 It leads to hyperactivity of the nervous system and painful muscular contractions (symptoms of tetany).; It decreases clotting and causes bleeding.

70 Calcium is nonionized; hypocalcemia occurs.	When the body fluids are alkaline, what happens to calcium? *_____ _____
	71 Acidosis (increases/decreases) _____ the ionization of calcium.
71 increases	
72 hypercalcemia	**72** The kidneys excrete approximately 50–250 mg/dL of calcium in the urine daily. If the kidneys excrete less than 50 mg/dL, what type of calcium imbalance is likely to occur? _____

73 Eat foods that are high in acid content (meat, fish, poultry, eggs, cheese, peanuts, cereals) and/or drink at least 1 pint (2 glasses) of cranberry juice daily. Orange juice does not make the urine acid.	**73**
	 The health intervention for a client with hypercalcemia is to prevent renal calculi. There are three ways this can be accomplished:
	   a. Drink at least 12 glasses of fluid a day.
	   b. Keep urine acid.
	   c. Prevent urinary tract infections.
	 How do you think the urine can be kept acid? *_____
	 _____

● Clinical Considerations

1. Administer an oral calcium supplement containing vitamin D. Vitamin D is necessary for intestinal absorption of calcium.

2. Oral calcium supplements with vitamin D should be given 30 minutes before meals to improve GI absorption.

3. Intravenous calcium salts should be diluted in 5% dextrose in water (D_5W). Do NOT dilute calcium salts in a saline solution; sodium promotes calcium loss.

4. The suggested IV flow rate for a calcium solution is 1–3 mL/min (average: 2 mL/min).

5. Infiltration of calcium solution, especially calcium chloride, can cause sloughing of the subcutaneous tissues.

6. An elevated serum calcium level can enhance the action of digoxin, causing digitalis toxicity.

7. Diuretics such as furosemide (Lasix) can decrease the serum calcium level, and thiazide diuretics tend to increase the serum calcium levels. Steroids decrease serum calcium levels.

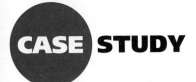

REVIEW

Mr. Morgan, age 58, has had a gastric upset for the past 6 weeks. He has been taking antacids and drinking several glasses of milk each day. His stomach discomfort was not relieved and he was admitted to the hospital to rule out a possible malignant tumor. His serum calcium was 5.9 mEq/L.

ANSWER COLUMN

1. hypercalcemia

2. 4.5–5.5 mEq/L, or 9–11 mg/dL

3. Decrease in ionized calcium for utilization. In alkaline fluids, calcium is nonionized and protein bound. An elevated serum calcium can result from large amounts of milk intake and from a malignant neoplasm. A variety of neoplasms (tumors) can cause hypercalcemia.

4. maintenance of normal cell permeability, formation of bone and teeth, normal clotting mechanism, and normal muscle and nerve activity.

5. elevated; Prolonged immobilization would increase the serum calcium by releasing calcium from the bones.

6. kidney stones

7. Drink at least 12 glasses of fluid a day, eat foods high in acid content to keep urine acid, and prevent urinary tract infections.

8. Hypercalcemia enhances the action of digoxin, making it more powerful.; decreased

9. hypocalcemia

1. His serum calcium level indicates what type of calcium imbalance? _____

2. The "normal" range for calcium balance is * _____ .

3. Explain what happens to body calcium when there is a decrease in gastric acidity and an increase in body alkaline fluids. * _____
_____

4. Give four functions of calcium in the body. * _____
_____
_____

5. If Mr. Morgan was bedridden, would you expect his serum calcium to be (elevated/decreased)? _____ Explain.
* _____
_____

6. Identify a health problem that can occur from immobilization. * _____

7. Identify three nursing interventions to prevent renal calculi resulting from hypercalcemia. _____
_____

8. Previously, Mr. Morgan had a "heart condition" and he was started on digoxin. What effect does hypercalcemia have on digoxin? * _____
Should his Digoxin dosage be (increased/decreased) _____ until his hypercalcemic state is corrected?

9. If Mr. Morgan's serum calcium became 3.9 mEq/L, what type of calcium imbalance would be present? _____

10. carpopedal spasm, twitching of the mouth, tingling of the fingers, spasm of the larynx, abdominal cramps, and muscle cramps

10. Identify five common signs and symptoms of hypocalcemia.
    *
    _____

    _____

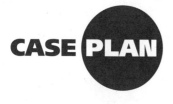

Client Management: Calcium

Hypocalcemia

Assessment Factors

▶ Obtain a health history to identify potential causes of hypocalcemia: insufficient diet in protein and calcium, lack of vitamin D intake, chronic diarrhea, hormonal influence [decreased parathyroid hormone (PTH)], drug influence, hypoparathyroidism, metabolic alkalotic state, and rapid administration of a blood transfusion that contains citrate.

▶ Assess for signs and symptoms of hypocalcemia, i.e., tetany symptoms (twitching around mouth, carpopedal spasms, laryngospasms), abdominal cramps, and muscle cramps.

▶ Obtain a serum calcium level that can be used as a baseline for comparison of future serum calcium levels. A serum calcium level below 4.5 mEq/L, or 9 mg/dL, or iCa <2.2 mEq/L indicates hypocalcemia.

▶ Check the ECG/EKG strips for changes in the QT interval. A prolonged QT interval may indicate a serum calcium deficit.

▶ Identify drugs the client is taking that may cause a serum calcium deficit, such as furosemide (Lasix), cortisone preparations, phosphate preparations, and massive use of antacids that can interfere with calcium absorption.

▶ Determine the acid-base status when hypocalcemia is present. In an acidotic state, calcium is ionized and can be utilized by the body even though there is a calcium deficit. This is not true when alkalosis occurs. Calcium is not ionized in an alkalotic state; and if a severe calcium deficit is present, tetany symptoms occur.

▶ Assess for positive Trousseau's and Chvostek's signs of hypocalcemia. For Trousseau's sign, inflate the blood pressure cuff for 3 minutes and observe for a carpopedal spasm. For Chvostek's sign, tap the facial nerve in front of the ear for spasms of the cheek and mouth.

Diagnosis 1

Altered Nutrition: less than body requirements, related to insufficient calcium intake, poor calcium absorption due to insufficient vitamin D and protein intake, or drugs (antacids, cortisone preparation) that interfere with calcium ionization.

Interventions and Rationale

1. Monitor serum calcium levels. A serum calcium level under 4.5 mEq/L or iCa <2.2 mEq/L can cause neuromuscular excitability. Tetany symptoms may occur.

2. Monitor ECG and note changes related to hypocalcemia, i.e., prolonged QT interval and lengthened ST segment.

3. Frequently monitor IV solutions containing calcium to prevent infiltration. Calcium is irritating to the subcutaneous tissues and can cause tissue sloughing.

4. Administer oral calcium supplements an hour before meals to enhance intestinal absorption.

5. Regulate IV 10% calcium gluconate or chloride in a liter of 5% dextrose in water (D_5W) to run 1–3 mL/min, or according to the order. Do not administer calcium salts in a normal saline solution (0.9% NaCl). The sodium encourages calcium loss.

6. Teach clients to eat foods rich in calcium, vitamin D, and protein, especially the older adult. Explain the importance of calcium in the diet to prevent osteoporosis and to aid normal clot formation. Tell the client that protein is needed to aid in calcium absorption. Nonfat dry milk can be used to meet calcium requirements.

7. Teach "bowel-conscious" persons that chronic use of laxatives can increase intestinal motility, which prevents calcium absorption from the intestine. Suggest fruits for bowel elimination, instead of laxatives.

8. Explain to persons using antacids that constant use of antacids can decrease calcium in the body. Antacids decrease acidity, which decreases calcium ionization.

9. Monitor the pulse regularly for bradycardia when the client is receiving digitalis and calcium, either orally or

intravenously. Increased serum calcium enhances the action of digitalis, and digitalis toxicity can result.

Diagnosis 2

Risk for injury: bleeding related to the interference with blood coagulation secondary to calcium loss.

Interventions and Rationale

1. Check for prolonged bleeding or reduced clot formation. A low serum calcium level inhibits the production of prothrombin, which is needed in clot formation.

2. Observe for symptoms of hypocalcemia in clients receiving massive transfusions of citrated blood. The serum calcium level may not be affected, but the citrates prevent calcium ionization.

Hypercalcemia
Assessment Factors

▶ Obtain a health history to identify probable causes of hypercalcemia, such as excessive use of calcium supplements, bone destruction due to cancer, cancer of the breast, lung, or prostate (ectopic PTH production), prolonged immobilization, multiple fractures, hormone influence (increased PTH, steroid therapy), hyperparathyroidism, and thiazide diuretics. Approximately 20–25% of hypercalcemia is due to continuous use of large doses of thiazide diuretics.

▶ Assess for signs and symptoms of hypercalcemia, i.e., flabby muscles, pain over bony areas, renal calculi, and pathologic fractures.

▶ Check ECG/EKG strips for changes in the QT interval. A shortened QT interval may indicate a serum calcium excess.

▶ Obtain a serum calcium level that can be used as a baseline for comparison of future serum calcium levels. A serum calcium level above 5.5 mEq/L, or 11 mg/dL, or iCa >2.5 mEq/L indicates hypercalcemia.

▶ Assess for fluid volume depletion and changes in the state of the client's sensorium. These changes may be indicators of hypercalcemia.

Diagnosis 1

Risk for injury related to pathologic fractures due to bone destruction from bone cancer, prolonged immobilization.

Interventions and Rationale

1. Monitor serum calcium levels. Report increased serum calcium levels. Levels exceeding 13.0 mg/dL can be life threatening.
2. Monitor ECG and note changes related to hypercalcemia, i.e., shortened QT interval and decreased ST segment.
3. Monitor client's state of sensorium. Extreme lethargy, confusion, and a comatose state may be the result of hypercalcemia. Safety precautions may be needed.
4. Promote active and passive exercise for bedridden clients. Immobilization promotes calcium loss from the bone.
5. Handle clients gently who have long-standing hypercalcemia and bone demineralization to prevent fractures.
6. Identify symptoms of digitalis toxicity. When the client has an elevated serum calcium level and is receiving a digitalis preparation such as digoxin, digitalis toxicity may occur. Elevated serum calcium enhances the action of digitalis. Symptoms of digitalis toxicity include bradycardia, nausea, and/or vomiting.

Diagnosis 2

Altered Nutrition: more than the body requirements, related to excess calcium intake.

Interventions and Rationale

1. Instruct clients with hypercalcemia to avoid foods rich in calcium and to avoid taking massive amounts of vitamin D supplements.
2. Teach clients with hypercalcemia to keep hydrated, in order to increase calcium dilution in the serum and urine and to prevent renal calculi formation.
3. Explain to clients with hypercalcemia that the purpose for maintaining an acid urine is to increase solubility of calcium. An acid-ash diet may be ordered that includes meats, fish,

poultry, eggs, cheese, cereals, nuts, cranberry juice, and prune juice. Orange juice will not change the urine pH.

Diagnosis 3

Altered urinary elimination related to causes of hypercalcemia.

Interventions and Rationale

1. Monitor urinary output and urine pH. Calcium precipitates in alkaline urine and renal calculi may result. Acid-ash foods and juices such as cranberry and prune juices should be encouraged to increase the acidity of the urine.

2. Instruct clients to increase fluid intake to dilute the serum and urine levels of calcium to prevent formation of renal calculi.

3. Administer prescribed loop diuretics to enhance calcium excretion. Thiazide diuretics inhibit calcium excretion and are not indicated in hypercalcemia.

Evaluation/Outcome

1. Evaluate the cause of calcium imbalance and document corrective measures taken.

2. Evaluate the effects of prescribed clinical management for hypocalcemia or hypercalcemia. Serum calcium and ionized calcium levels are within normal range.

3. Remain free of signs and symptoms of hypocalcemia. (Tetany signs and symptoms are absent. Vital signs are within normal range.)

4. Recognize risk factors related to hypocalcemia and hypercalcemia.

5. Include foods rich in calcium and take oral calcium supplements, containing Vitamin D, as prescribed.

6. Document compliance with the prescribed drug therapy—medical and dietary regimens.

7. Maintain a support system, i.e., health professionals, family, and friends.

8. Schedule follow-up appointment.

Magnesium Imbalances

CHAPTER

9

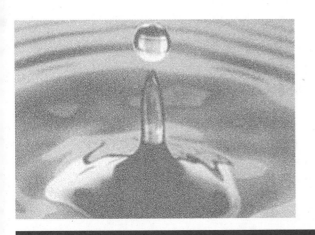

▶ INTRODUCTION

Magnesium (Mg), the second most plentiful intracellular cation, has similar functions, causes of imbalances, and clinical manifestations as potassium. Approximately one-half (50%) of the body's magnesium is contained in the bone, 49% in the body cells (intracellular fluid), and 1% in the extracellular fluid. The normal serum magnesium range is 1.5–2.5 mEq/L, or 1.8–3.0 mg/dL.

1

Magnesium is a(n) (anion/cation) _____ . Its highest concentration is found in what type of body fluid? _____

1 cation; intracellular

2

What other cation has its highest concentration in the intracellular fluid? _____

2 potassium

3

Magnesium is widely distributed throughout the body. Half of the body magnesium is in the bone. What other ion is found plentifully in the bone? _____

3 calcium

4

Magnesium has a higher concentration in the cerebrospinal fluid, also known as spinal fluid, than in the blood plasma. The serum concentration of magnesium is *_____ .

4 1.5–2.5 mEq/L, or 1.8–3.0 mg/dL

5

One-third of magnesium is protein bound and approximately two-thirds is ionized, free magnesium that can be utilized by the body. Magnesium is absorbed from the small intestine. Sixty percent of magnesium is excreted in the feces (magnesium that was not absorbed) and 40% is excreted through the kidneys.

Forty percent of magnesium is excreted via _____ and 60% is excreted via _____ .

5 kidneys; feces

6

The minimum daily magnesium requirement is 200–300 mg for an adult and 150 mg for an infant. Many of the same foods that are rich in potassium are also rich in magnesium. These foods include green vegetables, whole grains, fish and seafood, and nuts.

If your client has a magnesium deficit, name three foods rich in magnesium that the client should include in his or her diet.
*_____

_____

6 green vegetables, whole grains, and fish and seafood

7

A serum magnesium level of less than 1.5 mEq/L is known as (hypomagnesemia/hypermagnesemia) _____ . A serum magnesium level of greater than 2.5 mEq/L is called _____ .

7 hypomagnesemia; hypermagnesemia

▶ FUNCTIONS

Table 9-1 describes the various functions of magnesium. Study the table and refer to it as needed.

8

Magnesium plays an important role in enzyme activity. An *enzyme* is a catalyst capable of inducing chemical changes in other substances. Magnesium acts as a coenzyme in the metabolism of carbohydrates and protein.

Magnesium is also involved in maintaining neuromuscular stability. What other ion has this similar function? _____

8 calcium

9

Indicate which of the following are functions of magnesium:
( ) a. Neuromuscular activity
( ) b. Contraction of the myocardium
( ) c. Exchange of CO_2 and O_2
( ) d. Enzyme activity
( ) e. Responsibility (partial) for Na and K crossing cell membranes.

9 a, b, d, e

Table 9-1

Magnesium and Its Functions

Body Involvement	Functions
Neuromuscular	Transmits neuromuscular activity. Important mediator of neural transmission in the CNS.
Cardiac	Contracts the heart muscle (myocardium).
Cellular	Activates many enzymes for proper carbohydrate and protein metabolism. Responsible for the transportation of sodium and potassium across cell membranes. Influences utilization of potassium, calcium, and protein. Magnesium deficits are frequently accompanied by a potassium and/or calcium deficit.

10
When there is a magnesium deficit, what two other cations may also be decreased? _____

10 potassium and calcium

▶ PATHOPHYSIOLOGY

11
Magnesium maintains neuromuscular function. A serum magnesium deficit increases the release of acetylcholine from the presynaptic membrane of the nerve fiber. This increases neuromuscular excitability.

A serum magnesium excess has a sedative effect on the neuromuscular system that may result in a loss of deep tendon reflexes.

Indicate which neuromuscular function may occur from the magnesium imbalances listed on the left.

_____ 1. Hypomagnesemia   a. Hyperexcitability
_____ 2. Hypermagnesemia   b. Inhibition

11 1. a (due to increased release of acetylcholine); 2. b (causing a sedative effect)

12
Cardiac dysrhythmias can result from a serum magnesium deficit. Tachycardia, hypertension, and ventricular fibrillation may result from hypomagnesemia. Hypotension and heart block may result from hypermagnesemia.

What is the most serious cardiac dysfunction that might occur from hypomagnesemia? *_____
From hypermagnesemia? *_____

12 ventricular fibrillation; heart block

13
In the gastrointestinal tract, an increase in calcium absorption causes a decrease in magnesium absorption and an increase in magnesium excretion.

What is likely to occur with decreased calcium absorption?
*_____

13 increased magnesium absorption

14
Magnesium inhibits the release of the parathyroid hormone (PTH). A decrease in the release of PTH (increases/decreases) _____ the amount of calcium released from the bone. This can cause a calcium (excess/deficit) _____ .

14 decreases; deficit

15

Match the serum magnesium levels on the left with the type of magnesium imbalance or balance on the right.

_____ 1. 1.2 mEq/L	a. Normal serum magnesium
_____ 2. 2.0 mEq/L	level
_____ 3. 2.3 mEq/L	b. Hypomagnesemia
_____ 4. 2.9 mEq/L	c. Hypermagnesemia
_____ 5. 1.0 mEq/L	
_____ 6. 3.6 mEq/L	

15 1. b; 2. a; 3. a; 4. c; 5. b; 6. c

▶ ETIOLOGY

Hypomagnesemia is probably the most undiagnosed electrolyte deficiency. This is most likely due to the fact that hypomagnesemia is asymptomatic until the serum magnesium level approaches 1.0 mEq/L. The total serum magnesium concentration is not representative of the cellular magnesium levels. This is why many clients with hypomagnesemia are asymptomatic. Clients with hypokalemia or hypocalcemia who do not respond to potassium and/or calcium replacement may also have hypomagnesemia. Correction of the magnesium deficit is an important consideration when correcting serum potassium and serum calcium imbalances.

The causes of hypomagnesemia and hypermagnesemia are presented in two tables. Table 9-2 lists the etiology and rationale for hypomagnesemia and Table 9-3 lists the etiology and rationale for hypermagnesemia. After studying the tables, proceed to the questions. Refer to the tables as needed.

16

Magnesium is found in various foods; thus prolonged inadequate nutrient intake can cause (hypomagnesemia/hypermagnesemia) _____ .

16 hypomagnesemia

17

Chronic alcoholism is a leading cause and problem of hypomagnesemia. This results from GI losses due to diarrhea and poor absorption related to *_____ .

Chronic diarrhea is attributed to hypomagnesemia. Why?

*_____

_____

17 inadequate nutritional intake; because of impaired magnesium absorption

Table 9-2

Causes of Hypomagnesemia (Serum Magnesium Deficit)

Etiology	Rationale
Dietary Changes	
Inadequate intake, poor absorption, GI losses	Magnesium is found in various foods, e.g., green, leafy
Malnutrition, starvation	vegetables and whole grains.
	Inadequate nutrition can result in a magnesium deficit.
Total parenteral nutrition (TPN, hyperalimentation)	Continuous use of TPN without a magnesium supplement can cause a magnesium deficit.
Chronic alcoholism	Alcoholism promotes inadequate food intake and GI
Increased calcium intake	loss of magnesium.
	Calcium absorption promotes magnesium loss in feces.
Chronic diarrhea, intestinal fistulas, chronic use of laxatives	Chronic diarrhea impairs magnesium absorption. Prolonged use of laxatives can cause a magnesium deficit.
Renal Dysfunction	
Diuresis: diabetic ketoacidosis	Diuresis due to diabetic ketoacidosis causes magnesium loss via the kidneys.
Acute renal failure (ARF)	ARF in the diuretic phase promotes magnesium loss.
Cardiac Dysfunction	
Acute myocardial infarction (AMI)	Hypomagnesemia may occur from the first to the fifth day post-acute MI.
Congestive heart failure (CHF)	Prolonged diuretic therapy for CHF can cause a magnesium deficit.
Electrolyte Influence	
Hypokalemia	The cations potassium and calcium are interrelated
Hypocalcemia	with magnesium action.
	Hypomagnesemia can occur with hypokalemia and hypocalcemia.
Drug Influence	
Aminoglycosides, potassium-wasting diuretics, cortisone, amphotericin B, digitalis	These drugs promote the loss of magnesium. Hypomagnesemia enhances the action of digitalis; digitalis toxicity may result.

Table 9-3

Causes of Hypermagnesemia (Serum Magnesium Excess)

Etiology	Rationale
Dietary Changes Excessive administration of magnesium products IV magnesium sulfate Antacids with magnesium Laxatives with magnesium	Hypermagnesemia rarely occurs unless there is a prolonged excess use of magnesium-containing antacids (Maalox), laxatives (milk of magnesia), and IV magnesium sulfate.
Renal Dysfunction Renal insufficiency Renal failure	Renal insufficiency or failure inhibits the excretion of magnesium.
Severe Dehydration Diabetic ketoacidosis	Loss of body fluids due to diuresis from diabetic ketoacidosis causes a hemoconcentration of magnesium, which can result in an increased magnesium level.

18 potassium-wasting diuretics; during the diuretic phase of ARF

19 congestive heart failure (CHF); 1–5 days post-AMI

20 no; Large doses of potassium and calcium supplements do not fully correct hypokalemia and hypocalcemia unless the magnesium deficit is also corrected.

18
The diuretics that promote magnesium loss are the (potassium-wasting diuretics/potassium-sparing diuretics) *_____

_____ .
   When does acute renal failure (ARF) cause hypomagnesemia?
*_____ .

19
Two cardiac causes of hypomagnesemia are acute myocardial infarction (AMI) and *_____.
   During what period of time during the AMI does a serum magnesium deficit occur? *_____ .

20
Hypokalemia and hypocalcemia may be present along with hypomagnesemia. Can hypokalemia and hypocalcemia be corrected without correcting hypomagnesemia? _____ .
Explain. *_____

_____

21

Indicate which of the following are causes of hypomagnesemia.

( ) a. Chronic alcoholism

( ) b. Chronic use of laxatives

( ) c. Potassium-sparing diuretics

( ) d. Hyperkalemia

( ) e. Increased calcium intake

( ) f. Malnutrition

( ) g. Diuresis due to diabetic ketoacidosis

( ) h. Magnesium-containing antacids

( ) i. Continuous TPN or salt-free IV fluids

21 a, b, e, f, g, i

22

When magnesium-containing antacids and laxatives are taken continuously for a prolonged period of time, what type of magnesium imbalance is likely to occur? _____

Name an antacid that can cause a magnesium excess when used for a prolonged period of time or in conjunction with renal impairment? *_____

Name a laxative that if used constantly can cause a magnesium excess, especially if there is renal impairment? *_____

_____

22 hypermagnesemia, or magnesium excess; Maalox and Mylanta; milk of magnesia (MOM) and magnesium sulfate (Epsom salt)

23

Approximately one-half of magnesium is excreted via the kidneys. With renal insufficiency, the serum magnesium level is (increased/decreased) _____ .

What other electrolyte is primarily excreted in the urine?

_____

23 increased; potassium

24

Place a D for magnesium deficit and an E for magnesium excess in the following situations:

_____ a. Renal insufficiency

_____ b. Prolonged diuresis

_____ c. Constant use of Epsom salt or milk of magnesia

_____ d. Chronic alcoholism

_____ e. Malnutrition

_____ f. Prolonged inadequate nutrient intake

_____ g. Severe diarrhea

_____ h. Constant use of antacids with magnesium hydroxide

24 a. E; b. D; c. E; d. D; e. D; f. D; g. D; h. E

◗ CLINICAL MANIFESTATIONS

25

The normal serum magnesium range is *_____ .

A serum magnesium level less than _____ mEq/L is known as hypomagnesemia.

For hypermagnesemia to occur, the serum magnesium level should be greater than _____ mEq/L.

26

Severe magnesium imbalance occurs when the serum magnesium level is below 1.0 mEq/L and above 10.0 mEq/L. A cardiac arrest may result with a severe magnesium imbalance.

Severe serum magnesium deficit and excess are life threatening and need immediate action. Would a serum magnesium deficit of 1.3 mEq/L be life threatening? _____

For severe hypermagnesemia to be life threatening, the serum magnesium level is *_____ .

Table 9-4 lists the clinical manifestations of hypomagnesemia and hypermagnesemia according to the body area affected. The serum magnesium level and the ECG determine the severity of the magnesium imbalance. Study the table carefully and refer to it as needed.

27

Magnesium influences the nervous system; too much or too little magnesium affects the neuromuscular function.

Hyperirritability, tremors, and twitching of the face are signs and symptoms of _____ .

Lethargy, drowsiness, and loss of deep tendon reflexes are signs and symptoms of _____ .

28

Central nervous system depression, inhibited neuromuscular transmission, decreased respiration, and lethargy are signs and symptoms of _____ .

29

Match the cardiac signs and symptoms on the left to a magnesium deficit or excess on the right

25 1.5–2.5 mEq/L, or 1.8–3.0 mg/dL; 1.5; 2.5

26 no; greater than 10 mEq/L

27 hypomagnesemia; hypermagnesemia

28 hypermagnesemia

Table 9-4

Clinical Manifestations of Magnesium Imbalances

Body Involvement	Hypomagnesemia	Hypermagnesemia

Neuromuscular abnormalities	Hyperirritability
	Tetanylike symptoms
	  Tremors
	  Twitching of face
	  Spasticity
	Increased tendon reflexes
		CNS depression
		  Lethargy, drowsiness,
		    weakness, paralysis
		  Loss of deep tendon reflexes

Cardiac abnormalities	Hypertension
	Cardiac dysrhythmias
	  Premature ventricular
	  contractions
	  Ventricular tachycardia
	  Ventricular fibrillation
		Hypotension (if severe,
		  profound hypotension)
		Complete heart block

ECG/EKG	Flat or inverted T wave Depressed ST segment	Widened QRS complex Prolonged QT interval
Others		Flushing Respiratory depression

---

29 1. b; 2. a; 3. a; 4. b

_____ 1. Hypotension

_____ 2. Ventricular tachycardia

_____ 3. PVC (premature
ventricular contraction)

_____ 4. Heart block

a. Hypomagnesemia

b. Hypermagnesemia

30

Place a D for hypomagnesemia and an E for hypermagnesemia
beside the following signs and symptoms:

_____ a. Hyperirritability

_____ b. CNS depression

_____ c. Lethargy

_____ d. Tremors

_____ e. Twitching of the face

_____ f. Convulsion

_____ g. Decreased respiration

_____ h. Loss of deep tendon reflexes

_____ i. Ventricular fibrillation

30 a. D; b. E; c. E; d. D; e. D; f. D;
g. E; h. E; i. D

◗ CLINICAL MANAGEMENT

Clinical management of hypomagnesemia may be corrected by a diet consisting of green vegetables, legumes, nuts (peanut butter), and fruits. Oral or intravenous magnesium salts may be prescribed when there is a marked to severe magnesium deficit.

For hypermagnesemia, correcting the underlying cause and using intravenous saline or calcium salts decreases the magnesium level.

Magnesium Replacement

31

Oral magnesium comes as sulfate, gluconate, chloride, citrate, and hydroxide in liquid, tablet, and powder form.

For magnesium supplement for maintenance or replacement, magnesium gluconate/Magonate and magnesium-protein complex/Mg-PLUS may be ordered by the health professional.

For severe hypomagnesemia do you think the ordered magnesium replacement should be administered (orally/intramuscularly/intravenously)? _____ Why? *_____
_____

31 intravenously; It is a direct and quick method for correcting serum magnesium deficit.

32

Magnesium sulfate is the parenteral replacement for hypomagnesemia and can be administered intramuscularly or intravenously. The drug is available in strengths of 10, 12.5, and 50%. A suggested order for adults is 10 mL of a 50% solution.

For intramuscular injections the dosage is divided and for intravenous infusion the dosage is diluted into 1 liter of solution. The two injectable routes in which magnesium sulfate can be delivered to the body are *_____.

32 intramuscular and intravenous

Hypermagnesemia Correction

33

For a temporary correction of a serum magnesium excess, the intravenous electrolyte *_____ or *_____ may be prescribed.

33 saline (sodium chloride); calcium salt

If hypermagnesemia is due to renal failure, dialysis may be necessary. Ventilator assistance may be needed if respiratory distress occurs.

34

Intravenous calcium is an (agonist /antagonist) _____ to magnesium; therefore, calcium can (increase/decrease) _____ the symptoms of hypermagnesemia.

34 antagonist; decrease

35

If renal failure is the cause of the severe hypermagnesemia, what is the best course to correct this imbalance? _____

35 dialysis

Drugs and Their Effect on Magnesium Balance

36

Long-term administration of saline infusions may result in magnesium and calcium loss.

Can you explain why long-term or excessive use of saline infusions can cause magnesium and calcium deficits?

*_____

36 It expands the extracellular fluid (ECF), causes dilution, and inhibits tubular absorption of Mg and Ca.

Diuretics, antibiotics, laxatives, and digitalis are groups of drugs that promote magnesium loss (hypomagnesemia). Excess intake of magnesium salts is the major cause of serum magnesium excess (hypermagnesemia). Table 9-5 lists drugs that affect magnesium balance.

37

Place MD for magnesium deficit /hypomagnesemia and ME for magnesium excess/hypermagnesemia beside the following drugs:

_____ a. Furosemide/Lasix
_____ b. Tobramycin
_____ c. Magnesium hydroxide/MOM
_____ d. Digitalis
_____ e. Magnesium sulfate for toxemia
_____ f. Laxatives
_____ g. Cortisone
_____ h. Lithium

37 a. MD; b. MD; c. ME; d. MD; e. ME; f. MD; g. MD; h. ME

Table 9-5

Drugs Affecting Magnesium Balance

Magnesium Imbalance	Drugs	Rationale

Hypomagnesemia (serum magnesium deficit)	Diuretics
	  Furosemide/Lasix
	  Ethacrynic acid/Edecrin
	  Mannitol
		Diuretics promote urinary loss of magnesium.

	Antibiotics
	  Gentamicin
	  Tobramycin
	  Carbenicillin
	  Capreomycin
	  Neomycin
	  Polymyxin B
	  Amphotericin B
	Digitalis
	Calcium gluconate
	Insulin
		These agents can cause magnesium loss via kidney.

	Laxatives Cisplatin	Laxative abuse causes magnesium loss via GI.

	Corticosteroids
	  Cortisone
	  Prednisone
		Steroids can decrease serum magnesium levels.

Hypermagnesemia (serum magnesium excess)	Magnesium salts:
	Oral and enema
	  Magnesium hydroxide/MOM
	  Magnesium sulfate/Epsom salt
	  Magnesium citrate
	  Magnesium sulfate (maternity)
		Excess use of magnesium salts can increase serum magnesium levels.
		
		Use of excess $MgSO_4$ in treatment of toxemia can cause hypermagnesemia.

	Lithium	Hypermagnesemia can be associated with lithium therapy.

38

Excessive use of steroids (corticosteroids) can cause hypomagnesemia.

A decrease in the adrenal cortical hormone can cause (hypomagnesemia/hypermagnesemia). _____ .

38 hypermagnesemia

39

Hypomagnesemia enhances the action of digitalis and causes digitalis toxicity. Magnesium sulfate corrects hypomagnesemia and symptoms of digitalis toxicity.

Give at least three symptoms of digitalis toxicity.

*_____

What other electrolyte (cation) deficit can cause digitalis toxicity? _____

39 nausea and vomiting, anorexia, and bradycardia; potassium

▶ **CLINICAL APPLICATIONS**

Hypomagnesemia is frequently an undiagnosed problem that surfaces when the client is hospitalized, critically ill, or not responding to correction of hypokalemia or hypocalcemia. Approximately 65% of clients with normal renal function in intensive care units (ICUs) have a low serum magnesium level. Over 40% of the clients with hypomagnesemia also have hypokalemia. Twenty percent of the elderly have a decreased serum magnesium level.

40

When a client is being treated for hypokalemia and is not responding to therapy, the serum magnesium should be checked. If a magnesium deficit is present, hypokalemia (may/may not) _____ be completely corrected.

40 may not

41

The kidneys regulate the concentration of magnesium in the body. When there is a slight increase in the magnesium concentration, the kidneys excrete the excess. When there is a decreased serum magnesium level, what do you think the kidneys do? *_____

_____

If a client has renal insufficiency and is receiving magnesium sulfate, what type of magnesium imbalance can occur? _____ Why? *_____

41 Kidneys conserve Mg or Mg is reabsorbed from the kidney tubules—not excreted.; hypermagnesemia; Kidneys regulate Mg balance—do not excrete it.

42

For clients on prolonged hyperalimentation (TPN), the serum magnesium level should be checked.

What type of magnesium imbalance can occur when magnesium is not included in the solutions for TPN? _____

42 hypomagnesemia

43

Magnesium is needed by the heart for myocardial contractions. It is said that magnesium slows the rate of the atrial contractions and corrects atrial flutter.

Electrocardiographic changes due to magnesium imbalances are similar to potassium imbalances. With hypomagnesemia, the T wave may be *_____ and the ST segment _____ .

43 flat or inverted; depressed

44

In diabetic acidosis, magnesium leaves the cells. When insulin and dextrose are given intravenously, magnesium returns to the cells.

If the diabetic condition is corrected too fast, then (hypomagnesemia/hypermagnesemia) _____ occurs. Why? *_____

_____

44 hypomagnesemia; Magnesium leaves the ECF rapidly and returns to the cells.

● Clinical Considerations

1. Signs and symptoms of hypomagnesemia are similar to those of hypokalemia.

2. Excess use of laxatives and antacids that contain magnesium can cause hypermagnesemia.

3. A magnesium deficit is often accompanied by a potassium and calcium deficit (40% of clients with hypomagnesemia also have hypokalemia). If a potassium deficit does not respond to potassium replacement, hypomagnesemia should be suspected.

4. Severe hypomagnesemia can cause symptoms of tetany.

5. Intravenous magnesium sulfate diluted in IV solution should be administered at a slow rate. Rapid infusion can cause hot and flushed feelings.

6. In emergency situations, IV calcium gluconate is given to reverse hypermagnesemia.

7. Long-term administration of saline (NaCl) infusions can result in magnesium and calcium losses. Sodium inhibits renal absorption of magnesium and calcium.

8. A magnesium deficit enhances the action of digoxin.

9. Thiazides and loop (high-ceiling) diuretics decrease serum magnesium levels.

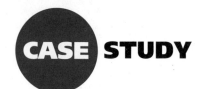

CASE STUDY

REVIEW

Mrs. Landis has had diuresis for several days. In the hospital her diagnoses were prolonged diuresis, severe dehydration, and malnutrition. She received 3 liters of 5% dextrose in 1/2 of normal saline (0.45% NaCl). Her serum magnesium was 1.3 mEq/L.

ANSWER COLUMN

1. 1.5–2.5 mEq/L

2. hypomagnesemia

3. It causes dilution of magnesium in the ECF.

4. renal insufficiency and use of Epsom salt (MgSO₄) as a laxative (also magnesium-containing antacids)

5. a. irregular pulse (dysrhythmia); b. tremors;, c. twitching of the face

6. calcium

7. CNS depression (lethargic, drowsiness) and decrease in respiration

1. What is the "normal" serum magnesium range?* _____

2. Name the type of magnesium imbalance present. _____

3. Mrs. Landis received fluids intravenously. Explain the relationship of IV fluids to magnesium deficit.* _____
   _____

4. Name two clinical causes of hypermagnesemia.* _____
   _____

Mrs. Landis's pulse was irregular. She developed tremors and twitching of the face. The physician ordered 10 mL of magnesium sulfate IV to be diluted in 1 liter of solution. Other drugs that she was receiving included digoxin and Lasix.

5. Name Mrs. Landis's clinical signs and symptoms of hypomagnesemia.
   a. * _____
   b. _____
   c. * _____

6. What cation, in a *hypo* state, causes CNS abnormalities similar to hypomagnesemia? _____

7. Name at least two symptoms of hypermagnesemia.* _____
   _____

8. Kidneys excrete excess magnesium and kidney impairment can cause hypermagnesemia.

9. Hypomagnesemia enhances the action of digitalis.

10. hypomagnesemia

8. The physician ordered IV magnesium sulfate diluted in 1 liter of IV fluids. The nursing implication is to first check Mrs. Landis's urinary output. Explain the rationale. * _____

_____

9. The nurse should be assessing digitalis toxicity while Mrs. Landis's serum magnesium is low. Explain. * _____

_____

10. Lasix can cause (hypomagnesemia/hypermagnesemia)

_____ .

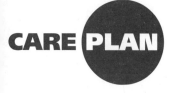

Client Management

Hypomagesemia
Assessment Factors

▶ Obtain a health history and identify which findings are associated with hypomagnesemia, such as malnutrition, chronic alcoholism, chronic diarrhea, laxative abuse, TPN with magnesium, and electrolyte imbalance (hypokalemia, hypocalcemia).

▶ Assess for signs and symptoms of hypomagnesemia (neuromuscular and cardiac abnormalities), i.e., tetanylike symptoms due to hyperexcitability (tremors, twitching of the face), cardiac dysrhythmias (ventricular tachycardia leading to ventricular fibrillation), and hypertension.

▶ Assess dietary intake and use of IV therapy without magnesium. Prolonged IV therapy including total parenteral nutrition (TPN, hyperalimentation) may be a cause of hypomagnesemia.

▶ Check the ECG/EKG strips for changes in the T wave (flat or inverted) and ST segment (depressed) that may indicate hypomagnesemia.

▶ Check serum magnesium level. Frequently the serum magnesium level is not ordered and is usually not part of the routine chemistry test. If a potassium deficit does not respond to potassium replacement, hypomagnesemia should be suspected.

Diagnosis 1

Altered nutrition: less than body requirements, related to poor nutritional intake, chronic alcoholism, chronic laxative abuse, and chronic diarrhea.

Interventions and Rationale

1. Instruct the client to eat foods rich in magnesium [green vegetables, fruits, fish and seafood, grains, and nuts (peanut butter)].

2. Report to health professionals when clients receive continuous magnesium-free IV fluids. Solutions for hyperalimentation should contain some magnesium.

3. Administer IV magnesium sulfate diluted in solution slowly unless the client has a severe deficit. Rapid infusion can cause a hot or flushed feeling.

4. Have IV calcium gluconate available for emergency to reverse hypermagnesemia from overcorrection of a magnesium deficit.

Diagnosis 2

Decreased cardiac output related to a serum magnesium deficit.

Interventions and Rationale

1. Monitor vital signs and ECG strips. Report abnormal findings to the physician.

2. Monitor serum electrolyte results. Report a low serum potassium and/or calcium level. A low serum magnesium level may be attributed to hypokalemia or hypocalcemia. When correcting a potassium deficit, potassium is not replaced in the cells until magnesium is replaced. A serum magnesium level of 1.0 mEq/L or less can cause cardiac arrest.

3. Check clients with hypomagnesemia who are taking digoxin for digitalis toxicity, e.g., nausea and vomiting, bradycardia. Magnesium deficit enhances the action of digoxin (digitalis preparations).

4. Report urine output of less than 25 mL/h or 600 mL/day when the client is receiving magnesium supplements. Magnesium excess is excreted by the kidneys. With a poor urine output, hypermagnesemia can occur.

5. Check for positive Trousseau's and Chvostek's signs of severe hypomagnesemia. Tetany symptoms occur in both magnesium and calcium deficits.

Hypermagnesemia
Assessment Factors

▶ Assess, via health history, for possible causes of hypermagnesemia, i.e., renal insufficiency or failure and chronic use of antacids and laxatives containing magnesium salts.

▶ Assess for signs and symptoms of hypermagnesemia, such as decreased neuromuscular activity, lethargy, decreased respiration, and hypotension.

▶ Obtain a serum magnesium level that can be used as a baseline for comparison of future serum magnesium levels. A serum magnesium level above about 2.5 mEq/L or 3.0 mg/dL is indicative of hypermagnesemia.

Diagnosis 1

Altered nutrition: more than body requirements, related to oral and IV magnesium supplements and chronic use of drugs containing magnesium.

Interventions and Rationale

1. Monitor urinary output for clients taking magnesium-containing drugs. Urine output, 600–1200 mL/day, allows for the excretion of magnesium. A poor urine output can result in hypermagnesemia.

2. Observe for signs and symptoms of hypermagnesemia, such as decreased neuromuscular activity, decreased reflexes, lethargy and drowsiness, decreased respirations, and hypotension.

3. Monitor serum magnesium levels. A serum magnesium level exceeding 10 mEq/L can precipitate cardiac arrest.

4. Monitor for ECG changes. A wide QRS complex and a prolonged QT interval can suggest hypermagnesemia.

5. Instruct the client to avoid prolonged use of antacids and laxatives containing magnesium. Suggest that the client check drug labels for magnesium.

6. Suggest that the client increase fluid intake unless contraindicated. Fluids dilute the serum magnesium level and should increase urine output.

Evaluation/Outcome

1. Evaluate that the cause of the magnesium imbalance has been corrected (serum potassium level within normal range). Because potassium and magnesium are cations and have similar functions, one electrolyte imbalance affects the other electrolyte balance.

2. Evaluate the effect of the therapeutic regimen for correcting magnesium balance (magnesium within normal range).

3. Remain free of clinical manifestations of hypomagnesemia and hypermagnesemia; ECG, vital signs, etc., return to the client's normal baseline patterns.

4. Diet includes foods rich in magnesium.

5. Maintain a support system.

Phosphorus Imbalances

CHAPTER 10

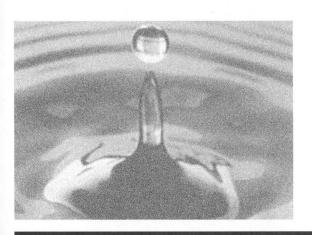

▶ INTRODUCTION

Phosphorus (P) is a major anion and has its highest concentration in the intracellular fluid. Phosphorus and calcium have similar and opposite effects. Both electrolytes need vitamin D for intestinal absorption. Phosphorus and calcium in their highest concentrations are in bones and teeth. The parathyroid hormone (PTH) acts on phosphorus and calcium differently. While PTH stimulates the renal tubules to excrete phosphorus, thus decreasing serum phosphorus levels, it increases serum calcium levels by pulling calcium from the bone.

The ions phosphorus (P) and phosphate (PO_4) are used interchangeably. Phosphorus is measured in the serum; in the cells it appears as a form of phosphate.

1

1 intracellular (highest
concentration)

Phosphorus is found in high concentration in the (extracellular/
intracellular) _____ fluid.

2

Approximately 85% of phosphorus is located in the bones and
the remaining 15% is located in the intracellular fluid. The
normal serum phosphorus range is 1.7–2.6 mEq/L, or
2.5–4.5 mg/dL.

   A serum phosphorus level below 1.7 mEq/L, or 2.5 mg/dL, is
identified as hypophosphatemia. A serum level above 2.6

2 hyperphosphatemia

mEq/L, or 4.5 mg/dL, is labeled _____ .

3

The normal serum phosphorus range in adults is _____

3 1.7–2.6; 2.5–4.5

mEq/L, or _____ mg/dL.

   The serum phosphorus level is usually higher in children:
4.0–7.0 mg/dL.

4

Like potassium, 90% of the phosphorus compound is excreted
by the kidneys and 10% is excreted by the gastrointestinal tract.

   Potassium is a(n) (anion/cation) _____ , and phosphorus
is a(n) (anion/cation) _____ . Both potassium and
phosphorus are most plentiful in the (extracellular/intracellular)

4 cation; anion; intracellular

_____ fluid.

5

Phosphorus balance is influenced by the parathyroid hormone
(PTH). PTH stimulates calcitriol, a vitamin D derivative, which
increases phosphorus absorption from the gastrointestinal tract.
PTH also stimulates the proximal renal tubules to increase
phosphate excretion.

   The two hormones that influence phosphorus/phosphate

5 calcitriol and parathyroid
hormone (PTH)

balance are *_____ .

❱ FUNCTIONS

Phosphorus has many functions. It is a vital element needed in bone formation, a component of the cell (nucleic acids and cell membrane), and is incorporated into the enzymes needed for metabolism, e.g., adenosine triphosphate (ATP), and acts as an acid-base buffer. Table 10-1 explains the functions of phosphorus according to the body system and structure it affects. Study the table carefully and refer to the table as needed.

6

An important function of phosphorus is neuromuscular activity. Name at least two cations that play an important role in neuromuscular activity. *_____

7

Phosphorus, like calcium, is needed for strong, durable teeth and _____ .

8

Intracellular ATP is needed for cellular energy.
    The red-blood-cell enzyme 2,3-DPG is responsible for
*_____ .

6   potassium and sodium
    (answer can also be
    calcium and magnesium)

7   bones

8   delivering oxygen to the
    tissues

Table 10-1

Phosphorus and Its Functions

Body Involvement	Functions
Neuromuscular	Normal nerve and muscle activity.
Bones and teeth	Bone and teeth formation, strength, and durability.
Cellular	Formation of high-energy compounds (ATP, ADP). Phosphorus is the backbone of nucleic acids and stores metabolic energy.
	Formation of the red-blood-cell enzyme 2,3-diphosphoglycerate (2,3-DPG) is responsible for delivering oxygen to tissues.
	Utilization of B vitamins.
	Transmission of hereditary traits.
	Metabolism of carbohydrates, proteins, and fats.
	Maintenance of acid-base balance in body fluids.

9

Other functions of phosphorus include which of the following:

( ) a. Utilization of vitamin A
( ) b. Utilization of B vitamins
( ) c. Metabolism of carbohydrates, proteins, and fats
( ) d. Maintenance of acid-base balance in body fluids
( ) e. Transmission of hereditary traits

9 b, c, d, e

▶ PATHOPHYSIOLOGY

10

Hypophosphatemia occurs approximately 3–4 days after an inadequate nutrient intake of foods rich in phosphorus. The kidneys compensate by decreasing urinary phosphate excretion; however, a continuous inadequate intake of phosphorus results in an extracellular fluid shift to the cells in order to replace the phosphorus loss.

What happens to the serum phosphorus level with this shift?

*_____

_____

10 The serum phosphorus level decreases, resulting in hypophosphatemia.

11

Indicate the type of phosphorus imbalance based upon the serum phosphorus level listed on the left:

_____ 1. 3.0 mg/dL	a. Hypophosphatemia
_____ 2. 6.8 mg/dL	b. Hyperphosphatemia
_____ 3. 1.5 mg/dL	c. Normal
_____ 4. 1.2 mEq/L	
_____ 5. 3.2 mEq/L	
_____ 6. 2.0 mEq/L	

11 1. c; 2. b; 3. a; 4. a; 5. b; 6. c

▶ ETIOLOGY

Table 10-2 lists the causes of hypophosphatemia and Table 10-3 lists the causes of hyperphosphatemia. Study the tables and then proceed to the questions that follow. Refer to the tables as needed.

Table 10-2

Causes of Hypophosphatemia (Serum Phosphorus Deficit)

Etiology	Rationale
Dietary Changes	
Malnutrition	Poor nutrition results in a reduction of phosphorus intake.
Chronic alcoholism	Alcoholism contributes to dietary insufficiencies and increased diuresis.
Total parenteral nutrition (TPN, hyperalimentation)	TPN is usually a phosphorus-poor or -free solution. IV concentrated glucose and protein given rapidly shift phosphorus into the cells, thus causing a serum phosphorus deficit.
Gastrointestinal Abnormalities	
Vomiting, anorexia Chronic diarrhea	Loss of phosphorus through the GI tract decreases cellular ATP (energy) stores.
Intestinal malabsorption	Vitamin D deficiencies inhibit phosphorus absorption. Phosphorus is absorbed in the jejunum in the presence of vitamin D.
Hormonal Influence	
Hyperparathyroidism (increased PTH)	Parathyroid hormone (PTH) production enhances renal phosphate excretion and calcium reabsorption.
Drug Influence	
Aluminum-containing antacids	Phosphate binds with aluminum to decrease the serum phosphorus level.
Diuretics	Most diuretics promote a decrease in the serum phosphorus level.
Cellular Changes	
Diabetic ketoacidosis	Glycosuria and polyuria increase phosphate excretion. A dextrose infusion with insulin causes a phosphorus shift into the cells; decreasing the serum phosphorus level.
Burns	Phosphorus is lost due to its increased utilization in tissue building.
Acid-base disorders	Respiratory alkalosis from prolonged hyperventilation decreases the serum phosphorus level by causing an intracellular shift of phosphorus. Metabolic alkalosis can also cause this shift.

Table 10-3

Causes of Hyperphosphatemia (Serum Phosphorus Excess)

Etiology	Rationale
Dietary Changes Oral phosphate supplements Intravenous phosphate	Excessive administration of phosphate-containing substances increases the serum phosphorus level.
Hormonal Influence Hypoparathyroidism (lack of PTH)	Lack of PTH causes a calcium loss and a phosphorus excess.
Renal Abnormalities Renal insufficiency	Renal insufficiency or shutdown decreases phosphorus excretion.
Drug Influence Laxatives containing phosphate	Frequent use of phosphate laxatives increases the serum phosphorus level.

12 hypophosphatemia; malnutrition and chronic alcoholism (also the use of phosphorus-poor or phosphorus-free IV solutions including those used for TPN)

13 a poor diet (malnutrition); diuresis

14 vitamin D

15 vomiting; anorexia; chronic diarrhea; intestinal malabsorption

12
A decreased serum phosphorus level is known as a phosphorus deficit or _____ .
  Name two dietary changes that can cause a decreased serum phosphorus level. *_____

_____

13
Alcoholism can cause severe hypophosphatemia. The phosphorus loss is the result of *_____ or _____ .

14
Name the vitamin that is necessary for phosphorus absorption via the small intestines. _____

15
Gastrointestinal abnormalities that may cause hypophosphatemia include _____ , _____ , *_____ , and _____ .

16

In parathyroid disorders the parathyroid hormone (PTH) influences phosphorus balance.

   Increased PTH secretion causes a phosphorus (loss/excess) _____ .

16 loss

17

An increased calcium level is usually accompanied by a decreased serum phosphorus level.

   Aluminum-containing antacids decrease the serum phosphorus level. Explain how. *_____

_____

17 Phosphate binds with aluminum.

18

A client in diabetic ketoacidosis may have severe hypophosphatemia. Give two reasons why the phosphorus deficit occurs.

   a. *_____

   b. *_____

18 a. Glycosuria and polyuria increase phosphorus excretion.; b. Dextrose infusions with insulin cause a phosphorus shift from the serum into cells.

19

Explain how hypophosphatemia occurs as a result of prolonged hyperventilation.

*_____

What type of acid-base imbalance can result from prolonged hyperventilation?

*_____

19 Phosphorus shifts into cells (intracellular fluid). respiratory alkalosis

20

An elevated serum phosphorus level is known as phosphorus excess or _____ .

   With a decrease in the serum calcium level, the serum phosphorus level (increases/decreases) _____ .

20 hyperphosphatemia; increases

21

Hypoparathyroidism causes a(n) (increase/decrease) _____ in the secretion of the parathyroid hormone (PTH).

   A decrease in PTH secretion causes a calcium (loss/excess) _____ and a phosphorus (loss/excess) _____ .

21 decrease; loss; excess

22

Certain groups of drugs affect phosphorus balance. Enter PD for phosphorus deficit and PE for phosphorus excess against the drug groups that can cause phosphorus imbalance.

_____ a. Aluminum antacids
_____ b. Phosphate-containing laxatives
_____ c. Thiazide diuretics
_____ d. Oral phosphate ingestion
_____ e. Intravenous phosphate administration

22 a. PD; b. PE; c. PD; d. PE; e. PE

▶ CLINICAL MANIFESTATIONS

23

Clinical manifestations of hypophosphatemia and hyperphosphatemia are determined by signs and symptoms of phosphorus imbalances, particularly neuromuscular irregularities, hematologic abnormalities, and an abnormal serum phosphorus level.

The normal serum phosphorus range is *_____ .

A serum phosphorus level of less than _____ mg/dL indicates hypophosphatemia, and one greater than _____ mg/dL indicates hyperphosphatemia.

23 1.7–2.6 mEq/L, or 2.5–4.5 mg/dL; 2.5; 4.5

Table 10-4 lists the clinical manifestations of hypophosphatemia and hyperphosphatemia according to the body areas that are affected. Study the table carefully and refer to it as needed.

24

Indicate which of the following signs and symptoms relate to hypophosphatemia:

( ) a. Muscle weakness
( ) b. Paresthesia
( ) c. Bone pain
( ) d. Flaccid paralysis
( ) e. Tissue hypoxia
( ) f. Tachycardia
( ) g. Hyporeflexia

24 a (also could occur with hyperphosphatemia), b, c, e, g

25

Indicate which of the following signs and symptoms relate to hyperphosphatemia:

Table 10-4

Clinical Manifestations of Phosphorus Imbalances

Body Involvement	Hypophosphatemia	Hyperphosphatemia
Neuromuscular Abnormalities	Muscle weakness Tremors Paresthesia Bone pain Hyporeflexia Seizures	Tetany (with decreased calcium) Hyperreflexia Flaccid paralysis Muscular weakness
Hematologic Abnormalities	Tissue hypoxia (decreased oxygen-containing hemoglobin and hemolysis) Possible bleeding (platelet dysfunction) Possible infection (leukocyte dysfunction)	
Cardiopulmonary Abnormalities	Weak pulse (myocardial dysfunction) Hyperventilation	Tachycardia
GI Abnormalities	Anorexia Dysphagia	Nausea, diarrhea Abdominal cramps
Laboratory Values Milliequivalents per liter Milligrams per deciliter	<1.7 mEq/L <2.5 mg/dL	>2.6 mEq/L >4.5 mg/dL

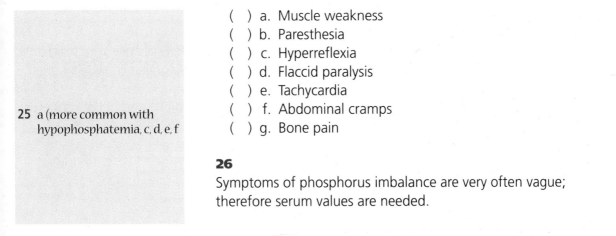

( ) a. Muscle weakness
( ) b. Paresthesia
( ) c. Hyperreflexia
( ) d. Flaccid paralysis
( ) e. Tachycardia
( ) f. Abdominal cramps
( ) g. Bone pain

25 a (more common with hypophosphatemia, c, d, e, f

26
Symptoms of phosphorus imbalance are very often vague; therefore serum values are needed.

26 1.7; 2.5; 2.6; 4.5

Hypophosphatemia is present when the serum phosphorus level is less than _____ mEq/L, or _____ mg/dL. Hyperphosphatemia is present when the serum phosphorus level is greater than _____ mEq/L, or _____ mg/dL.

▶ CLINICAL MANAGEMENT

When the serum phosphorus level falls below 1.5 mEq/L, or 2.5 mg/dL, oral and/or IV phosphate-containing solutions are usually ordered.

If the serum phosphorus level falls below 0.5 mEq/L, or 1 mg/dL, severe hypophosphatemia occurs. Intravenous phosphate-containing solutions are indicated.

Phosphorus Replacement

27

27 sodium phosphate/ Phospho-Soda and potassium phosphate/Neutra-Phos K

Name two drugs, oral or IV, that are administered to replace the phosphorus deficit (refer to Table 10-5 on pages 214 and 215).
*_____

28

28 Necrosis or sloughing of tissue. Potassium is extremely irritating to subcutaneous tissue.

Concentrated IV phosphates are hyperosmolar and must be diluted. If IV potassium phosphate (KPO_4) is given in IV solution, the IV rate should be no more than 10 mEq/h to avoid phlebitis.

If an IV potassium phosphate solution infiltrates, what happens to the tissue? *_____

_____

29

Foods rich in phosphorus include milk (especially skim milk), milk products, meat (beef and pork), whole grain cereals, and dried beans.

Phosphorus-rich foods are indicated if the serum phosphorus level is which of the following:

( ) a. 0.3 mEq/L, or 1 mg/dL
( ) b. 0.9 mEq/L, or 1.5 mg/dL

29 c

( ) c. 1.6 mEq/L, or 2.4 mg/dL

Drugs and Their Effect on Phosphorus Balance

The major drug group that causes hypophosphatemia is aluminum antacids; other drug groups responsible for hyperphosphatemia are phosphate laxatives, phosphate enemas, and oral and IV phosphates. Table 10-5 lists the names and rationales for drugs that affect phosphorus balance.

30
Prolonged intake of aluminum antacids, with or without magnesium, decreases the serum phosphorus level. Why?
*_____
The phosphorus imbalance that results is _____ .

31
Aluminum antacids may be ordered for hyperphosphatemia. Do you know why? *_____
_____

32
Enter PD for phosphorus deficit and PE for phosphorus excess beside the drugs that can cause a phosphorus imbalance:

_____ a. Amphojel
_____ b. Cortisone
_____ c. Phospho-Soda
_____ d. Fleet's sodium phosphate
_____ e. Epinephrine/adrenalin
_____ f. Diuretics
_____ g. IV potassium phosphate

▶ CLINICAL APPLICATIONS

33
Severe hypophosphatemia can result from hyperalimentation/TPN. Two reasons for a serum phosphorus deficit related to hyperalimentation are
a. *_____
b. *_____

Margin answers:

30 Aluminum-containing antacids bind with phosphorus.; hypophosphatemia

31 Aluminum binds with phosphorus to decrease the serum phosphorus level.

32 a. PD; b. PD; c. PE; d. PE; e. PD; f. PD; g. PE

33 a. phosphate-poor or phosphate-free solution; b. Concentrated glucose and/or protein, given too rapidly, causes phosphorus to shift from serum into cells.

Table 10-5

Drugs That Affect Phosphorus Balance

Phosphorus Imbalance	Drugs	Rationale

Hypophosphatemia (serum phosphorus deficit)	Sucralfate
	Aluminum antacids
	  Amphojel
	  Basaljel
	Aluminum/magnesium antacids
	  Di-Gel
	  Gelusil
	  Maalox
	  Maalox Plus
	  Mylanta
	  Mylanta II
	
	Calcium antacids
	  Calcium carbonate
		Aluminum-containing antacids bind with phosphorus; therefore the serum phosphorus level is decreased. Calcium promotes phosphate loss.

	Diuretics
	  Thiazide
	  Loop (high ceiling)
	  Acetazolamide
		Phosphorus can be lost when diuretics are used.

	Androgens
	Corticosteroids
	  Cortisone
	  Prednisone
	Glucagon
	Gastrin
	Epinephrine
	Mannitol
	
	Salicylate overdose
	Insulin and glucose
		These agents have a mild to moderate effect on phosphorus loss.

continues on the following page

34 slow; hypophosphatemia; Concentrated glucose tends to shift phosphorus into cells; the result is a serum phosphorus deficit.

34
If a severely malnourished patient is receiving a 25% dextrose solution (TPN), the infusion rate should be (fast/slow) _____ when first administered? What type of serum phosphorus imbalance can occur if the infusion rate is faster than 80 mL/h? _____ Why? * _____
_____

Table 10-5

(Continued)

Phosphorus Imbalance	Drugs	Rationale

Hyperphosphatemia (serum phosphorus excess)	Oral phosphates
	  Sodium phosphate/
	    Phospho-Soda
	  Potassium phosphate/
	    Neutra-Phos K
		Excess oral ingestion and IV infusion can increase the serum phosphorus level.

	Intravenous phosphates
	  Sodium phosphate
	  Potassium phosphate	

	Phosphate laxatives
	  Sodium phosphate
	  Sodium biphosphate/
	    Phospho-Soda
	  Phosphate enema
	  Fleet sodium phosphate
		Continuous use of phosphate laxatives and enemas can increase the serum phosphorus level.

	Excessive vitamin D
	Antibiotics
	  Tetracyclines
	  Methicillin	

35

Any carbohydrate-loading diet can cause a phosphorus shift from the serum into the cells.

During tissue repair following trauma, phosphorus shifts into the cells. The serum phosphorus imbalance that occurs is called _____ .

35 hypophosphatemia

● Clinical Considerations

1. Phosphorus is needed for durable bones and teeth, formation of ATP (high-energy compound for cellular activity), metabolism of carbohydrates, proteins, and fats, utilization of B vitamins, transmission of hereditary traits, and others.

2. Phosphorus and calcium are similar and yet differ in action. Both need vitamin D for intestinal absorption. PTH promotes renal excretion of phosphorus (phosphate) and calcium reabsorption from the bones.

3. Vomiting and chronic diarrhea cause a loss of phosphorus.

4. Concentrated IV phosphates are hyperosmolar and must be diluted. If IV potassium phosphate is given in IV solution, the IV rate should be no more than 10 mEq/h to avoid phlebitis and a potassium overload.

5. Aluminum-containing antacids decrease the serum phosphorus level; phosphate binds with the aluminum.

6. Continuous use of phosphate laxatives can cause an elevated serum phosphorus level.

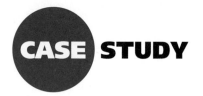

CASE STUDY REVIEW

Mrs. Peterson had a history of alcohol abuse. She was admitted for GI bleeding. In her own words she had not eaten a balanced diet for 2 months and had been taking Amphojel to relieve an "upset stomach." Mrs. Peterson complained of hand paresthesias and "overall" muscle weakness.

ANSWER COLUMN

1. hypophosphatemia

2. 1.7–2.6; 2.5–4.5

3. poor diet (possible malnutrition) and ingestion of aluminum hydroxide antacid, Amphojel

4. a. hand paresthesias; b. muscle weakness

5. bone pain, tissue hypoxia, weak pulse, and hyperventilation

6. Phosphorus binds with aluminum, thus lowering the serum phosphorus level.

1. What type of phosphorus imbalance does Mrs. Peterson have? _____

2. Give the "normal" serum phosphorus range: _____ mEq/L, or _____ mg/dL.

3. Give two reasons for Mrs. Peterson's imbalance: * _____
_____

4. What among Mrs. Peterson's signs and symptoms indicated a phosphorus deficit?
   a. * _____
   b. * _____

5. Name four other clinical signs and symptoms of hypophosphatemia. * _____
_____

6. Explain how aluminum hydroxide lowers the serum phosphorus level. * _____
_____

Mrs. Peterson was given a 10% dextrose solution intravenously. Her serum phosphorus level was 1.5 mg/dL and her potassium level, 3.0 mEq/L. Several hours later potassium phosphate was added to her intravenous solution.

7. Concentrated glucose causes a shift of phosphorus from the serum into the cells.
8. monitor IV rate so Mrs. Peterson receives approximately 10 mEq/h of KPO_4; check infusion site frequently for signs of infiltration
9. sodium phosphate/ Phospho-Soda and potassium phosphate/ NeutraPhos K

7. What effect does concentrated dextrose (glucose) solution have on the serum phosphorus level? * _____
_____

8. What is the responsibility of the nurse who is attending Mrs. Peterson while she is receiving IV potassium phosphate diluted in this solution?
* _____

9. Name two oral phosphate drugs. * _____
_____

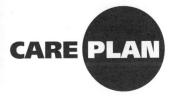

Client Management

Hypophosphatemia
Assessment Factors

▶ Obtain a history of clinical problems. Note if the health problem is related to hypophosphatemia, i.e., malnutrition, chronic alcoholism, chronic diarrhea, vitamin D deficit, continuous use of IV solutions without a phosphate additive (including TPN), hyperparathyroidism, continuous use of aluminum-containing antacids, and alkalotic state due to hyperventilation (respiratory alkalosis).

▶ Assess for signs and symptoms of hypophosphatemia, i.e., muscle weakness, paresthesia, hyporeflexia, weak pulse, and overbreathing (tachypnea).

▶ Check serum phosphorus level. The serum phosphorus level can act as a baseline level for assessing future serum phosphorus levels.

▶ Check serum calcium level and, if elevated, report findings to the health care provider. An elevated calcium level causes a decreased phosphorus level.

Diagnosis

Altered nutrition: less than body requirements, related to inadequate nutritional intake, chronic alcoholism, vomiting, chronic diarrhea, lack of vitamin D intake, intravenous fluids, including TPN with lack of phosphate additive.

Interventions and Rationale

1. Monitor neuromuscular and cardiopulmonary abnormalities related to a decreased phosphorus level, such as muscle weakness, tremors, paresthesia, hyporeflexia, bone pain, weak pulse, and tachypnea.

2. Monitor serum phosphorus and calcium levels. Report abnormal findings to the health care provider. An increase in the serum calcium level results in a decrease in the serum phosphorus level and vice versa.

3. Monitor oral and IV phosphorus replacements. Some of the oral phosphate salts (Neutrophos) come in capsules, which are indicated if nausea is present. Administer IV phosphate [potassium phosphate (KPO_4)] slowly to prevent hyperphosphatemia and irritation of the blood vessel. The suggested amount of KPO_4 to be administered per hour is 10 mEq. Rapidly administered KPO_4 and/or high concentrations of phosphate can cause phlebitis.

4. Check for signs of infiltration at the IV site; KPO_4 is extremely irritating to subcutaneous tissue and can cause sloughing of tissue and necrosis.

5. Inform the health care provider (HCP) if your client is receiving a phosphorus-poor or phosphorus-free solution for TPN.

6. Instruct the client to eat foods rich in phosphorus, i.e., meats (beef, pork, turkey), milk, whole grain cereals, and nuts. Most carbonated drinks are high in phosphates.

7. Instruct the client not to take antacids that contain aluminum hydroxide (Amphojel). Phosphorus binds with aluminum products; a low serum phosphorus level results.

Hyperphosphatemia
Assessment Factors

▶ Obtain a history of clinical problems; associate the health problems to hyperphosphatemia, i.e., continuous use of phosphate-containing laxatives, hypoparathyroidism, and renal insufficiency.

▶ Assess for signs and symptoms of hyperphosphatemia, i.e., hyperreflexia, tachycardia, abdominal cramps, and tetany symptoms, which can also indicate a low serum calcium level.

▶ Check serum phosphorus level. A serum phosphorus level greater than 4.5 mg/dL or greater than 2.6 mEq/L indicates hyperphosphatemia. A serum phosphorus level exceeding 10 mg/dL can result in cardiac distress.

▶ Check urinary output. A decrease in urine output, <25 mL (cc) per hour or <600 mL/day, increases the serum phosphorus level. This is especially true if the client is receiving a phosphate-containing product.

Diagnosis

Altered nutrition: more than body requirements, related to excess intake of phosphate-containing compounds such as some laxatives, intravenous potassium phosphate, and others.

Interventions and Rationale

1. Monitor neuromuscular, cardiac, and GI abnormalities related to an increased phosphorus level.

2. Monitor serum phosphorus and calcium levels. A decreased calcium level can result in an increase in the phosphorus level. Report abnormal findings to the HCP.

3. Observe the client for signs and symptoms of hypocalcemia (e.g., tetany) when phosphate supplements are being administered. An increase in the serum phosphorus level decreases the calcium level.

4. Instruct the client to eat foods that are low in phosphorus, such as vegetables. Instruct the client to avoid drinking carbonated beverages that contain phosphates.

5. Instruct client with hyperphosphatemia or poor renal output to read labels on over-the-counter medications and canned foods that may contain phosphate ingredients.

6. Monitor urine output. Report inadequate urine output. Phosphorus is excreted by the kidneys and poor renal function can cause hyperphosphatemia.

Evaluation/Outcome

1. Evaluate that the cause of phosphorus imbalance has been eliminated.

2. Evaluate the effect of clinical management in correcting the phosphorus imbalance (phosphorus level within normal range).

3. Determine that the signs and symptoms of phosphorus imbalance are absent. The client is free of neuromuscular abnormalities such as muscle weakness and tetany symptoms.

4. Document compliance with prescribed drug therapy and medical and dietary regimen.

5. Maintain a support system.

ACID-BASE BALANCE AND IMBALANCE

OBJECTIVES

Upon completion of this unit, the reader should be able to:

- Explain the influence of the hydrogen ion (H^+) on body fluids.
- Identify the pH ranges for acidosis and alkalosis.
- Discuss the four regulatory mechanisms for pH control and how the regulatory mechanisms can maintain acid-base balance.
- Identify metabolic acidosis and alkalosis and respiratory acidosis and alkalosis through use of arterial blood gases.
- Explain how various clinical conditions can cause metabolic acidosis and alkalosis and respiratory acidosis and alkalosis.
- Identify clinical symptoms of metabolic acidosis and alkalosis and respiratory acidosis and alkalosis.
- Discuss the body's defense action and the clinical management for acid-base balance and be able to apply this information to various clinical situations.
- Explain the health interventions for clients in metabolic and respiratory acidosis and alkalosis states.

▌ INTRODUCTION

Our body fluid must maintain a balance between acidity and alkalinity in order for life to be maintained. *Acid* comes from the Latin word meaning "sharp," and acid is frequently referred to as being sour. On the other hand, alkaline is referred to as being sweet. According to the Bronsted-Lowry concept of acids and bases, an "*acid* is any molecule or ion that can *donate a proton* to any other substance, whereas a *base* is any molecule or ion that can *accept a proton.*" The more readily an acid gives up its protons, the stronger it is as an acid. Acids and bases are not synonymous with anions and cations.

Other theories state that the concentration of hydrogen ions (plus or minus) determine either the acidity or the alkalinity of a solution. The amount of ionized hydrogen in extracellular fluid is extremely small; around 0.0000001 g/L. Instead of using this cumbersome figure, the symbol pH is used, which stands for the negative logarithm (exponent) of the hydrogen ion concentration. Mathematically, it is expressed as 10^{-7}, the base being 10 and the power -7, the logarithm of the number. In this example the minus sign is dropped and the symbol used to designate the hydrogen ion concentration is pH 7. As the hydrogen ion concentration rises (in solution), the pH value falls, indicating a decreased negative logarithm of the hydrogen ion concentration, thus indicating increased acidity. As the hydrogen concentration falls, the pH rises, thus indicating increased alkalinity.

The hydroxyl ions (OH^-) are base ions and, when in excess, increase the alkalinity of the solution. A solution of pH 7 is neutral since at this concentration the number of hydrogen ions (H^+) is exactly balanced by the number of hydroxyl ions (OH^-). It should be noted that being balanced does not mean that the hydrogen and hydropyl ions are the same concentration.

The above information will help you in the basic understanding of acidity and alkalinity. This information will aid in the understanding of the regulatory mechanism for pH control; the determination of acid-base imbalances including metabolic acidosis and alkalosis; and respiratory acidosis and alkalosis.

Refer to the Introduction as needed to answer the first five frames. An asterisk (*) on an answer line indicates a multiple-word answer. The meanings for the following symbols are: ↑ increased, ↓ decreased, > greater than, < less than.

1

According to the Bronsted-Lowry concept of acids and bases, an acid is a proton (donor/acceptor) _____ and a base is a proton (donor/acceptor) _____ .

1   donor; acceptor

2

For our purposes, consider that the acidity or alkalinity of a solution depends on the concentration of the *_____ .

An increase in concentration of the hydrogen ions makes a solution more _____ and a decrease in the concentration of hydrogen ions makes it more _____ .

2   hydrogen ions; acid; alkaline

3

Explain the meaning of the pH symbol. *_____ .
The pH determines the *_____ of a solution.

3   negative logarithm of the hydrogen ion; acidity or alkalinity

4

As the hydrogen ion concentration increases, the pH value _____ . What does this indicate? _____ .
As the hydrogen ion concentration falls, the pH value _____ . What does this indicate? _____ .

4   falls, or decreases; acidity; rises, or increases; alkalinity

5

A solution at pH 7 is neutral. Why? *_____

_____

The symbol for the hydrogen ion is _____ and the symbol for the hydroxyl ion is _____ .
A hydroxyl ion and CO_2 yields _____ , which is known as a _____ .

5   The number of hydrogen ions is balanced by the number of hydroxyl ions.; H^+; OH^-; HCO_3; bicarbonate

6

The pH of extracellular fluid in health is maintained at a level between 7.35 and 7.45. With a pH higher than this range (7.35–7.45), the body is considered to be in a state of alkalosis.

What would you call a state in which the pH is below 7.35? _____ .

6   acidosis

7

7 7.35–7.45

The pH norm of blood serum is 7.4; a variation of 0.4 of a pH unit in either direction can be fatal.

In a healthy individual, the pH range of blood serum is

_____ .

8

8 acidic; The pH is below 7.35.; a, b, c

Within our bodies the pH concentration of different fluids varies. The normal pH for urine is 6.0; for gastric juice, 1.0–2.0; for bile, 5.0–6.0; and for intracellular fluid, 6.9–7.2. These body fluids are (acidic/alkaline) _____ .

Why? * _____ .

The normal pH for intestinal juice is 6.5–7.6. The fluids from the intestinal tract can be which of the following:

(   ) a. Acidic

(   ) b. Alkaline

(   ) c. Neutral

9

9 hydrogen

Whether a substance is acid, neutral, or alkaline depends on the number of _____ ions present in a given weight or volume.

10

10 acid; alkaline

When the number of hydrogen ions increases in the body fluid, the body fluid becomes _____ .

When the number of hydrogen ions decreases, the body fluid becomes _____ .

11

11 balance

In health, there are $1\frac{1}{3}$ mEq/L of acid to each 27 mEq of alkali for each liter of extracellular fluid, which represents a ratio of 1 part of acid to 20 parts of alkali.

If the ratio of 1:20 is maintained, the client is said to be in acid-base (balance/imbalance) _____ .

Figure U4-1 demonstrates by the arrow that the body is in acid-base balance when there is 1 part acid to 20 parts alkali. A pH of 7.4 represents this balance. If the arrow tilts left due to an alkali deficit or acid excess, then acidosis occurs, and if the arrow

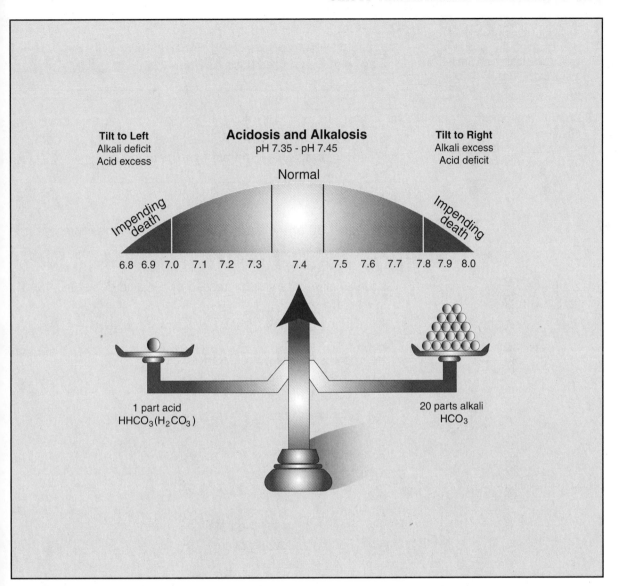

Figure U4-1 Acidosis and alkalosis.

tilts right due to an alkali excess or acid deficit, then alkalosis occurs. Carbonic acid is H_2CO_3.

Study this diagram carefully. Know what happens when the arrow tilts either left or right. Refer to the figure when needed.

12 An acidotic condition has occurred. It is due to either too much acid or too little alkali in the extracellular fluid.

13 Disturbance causing alkalosis. It is due to too much alkali or to too little acid. Borderline on impending death.

14 acidosis; alkalosis

15 left; a, d; < 7.35

16 right; b, c; > 7.45

12

Your client's serum pH is 7.1. Tell everything you can about the client's condition on the basis of Figure U4-1. *_____

_____ .

13

Another client's serum pH is 7.8. Tell everything you can about the client's condition on the basis of the diagram. *_____

_____ .

14

If the ratio 1:20 of the extracellular fluid is no longer present and the acid is increased or the alkali is decreased, then we say the client suffers from _____ .

  If the alkaline reserve is increased or the acid decreases, then he suffers from _____ .

15

When there is acidosis, the balance is tilted _____ .
  Which of the following occur:
  ( ) a. Alkali deficit
  ( ) b. Alkali excess
  ( ) c. Acid deficit
  ( ) d. Acid excess
  The pH is _____ .

16

When there is alkalosis, the balance is tilted _____ .
  Which of the following occur:
  ( ) a. Alkali deficit
  ( ) b. Alkali excess
  ( ) c. Acid deficit
  ( ) d. Acid excess
  The pH is _____ .

Regulatory Mechanisms for pH Control

CHAPTER 11

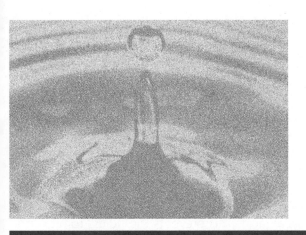

▌ INTRODUCTION

The regulatory mechanisms for pH control consist of four mechanisms; (1) buffer systems, (2) ion exchange, (3) respiratory regulation, and (4) renal regulation. Each of the regulatory mechanisms is discussed individually and is accompanied with illustrations. This chapter is not a clinical chapter and does not include assessment factors, diagnoses, interventions, and evaluation.

1 buffer system, ion exchange, respiratory regulation, and renal regulation

1

Name the four regulatory mechanisms for pH control. *_____

_____

Table 11-1 is divided into three parts. Part A explains the buffer system. Buffers maintain the acid-base balance of body fluids by protecting the fluids against changes in pH. They act like chemical sponges, by either soaking up surplus hydrogen ions or releasing them.

There are four main examples of the buffer system, including bicarbonate–carbonic acid; phosphate; hemoglobin-oxyhemoglobin; and protein. They are shown in Table 11-1A along with their interventions—their action as a buffer—and the rationale—the reason for their action. The bicarbonate–carbonic acid buffer system is more readily available and acts within a fraction of a second to prevent excessive changes in H^+ concentration, and therefore it is the principal buffer system of the body. Strong acids, when added, combine with the bicarbonate ion to form carbonic acid, which is a weak acid. This prevents the fluids from becoming strongly acid.

Remember that bicarbonate and phosphates are anions. Refer to the glossary for unknown words. Study the table carefully and refer to it as needed.

2 They protect fluids against changes in pH.; They soak up surplus H^+ and release them as needed.

2

Explain the purpose of the buffer systems. *_____
How do the buffer systems accomplish their purpose? *_____

_____

3 the bicarbonate–carbonic acid buffer system

3

What is the principal buffer system of the body? *_____

4 carbonic acid (H_2CO_3); water (H_2O) and bicarbonate (HCO_3)

4

When acid enters the body, the H^+ is picked up by the bicarbonate, changing it to *_____ .

A base added to the body is neutralized by carbonic acid to form _____ and _____ .

Table 11-1A

Regulatory Mechanism for pH Control: Buffer Systems

Regulatory Mechanism	Intervention	Rationale
a. Bicarbonate–carbonic acid buffer system (principal buffer system of body)	Acids combine with bicarbonates in blood to form neutral salts (bicarbonate salt) and carbonic acid (weak acid). Carbonic acid (H_2CO_3) is weak and unstable acid, changing to water and carbon dioxide in fluid ($H_2CO_3 \rightleftharpoons H_2O + CO_2$). A strong base combines with weak acid, e.g., H_2CO_3	When a strong acid such as HCl enters the body, H^+ ions combine with HCO_3^- ions of $NaHCO_3$, yielding carbonic acid and neutral salt (HCl + Na<u>HCO</u>$_3$ → $H_2\underline{CO}_3$ + NaCl). Weak acid, e.g., H_2CO_3, does not release H^+ as readily as does a strong acid, e.g., HCl, and thus ionizes less effectively. When a strong base such as NaOH is added to the system, it is neutralized by carbonic acid, yielding water and HCO_3^- from a salt (Na<u>OH</u> + $H_2\underline{CO}$ → $\underline{H_2}O$ + NA<u>HCO</u>$_3$).
b. Phosphate buffer system	The phosphate buffer system increases the amount of sodium bicarbonate ($NaHCO_3$) in extracellular fluids, making extracellular fluids more alkaline. The H^+ is excreted as NaH_2PO_4 and Na and bicarbonate ions combine.	Excess H^+ combines in renal tubules with Na_2HPO_4 (disodium phosphate), forming NaH_2PO_4 (H^+ + Na_2HPO_4 → Na^+ + NaH_2PO_4); Na^+ is reabsorbed (Na^+ + HCO_3^- → $NaHCO_3$) and H^+ is passed into urine.
c. Hemoglobin-oxyhemoglobin buffer system	Maintains same pH level in venous blood as in arterial blood.	Venous blood has higher CO_2 content and bicarbonate ion concentration than arterial blood. The pH is the same since oxyhemoglobin (acid) in erythrocyte has taken over some anion function that was provided by excess bicarbonate in venous plasma.
d. Protein buffer system	Proteins can exist in form of acids (H protein) or alkaline salts (B protein) and in this way are able to bind or release excess hydrogen as required.	Proteins are amphoteric, carrying both acidic and basic charge.

5 HCl + NaHCO$_3$ → H$_2$CO$_3$ +
NaCl; NaOH + H$_2$CO$_3$ → H$_2$O
+ NaHCO$_3$

6 NaH$_2$PO$_4$; urine; excretes

7 It maintains the same pH
level in the venous blood
and the arterial blood.

8 It is amphoteric—it has the
ability to bind or release
excess H$^+$; acidic; basic

9 bicarbonate–carbonic acid,
phosphate, hemoglobin-
oxyhemoglobin, and
protein

5
The bicarbonate–carbonic acid buffer system is the most
important buffer system in the body. It maintains acid-base
balance 55% of the time. Give an example with a formula of
how a strong acid combines with a bicarbonate to yield a weak
acid. *_____

    Write an example with a formula of how a strong base is
neutralized by a weak acid to yield water and bicarbonate from
a weak salt. *_____

6
The phosphate buffer system maintains the acid-base balance by
combining the excess H$^+$ with sodium salts, forming
*_____ .

    The H$^+$ is excreted in _____ .
    This system (excretes/retains) _____ excess acid in the
body.

7
What is the function of the hemoglobin-oxyhemoglobin buffer
system? *_____

_____

8
What is unique about the protein buffer system? *_____

_____

    This system carries a(n) _____ and a(n) _____
charge.

9
The four buffer systems in the body are *_____

_____ .

    Table 11-1B gives an explanation of the ion exchange in the
respiratory regulation of ions as regulatory mechanisms for pH
control. The ion exchange is frequently referred to as the *chloride
shift.* The respiratory regulation depends on the lungs to exhale
CO$_2$ or retain CO$_2$ for the control of pH. Again, the interventions
refer to the action, and the rationale refers to the reason.
    Study this table carefully and refer to it as needed.

Table 11-1B

Regulatory Mechanism for pH Control:
Ion Exchange and Respiratory Regulation

Regulatory Mechanism	Intervention	Rationale
Ion exchange	Ion exchange of HCO_3 and Cl occurs in red blood cells (RBCs) as result of O_2 and CO_2 exchange. There is redistribution of anions in response to increase in CO_2. Chloride ion enters RBCs as bicarbonate ion and diffuses into plasma in order to restore ionic balance.	Increase in serum carbon dioxide causes CO_2 to diffuse into RBCs combining with H_2O to form H_2CO_3. This weak acid dissociates, forming acid and base ions, $H_2CO_3 \rightarrow H^+ + HCO_3^-$. Hydrogen ion is buffered by hemoglobin, and HCO_3^- ion moves into plasma as chloride ion (Cl^-) shifts into cell to replace it.

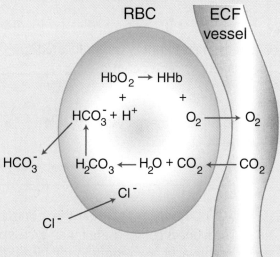

Respiratory regulation (acts quickly in case of emergency)	For regulation of acid balance, the lungs blow off more CO_2, and for regulation of alkaline balance, the respiratory center depresses respirations in order to retain CO_2. It takes 1–3 minutes for the respiratory system to readjust H^+ concentration.	Respiratory center in medulla controls the rate and depth of respiration and is sensitive to changes in blood pH or CO_2 concentration. When pH is decreased, carbonic acid is exhaled in the form of carbon dioxide and moist air ($H_2CO_3 \rightarrow H_2O + CO_2$); thus acid is eliminated.

Note: Illustration from "Blood-Gases and Blood-Gas Transport," by J. L. Keyes, 1974, *Heart and Lung,* pp. 945–954. Copyright 1982. Adapted by permission.

10 Bicarbonate diffuses out of the cell and the chloride ion enters the cell.; chloride shift

11 bicarbonate (HCO_3); chloride (Cl); bicarbonate (HCO_3)

12 When the serum pH is decreased, the lungs blow off CO_2. With an increased pH, the lungs retain CO_2.

13 medulla; rate and depth of respirations

14 a. As the CO_2 enters the red blood cells, HCO_3 leaves the red blood cells and Cl enters.; b. The lungs blow off more CO_2.

15 acidification of phosphate buffer salts, reabsorption of bicarbonate, and secretion of ammonia

---

10

When carbon dioxide enters red blood cells, what happens to the bicarbonate and chloride anions? * _____

_____

This ion exchange is frequently called the * _____ .

11

When the red blood cells are oxygenated, what anion is commonly present? _____

When carbon dioxide enters the red blood cells, what anion also enters? _____

What anion leaves as carbon dioxide enters? _____

12

How does the respiratory regulatory mechanism control the serum pH? * _____

_____

13

Where is the respiratory center located? _____ What does the respiratory center control? * _____

14

How do the two mechanisms in Table 11-1B deal with an increased CO_2?

a. * _____

b. * _____

Table 11-1C describes how the kidneys regulate pH in the body. The kidneys compensate for an excess production of acid by excreting the acid and returning the bicarbonate to the extracellular fluid. The acid occurs as the result of normal metabolism.

Study the table carefully, noting how, in each instance, the excess H^+ ions are neutralized. When you think you understand the renal regulatory mechanism described in the table, answer the questions that follow. Refer to the table when needed.

15

Name the three renal regulatory mechanisms for pH control.

* _____

_____

Table 11-1C

Regulatory Mechanism for pH Control: Renal Regulation

Regulatory Mechanism	Intervention	Rationale
a. Acidification of phosphate buffer salts	Exchange mechanism occurs between H^+ of renal tubular cells and disodium salt (Na_2HPO_4) in tubular urine.	Sodium salt (Na_2HPO_4) dissociates into Na^+ and $NaHPO_4^-$; Na^+ moves into tubular cell and hydrogen unites with $NaHPO_4$, forming dihydrogen phosphate salt, NaH_2PO_4, which is excreted.

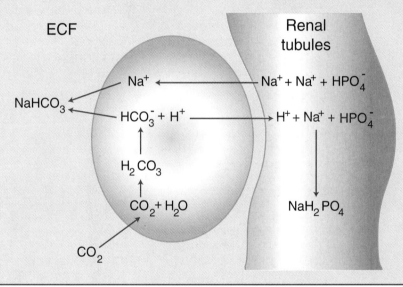

Note: Illustrations from *Textbook of Medical Physiology,* (8th ed.), by A. C. Guyton, 1991, Philadelphia: W. B. Saunders Co. Copyright 1991 by W. B. Saunders Co. Adapted by permission.

continues on the following page

16 The H^+ replaces a Na^+, forming a dihydrogen phosphate salt, NaH_2PO_4. This salt is excreted.

16
Hydrogen ions exist largely in the renal tubules in the buffered state. They are excreted indirectly by replacing a cation in excretion.
  Explain how the hydrogen ion is excreted after it combines with the sodium salt Na_2HPO_4. * _____

_____

Table 11-1C

Regulatory Mechanism for pH Control: Renal Regulation *(Continued)*

Regulatory Mechanism	Intervention	Rationale
b. Reabsorption of bicarbonate	Carbon dioxide is absorbed by tubular cells from blood and combines with water present in cells to form carbonic acid, which in turn ionizes, forming H^+ and HCO_3^-. Na^+ of tubular urine exchanges with H^+ of tubular cells and combines with HCO_3^- to form sodium bicarbonate and is reabsorbed into blood.	The enzyme carbonic anhydrase is responsible for formation of carbonic acid H_2CO_3. Ionization of $H_2CO_3 \rightarrow H^+ + HCO_3^-$. Free H^+ exchanges with Na^+. Exchange of H^+ and Na^+ permits reabsorption of bicarbonate with sodium. ($NaHCO_3$) and excretion of an acid or H^+.

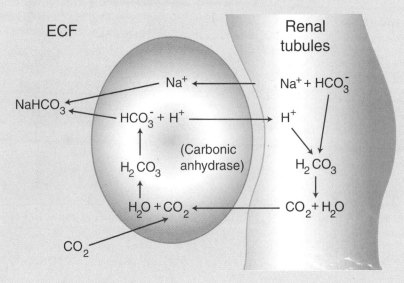

continues on the following page

17 by the ionization of H_2CO_3 $\rightarrow H^+ + HCO_3^-$
The Na^+ exchanges with the H^+ in renal tubules and the Na^+ combines with HCO_3^- and is reabsorbed into the blood.

17
The kidneys regulate the H^+ levels in the body by varying the excretion and reabsorption of H^+ and HCO_3^-.
　　Explain how the H^+ is derived from carbonic acid. *_____
　　Explain how the bicarbonate ion is reabsorbed. *_____

Table 11-1C

(Continued)

Regulatory Mechanism	Intervention	Rationale
c. Secretion of ammonia	Ammonia (NH_3) unites with HCl in renal tubules and H^+ is excreted as NH_4Cl (ammonium chloride).	Almost half of H^+ excretion is from this method: $HCl + NH_3 \rightarrow NH_4Cl$. Ammonia is formed in renal tubular cells by oxidative breakdown of amino acid glutamine in presence of enzyme glutaminase. Ammonia can also be converted into urea by the liver and excreted as urea by the kidneys.

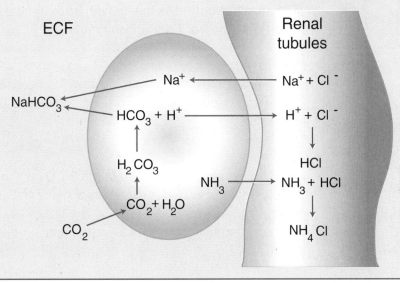

ECF

Renal tubules

Na^+ ← $Na^+ + Cl^-$

$NaHCO_3$ ← $HCO_3 + H^+$ → $H^+ + Cl^-$

↓

HCl

H_2CO_3

NH_3 → $NH_3 + HCl$

↑

↓

$CO_2 + H_2O$

NH_4Cl

CO_2

---

18 It is formed from the breakdown of amino acid glutamine.; NH_3 unites with HCl and is excreted as NH_4Cl (ammonium chloride).

18

Explain the formation of ammonia in the renal tubular cells.

*_____

_____

How does ammonia aid in the excretion of the hydrogen ion?

*_____

_____

19

Which one of the three methods in Table 11-1C is responsible for nearly half of the hydrogen ion excretion? *_____

The three major mechanisms that regulate pH or the hydrogen ion concentration in the body fluids are chemical buffers, pulmonary (respiration) exchange, and renal (kidney) regulation. The action time that it takes to maintain acid-base balance (homeostasis) varies.

Regulatory Mechanisms	Action Time
Chemical buffers	Immediate
Pulmonary exchange	Minutes
Renal regulation	Hours to days (effective and lasting)

20

The chemical buffers combine with acids or bases to maintain acid-base balance. Their action time is _____ .

21

The lungs control the carbon dioxide (CO_2) concentration by increasing or decreasing the rate of respirations. The action time occurs in _____ .

22

The kidneys control bicarbonate ion (HCO_3^-) concentration by reabsorption of HCO_3 or excretion of hydrogen ion (H^+) and the production of ammonia.

The action time for the kidneys to maintain this acid-base balance is *_____ .

23

Match the regulatory mechanisms on the left according to their action times for maintaining acid-base balance.

_____ 1. Chemical buffers   a. Minutes
_____ 2. Respiratory action   b. Hours to days
_____ 3. Kidney action   c. Immediate

19 secretion of ammonia

20 immediate

21 minutes

22 hours to days

23 1. c; 2. a; 3. b

Determination of Acid-Base Imbalances

CHAPTER

12

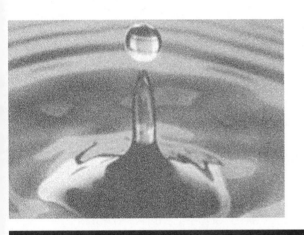

▶ INTRODUCTION

Hydrogen ions circulate throughout the body fluids in two forms: *volatile acid* and *nonvolatile acid*. Volatile acid is excreted as a gas. Nonvolatile acid, a fixed acid, results from various organic acids and is excreted in the urine. Accurate assessments of acid-base imbalances are identified with the use of arterial blood gases. The determinant blood gas factors used to assess the extent of acid-base imbalance include pH, $PaCO_2$, and HCO_3. Compensatory mechanisms discussed in this chapter positively influence pH control. Because this chapter describes the process for determining acid-base imbalance, assessment factors, diagnoses, interventions, and evaluation are not included.

1

A volatile acid (carbonic acid—H_2CO_3) circulates as CO_2 and H_2O and is excreted as a gas. The gas excreted is (HCO_3/CO_2) _____ , which helps maintain acid-base balance.

A nonvolatile acid (fixed acid, e.g., lactic, pyruvic, sulfuric, phosphoric acid) is produced as the result of various organic acids within the body. It must be excreted from the body in water, e.g., urine. What regulatory mechanism is responsible for excreting nonvolatile acids? _____

1   CO_2; kidney or renal

2

The lungs excrete (volatile/nonvolatile) _____ acids and the kidneys excrete (volatile/nonvolatile) _____ acids.

2   volatile; nonvolatile

Renal Regulation		*Respiratory Regulation*
$H^+ + HCO_3^- \rightleftharpoons$	$[H_2CO_3]$	$\rightleftharpoons H_2O + CO_2$
(excreted as nonvolatile acid)		(excreted as volatile acid)

3

The kidneys and lungs aid in acid-base balance. Label the chemical formula according to the organ that is responsible for acid-base regulation:

3   kidneys; lungs

_____ $H^+ + HCO_3^- \rightleftharpoons [H_2CO_3] \rightleftharpoons H_2O + CO_2$ _____
   (organ)   (organ)

To determine the type of acid-base imbalance, the blood tests described in Table 12-1 are essential.

4

To determine the presence of acid-base imbalance, the pH is first checked. If the pH of the arterial blood gas is less than 7.35 (acidosis/alkalosis) _____ is present.

If the pH of the arterial blood gas is more than 7.45, (acidosis/alkalosis) _____ is present.

4   acidosis; alkalosis

5

To determine if acidosis or alkalosis is present, the nurse should *first* check for the (pH/$PaCO_2$/HCO_3) _____ of the arterial blood gas results.

5   pH

Table 12-1

Determination of Acid-Base Imbalance

Blood Tests	Normal Values	Imbalance
pH	Adult: 7.35–7.45 Newborn: 7.27–7.47 Child: 7.33–7.43	Adult: <7.35 = acidosis >7.45 = alkalosis

$PaCO_2$
(respiratory component)
	Adult and child:
	  35–45 mm Hg
	Newborn: 27–41 mm Hg
		Adult and child:
		  <35 mm Hg = respiratory alkalosis
		    (hyperventilation)
		  >45 mm Hg = respiratory acidosis
		    (hypoventilation)

HCO_3^-
(metabolic and renal component)
	Adult and child:
	  24–28 mEq/L
	Newborn: 22–30 mEq/L
		Adult and child:
		  <24 mEq/L = metabolic acidosis
		  >28 mEq/L = metabolic alkalosis

Base excess (BE)
(metabolic and renal component)
	Adult and child
	  +2 to −2
		Adult and child
		  <−2 = metabolic acidosis
		  >+2 = metabolic alkalosis

CO_2*
(metabolic and renal component)
	Adult and child:
	  22–32 mEq/L
		Adult and child:
		  <22 mEq/L = metabolic acidosis
		  >32 mEq/L = metabolic alkalosis

*Serum CO_2 is a serum bicarbonate determinant and is frequently called CO_2 *combining power.* It refers to the amount of cations, e.g., H^+, Na^+, K^+, etc., available to combine with HCO_3^-. The level of HCO_3^- in the blood is determined by the amount of CO_2 dissolved in the blood.

6
To determine if the acid-base imbalance is respiratory acidosis or alkalosis, the $PaCO_2$ should be checked. If the $PaCO_2$ is within the normal range, the imbalance is not respiratory.

  If the $PaCO_2$ is greater than 45 mm Hg and the pH is less than 7.35, the type of acid-base imbalance is *_____ .

  If the $PaCO_2$ is less than 35 mm Hg and the pH is greater than 7.45, the type of acid-base imbalance is *_____ .

6 respiratory acidosis;
    respiratory alkalosis

7
The third step to determine the type of acid-base imbalance is to check the bicarbonate (HCO_3^-) and base excess (BE) levels of the arterial blood gas and the serum CO_2 level (either one of the levels or all of them if available).

If the HCO_3 is less than 24 mEq/L, the BE is less than −2, or the serum CO_2 is less than 22 mEq/L and pH is less than 7.35, the type of acid-base imbalance is *_____ .

If the HCO_3 is greater than 28 mEq/L, the BE is greater than +2, or the serum CO_2 is greater than 32 mEq/L and pH is greater than 7.45, the type of acid-base imbalance is *_____ .

7 metabolic acidosis; metabolic alkalosis

8

The normal range for pH in blood is _____ . The normal range for $PaCO_2$ in arterial blood is *_____ . The normal range of HCO_3 in arterial blood is *_____ . The normal range of serum CO_2 in venous blood is *_____ .

8 7.35–7.45; 35–45 mm Hg; 24–28 mEq/L; 22–32 mEq/L

9

To determine acidotic and alkalotic states, the nurse must first assess the _____ level; second the _____ of arterial blood; and third the _____ of arterial blood or _____ of venous blood.

9 pH; $PaCO_2$; HCO_3; serum CO_2

10

Respiratory acidosis and alkalosis are determined by which of the following:

( ) a. pH
( ) b. $PaCO_2$
( ) c. HCO_3
( ) d. BE

10 a, b

11

Metabolic acidosis and alkalosis are determined by which of the following:

( ) a. pH
( ) b. $PaCO_2$
( ) c. HCO_3
( ) d. BE
( ) e. serum CO_2

11 a, c, d, e

12

Place R. Ac for respiratory acidosis, R. Al for respiratory alkalosis, M. Ac for metabolic acidosis, and M. Al for metabolic alkalosis beside the following laboratory determinants.

_____, _____   a. pH ↑

_____, _____   b. pH ↓

_____   c. $PaCO_2$ ↑

_____   d. HCO_3 ↑

_____   e. $PaCO_2$ ↓

_____   f. HCO_3 ↓

_____   g. serum CO_2 ↓

_____   h. serum CO_2 ↑

12 a. R. Al, M. Al; b. R. Ac, M. Ac; c. R. Ac; d. M. Al; e. R. Al; f. M. Ac; g. M. Ac; h. M. Al

▶ COMPENSATION FOR pH BALANCE

There are specific compensatory reactions in response to metabolic acidosis and alkalosis and respiratory acidosis and alkalosis. The pH returns to normal or close to normal by changing the component, e.g., $PaCO_2$ or HCO_3 and/or BE, that originally was not affected.

The respiratory system can compensate for metabolic acidosis and alkalosis, and the metabolic/renal system can compensate for respiratory acidosis and alkalosis. With metabolic acidosis, the lungs (stimulated by the respiratory center) hyperventilate to decrease CO_2 level.

A pH of 7.33, $PaCO_2$ of 24, and HCO_3 of 15 indicate metabolic acidosis, since the pH is slightly acid and the HCO_3 is definitely low (acidosis). The $PaCO_2$ should be normal (35–45); however, it is low since the respiratory center compensates for the acidotic state by "blowing off" CO_2 (hyperventilating); thus, respiratory compensation exists. Without compensation, the pH could be extremely low, e.g., pH 7.2.

13

For metabolic acidosis, the lungs (hypoventilate/hyperventilate) _____ to blow off _____ .

With a pH of 7.32, $PaCO_2$ of 27, and HCO_3 of 14, the pH and HCO_3 indicate *_____ .

The $PaCO_2$ indicates respiratory compensation. Explain.

* _____

_____

13 hyperventilate; CO_2; metabolic acidosis; The lungs compensate for the acidotic state by blowing off CO_2 (respiratory compensation).

14

For metabolic alkalosis, the lungs (hypoventilate/hyperventilate) _____ to conserve _____ .

    With a pH of 7.48, $PaCO_2$ of 46, and HCO_3 of 39, the pH and HCO_3 indicate *_____ .

    The $PaCO_2$ indicates respiratory compensation. Explain.

*_____

_____

15

With respiratory acidosis, the kidneys excrete more acid, H^+, and conserve HCO_3^-.

    With a pH of 7.35, $PaCO_2$ of 68, and HCO_3 of 35, the pH is low normal, borderline acidosis, and the $PaCO_2$ is highly elevated, indicating CO_2 retention—respiratory acidosis. The HCO_3 indicates *_____

_____.

16

With respiratory alkalosis, the kidneys excrete _____ ions and conserve _____ ions.

    A pH of 7.46, $PaCO_2$ of 20, and HCO_3 of 18, the pH and $PaCO_2$ indicate *_____ . The HCO_3 indicates renal or metabolic compensation.

    Explain how. *_____

_____

17

When the body is in a state of metabolic acidosis, an excess of nonvolatile acid is retained in body fluids.

    What do you suppose occurs in metabolic alkalosis?

*_____

_____

    How is a nonvolatile acid excreted from the body? _____

18

With respiratory acidosis, there is an excess of volatile acid. How is a volatile acid excreted from the body? *_____

    With respiratory alkalosis, there is a(n) (increase/decrease) _____ in volatile acid.

---

14 hypoventilate; CO_2; metabolic alkalosis; The lungs compensate for the alkalotic state by conserving CO_2 (respiratory compensation).

15 Kidney or metabolic compensation. Without this compensation the pH is lower.

16 bicarbonate (HCO_3^-); acid (H^+); respiratory alkalosis; The kidneys compensate for the alkalotic state by excreting HCO_3 (metabolic compensation).

17 a decrease in nonvolatile acid in body fluids; in the urine

18 as a gas (via lungs); decrease

19 a. respiratory acidosis with metabolic compensation;
b. respiratory alkalosis with NO compensation;
c. respiratory acidosis with NO compensation; d. metabolic acidosis with NO compensation; e. metabolic alkalosis with NO compensation; f. normal arterial blood gases and acid-base balance; g. respiratory acidosis with metabolic compensation; h. metabolic acidosis with respiratory compensation;
i. metabolic alkalosis with respiratory compensation;
j. metabolic acidosis with respiratory compensation

19

Identify the type of acid-base imbalance, and if there is compensation, indicate which kind, metabolic or respiratory. Memorize the norms for pH, $PaCO_2$, and HCO_3.

	pH	$PaCO_2$	HCO_3	Type	Compensation Metabolic/Renal	Respiratory
a.	7.33	62	32	_____	_____ _____	_____
b.	7.50	29	26	_____	_____ _____	_____
c.	7.26	59	27	_____	_____ _____	_____
d.	7.21	40	19	_____	_____ _____	_____
e.	7.53	39	36	_____	_____ _____	_____
f.	7.40	40	26	_____	_____ _____	_____
g.	7.32	79	41	_____	_____ _____	_____
h.	7.1	16	6	_____	_____ _____	_____
i.	7.57	48	40	_____	_____ _____	_____
j.	7.23	23	10	_____	_____ _____	_____

CHAPTER 13

Metabolic Acidosis and Alkalosis

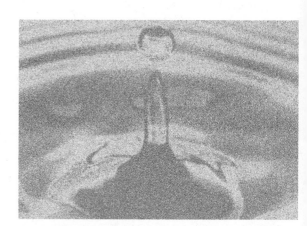

▶ INTRODUCTION

Two types of metabolic acid-base imbalance are *metabolic acidosis* and *metabolic alkalosis.* With metabolic acidosis, there is either an excess acid production, e.g., excess hydrogen ions and ketone bodies, or a base (bicarbonate) deficit. With metabolic alkalosis, there is an acid (hydrogen ion) deficit or more likely a base (bicarbonate) excess. Metabolic acidosis and metabolic alkalosis are discussed separately in this chapter.

1 pH, or hydrogen ion deficit or excess

2 pH; $PaCO_2$; HCO_3^- (bicarbonate)

3 bicarbonate and base excess; $PaCO_2$

4 acidotic; alkalotic

5 decreased; increased

6 decreased; increased

1
Acidosis and alkalosis can be determined by the _____ .

2
As discussed in Chapter 12, Table 12-1, the type of acid-base imbalance can be determined by the arterial blood gases _____ , _____ , and _____ .

3
The metabolic/renal components for metabolic acidosis and alkalosis include _____ and _____ .
    The respiratory component for respiratory acidosis and alkalosis is _____ .

    Acid-base balance is maintained by 1 part of acid and 20 parts of base. Figure 13–1 demonstrates the normal acid-base balance, and the blood tests pH, HCO_3^-, base excess (BE), and serum CO_2 are utilized in determining metabolic acidosis and alkalosis.

4
When the acid-base scale tips to the left, it is an indication that an (acidotic/alkalotic) _____ state is present.
    When the scale tips to the right, the type of acid-base imbalance is an (acidotic/alkalotic) _____ state.

5
With metabolic acidosis, the pH is _____ .
    With metabolic alkalosis, the pH is _____ .

6
In metabolic acidosis, the bicarbonate and base excess are _____ .
    In metabolic alkalosis, the bicarbonate and base excess are _____ .

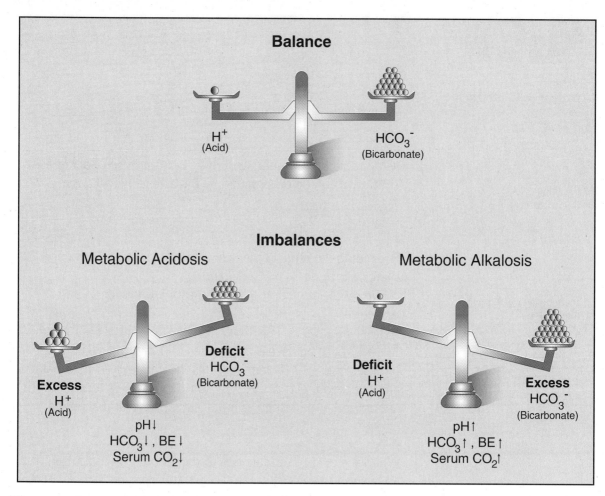

Figure 13-1 Acid-base balance and metabolic imbalances.

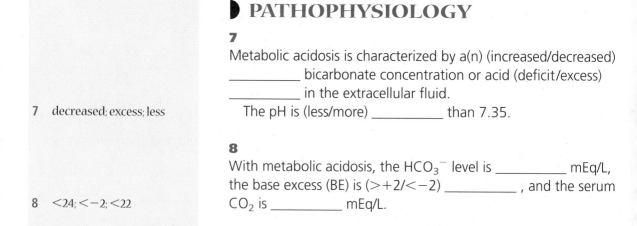

❱ PATHOPHYSIOLOGY

7

Metabolic acidosis is characterized by a(n) (increased/decreased) _____ bicarbonate concentration or acid (deficit/excess) _____ in the extracellular fluid.
  The pH is (less/more) _____ than 7.35.

8

With metabolic acidosis, the HCO_3^- level is _____ mEq/L, the base excess (BE) is ($>+2/<-2$) _____ , and the serum CO_2 is _____ mEq/L.

7 decreased; excess; less

8 $<24; <-2; <22$

9

Metabolic alkalosis is characterized by a(n) (increased/decreased) _____ bicarbonate concentration or loss of the hydrogen ion (strong acid) in the extracellular fluid.

The pH is *_____ .

9 increased; greater than 7.45

10

With metabolic alkalosis, the bicarbonate level is _____ mEq/L; BE is _____; and the serum CO_2 is _____ mEq/L.

10 >28; >+2; >32

▶ ETIOLOGY

The causes of metabolic acidosis and metabolic alkalosis are described in Tables 13–1 and 13–2. The rationale is given with each of the causes. Study the tables and then proceed to the questions. Refer to the tables as needed.

11

With severe or chronic diarrhea, the anion that is lost from the small intestine is _____ . The sodium ion is also lost in excess of the chloride ion. The chloride ion combines with the hydrogen ion to produce _____ acid.

11 bicarbonate; hydrochloric

12 Nonvolatile acids such as lactic acid result from cellular breakdown.

12

How does starvation cause metabolic acidosis? *_____ .

13 The liver produces fatty acids, which leads to ketone body production.

13

With uncontrolled diabetes mellitus, glucose cannot be metabolized; therefore, what occurs? *_____ _____ .

14

Shock, trauma, severe infection, and fever can cause cellular (anabolism/catabolism) _____ . The acid products frequently released from the cells are *_____ _____ .

14 catabolism; nonvolatile acids such as lactic acid

Table 13-1

Causes of Metabolic Acidosis

Etiology	Rationale
Gastrointestinal Abnormalities	
Starvation	Nonvolatile acids, i.e., lactic and pyruvic acids, occur as the
Severe malnutrition	result of an accumulation of acid products from cellular
	breakdown due to starvation and/or severe malnutrition.
Chronic diarrhea	Loss of bicarbonate ions in the small intestines is in excess. Also, the loss of sodium ions exceeds that of chloride ions. Cl^- combines with H^+, producing a strong acid (HCl).
Renal Abnormalities	
Kidney failure	Kidney mechanisms for conserving sodium and water and for excreting H^+ fail.
Hormonal Influence	
Diabetic ketoacidosis	Failure to metabolize adequate quantities of glucose causes the liver to increase metabolism of fatty acids. Oxidation of fatty acids produces ketone bodies, which cause the ECF to become more acid. Ketones require a base for excretion.
Hyperthyroidism, thyrotoxicosis	An overactive thyroid gland can cause cellular catabolism (breakdown) due to a severe increase in metabolism, which increases cellular needs.
Others	
Trauma, shock	Trauma and shock cause cellular breakdown and the release of nonvolatile acids.
Excess exercise, severe infection, fever	Excessive exercise, fever, and severe infection can cause cellular catabolism and acid accumulation.

15

Indicate which of the following conditions can cause metabolic acidosis:

( ) a. Starvation
( ) b. Gastric suction
( ) c. Excessive exercise
( ) d. Shock
( ) e. Uncontrolled diabetes mellitus (ketoacidosis)

15 a, c, d, e

16

Name the anion that is lost in great quantities due to vomiting or gastric suction. _____

16 chloride

Table 13-2

Causes of Metabolic Alkalosis

Etiology	Rationale
Gastrointestinal Abnormalities	
Vomiting, gastric suction	With vomiting and gastric suctioning, large amounts of chloride and hydrogen ions that are plentiful in the stomach are lost. Bicarbonate anions increase to compensate for chloride loss.
Peptic ulcers	Excess of alkali in ECF occurs when a client takes excessive amounts of acid neutralizers such as $NaHCO_3$ to ease ulcer pain.
Hypokalemia	Loss of potassium from the body is accompanied by loss of chloride.

17 overtreated peptic ulcer, vomiting, gastric suction, and loss of potassium

18 a. M. Ac; b. M. Al; c. M Ac; d. M. Ac; e. M. Al; f. M. Ac; g. M. Ac

17

Name the conditions that cause metabolic alkalosis.
*_____ , _____ , *_____ , and *_____

18

For causes of metabolic acidosis and alkalosis, place M. Ac for metabolic acidosis and M. Al for metabolic alkalosis for the appropriate condition.

_____ a. Diabetic ketoacidosis
_____ b. Overtreated peptic ulcer
_____ c. Severe diarrhea
_____ d. Shock, trauma
_____ e. Vomiting, gastric suction
_____ f. Fever, severe infection
_____ g. Excessive exercise

▶ CLINICAL APPLICATIONS

Anion gap is a useful indicator for determining the presence or absence of metabolic acidosis.

Anion gap can be obtained by completing the following steps:
1. Adding the serum chloride/Cl and serum CO_2 values
2. Subtracting the sum of serums Cl and CO_2 from the serum sodium/Na value

The difference is the anion gap.

19

If the anion gap is greater than 16 mEq/L, metabolic acidosis is suspected.

Which of the following acid-base imbalances are indicated by an anion gap that exceeds 16 mEq/L:

( ) a. Metabolic acidosis

( ) b. Metabolic alkalosis

( ) c. Respiratory acidosis

20

A client's serum values are Na, 142 mEq/L; Cl, 102 mEq/L; and CO_2, 18 mEq/L.

The anion gap is *_____ .

Is metabolic acidosis present? _____ Why? *_____

_____ .

21

Conditions associated with an anion gap that is greater than 16 mEq/L are diabetic ketoacidosis, lactic acidosis, poisoning, and renal failure.

Indicate which of the following conditions might apply to an anion gap of 25 mEq/L:

( ) a. Diabetic ketoacidosis

( ) b. Chronic obstructive pulmonary disease (COPD)

( ) c. Respiratory failure

( ) d. Renal failure

( ) e. Poisoning

( ) f. Lactic acidosis

22

When a client takes excessive amounts of baking soda or commercially prepared acid neutralizers to ease indigestion or stomach ulcer pain, what imbalance will most likely occur?

*_____ Why? *_____

▶ CLINICAL MANIFESTATIONS

When metabolic acidosis occurs, the central nervous system (CNS) is depressed and symptoms can include apathy, disorientation, weakness, and stupor. Deep, rapid breathing is a respiratory

---

19 a

20 142 − 120 = 22 mEq/L; yes; The anion gap is greater than 16 mEq/L.

21 a, d, e, f

22 metabolic alkalosis; There is excess alkali in the extracellular fluid.

compensatory mechanism for the purpose of decreasing acid content in the blood.

With metabolic alkalosis, excitability of the CNS occurs. These symptoms may include irritability, mental confusion, tetanylike symptoms, and hyperactive reflexes. Hypoventilation may occur, and it acts as a compensatory mechanism for metabolic alkalosis and conserves the hydrogen ions and carbonic acid.

Table 13-3 lists the clinical manifestations related to metabolic acidosis and alkalosis. Study the table and refer to it as needed when answering the questions.

23
With metabolic acidosis, the CNS is (depressed/excited)
_____ .

With metabolic alkalosis, the CNS is (depressed/excited)
_____ .

23 depressed; excited

Table 13-3

Clinical Manifestations of Metabolic Acidosis and Metabolic Alkalosis

Body Involvement	Metabolic Acidosis	Metabolic Alkalosis
CNS Abnormalities	Restlessness, apathy, weakness, disorientation, stupor, coma	Irritability, confusion, tetanylike symptoms, hyperactive reflexes
Respiratory Abnormalities	Kussmaul breathing: deep, rapid, vigorous breathing	Shallow breathing
Skin Changes	Flushing and warm skin	
Cardiac Abnormalities	Cardiac dysrhythmias, decrease in heart rate and cardiac output	
Gastrointestinal Abnormalities	Nausea, vomiting, abdominal pain	Vomiting with loss of chloride and potassium
Laboratory Values		
pH	<7.35	>7.45
HCO_3, BE	<24 mEq/L; <−2	>28 mEq/L; >+2
Serum CO_2	<22 mEq/L	>32 mEq/L

24

Indicate which of the following CNS abnormalities are associated with metabolic acidosis (M. Ac) and metabolic alkalosis (M. Al).

_____ a. Irritability
_____ b. Apathy
_____ c. Disorientation
_____ d. Tetanylike symptoms
_____ e. Hyperactive reflexes
_____ f. Stupor

24 a. M. Al; b. M. Ac; c. M. Ac; d. M. Al; e. M. Al; f. M. Ac

25

Metabolic acidosis results from a *_____ .
   In metabolic acidosis, the HCO_3 and BE are (decreased/ increased) _____ and the serum CO_2 is (decreased/ increased) _____ .

25 bicarbonate deficit or acid excess; decreased; decreased

26

With metabolic acidosis, the renal and respiratory mechanisms try to reestablish pH balance.
   Explain how the renal mechanism works to reestablish balance.
   *_____

   Explain how the respiratory mechanism works to reestablish balance.
   *_____

   When these two mechanisms fail, what happens to the plasma pH?
   *_____

26 The H^+ exchange with the Na^+ and thus H^+ is excreted.; As the result of the Kussmaul breathing, CO_2 is blown off, decreasing carbonic acid (H_2CO_3). It decreases.

27

Metabolic alkalosis results from a *_____ .
   In metabolic alkalosis, the HCO_3^- and BE are (decreased/ increased) _____ , and the serum CO_2 is (decreased/ increased) _____ .

27 bicarbonate excess; increased; increased

28

With metabolic alkalosis, the buffer, renal, and respiratory mechanisms try to reestablish balance. With the buffer mechanism, the excess bicarbonate reacts with buffer acid salts; thus, there is a decrease in bicarbonate ions in the extracellular fluid and an increase in the concentration of carbonic acid.

Explain how the renal mechanism works to reestablish balance.
* _____ .

Explain how the respiratory mechanism works to reestablish balance.
* _____ .

When these three mechanisms fail, what happens to the plasma pH?
* _____ .

28 H^+ is conserved and Na^+ and K^+ are excreted with HCO_3.; Pulmonary ventilation is decreased; therefore, CO_2 is retained, increasing H_2CO_3. It increases.

▶ CLINICAL MANAGEMENT

Figure 13-2 outlines the body's normal defense actions and various methods of treatment for restoring balance in metabolic acidosis and alkalosis. Study this figure carefully, with particular attention to the cause of each imbalance, the body's defense action, the pH of the urine as to whether it is acidic or alkaline, and the treatment for these imbalances. Refer to the figure whenever you find it necessary.

29
What is metabolic acidosis? * _____
  The urine is (acid/alkaline) _____ .
  What are the body's defense actions against it?
  a. * _____
  b. * _____

29 bicarbonate deficit or acid excess; acid; a. Lungs blow off CO_2 or acid.; b. Kidneys excrete acid or H^+ and conserve alkali.

30
Identify three treatment modalities for metabolic acidosis.
* _____

30 remove cause, administer IV alkali solution (e.g., $NaHCO_3$), and restore H_2O and electrolyte

31
What is metabolic alkalosis? * _____
  The urine is (acid/alkaline) _____ .
  What are the body's defense actions against it?
  a. * _____
  b. * _____

31 bicarbonate excess; alkaline; a. Breathing is suppressed.; b. Kidneys excrete alkali ions (e.g., HCO_3) and retain H^+ and nonbicarbonate ions.

32
Identify three treatment modalities for metabolic alkalosis.
* _____
_____

32 remove cause, administer IV chloride solution (e.g., NaCl), and replace K deficit

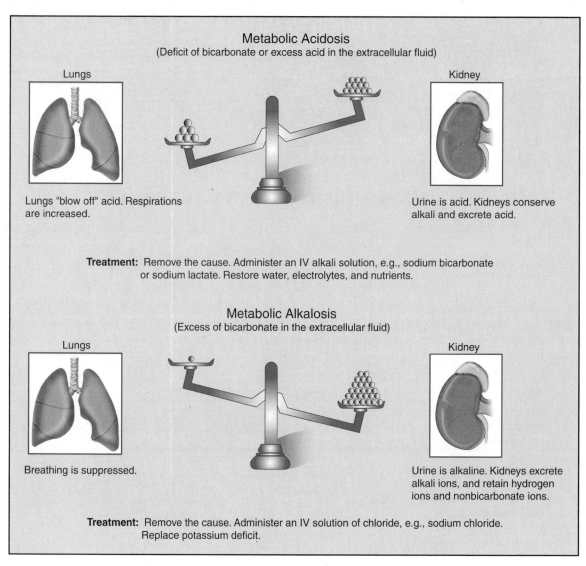

Metabolic Acidosis
(Deficit of bicarbonate or excess acid in the extracellular fluid)

Lungs

Kidney

Lungs "blow off" acid. Respirations are increased.

Urine is acid. Kidneys conserve alkali and excrete acid.

Treatment: Remove the cause. Administer an IV alkali solution, e.g., sodium bicarbonate or sodium lactate. Restore water, electrolytes, and nutrients.

Metabolic Alkalosis
(Excess of bicarbonate in the extracellular fluid)

Lungs

Kidney

Breathing is suppressed.

Urine is alkaline. Kidneys excrete alkali ions, and retain hydrogen ions and nonbicarbonate ions.

Treatment: Remove the cause. Administer an IV solution of chloride, e.g., sodium chloride. Replace potassium deficit.

Figure 13-2 Body's defense action and treatment for metabolic acidosis and alkalosis.

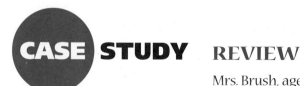

CASE STUDY REVIEW

Mrs. Brush, age 56, has chronic renal disease. Her respirations are rapid and vigorous. She is restless. Her urine pH is 4.5 and urine output is decreased. Her laboratory results are pH of 7.2, $PaCO_2$ of 38, and HCO_3 of 14.

ANSWER COLUMN

1. 7.35–7.45; 36–44 mm Hg; 24–28 mEq/L

2. metabolic acidosis

3. no

4. rapid, vigorous breathing and restlessness

5. b

6. rapid, vigorous breathing and excretion of acid urine

7. retention or buildup of nonvolatile acids

8. metabolic acidosis

9. yes; Lungs were blowing off CO_2 [$CO_2 + H_2O \rightarrow H_2CO_3$ (acid)].

10. Sodium bicarbonate restores the bicarbonate level in ECF.

1. The "normal" extracellular level of pH is _____ . The average range of $PaCO_2$ is *_____ , and that of HCO_3 is *_____ .

2. According to Mrs. Brush's pH and HCO_3, her acid-base imbalance is *_____ .

3. Is there effective respiratory compensation? _____

4. Identify two symptoms related to her acid-base imbalance. *_____

5. Identify the source of the imbalance.
   ( ) a. Bicarbonate excess
   ( ) b. Bicarbonate deficit
   ( ) c. Carbonic acid excess
   ( ) d. Carbonic acid deficit

6. How are Mrs. Brush's lungs and kidneys compensating for the acid-base imbalance? *_____ and _____ .

7. Her chronic renal disease (failure) can cause an acid-base imbalance due to *_____ .

Later Mrs. Brush's pH is 7.34, $PaCO_2$ is 31, and HCO_3 is 20. Fluid with sodium bicarbonate was given IV. As a nurse, you should reassess her laboratory findings.

8. Her pH and HCO_3 indicate *_____ .

9. Is there effective respiratory compensation? _____ Explain how. *_____ _____

10. Why are IV fluids with sodium bicarbonate administered? *_____

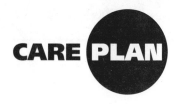

Client Management: Metabolic Acidosis and Metabolic Alkalosis

Assessment Factors

▶ Obtain a client history of clinical problems that are occurring. Recognize the client's health problems that are associated with metabolic acidosis, i.e., starvation, severe or chronic diarrhea, kidney failure, diabetic ketoacidosis, severe infection, trauma, and shock, and with metabolic alkalosis, i.e., vomiting, gastric suction, peptic ulcer, and electrolyte imbalance (hypokalemia, hypochloremia).

▶ Check the arterial bicarbonate and serum CO_2 levels for metabolic acid-base imbalance. Decreased HCO_3 (<24 mEq/L) and serum CO_2 (<22 mEq/L) are indicative of metabolic acidosis, and increased HCO_3 (>28 mEq/L) and serum CO_2 (>32 mEq/L) are indicative of metabolic alkalosis.

▶ Obtain baseline vital signs for comparison with future vital signs. Note if there are any cardiac dysrhythmias and/or bradycardia that may result from a severe acidotic state. Check respirations for Kussmaul breathing. This is a sign of metabolic acidosis; also may be due to diabetic ketoacidosis.

▶ Check laboratory results, especially blood sugar and electrolytes.

Metabolic Acidosis
Diagnosis 1

Altered nutrition: less than body requirements, related to starvation, diabetic ketoacidosis.

Interventions and Rationale

1. Monitor dietary intake and report inadequate nutrient and fluid intake.

2. Check the laboratory results regarding electrolytes, blood sugar, and arterial blood gases (ABGs). Some abnormal findings associated with metabolic acidosis are hyperkalemia, decreased serum CO_2, elevated blood sugar (slightly elevated with trauma and shock and highly elevated with uncontrolled diabetes mellitus), and decreased arterial bicarbonate level and pH (HCO_3 <24 mEq/L and pH <7.35).

3. Monitor vital signs. Report the presence of Kussmaul respirations that relate to diabetic ketoacidosis or severe shock. Compare results of vital signs with baseline findings.

4. Monitor signs and symptoms related to metabolic acidosis, i.e., CNS depression (apathy, restlessness, weakness, disorientation, stupor); deep, rapid, vigorous breathing (Kussmaul respirations); and flushing of the skin (vasodilation resulting from sympathetic nervous system depression).

5. Administer adequate fluid replacement with sodium bicarbonate as prescribed by the physician to correct severe acidotic state.

Diagnosis 2

Decreased cardiac output related to severe metabolic acidotic state.

Interventions and Rationale

1. Monitor the heart rate closely and note any cardiac dysrhythmia. During severe acidosis, the heart rate decreases and dysrhythmias can occur, causing a decrease in cardiac output.

2. Provide comfort and alleviate anxiety when possible.

Diagnosis 3

Risk for injury related to disorientation, weakness, and stupor.

Interventions and Rationale

1. Monitor client's sensorium and note changes, i.e., increased disorientation and stupor.

2. Provide safety measures such as bedside rails.

3. Assist the client in meeting physical needs.

Metabolic Alkalosis
Diagnosis 1

Fluid volume deficit related to vomiting or nasogastric suctioning.

Interventions and Rationale

1. Monitor fluid intake and output. Record the amount of fluid loss via vomiting and gastric suctioning. Hydrogen and

chloride are lost with the gastric secretions, which increases the pH level, causing metabolic alkalosis.

2. Administer IV fluids as ordered; fluids should contain 0.45–0.9% sodium chloride (normal saline). Encourage oral fluids if able to retain and as prescribed by the physician.

3. Monitor the serum electrolytes. If the serum chloride is decreased and the serum CO_2 is decreased, an alkalotic state is present.

4. Monitor vital signs. Note if the respirations remain shallow and slow.

5. Report if the client is consuming large quantities of acid neutralizers that contain bicarbonate compounds such as Bromo-Seltzer.

6. Monitor signs and symptoms of metabolic alkalosis, i.e., CNS excitability (tetanylike symptoms, irritability, confusion, hyperactive reflexes) and shallow breathing.

Diagnosis 2

Risk for injury related to CNS excitability secondary to metabolic alkalosis.

Interventions and Rationale

1. Provide safety measures while the client is confused and irritable, such as bedside rails and assistance with basic needs.

2. Monitor the client's state of CNS excitability. Report tetany-like symptoms.

Evaluation/Outcome

1. Evaluate that the cause of metabolic acidosis or metabolic alkalosis has been corrected or controlled.

2. Evaluate the therapeutic effect in correcting metabolic acidosis or metabolic alkalosis. Client's ABGs are returning to or have returned to normal range.

3. Remain free of signs and symptoms of metabolic acidosis and metabolic alkalosis; vital signs returned to normal range, especially respiration.

4. Client is able to perform activities of daily living.

5. Maintain follow-up appointments.

6. Maintain a support system for the client.

Respiratory Acidosis and Alkalosis

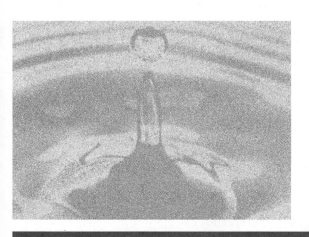

▶ INTRODUCTION

Two types of respiratory acid-base imbalance are *respiratory acidosis* and *respiratory alkalosis*. Respiratory acidosis is mainly due to acid excess, particularly carbonic acid (H_2CO_3). The major problem causing respiratory acidosis is carbon dioxide (CO_2) retention due to a respiratory disorder. With respiratory alkalosis, there is a bicarbonate deficit. The result of respiratory alkalosis is mostly due to a loss of carbonic acid. Blowing off of CO_2 can be due to hysteria (overbreathing), excess exercise, etc. Respiratory acidosis and respiratory alkalosis are discussed separately in this chapter.

1

The pH of arterial blood gases (ABGs) can determine the presence of _____ and _____ .

1   acidosis; alkalosis

2

The respiratory component from the ABGs for determining respiratory acidosis and alkalosis is _____ .

2   $PaCO_2$

Acid-base balance is maintained by 1 part of acid and 20 parts of base. Figure 14-1 demonstrates the normal acid-base balance. The blood tests pH and $PaCO_2$ are utilized in determining respiratory acidosis and alkalosis.

3

With respiratory acidosis, the pH is _____ .
With respiratory alkalosis, the pH is _____ .

3   decreased; increased

4   increased; decreased; With acidosis, the pH is always decreased and with alkalosis, it is increased. In respiratory acidosis, the CO_2 is conserved; mixes with $H_2O = H_2CO_3$. The $PaCO_2$ would be increased.

4

In respiratory acidosis, the $PaCO_2$ is _____ .
In respiratory alkalosis, the $PaCO_2$ is _____ .
Explain why the pH and $PaCO_2$ values differ. *_____

_____

▶ PATHOPHYSIOLOGY

5

Respiratory acidosis is characterized by a(n) (increase/decrease) _____ of carbon dioxide (CO_2) and carbonic acid ($CO_2 + H_2O \rightarrow H_2CO_3$) concentration in the extracellular fluid.
   The pH is (<7.35/>7.45) _____ .

5   increase; <7.35

6

Respiratory alkalosis is characterized by a decrease in the *_____ concentration in the extracellular fluid. The pH is _____ .

6   carbonic acid; >7.45

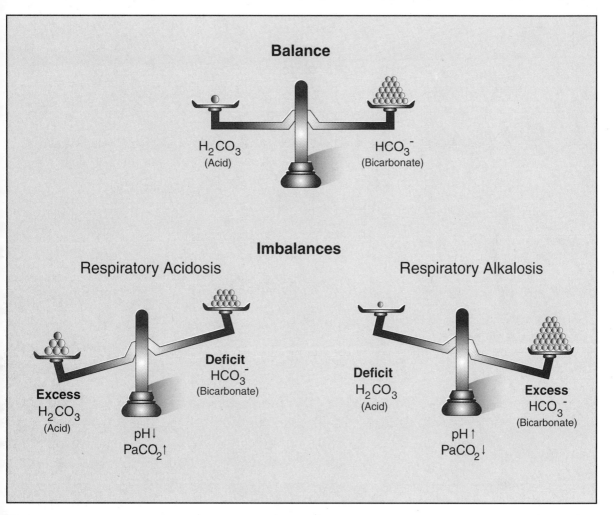

Figure 14-1 Acid-base balance and respiratory imbalances.

7

With respiratory acidosis, the $PaCO_2$ is _____ mm Hg.
With respiratory alkalosis, the $PaCO_2$ is _____ mm Hg.

7 >45; <35

▶ ETIOLOGY

The causes of respiratory acidosis and alkalosis are described in Tables 14-1 and 14-2. Study the tables and then proceed to the questions. Refer to the tables as needed.

Table 14-1

Causes of Respiratory Acidosis

Etiology	Rationale
CNS Depressants Drugs: narcotics [morphine, meperidine (Demerol)], anesthetics, barbiturates	These drugs depress the respiratory center in the medulla, causing retention of CO_2 (carbon dioxide), which results in hypercapnia (increased partial pressure of CO_2 in the blood).
Pulmonary Abnormalities Chronic obstructive pulmonary disease (COPD: emphysema, severe asthma)	Inadequate exchange of gases in the lungs due to a decreased surface area for aeration causes retention of CO_2 in the blood.
Pneumonia, pulmonary edema	Airway obstruction inhibits effective gas exchanges, resulting in a retention of CO_2.
Poliomyelitis, Guillain-Barré syndrome, chest injuries	Weakness of the respiratory muscles decreases the excretion of CO_2, thus increasing carbonic acid concentration.

Table 14-2

Causes of Respiratory Alkalosis

Etiology	Rationale
Hyperventilation Psychologic effects: anxiety, hysteria, overbreathing Pain Fever Brain tumors, meningitis, encephalitis Early salicylate poisoning Hyperthyroidism	Excessive blowing off of CO_2 through the lungs results in hypocapnia (decreased partial pressure of CO_2 in the blood). Overstimulation of the respiratory center in the medulla results in hyperventilation.

8

It causes a retention of CO_2 in the blood: $H_2O + CO_2 \rightarrow H_2CO_3$.

8

Explain how an inadequate exchange of gases in the lungs can cause respiratory acidosis. *_____

_____

9

Narcotics, sedatives, chest injuries, respiratory distress syndrome, pneumonia, and pulmonary edema can cause acute respiratory acidosis (ARA). ARA results from the rapidly increasing CO_2 level and retention of CO_2 in the blood.

With chronic obstructive pulmonary disease (COPD), the body compensates for CO_2 accumulation by excreting excess hydrogen ions and conserving the bicarbonate ion. The type of respiratory acidosis that occurs with COPD is (acute/chronic)

_____ .

9 chronic

10 These conditions weaken the respiratory muscles, thus inhibiting CO_2 excretion.

10

Explain how poliomyelitis and Guillain-Barré syndrome can cause CO_2 retention. *_____

_____

11

Respiratory alkalosis occurs as the result of a carbonic acid deficit due to *_____

_____ .

The kidneys compensate for the alkalotic state by (excreting/retaining) _____ bicarbonate ions in the plasma to maintain the bicarbonate-to-carbonic-acid ratio.

11 blowing off of CO_2, which results in a lack of H_2CO_3, excreting

12

Indicate which of the following conditions can cause respiratory alkalosis:

_____ a. Early aspirin toxicity
_____ b. Emphysema
_____ c. Anxiety
_____ d. Encephalitis
_____ e. Narcotics
_____ f. Pneumonia
_____ g. Pain and fever

12 a, c, d, g

13 respiratory alkalosis ↓ $PaCO_2$, carbonic acid deficit; respiratory acidosis ↑ $PaCO_2$, carbonic acid excess

13
Explain the difference between respiratory alkalosis and respiratory acidosis according to $PaCO_2$ and carbonic acid levels.
*_____

_____

▶ CLINICAL APPLICATIONS

14 chronic obstructive pulmonary disease

14
For 25 years your client has been a heavy smoker. The client has been diagnosed as having COPD, which stands for
*_____ .

15 chronic

15
COPD frequently causes (acute/chronic) _____ respiratory acidosis.

16 respiratory acidosis; Yes, there is metabolic compensation (bicarbonate is conserved).

16
The client's blood gases are pH 7.21, $PaCO_2$ 98 mm Hg, and HCO_3 40 mEq/L. The type of acid-base imbalance is
*_____ . Is there metabolic (renal) compensation?
*_____ . (For acid-base compensation, see Chapter 12.)

17 Encourage the client to breathe slowly and deeply. There is a lack of CO_2, so giving CO_2 (e.g., rebreathing CO_2 from a paper bag) stimulates the lungs to breathe more deeply and then more slowly.

17
Frequently, with respiratory alkalosis, you notice that sufferers are very apprehensive and anxious. They hyperventilate to overcome their anxiety. Many times this occurs for a psychologic reason, e.g., giving a speech for the first time or fear of failing an exam. How do you think you might help with respiratory compensation for this imbalance? *_____

_____

▶ CLINICAL MANIFESTATIONS

With respiratory acidosis, an increase in hypercapnia causes dyspnea (difficulty in breathing), an increased pulse rate, and an elevated blood pressure. The skin may be warm and flushed due to vasodilation from the increased CO_2 concentration.

Table 14-3

Clinical Manifestations of Respiratory Acidosis and Respiratory Alkalosis

Body Involvement	Respiratory Acidosis	Respiratory Alkalosis
Cardiopulmonary Abnormalities	Dyspnea Tachycardia Blood pressure	Rapid, shallow breathing Palpitations
CNS Abnormalities	Disorientation Depression, paranoia Weakness Stupor (later)	Tetany symptoms: numbness and tingling of fingers and toes, positive Chvostek and Trousseau signs Hyperactive reflexes Vertigo (dizziness) Unconsciousness (later)
Skin	Flushed and warm	Sweating may occur
Laboratory Values pH	<7.35 (when compensatory mechanisms fail)	>7.45 (when compensatory mechanisms fail)
$PaCO_2$	>45 mm Hg	<35 mm Hg

When respiratory alkalosis occurs, there is CNS hyperexcitability and a decrease in cerebral blood flow. Tetanylike symptoms and dizziness frequently result.

Table 14-3 lists the clinical manifestations related to respiratory acidosis and alkalosis. Study the table carefully. Refer to the table as needed when answering the questions.

18

Respiratory patterns of breathing are clues to the type of respiratory acid-base imbalance.

The characteristic breathing pattern associated with respiratory acidosis is _____ , and for respiratory alkalosis, the breathing pattern is *_____

_____ .

18 dyspnea (labored or
difficulty in breathing);
rapid, shallow breathing
(hyperventilating or
overbreathing)

19

Indicate which CNS abnormalities are associated with respiratory acidosis (R. Ac) and respiratory alkalosis (R. Al).

_____ a. Tetanylike symptoms
_____ b. Disorientation
_____ c. Dizziness or lightheadedness
_____ d. Depression, paranoia
_____ e. Hyperactive reflexes
_____ f. Positive Chvostek's sign

20
Respiratory acidosis results from a(n) (deficit/excess) _____ of carbonic acid.
    The PaCO$_2$ is * _____ .

21
With respiratory acidosis, the buffer, renal, and respiratory mechanisms try to reestablish balance. As a result of the chloride shift, bicarbonate ions are released to neutralize carbonic acid excess.
    With an increased CO$_2$, explain how the respiratory mechanism works to compensate for this imbalance. * _____

_____
    Explain how the renal mechanism works to compensate for this imbalance.
    a. * _____
    b. * _____
    When these mechanisms fail, what happens to the blood pH?
    * _____

22
Respiratory alkalosis results from a(n) (deficit/excess) _____ of carbonic acid.
    The PaCO$_2$ is * _____ .

23
The buffer mechanism produces more organic acids, in respiratory alkalosis, which react with the excess bicarbonate ions.
    How do you think the renal mechanism works to compensate for this imbalance? * _____
    When these mechanisms fail, what happens to the blood pH?
    * _____

---

19 a. R. Al; b. R. Ac; c. R. Al; d. R. Ac; e. R. Al; f. R. Al

20 excess; greater than (>) 45 mm Hg

21 CO$_2$ stimulates the respiratory center to increase the rate and depth of respiration. CO$_2$ is blown off with water. H$_2$O + CO$_2$ → H$_2$CO$_3$. (However, usually in respiratory acidosis, the respiratory system is affected and not able to accomplish this.); a. the H$^+$ exchanges with Na$^+$, and the Na$^+$ is reabsorbed with the HCO$_3$; b. an increased secretion of ammonium chloride; It is decreased.

22 deficit; <35 mm Hg

23 an increased HCO$_3$ excretion and a H$^+$ retention; It increases.

▶ CLINICAL MANAGEMENT

Figure 14-2 outlines the body's normal defense actions and various methods of treatment for restoring balance in respiratory acidosis and alkalosis. Study the figure carefully, with particular attention to the factors causing the acid-base imbalances, the pH of the urine as to whether it is acid or alkaline, and the treatment for these imbalances. Refer to the figure as needed.

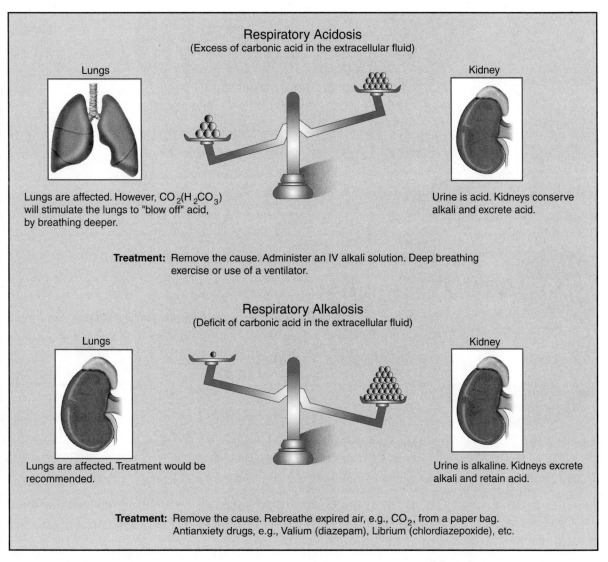

Respiratory Acidosis
(Excess of carbonic acid in the extracellular fluid)

Lungs

Kidney

Lungs are affected. However, $CO_2(H_2CO_3)$ will stimulate the lungs to "blow off" acid, by breathing deeper.

Urine is acid. Kidneys conserve alkali and excrete acid.

Treatment: Remove the cause. Administer an IV alkali solution. Deep breathing exercise or use of a ventilator.

Respiratory Alkalosis
(Deficit of carbonic acid in the extracellular fluid)

Lungs

Kidney

Lungs are affected. Treatment would be recommended.

Urine is alkaline. Kidneys excrete alkali and retain acid.

Treatment: Remove the cause. Rebreathe expired air, e.g., CO_2, from a paper bag. Antianxiety drugs, e.g., Valium (diazepam), Librium (chlordiazepoxide), etc.

Figure 14-2 Body's defense action and treatment for respiratory acidosis and respiratory alkalosis.

24 carbonic acid excess; acidic;
a. Excess CO_2 accumulation
stimulates the lung to
blow off CO_2 or acid;
b. Kidneys conserve alkali
and excrete H^+ or acid
urine.

25 removal of cause, deep
breathing exercise, airway
management, and
ventilator

26 carbonic acid deficit;
alkaline; Kidneys excrete
alkaline HCO_3 and retain
acid, H^+.

27 removal of cause,
rebreathing expired air,
and antianxiety drugs, e.g.,
chlordiazepoxide (Librium)
and diazepam (Valium)

24
What is the basic cause of respiratory acidosis? *_____
    The urine is (acidic/alkaline) _____ .
What are the body's defense actions (lung and kidney)?
    a. *_____
    b. *_____

25
Identify three treatment modalities for respiratory acidosis.
*_____

26
What is the basic cause of respiratory alkalosis? *_____
    The urine is (acidic/alkaline) _____ .
    Identify the body's defense action against it? *_____
_____

27
Identify three treatment modalities for respiratory alkalosis.
*_____
_____

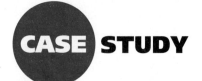

CASE STUDY REVIEW

Mr. Swift, age 46, has a history of respiratory problems. His latest
problem was pneumonia. He smokes two or three packs of ciga-
rettes a day. His condition indicates an acid-base imbalance.

**ANSWER
COLUMN**

1. hydrogen

2. hyperventilating;
hypoventilating

3. hydrogen; bicarbonate;
bicarbonate; hydrogen

1. The acidity or alkalinity of a solution depends on the concentration of the (hydrogen/bicarbonate) _____ ions.

2. With respiratory regulation, for acid-base balance the lungs
   blow off or conserve CO_2 by _____ or _____ .

3. The kidney maintains the acid-base balance by excreting
   _____ or _____ and by retaining _____ or
   _____ .

4. lungs

5. excess; deficit

6. respiratory acidosis
7. no
8. Hypoventilating. It causes CO_2 retention—respiratory acidosis.
9. Yes. If compensation was not present, the pH would be greatly decreased, causing more H^+ concentration.
10. *Metabolic Acidosis*
pH↓
$PaCO_2$ —
HCO_3 or serum CO_2↓
Metabolic Alkalosis
pH↑
$PaCO_2$ —
HCO_3 or serum CO_2↑
Respiratory Acidosis
pH↓
$PaCO_2$ ↑
HCO_3 or serum CO_2 —
Respiratory Alkalosis
pH↑
$PaCO_2$↓
HCO_3 or serum CO_2 —

4. Which acts faster in regulating or correcting acid-base imbalance (kidneys/lungs)? _____

5. Respiratory acidosis has a carbonic acid (excess/deficit) _____ , whereas respiratory alkalosis has a carbonic acid (excess/deficit) _____ .

Mr. Swift's blood gases are a pH of 7.29, $PaCO_2$ of 54, and HCO_3 of 25.

6. Mr. Swift's pH and $PaCO_2$ indicate * _____ .

7. Is there any renal (metabolic) compensation? _____

Two days later Mr. Swift's blood gases had a pH of 7.34, $PaCO_2$ of 62, and HCO_3 of 30.

8. Mr. Swift has been (hyperventilating/hypoventilating)? _____ .

9. Is there metabolic (renal) compensation? _____ .

10. Complete the following chart on acid-base imbalance as to pH, $PaCO_2$, and HCO_3. Use the arrow pointed upward for increase, the arrow pointed downward for decrease, and — for not involved (except with compensation).

Metabolic Acidosis	*Metabolic Alkalosis*
pH	pH
$PaCO_2$	$PaCO_2$
HCO_3 or serum CO_2	HCO_3 or serum CO_2
Respiratory Acidosis	*Respiratory Alkalosis*
pH	pH
$PaCO_2$	$PaCO_2$
HCO_3 or serum CO_2	HCO_3 or serum CO_2

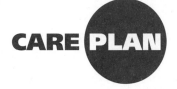

Client Management: Respiratory Acidosis and Respiratory Alkalosis

Assessment Factors

▶ Obtain a client history of clinical problems. Recognize the client's health problems that are associated with respiratory acidosis, i.e., CNS depressant drugs (narcotics, sedatives, anesthetics), pneumonia, pulmonary edema, and chronic obstructive pulmonary (lung) disease (COPD or COLD) such as emphysema, chronic bronchitis, bronchiectasis, and severe asthma, and those associated with respiratory alkalosis, i.e., anxiety, hysteria, fever, severe infection, aspirin toxicity, and deliberate over-breathing.

▶ Check for signs and symptoms of respiratory acidosis, i.e., dyspnea, tachycardia, disorientation, weakness, stupor, and flushed and warm skin, and signs and symptoms related to respiratory alkalosis, i.e., apprehension, rapid, shallow breathing, palpitations, tetanylike symptoms such as numbness and tingling of the toes and fingers, hyperactive reflexes, and dizziness.

▶ Obtain vital signs for a baseline record to compare with future vital signs.

▶ Check arterial blood gas report, particularly the $PaCO_2$ result. An increased $PaCO_2$ that exceeds 45 mm Hg is indicative of respiratory acidosis and a decreased $PaCO_2$ of less than 35 mm Hg is indicative of respiratory alkalosis. Report abnormal findings.

Respiratory Acidosis
Diagnosis 1

Impaired gas exchange related to inadequate ventilation (hypoventilation) secondary to COPD.

Interventions and Rationale

1. Monitor client's respiratory status for changes in respiratory rate, distress, and breathing pattern.

2. Monitor arterial blood gases (ABGs), especially the pH, $PaCO_2$, and HCO_3. A pH of less than 7.35 indicates acidosis and a $PaCO_2$ of greater than 45 mm Hg indicates respiratory acidosis. If the bicarbonate level (HCO_3) is greater than 28 mEq/L, then there is metabolic (renal) compensation. With compensation, the respiratory acidotic state is most likely to be chronic rather than acute.

3. Auscultate breath sounds periodically to determine wheezing, rhonchi, or crackles (rales) that indicate poor gas exchange.

4. Monitor vital signs for tachycardia or cardiac dysrhythmias associated with hypercapnia and hypoxemia (oxygen deficit in the blood).

5. Monitor mechanical ventilator use for a client having respiratory distress due to impaired gas exchange.

6. Maintain adequate airway clearance by suctioning, chest physical therapy, etc., as needed.

Diagnosis 2

Ineffective airway clearance related to thick bronchial secretions and/or bronchial spasms.

Interventions and Rationale

1. Assist client with self-care.

2. Encourage client to deep breathe and cough. This helps to eliminate bronchial secretions and improve gas exchange.

3. Assist the client with use of an inhaler containing a bronchodilator drug. Explain the use and frequency of medications.

4. Administer chest clapping on COPD clients or others to break up mucous plugs and secretions in the alveoli.

5. Teach breathing exercises and postural drainage to clients with chronic obstructive pulmonary disease (COPD). Mucous secretions are trapped in overextended alveoli (air sacs), and breathing exercises and postural drainage help to remove secretions and restore gas exchange (ventilation).

6. Monitor oxygen administration. Too high a concentration of oxygen intake such as greater than 3 liters may depress respirations and increase the severity of the respiratory acidosis. Hypercapnia (increased partial pressure of carbon dioxide) stimulates the respiratory center in the brain; however, after the $PaCO_2$ level becomes highly elevated, it is no longer a stimulus. The hypoxemia continues to stimulate the respiratory center. Too much oxygen inhibits the respiratory stimulus effect.

7. Encourage the client to increase fluid intake in order to decrease tenacity of the secretions.

Diagnosis 3

Risk for injury related to hypoxemia and hypercapnia.

Interventions and Rationale

1. Monitor the client's state of sensorium for signs of disorientation due to a lack of oxygen to the brain.

2. Provide safety measures, such as bedside rails when the client is disoriented or in a stuporous state.

Diagnosis 4

Activity intolerance related to dyspnea secondary to poor gas exchange.

Interventions and Rationale

1. Assist the client with activities of daily living.
2. Plan daily activities that follow his or her breathing exercises as indicated by the physician.
3. Encourage the client to participate in a pulmonary rehabilitation program.

Other Diagnoses to Consider

Ineffective breathing pattern related to inadequate ventilation.

Respiratory Alkalosis
Diagnosis 1

Anxiety related to hyperventilation secondary to behaviorial problems and stressful situations.

Interventions and Rationale

1. Encourage the client who is overanxious and hyperventilating to take deep breaths and breathe slowly. Proper breathing prevents respiratory alkalosis.
2. Listen to client who is emotionally distressed. Encourage the client to seek professional help for psychologic problems.

Diagnosis 2

Ineffective breathing pattern related to hyperventilation and anxiety.

Interventions and Rationale

1. Demonstrate a slow, relaxed breathing pattern to decrease overbreathing, which causes respiratory alkalosis.
2. Administer a sedative as prescribed to relax client and restore a normal breathing pattern.

Diagnosis 3

Risk for injury related to dizziness, lightheadedness, and syncope or unconsciousness.

Interventions and Rationale

1. Instruct the client to be seated when feeling dizzy or light-headed.
2. Remove objects that may harm the client if dizziness leads to syncope (fainting).
3. Provide side rails if unconsciousness occurs due to severe respiratory alkalosis.

Evaluation/Outcome

1. Evaluate that the cause of respiratory acidosis or respiratory alkalosis is corrected or is controlled. Client's ABGs are returning to or have returned to normal ranges.
2. Remain free of signs and symptoms of respiratory acidosis or respiratory alkalosis; vital signs are within normal ranges.
3. Client exhibits a patent airway and breath sounds have improved.
4. Ambulates with little to no assistance and without breathlessness.
5. Document compliance with prescribed drug therapy and medical regimen.
6. Maintain a support system for the client.
7. Keep scheduled follow-up appointments.

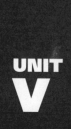

UNIT V

INTRAVENOUS THERAPY

▶ INTRODUCTION

This unit consists of three chapters that discuss general purposes for intravenous (IV) therapy, selected IV therapy solutions, the classification of IV fluids including transfusion of blood and blood products, calculation of prescribed flow rates for IV infusions, types of IV infusion devices, and total parenteral nutrition (TPN). The assessment of clients receiving IV therapy, diagnoses associated with IV therapy, and important interventions with rationale are summarized at the end of each chapter. Clinical applications throughout the chapter allow students to apply selected knowledge and skills with specific clients receiving IV therapies.

Refer to the text as needed.

An asterisk (*) indicates a multiple-word answer. The meaning of the following symbols are: ↑ increased, ↓ decreased, > greater than, < less than.

Intravenous Solutions

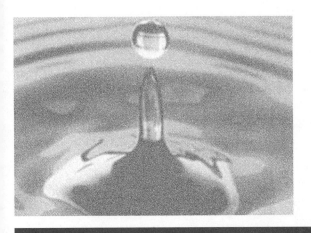

OBJECTIVES

Upon completion of this chapter, the reader should be able to:

● Discuss the implications for the selection of each type of IV solution.

● List four important considerations associated with the transfusion of blood and blood components.

● List selected diagnoses and corresponding clinical interventions for clients receiving IV solutions.

▶ INTRODUCTION

This chapter discusses the basic classifications of IV solutions in terms of their osmolality, implications for use, special considerations associated with the transfusion of blood and blood products, and selected health care considerations for clients receiving IV solutions. Many of the solutions used for IV therapy are produced commercially to meet client needs associated with specific types of fluid and electrolyte or acid-base imbalances. IV solutions are classified as being hypotonic, isotonic, or hypertonic. The osmolality of a solution is determined by the concentration or the number of particles (osmols) suspended in the solution. The greater the number of particles in the solution, the higher the osmolality of the solution.

Tables 15–1 and 15–2 list commonly used IV solutions, their tonicity, the types of particles suspended in the solution, and the rationale for their selection. Study these tables carefully before proceeding to the questions that follow them. Feel free to refer to the tables as often as necessary to complete each question. Remember: hypo-osmolar solutions have less than 240 mOsm/L, iso-osmolar solutions have approximately 240–340 mOsm/L, and hyperosmolar solutions have greater than 340 mOsm/L.

▶ BASIC CLASSIFICATIONS OF IV SOLUTIONS

The five basic classifications of IV solutions are (1) sources of free water and calories, (2) crystalloids, (3) colloids, (4) blood and blood components, and (5) hypertonic-hyperosmolar solutions.

ANSWER COLUMN

1 source of free water and calories, crystalloids, colloids, blood and blood components, and hypertonic-hyperosmolar solutions

1

The five basic classifications of intravenous solutions are

*_____

_____ .

Table 15-1

Protein and Plasma Solutions Commonly Used in IV Therapy

Solution Classifications	Osmolality (Tonicity)	Caloric Units	mEq/L			Miscellaneous	Rationale for Use of Selected IV Fluids
			Na$^+$	K$^+$	Cl$^+$		
Protein Solutions							
Aminosyn RF 5.2%	Hyper	175	0	5.4	0	Amino acids	Provides protein and fluid for the body and promotes wound healing.
Aminosyn II 3.5% with dextrose 5%	Hyper	345	18	0	—	Amino acids	Provides protein, calories, and fluid; especially helpful for clients who are elderly and malnourished and for clients with hypoproteinemia due to other causes. Not to be used in severe liver damage.
Plasma Expander							
Dextran 40 10% in normal saline (0.9%) or 5% dextrose in water (500-mL bottle)	Iso						Dextran is a colloidal solution used to increase plasma volume. Dextran 40 is a short-lived plasma volume expander (4–6 h). It is useful in early shock by helping to correct hypovolemia, increasing arterial pressure, pulse pressure, and cardiac output. It improves microcirculation by reducing red blood cell (RBC) aggregation in the capillaries (increases small-vessel perfusion). *Caution:* It should not be used for clients who are severely dehydrated, have renal disease, have thrombocytopenia, or are actively hemorrhaging.
Dextran 70 6% in normal saline (0.9%)	Iso						Dextran 70 is a long-lived plasma volume expander (20 h). It is useful for shock or impending shock due to hemorrhage, surgery, or burns. It can interfere with platelet function causing prolonged bleeding. Blood for type and cross-match should be drawn before starting dextran because dextran coats RBCs, making the blood type difficult to obtain. Overhydration may occur if oliguria or heart failure is present. Allergic reactions can occur, i.e., nausea, vomiting, dyspnea, wheezing, hypotension.

Table 15-2

Hydrating and Replacement Solutions Commonly Used in IV Therapy

Solution	Osmolality (Tonicity)	Caloric Units	mEq/L							Rationale for Use of Selected IV Fluids
			Na^+	K^+	Ca^{2+}	Cl	Lactate	Mg^{2+}	P	
Hydrating Solution										
Sodium chloride 0.45%	Hypo	—	77	—	—	77	—	—		Useful for daily maintenance of body fluid but not for replacement therapy. It is helpful for establishing renal function.
Dextrose 2.5% in 0.45% saline	Iso	85	77	—	—	77	—	—		Helpful in establishing renal function/urine output.
Dextrose 5% in 0.2% saline	Iso	170	38	—	—	38	—	—		Useful for daily maintenance of body fluids when Na and Cl replacement therapy is not required.
Dextrose 5% in 0.33% saline	Hyper	170	51	—	—	51	—	—		Useful for daily maintenance of body fluids and nutrition and for treating fluid volume deficits.
Dextrose 5% in 0.45% saline	Hyper	170	77	—	—	77	—	—		
Dextrose 5% in water (50 g) (dextrose 10% is occasionally used)	Iso	170	—	—	—	—	—	—		Helpful in rehydration and elimination. May cause urinary sodium loss. Good vehicle for IV potassium.
Replacement Solutions										
Dextrose 5% in saline 0.9%	Hyper	170	154	—	—	154	—	—		Replacement of fluid, sodium, chloride, and calories.
Dextrose 10% in saline 0.9%	Hyper	340	154	—	—	154	—	—		Replacement of fluid, sodium, chloride, and calories.
Lactated Ringer's	Iso	0	130	4	3	109	28	—		This solution resembles the electrolyte composition of normal blood serum and plasma. The amount of potassium available is not sufficient for the body's daily potassium requirement.

Solution	Tonicity									Comments
Dextrose 5% in lactated Ringer's solution	Hyper	180	130	4	3	109	28	—	—	Same contents as lactated Ringer's plus calories.
Ringer's solution	Iso	—	147	4	5	156	—	—	—	Does not contain lactate, which can be harmful to people who lack enzymes essential to metabolize lactic acid.
Dextrose 5% Ringer's solution	Hyper	170	147	4	4	156	—	—	—	Same contents as Ringer's solution plus calories.
M/6 sodium lactate	Iso	56	167	—	—	—	167	—	—	Supplies sodium without chloride. Lactate has some caloric value and is metabolized into CO_2 for excretion or increases bicarbonate in alkalosis.
Normal saline (0.9%)	Iso	—	154	—	—	154	—	—	—	Restores extracellular fluid volume and replaces sodium chloride deficit.
Hyperosmolar saline 3% and 5% NaCl	Hyper	—	856	—	—	856	—	—	—	Helpful in hyponatremia by raising Na osmolality of the blood. Helpful in eliminating intracellular fluid excess.
Ionosol B with dextrose 5%	Hyper	178	57	25	—	49	25	5	7	Useful in treating clients requiring polyionic parenteral replacement, e.g., alkalosis due to vomiting, diabetic acidosis, fluid losses due to burns, and postoperative fluid volume deficits.
Ionosol D-CM with dextrose 5%	Hyper	186	138	12	5	108	50	3	—	Useful for electrolyte replacement of duodenal fluid losses related to intestinal suction and biliary or pancreatic drainage. Helps to correct mild acidosis.

Source: Solution chart reviewed by Abbott Laboratories Clinical Research Associate and Baxter Laboratories Clinical Information Manager. Selected portions from *Wall Chart, Intravenous and Other Solutions* by Abbott Laboratories, October 1968, Chicago: Author; *Guide to Fluid Therapy* by Travenol Laboratories, Inc., 1981, Deerfield, IN: Author; *Fluid and Electrolyte Balance: Nursing Considerations* (3rd ed.) by N. Methany, 1996, Philadelphia: Saunders; *A Primer of Water, Electrolyte and Acid-Base Syndromes* (8th ed.), Philadelphia: Davis.

2

The most commonly used free water and caloric solution is the isotonic solution of dextrose 5% and water (D_5W). When the glucose in D_5W is metabolized, free water is available to the body. Solutions used to provide free water and calories are often referred to as hydrating solutions.

Dextrose 5% in water is an example of an (isotonic/hypotonic/hypertonic) _____ solution. It provides the client with
* _____ .

Commonly used crystalloid solutions include sodium chloride and lactated Ringer's (or Ringer's lactate). Crystalloid solutions can be isotonic (approximately equal to the sodium chloride concentration of blood, which is 0.9%), hypotonic (less than the sodium chloride concentration of blood), and hypertonic (greater than the sodium chloride concentration of blood). Sodium chloride 0.9% or normal physiologic saline (NS) is an example of an isotonic saline solution. Hypotonic solutions include 0.2% or ¼ NS, 0.33% or ⅓ NS, and 0.45% or ½ NS. Hypertonic saline solutions include 3 and 5% sodium chloride. Saline solutions may or may not include dextrose.

3

Crystalloid solutions can be (isotonic/hypotonic/hypertonic)
* _____ in nature.

Two common examples of isotonic crystalloid solutions are
* _____ .

Identify three examples of hypotonic crystalloid solutions.
* _____

Identify two examples of hypertonic crystalloid solutions.
* _____

Saline solutions (may/may not) * _____ include dextrose.

Colloids are frequently called volume expanders or plasma expanders; they physiologically function like plasma proteins in blood by maintaining oncotic pressure. Commonly used colloids include albumin, dextran, Plasmanate, and hetastarch (artificial blood substitute). Hypotension and allergic reactions can occur with the use of colloid solutions.

Margin answers:

2 isotonic; free water and calories

3 isotonic, hypotonic, or hypertonic; 0.9% NS and lactated Ringer's; 0.2% or 1/4 NS, 0.33% or 1/3 NS, and 0.45% or 1/2 NS; 3% and 5% NS, 10% dextrose in water ($D_{10}W$), also D_5/0.9% NS; may or may not

4
Colloids function like _____ and are often called volume or plasma _____ .
  Identify four examples of commonly used colloid solutions.
* _____

  Identify two possible adverse reactions to colloid solutions.
* _____

  Total parenteral nutrition (TPN) utilizes hypertonic IV solutions. TPN is designed to meet the complete nutritional needs of selected clients who cannot maintain their nutrition via the enteral route. TPN is a mixture of a 25% glucose solution containing proteins, selected electrolytes, vitamins, and trace elements. TPN therapy is covered more extensively later.

5
Hypertonic solutions are used in _____ therapy.
  Four major components of TPN solutions are * _____
_____ .

6
Blood and blood components are another type of IV therapy. Whole blood, packed red cells (whole blood minus the plasma), plasma, and platelets can be administered intravenously. Intravenous therapy in relation to blood and blood components is covered more extensively later in this chapter.
  Four examples of commonly used blood products are * _____
_____ .

7
Successful fluid and electrolyte therapy often depends upon satisfying all five purposes of IV therapy, which are to * _____
_____
_____ .

8
The five main classifications of parenteral solutions designed to address these purposes are * _____
_____ .

---

4 plasma; expanders; albumin, dextran, Plasmanate, and hetastarch; hypotension and allergic reactions

5 TPN (total parenteral nutrition); glucose, proteins (amino acids), electrolytes, and vitamins. Trace elements are a small part of these solutions.

6 whole blood, packed cells (whole blood minus the plasma), plasma, and platelets

7 provide maintenance requirements, replace previous losses, replace current losses, provide a mechanism for administering medications and/or blood or blood products, and provide nutrition

8 sources of free water and calories, crystalloids, colloids, blood and blood products, and hypertonic solutions

9   plasma volume; 4–6; 20

10   increases arterial blood pressure and increases cardiac output (also increases pulse pressure); reduces red blood cell (erythrocyte) aggregation in the capillaries

11   Severe dehydration: Dextran 40 increases dehydration by pulling more fluid from the cells and tissue space and into the vascular space. If urine output is good, the vascular fluid is excreted. Both cellular and extracellular dehydration can occur.; Renal disease: If oliguria is due to hypovolemia, dextran 40 may improve urine output; but if renal damage is present, dextran 40 may cause renal failure.; Thrombocytopenia: Dextran 40 tends to clot platelets and prolong bleeding time.; Active hemorrhaging: Dextran 40 improves microcirculation, which can cause additional blood loss from the capillaries if hemorrhage is prolonged.

12   Dextran 70 tends to coat red blood cells, which makes it difficult to accurately type and cross-match the blood specimen; urticaria (hives) and wheezing (also dyspnea, hypotension, nausea, and vomiting)

13   lactated Ringer's or Ringer's solution

9

Dextran is a colloidal solution that is used to expand the
*_____ . Dextran 40 remains in the circulatory system
_____ hours and dextran 70 remains in the circulation for
_____ hours.

10

Identify two ways that dextran 40 is useful in correcting
hypovolemia in early shock. *_____

_____

   How does dextran 40 improve the microcirculation? *_____

_____

11

Identify three clinical conditions in which dextran 40 is
contraindicated. Provide a rationale related to each condition:
   *_____

_____

   *_____

_____

   *_____

_____

12

Discuss why blood is typed and cross-matched before
administering dextran 70. *_____

_____

   The health professional should stay with the client receiving
dextran 70 for 30 minutes to observe for allergic reactions.
Name two allergic reactions. *_____

_____

13

Identify an IV solution resembling the electrolyte composition of
plasma. *_____

_____

14

Hydrating solutions are helpful for daily maintenance of body
fluid, rehydration, and establishing effective renal output.

Indicate which of the following are hydrating solutions:

( ) a. Dextrose 2 1/2% in 0.45% saline
( ) b. Ringer's solution
( ) c. Dextrose 5% in water
( ) d. Sodium chloride 5%
( ) e. Dextrose 5% in 0.45% saline
( ) f. Sodium chloride 0.45%
( ) g. Dextrose 5% in 0.2% saline

15

Dextrose solutions for IV therapy are prepared in two strengths: 5 and 10%. Five percent dextrose means that there are 5 g of dextrose in 100 mL of solution. If the IV container contains 1000 mL of 5% dextrose, how many grams are in this solution?

_____

16

Potassium is often administered intravenously by diluting the potassium chloride in an IV solution. A good vehicle for IV potassium is the hydrating solution *_____ .

17

Replacement solutions are used to replace fluid, calories, and electrolyte deficits resulting from injury or illness.

Indicate which of the following solutions are considered to be replacement solutions:

( ) a. Sodium chloride 0.45%
( ) b. Dextrose 5% in normal saline
( ) c. Lactated Ringer's
( ) d. Ringer's
( ) e. Dextrose 5% in water
( ) f. M/6 sodium lactate
( ) g. Hypertonic (3 or 5%) saline
( ) h. Dextrose 5% in 0.45% saline
( ) i. Multiple electrolyte or polyionic solutions (Ionosol B or D-CM solutions and Isolyte E)

18

Identify an IV solution that contains sodium but not chloride.
*_____

---

14 a, c, e, f, g

15 Ratio: $5 : 100 :: X : 1000$
$$100X = 5000$$
$$X = 50 \text{ g}$$
Fraction:
$$\frac{5}{100} = \frac{X}{1000}$$
$$100X = 5000$$
$$X = 50 \text{ g}$$

16 5% dextrose in water

17 b, c, d, f, g, i

18 M/6 sodium lactate

19 hyponatremia; osmolality

20 Ionosol B with 5% dextrose or Isolyte E with 5% dextrose (Ionosol B and Isolyte E come without dextrose)

21 Ionosol D-CM; The electrolyte content of this solution is similar to the gastrointestinal fluid.

22 No. The amount of potassium in lactated Ringer's is not sufficient to replace potassium deficits.

23 daily maintenance, rehydration, and maintenance of renal output

24 fluid; electrolyte

25 crystalloids

19

Hypertonic saline (3 or 5%) may be used when treating a client with severe (hypernatremia/hyponatremia) _____ . It is not usually administered unless the serum Na is below 115 mEq/L.

This solution raises the _____ of sodium in the blood.

20

The multiple electrolyte replacement solution useful in the treatment of severe vomiting, diabetic acidosis, postoperative dehydration, and fluid loss due to burns is *_____

_____ .

21

The multiple electrolyte replacement solution useful in correcting an electrolyte imbalance due to losses from the gastrointestinal tract is *_____ . Explain why?

*

22

Should lactated Ringer's solution be administered to replace a potassium deficit? Why or why not? *_____

_____

23

Name three purposes of hydrating solutions. *_____

_____

24

The health professional must determine a client's current _____ and _____ status before deciding which type of IV solution should be administered.

25

Three types of IV fluids that are used in restoring body fluids are:
Crystalloids (lactated Ringer's, saline, and dextrose)
Blood (whole blood and red blood cells)
Colloids (albumin, plasma, Plasmanate, and dextran)

Dextrose, saline, and lactated Ringer's are considered (crystalloids/colloids) _____ .

26

The first step in the treatment of fluid and electrolyte imbalances is the reconstitution of the interstitial extracellular fluid and intravascular blood volume. This can best be accomplished by using isotonic saline (normal saline), lactated Ringer's, or M/6 sodium lactate solutions.

The isotonic solutions used in the reconstitution of the extracellular fluid and blood volume are *_____

_____ .

27

Does the volume of urine increase or decrease following the administration of these isotonic solutions? _____ Why?
*_____

▶ WHOLE BLOOD AND BLOOD PRODUCTS

28

The hematocrit measures the volume of red blood cells (RBCs) in proportion to the extracellular fluid. A rise or drop in the hematocrit can indicate a gain or loss of intravascular extracellular fluid. An increased hematocrit reading can indicate an extracellular fluid loss. Why? *_____

_____

29

The concentration of red blood cells is known as *hemoconcentration*.

A high hematocrit reading can be an indication of an intravascular extracellular fluid volume (deficit/excess)

_____ .

30

The transfusion of whole blood or plasma decreases the hemoconcentration, lowers the hematocrit, raises the blood pressure, and establishes renal flow. The treatment of choice to decrease osmolality is the transfusion of plasma or crystalloids.

Does whole blood dilute the hemoconcentration? _____
Why? *_____

---

26 normal saline, lactated Ringer's, and M/6 lactated sodium

27 increase; There is more fluid in the body to be excreted.

28 Extracellular fluid loss increases the number of RBCs in proportion to the fluid volume.

29 deficit

30 Yes.; These products increase the extracellular fluid volume since 55% of whole blood is plasma; however, plasma or crystalloids may be a better choice depending on the cause of the hemoconcentration.

31 It aids in extracellular dilution and helps to prevent clotting of the blood.

31

For best results when transfusing whole blood to reduce hemoconcentration, it should be given after an initial dilution by an isotonic solution.

Explain why you think an isotonic solution might be given for hemoconcentration before blood is administered. *_____

_____

32

Various components of whole blood can be fractionated and transfused separately. These components include RBCs, plasma, platelets, white blood cells (WBCs) (leukocytes), albumin, and blood factors II, VII, VIII, IX, and X.

Name three blood components that can be fractionated from whole blood. *_____

_____

32 RBCs, plasma, and platelets (also WBCs, albumin, and blood factors)

33

Red blood cells are known as *packed* cells. A unit (200–250 mL) of RBCs (packed cells) is composed of whole blood minus the plasma.

Should a unit of RBCs be administered to dilute hemoconcentration? _____ When are packed RBCs used instead of whole blood? *_____

_____

33 no; to restore RBCs and not the fluid volume

34

The shelf life of refrigerated whole blood is 42 days. Red blood cells and plasma can be frozen to extend their shelf life up to 10 years for RBCs and 1 year for plasma. Platelets must be administered within 5 days after they have been extracted from whole blood.

As whole blood ages, potassium leaves the RBCs (increasing the K level in the serum). The platelets and RBCs are destroyed. After 3 weeks of shelf life, serum potassium (in whole blood) can be increased to 20–25 mEq/L.

The shelf life of refrigerated whole blood is _____ days; the shelf life of frozen RBCs is _____ years; the shelf life of platelets is _____ days; and the shelf life of plasma is _____ year/s.

34 42; 10; 5; 1

35 match/type, purpose, age/shelf life, osmolality, and electrolytes (Na, K)

36 increases; cardiac arrest or extreme hyperkalemia; No. The serum potassium level of old blood is increased and a further increase in the client's serum potassium level can cause cardiac dysrhythmias or a cardiac arrest.

37 No. Body sodium is further diluted.

38 albumin, plasma, Plasmanate, and dextran

39 body protein; plasma volume expander; lung sounds for fluid congestion (rales)

35
Identify four important considerations when administering blood products. *_____

_____

36
The serum potassium level in 3-week-old whole blood (increases/decreases) _____ .

What can happen if a critically ill client with poor renal function is given 3 or more units (pints) of "aging" whole blood? *_____

If a client has a serum potassium of 6.0 mEq/L, should the client receive a transfusion of 3-week-old whole blood? _____ Why? *_____

_____

37
As blood volume is being restored, attention is directed to the osmolal changes and correcting the osmolality of body fluids. A solution of 5% dextrose in water is effective in correcting a water deficit.

Should 5% dextrose be administered to a client with hyponatremia? _____ Why or why not? *_____

_____

▶ COLLOIDS

38
Name four colloids used to restore body fluids. (Refer to question 4.) *_____

_____

39
Albumin concentrate is helpful in restoring body protein. It is considered to be a plasma volume expander. Too much albumin, or albumin administered too rapidly, can cause fluid to be retained in the pulmonary vasculature.

Albumin is used to restore *_____ and is considered a
*_____ .

What should the nurse assess when the client is receiving albumin? *_____

40

Dextran, in saline or dextrose, is another plasma volume expander. Dextran comes in two concentrations, dextran 40 and 70. The stronger concentration is a colloid hyperosmolar solution. If large quantities are administered too rapidly, fluid leaves the cells and intestine, thus causing an intracellular fluid volume deficit.

Dextran can affect clotting by coating the platelets, which reduces their ability to clot. Dextran also interferes with blood typing and cross-matching.

If your client is to receive dextran and his blood is to be typed and cross-matched, what is the corresponding nursing action?
*_____

_____

40 Draw blood for type and cross-match before administering dextran.

41

Plasmanate is a commercially prepared protein product that is used instead of plasma and albumin to replace body protein.

Name the commercially prepared solution that resembles plasma and albumin. _____

41 Plasmanate

CASE STUDY REVIEW

Mrs. Ryan, age 60, was admitted to the hospital for a possible intestinal obstruction. Diagnostic studies were ordered. Food, except for soup and tea, nauseated her. She had not had a bowel movement for a week. An IV infusion of 2000 mL of 5% dextrose/0.33% saline with 20 mEq/L of KCl in 1 liter (1000 mL) was ordered for the first 24 hours.

ANSWER COLUMN

1. to provide fluid maintenance requirements

1. The purpose of Mrs. Ryan's IV therapy was *_____
   _____ .

2. hydrating solution/ crystalloid

2. Five percent (5%) dextrose/0.33% saline is what type of solution? *_____
   _____

3. daily maintenance of body fluid when minimal sodium and chloride are required

4. No. She was taking soup and tea.

5. a. hydrating solution/free water and calories;
   b. replacement solution/crystalloid

6. Lactated Ringer's resembles the electrolyte structure of normal blood serum plasma.

7. No. The potassium is 4 mEq/L. Daily requirement is approximately 40–45 mEq/L.

8. Renal dysfunction can result in electrolyte retention.

9. hypertonic

10. TPN increases the intestine's ability to absorb nutrients and allows the intestines to rest.

11. Central vein: subclavian or internal jugular veins. Femoral vein cutdown: high concentration of glucose is not as irritating to large veins and there is a decreased risk of phlebitis.

---

3. What is the rationale for using 5% dextrose/0.33% saline?
   *_____

4. Was Mrs. Ryan's fluid and nutrient intake completely dependent on IV therapy? _____ Explain *_____
   _____

   After 2 days, Mrs. Ryan vomited when she took any oral fluid. Her IV fluid order for the day was 1 liter of 5% dextrose in lactated Ringer's, followed by 1 liter of 5% dextrose in water.

5. Identify the classifications of solutions ordered:
   a. 5% dextrose in water: *_____
   b. 5% dextrose in lactated Ringer's: *_____

6. Explain the relationship of lactated Ringer's to body fluids.
   *_____

7. Is the potassium in lactated Ringer's sufficient to meet the daily requirement? _____ Explain. *_____
   _____
   _____

8. During IV administration of fluid and electrolytes, adequate kidney function is extremely important. Why? *_____
   _____
   _____

   Mrs. Ryan's clinical condition did not improve. Her x-ray showed a complete intestinal obstruction. The following day, a major bowel resection was performed. TPN was started with a hypertonic solution containing dextrose 25% per liter, protein hydrolysate, vitamins, and electrolytes.

9. One liter of dextrose 25% has 850 mOsm. The osmolality of this solution is (hypotonic/hypertonic) _____ (mOsm and osmolality are explained in Unit 1).

10. Why is TPN indicated following a major bowel resection?
    *_____

11. Mrs. Ryan should receive TPN therapy in what blood vessel?
    *_____
    Explain your reason. *_____
    _____
    _____

12. air embolism, infection, hyperglycemia, and hypoglycemia (also fluid overload or fluid volume excess)

13. a. Observe for sepsis due to infection. Nutrient-rich TPN solution provides a good medium for growth of bacteria and yeast.; b. Monitor blood glucose level with Dextrostix or chemstrip bg. A rapid rate of infusion can cause hyperglycemia.; Others: Observe for electrolyte imbalance, prevent air embolus, and use strict aseptic technique when dressing and tubing or infusion containers are changed.

14. Valsalva maneuver: taking a breath, holding it, and bearing down

12. Name four major complications that can result from TPN therapy. *_____
   _____

13. Name at least two interventions that are necessary when caring for Mrs. Ryan as she receives TPN.
   a. *_____
   b. *_____

14. How can an air embolus be prevented? *_____
   _____
   _____

Total Parenteral Nutrition (TPN)

CHAPTER

16

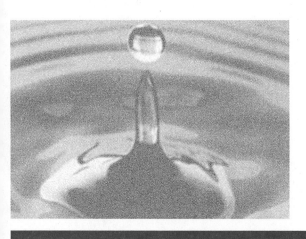

OBJECTIVES

Upon completion of this chapter, the reader should be able to:

● Describe the preparation of solutions used in total parenteral nutrition (TPN).
● Discuss the purpose of TPN.
● List four health indications for the use of TPN.
● Discuss five potential complications of TPN.
● List selected nursing diagnoses and corresponding clinical interventions for clients receiving TPN therapy.
● Discuss relevant clinical assessment factors for clients receiving TPN therapy.

❱ INTRODUCTION

Total parenteral nutrition, sometimes referred to as hyperalimentation, is the infusion of amino acids, hypertonic glucose, and additives such as vitamins, electrolytes, minerals, and trace elements. TPN can meet a client's total nutritional needs and is commonly used for clients whose caloric intake is insufficient. Clients with severe burns who are in negative nitrogen balance, clients who cannot take enteral feedings, and clients with gastrointestinal disorders such as ulcerative colitis, gastrointestinal fistulas, and other conditions where the GI track needs complete rest are prime candidates for TPN. Table 16-1 identifies selected indications with rationale for using TPN.

ANSWER COLUMN

1 hypertonic; It can pull fluid from the intracellular compartment (cells) into the extracellular compartment, thus causing a cellular fluid volume deficit.

1

Nutritional solutions for TPN contain glucose, amino acids, trace elements, vitamins, minerals, lipids, and electrolytes.

Are hyperalimentation solutions (hypotonic/hypertonic)?

_____

Explain the effects that this concentration can have on body cells. * _____

_____

2

A solution of 2500 mL of 10% dextrose in water provides 1000 calories. Concentrations of sugar higher than 10% dextrose can cause severe peripheral vein damage. Continuous use of 10% dextrose in water or dextrose solutions >10% increases the risk for developing phlebitis and should be administered via a central venous line.

2 No; Following surgical treatment 2500–3500 calories is needed daily. One thousand (1000) calories does not meet daily maintenance requirements for the client following major surgery.

Is 1000 calories daily sufficient for a client following major surgery? _____ Explain why/why not. * _____

_____

3

Glucose concentrations higher than 10% can cause venous damage when infused peripherally. Identify the type of vein

Table 16-1

Indications for TPN (Hyperalimentation)

Indications	Rationale
Oral or nasogastric feedings are contraindicated or not tolerated	Long-term use of IV glucose solutions can cause protein wasting. TPN maintains a positive nitrogen balance.
Severe malnutrition	Malnutrition can cause severe protein loss and wasting syndrome. Negative nitrogen (protein) balance occurs. TPN restores positive nitrogen balance.
Malabsorption syndrome	The inability to absorb nutrients in the small intestine requires nutrients to be offered intravenously.
Dysphagia	Difficulty in masticating and swallowing due to pharyngeal radiation treatment prevents clients from breaking down food sufficiently for digestion.
Gastrointestinal fistula	Fistulas promote protein losses. TPN allows the intestine to rest and decreases gall bladder, pancreas, and small intestine secretions.
Major bowel resection and ulcerative colitis	These disorders reduce the absorptive area of the small intestine. TPN increases the intestine's ability to absorb nutrients more quickly than oral feedings and it permits the bowel to rest.
Extensive surgical trauma and stress	Extensive surgery requires 3500–5000 calories a day to maintain protein balance. TPN lowers the chance for infection and provides a positive nitrogen balance to aid in wound healing. TPN before surgery improves the nutritional status so that the client can withstand surgery and its stresses.
Extensive burns	Extensive burns require 7500–10,000 calories daily. TPN improves wound healing and formation of granulation tissue and promotes successful skin grafting.
Metastatic cancer or AIDS with anorexia and weight loss	Clients with wasting syndrome and debilitating diseases, such as cancer or AIDS, frequently are in negative nitrogen balance. TPN restores protein balance and tissue synthesis.

3   phlebitis or thrombophlebitis (clots)

damage that occurs with irritating concentrations of glucose.
*_____

Subclavian veins, internal jugular veins, femoral veins, and venous cutdowns are used when administering hyperosmolar solutions.

4

Indicate which veins can be used for hyperalimentation.

( ) a. Peripheral arm veins
( ) b. Internal jugular veins
( ) c. Leg veins
( ) d. Subclavian veins
( ) e. Femoral veins
( ) f. Venous cutdowns

4 b, d, e, f

When clients do not receive enough protein-sparing calories in the form of amino acids, fat, and carbohydrates (CHO), the body's protein and fat are converted into carbohydrates. To prevent this conversion, the body needs 600–800 calories daily during the resting state, approximately 1600 calories daily for the sitting state, and 2500–3500 calories daily following major surgical procedures.

If a client receives 2500 mL ($2\frac{1}{2}$ liters) of 5% dextrose in water, the caloric intake is 500 calories (CHO: 1 g = 4 calories; 50 g = 5% dextrose per 1000 mL):

$$1000 \text{ mL } 5\% \text{ dextrose} = 50 \text{ g} \times 4 = 200 \text{ calories}$$

$$200 \times 2\frac{1}{2} \text{ liters} = 500 \text{ calories}$$

5

Is this a sufficient number of calories for the resting state? _____
Why? * _____

5 No.; In the resting state
   600–800 calories is needed.

6

The average percentage of dextrose used in TPN is between 25 and 30%. This high glucose concentration is mixed with commercially prepared protein sources. Vitamins and electrolytes are added prior to administration. Electrolytes are frequently added immediately before the infusion according to the client's serum electrolyte levels.

Since high glucose concentrations are irritating to peripheral veins, such concentrations are administered through * _____ . Identify two large veins commonly used in the administration of TPN. * _____

6 central venous lines;
   subclavian and internal
   jugular

7
The amount of electrolytes needed is determined by the client's daily serum electrolyte levels. Frequently, electrolytes are added with the other nutrients, 12–24 hours before infusion, according to the client's serum electrolyte levels.

8 a, c, d, e, g, h, i, j

9 a positive nitrogen balance

10 reduced absorptive area of the intestine

11 It allows the intestine (bowel) to rest.

7
Why is it recommended that electrolytes be added to the solution immediately before administration ? *_____
_____

　　Table 16-1 gives the indications for TPN. Study the table carefully before proceeding. Refer to the table as needed.

8
Indications for hyperalimentation, or TPN, include which of the following:
　( ) a. Major bowel resection
　( ) b. Minor surgical procedures
　( ) c. Gastrointestinal fistula
　( ) d. Severe malnutrition
　( ) e. Contraindicated or intolerable oral and gastric feedings
　( ) f. Severe congestive heart failure
　( ) g. Extensive burns
　( ) h. Metastatic cancer with weight loss
　( ) i. Malabsorption syndrome
　( ) j. Acquired immunodeficiency syndrome (AIDS) with wasting syndrome

9
In clients who are unable to tolerate oral or gastric feeding and suffer from severe malnutrition, TPN helps in restoring *_____ .

10
What happens to the intestinal area in relationship to nutrient absorption following major bowel resection? *_____
_____

11
What benefit does TPN provide for clients who have a gastrointestinal fistula and/or a major bowel resection?
*_____

12 increases; No.; One liter of 10% dextrose is 400 calories, 3 liters is 1200 calories, thus less than the caloric need of clients undergoing stress.

13 It improves the client's nutritional status so that he or she can withstand the surgical procedure and its stresses.

14 7500–10,000 calories daily; It promotes wound healing and formation of granulation tissue and enhances successful skin grafting.

15 Protein replacement restores the positive nitrogen (protein) balance and promotes tissue synthesis.

12

The trauma and stress related to an extensive surgical procedure (increases/decreases) _____ the body's daily caloric needs. Is 3000 mL (3 liters) of 10% dextrose in saline adequate to meet the client's daily caloric requirement following an extensive surgical procedure? _____ Explain why. *_____

_____

13

What purpose does TPN provide prior to surgery *_____

_____

14

What is the caloric need of clients with extensive burns?
*_____

Give two ways that TPN aids in healing extensive burns.
*_____

_____

15

Clients suffering from metastatic cancer with anorexia and weight loss frequently experience a negative nitrogen balance. Explain how TPN helps to remedy this clinical problem. *_____

_____

▶ COMPLICATIONS OF TPN

Major complications that can result from TPN therapy are air emboli, phlebitis, thrombus, infection, hyper/hypoglycemia, and a fluid overload.

TPN is an excellent medium for organisms, bacteria, and yeast to grow. Strict asepsis is necessary when medications are added to the solution and when IV tubing and dressings are changed. Most hospitals have a procedure for changing dressings in which strict aseptic technique (i.e., gloves, masks, and antibiotic ointment) is mandated.

When IV tubing is changed at the central venous catheter site, the client must lie flat and perform the Valsalva maneuver (take a breath, hold it, and bear down) to prevent air from being sucked into the circulation. The Valsalva maneuver increases intrathoracic pressure.

Increased blood glucose (hyperglycemia) occurs as a result of rapid infusion of hypertonic dextrose solutions used in TPN. An elevated blood glucose level may occur during early TPN until the pancreas adjusts to the hyperglycemic load. Regular insulin, either in the IV solution or by subcutaneous injection, may be required to prevent or control hyperglycemia. Other complications that can occur include hypoglycemia from abruptly discontinuing hyperosmolar dextrose solutions, fluid volume excess from the infusion of an excessive volume of fluid, or a fluid shift from intracellular to extracellular compartments.

Table 16-2 lists the five major complications associated with TPN therapy (hyperalimentation), their related causes, symptoms, and corresponding clinical interventions.

16

To prevent an air embolism when changing IV tubing with clients receiving TPN therapy, the Valsalva maneuver is performed. Explain how it is done (see introduction to TPN).

* _____

_____

16 Take a deep breath, hold it, and bear down.

17

Identify two immediate interventions when an air embolism is suspected.

* _____

_____

17 clamp catheter and position client on left side with head down

18

Hypertonic dextrose in a protein hydrolysate solution promotes yeast and bacteria growth. It has been reported that these organisms do not grow as rapidly in a crystalline amino acid solution as they do in protein hydrolysate solution.

Name three symptoms indicative of infection. *_____

_____

_____

18 elevated temperature; chills; redness, swelling, and drainage at insertion site; and sweating and pain in arm or shoulder

19

Usually 1 liter of solution is ordered for the first 24 hours when initiating TPN therapy. This allows the pancreas to accommodate to the increased glucose concentration of the solution.

Table 16-2

Complications of TPN

Complications	Causes	Symptoms	Interventions

Air embolism	IV tubing disconnected
	Catheter not clamped
	Injection port fell off
	Improper changing of
	  IV tubing (no Valsalva
	  procedure)
		Coughing
		Shortness of breath
		Chest pain
		Cyanosis
			Clamp catheter
			Client must lie on left
			  side with head down
			Check vital signs (VS)
			Notify health care
			  provider

Infection	Poor aseptic technique
	  when catheter
	  inserted
	Contamination when
	  changing tubing
	Contamination when
	  solution mixed
	Contamination when
	  dressing changed
		Temperature above
		  100° (37.7°C)
		Pulse increased
		Chills
		Sweating
		Redness, swelling,
		  drainage at insertion
		  site
		Pain in neck, arm, or
		  shoulder
		Lethargy
		Urine: glycosuria
		Bacteria
		Yeast growth
			Notify health care
			  provider
			Change dressing every
			  24–48 h according to
			  agency policy
			Change solution every
			  24 h
			Change tubing every
			  24 h according to
			  agency policy
			Check VS every 4 h

Hyperglycemia	Fluids rapidly infused
	Insufficient insulin
	  coverage
	Infection
		Nausea
		Weakness
		Thirst
		Headache
		Blood glucose elevated
			Monitor blood glucose
			Notify health care
			  provider
			Decrease infusion rate
			Regular insulin as
			  required
			Monitor blood glucose
			  every 4 h and prn

(continues on the following page)

Additional daily increases of 500–1000 mL per day are ordered until the desired daily volume is reached.

A usual maintenance volume of $2\frac{1}{2}$–3 liters of the hypertonic dextrose solution for TPN is administered over 24 hours. A continuous infusion rate is important to prevent fluctuations in blood glucose levels.

Table 16-2

(Continued)

Complications	Causes	Symptoms	Interventions
Hypoglycemia	Fluids abruptly discontinued Too much insulin infused	Nausea Pallor Cold, clammy Increased pulse rate Shaky feeling Headache Blurred vision	Notify health care provider Increase infusion rate with NO insulin, as per order or hospital policy or Orange juice with 2 teaspoons of sugar if client can tolerate fluids or Glucose IV, as per order or hospital policy or Glucagon, as per order or hospital policy
Fluid overload (hypervolemia)	Increased rate of IV infusions Fluid shift from cellular to vascular due to hyperosmolar solutions	Cough Dyspnea Neck vein engorgement Chest rales Weight gain	Check VS every 4 h Weigh daily Monitor intake and output Check neck veins for engorgement Check chest sounds Monitor electrolytes Monitor BUN and creatinine

Source: Adapted from "Helping Your Client Settle in with TPN" by L. Wilhelm, 1985, *Nursing 85, 15*(4), p. 63. Copyright 1985 by Springhouse Corporation. Reprinted with permission.

---

19 finger stick for blood sugar level (Chemistrip bG); every 4–6 hours

What test is suggested to assess, prevent, and control hyperglycemia? *_____

How often should the test be performed? *_____

20

It is suggested that an isotonic dextrose solution be administered for 12–24 hours after TPN therapy is discontinued. A

20 hypoglycemia; pallor; cold
    and clammy skin;
    increased pulse; shakiness
    (also nausea and blurred
    vision)

21 start an additional
    peripheral site or use a
    multilumen central venous
    catheter

22 TPN solution or hypertonic
    dextrose/protein solutions
    and fat emulsion solutions

gradual decrease in the hourly infusion rate of TPN may also be used to discontinue TPN therapy.

If the hypertonic dextrose solution is discontinued abruptly, what complication may develop? _____

What are the signs and symptoms of this complication? _____ , *_____ , *_____ , and _____ .

21

Medications should not be administered in TPN solutions. A multilumen catheter or additional peripheral site must be used if the client requires IV fluids, TPN, blood products, and/or medications.

What must be done when medications are given parenterally with TPN? *_____

22

Fat emulsion supplement therapy provides an increased number of calories and is a carrier of fat-soluble vitamins.

The two solutions that can provide nutrients, calories, and vitamins for TPN are *_____ .

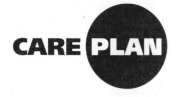

Client Management: Clients Receiving TPN

Assessment Factors

Total parenteral nutrition is a complex form of IV therapy intended to meet the complete nutritional needs of selected clients. Health professionals are responsible for the coordination of activities needed to ensure the proper use of therapy solutions, maintain a continuous infusion, and monitor the effectiveness of TPN therapy. Administration of TPN requires keen assessment skills and a thorough understanding of the physiologic factors related to nutrition and the fluid and electrolyte needs of clients receiving hypertonic solutions over an extended period of time. Before beginning TPN therapy, the placement of the central venous catheter must be confirmed with an x-ray report. Assessment factors for TPN therapy include the various observations with any IV therapy as well as some specific assessments focused on issues important to TPN therapy. Assess fluid balance; monitor intake and output closely to assess for signs of fluid (volume excess or volume deficit) retention or overload. Daily weights provide a good measure of the effectiveness of treatment, and any sudden weight gain or loss can be an alert to problems related to fluid volume retention or deficits.

▶ Monitor laboratory studies. Laboratory studies provide essential information about electrolyte and blood glucose levels associated with fluid balance. Important laboratory values include Na, K, HCO_3, Cl, Ca, P, Mg, serum glucose, serum creatinine, and total protein level. Glucose levels can be monitored with the blood Dextrostix or blood glucose scanner. Blood glucose levels should be measured every 4 hours in the acute stages of illness. Serum albumin and globulin should be monitored every 72 hours or per the health care professional's orders.

▶ Monitor vital signs. Temperature, pulse, respirations, and blood pressure readings alert the health care provider to potential fluid volume problems and impending infections.

▶ Monitor TPN solutions and maintain infusion lines. TPN solutions are usually prepared by the pharmacy under a laminar airflow hood. TPN lines are not to be interrupted except for lipids that may be piggybacked into the TPN line. All solutions must be verified before hanging. Solution containers should be checked for leaks and for clarity. Cloudy solutions may be defective and must be approved before hanging (unless lipids are added directly to the TPN solution). Strict aseptic techniques must be maintained when changing solutions and tubing. The health care provider prescribes the amount of fluid per 24 hours, and the health professional calculates the related flow rate depending upon the type of drip chamber and company specifications for number of drops per milliliter. It is highly recommended that flow rates be maintained by an electronic infusion pump (EIP); some literature states this as mandatory. Infusion rates must remain constant. The TPN port is not used for anything except TPN and lipid infusions. If TPN therapy is interrupted for any reason, infuse 10% D/W at the same rate ordered for the TPN therapy.

▶ Intravenous tubing is changed according to agency policy (usually every 24–48 hours). To prevent an air embolus when changing the IV tubing, either clamp the central venous line using plastic or padded clamps only or have the client perform the Valsalva maneuver while tubing is being changed. Assist the client if necessary by pressing down on the abdomen. If an air embolus is suspected, immediately place the client in a Trendelenburg position on his or her left side. Additional precautions to prevent an air embolism include using leur-lock connections on all-IV tubing, taping catheter and tubing connections securely, and suturing the central venous line in place. The tubing or filter should be anchored to prevent pulling on the central venous line, skin sutures, and catheter.

▶ Central venous line dressings are changed according to hospital policy, usually every 24–72 hours (regular IVs are changed every 48 hours), using strict sterile technique. Never use an existing TPN line for blood samples. All bags, IV lines, and dressings are to be labeled and dated accordingly with documentation on the client's chart.

▶ Each agency usually develops its own procedure for monitoring TPN therapy. Prepared solutions not in use are usually refrigerated and should be removed 2 hours before hanging. TPN is usually started at 1000 mL for the first 24 hours and is increased at a rate of 500–1000 mL daily until the desired volume is reached. When discontinuing TPN, decrease the daily rate gradually over 12–72 hours according to the volume prescribed and the health care provider's orders.

▶ Observe client and central venous line infusion site for signs of infection. Generalized symptoms of infection can indicate sepsis, requiring the discontinuation of the solutions along with the removal of cannulas. Complaints of pain, numbness, or tingling in the fingers, neck, or arm on the same side as the catheter may indicate thrombus formation and must be reported immediately.

▶ Monitor nutritional status—daily weights, physical assessment observations of skin, energy level, nitrogen balance (healing/tissue growth), etc.—as needed to determine adequacy of prescribed solutions.

TPN is a complex medical intervention requiring astute observations and reporting skills. Many complications of this complex treatment modality are life threatening.

Diagnoses

Diagnoses related to nutritional status associated with TPN are collaborative problems since the health care provider manages the fluid and nutritional replacement therapy.

Diagnosis 1

Risk for infection related to TPN therapy, concentrated glucose solutions, and invasive lines requiring dressing and tubing changes.

Interventions and Rationale

1. Assess source and extent of infection. TPN solutions are a prime medium for bacteria growth. Observe bags for leaks and solutions for clarity to provide clues to the source of infection when the solution is the medium. Infusion sites must be observed for signs of redness, swelling, and drainage that may indicate an infection. When an infection is suspected, cannulas are removed and may be cultured according to agency procedure. Environmental and personal contacts must be assessed as other sources of infection.

2. Reduce risks for infection. Use good surgical asepsis when changing solutions and tubing. Use sterile techniques with dressing changes. Invasive therapies increase the client's risk of infection; thus sterile technique must be maintained when providing invasive treatments.

3. Monitor vital signs. Assess for symptoms of infection. Elevated temperature, pulse, and respiration may indicate an impending infection.

4. Refrigerate TPN solutions not in use. High glucose concentration is an excellent medium for bacteria growth.

Diagnosis 2

Altered nutrition: less than body requirements, related to inadequate intake of calories and proteins.

Interventions and Rationale

1. Monitor client's caloric intake in relation to changes in exercise and supplemental nutritional intake in addition to TPN calories and proteins. Infections, tissue healing, exercise, and other factors that affect the client's metabolic rate have implications for the total nutritional status. Change and additional stresses must be factored into the TPN formula for meeting nutritional needs. Maintain TPN at prescribed rates without interruption.

2. Assess skin condition of pressure sites according to physical status. Immobile clients need close observation to prevent pressure sores, especially if the client is emaciated or receiving less than total caloric and protein needs.

Diagnosis 3

Fluid volume excess related to the risk of runaway TPN infusion, IV infusions, and client's physical condition.

Interventions and Rationale

For a fluid volume excess with TPN therapy interventions are similar to those with fluid volume excess with other parenteral therapies. Interventions addressed here are specific to TPN and central venous catheters.

1. Observe for signs and symptoms of fluid overload with TPN infusion (cough, dyspnea, engorged neck veins, chest rales, weight gain) that reflect a fluid shift from the cellular to the vascular system (a complication of hyperosmolar solutions) or occur as the result of a misplaced central venous catheter.

2. Monitor solutions and fluid volume closely. Verify all solutions with orders. Maintain a consistent flow rate as calculated. Catch-up or slowdown with TPN volumes is contraindicated and dangerous. Electronic infusion pumps are frequently used to maintain accurate flow rates. Medications are not to be added to or mixed with TPN infusions. Document hanging and completion times. Do not interrupt TPN solutions. Mark containers to monitor hourly infusion expectations.

Diagnosis 4

Altered comfort related to parenteral therapy using central venous lines.

Interventions and Rationale

1. Identify type and severity of discomfort. Complaints of pain, numbness, or tingling of the fingers, arm, and neck on the side of the central venous line may indicate thrombus formation. Report these symptoms to the health care provider. Chest pain and/or respiratory difficulty may indicate a pulmonary embolus resulting from lipid infusions or a dislodged thrombus. This pain indicates an emergency situation.

2. Assess client's physical status. Note for signs and symptoms of infection that may promote discomfort (elevated temperature, labored/rapid breathing). Note changes in condition of infusion site. Observe client for reactions to solutions and ad-

ditives or symptoms of overhydration. Clients are often apprehensive about infusions through central venous lines.

3. Observe for signs and symptoms of reactions to lipid solutions. Signs and symptoms of immediate reactions include elevated temperature, flushing, sweating, pressure sensation over eyes, nausea/vomiting, headache, chest pain, back pain, dyspnea, and cyanosis, while signs and symptoms of delayed reactions include hepatomegaly, thrombocytopenia, splenomegaly, hyperlipidemia, hepatic damage, and jaundice.

Diagnosis 5

Gas exchange: impaired, related to air embolism when inserting or removing the central venous line, when changing the central line, and when changing TPN solutions.

Interventions and Rationale

1. Place client on left side with head down and have her perform Valsalva maneuver when inserting central lines or changing tubing. Assist client by applying abdominal pressure if necessary. The Valsalva maneuver increases the intrathoracic pressure and reduces the risk of developing an air embolus.

Other nursing diagnoses for which the risks are increased during TPN therapy include:

High risk for fluid volume deficit, related to inadequate fluid intake and osmotic diuresis.
Breathing pattern: ineffective, related to complications of central venous lines and fluid volume excess.
Tissue perfusion (renal, cardiopulmonary, and peripheral): impaired, related to fluid volume deficit and osmotic diuresis.
Knowledge deficit, related to unfamiliarity with TPN therapy and procedures, specific to IV therapy equipment.

Evaluation/Outcome

1. Evaluate the effects of TPN on providing adequate/increased nutrition; weight increased, fluid and electrolyte balance determined by serum electrolyte and osmolality levels.

2. Remain free of complications: infection, air embolism, pulmonary embolism.

3. Maintain a support system.

Intravenous Administration

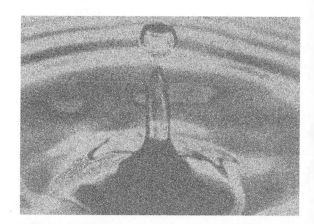

OBJECTIVES

Upon completion of this chapter, the reader should be able to:

- Explain the five purposes of IV therapy.
- Discuss two laboratory tests that assist health professionals in determining the need for IV therapy.
- Calculate the flow rate for IV fluids using macro- and mini-drip administration sets.
- Discuss the three most common infusion devices used for short-term IV therapy.
- Describe central venous catheters and four common reasons for their use.

(continued on next page)

OBJECTIVES (Continued)

● **Describe complications that can occur with central venous line placement and long-term maintenance of central venous lines.**

● **Identify important clinical assessment factors for IV therapy.**

● **Recognize various complications associated with different modes of IV therapy.**

● **List selected diagnoses and corresponding clinical interventions for clients receiving IV therapy.**

▶ INTRODUCTION

This chapter discusses the five basic purposes of IV therapy and describes procedural factors and infusion devices related to the administration of IV solutions. It explains tests that may indicate the need for IV therapy, assessment factors for monitoring IV therapy, and complications that may arise from the administration of IV solutions. Case examples of selected diagnoses and corresponding interventions focused on IV therapy are presented at the end of the chapter to reinforce learning.

▶ BASIC PURPOSES OF IV THERAPY

The five purposes of IV therapy are to:

1. Provide maintenance requirements for fluids and electrolytes
2. Replace previous losses
3. Replace concurrent losses
4. Provide nutrition
5. Provide a mechanism for the administration of medications and/or the transfusion of blood and blood components

Healthy persons can normally preserve their fluid and electrolyte balance; however, certain illnesses and conditions compromise the body's ability to adapt to fluid changes. When a client cannot maintain this balance, IV therapy may be indicated.

1 to provide maintenance requirements for fluids and electrolytes, replace previous fluid losses, meet current fluid losses, provide nutrition, and provide a mechanism for the administration of medications and/or blood and blood products

1

List the five basic purposes of administering fluids and electrolytes by IV therapy.

*_____

_____

_____

_____

_____

2

People requiring IV therapy may depend on this route to meet daily maintenance needs for water, electrolytes, calories, vitamins, and other nutritional substances.

 The first purpose in administering IV therapy is to

*_____ .

2 provide daily maintenance requirements

3

It is desirable for a client to have sufficient kidney function while receiving IV fluids and electrolytes. Renal dysfunction may result in electrolyte (retention/excretion) _____ .

3 retention

4

Multiple electrolyte solutions are helpful in accomplishing the second purpose for IV therapy. The second purpose for IV therapy is *_____ .

4 to replace previous fluid losses

5

Fluid and electrolyte losses that occur from diarrhea, vomiting, and/or gastric suction are an indication for the third purpose of administering fluids and electrolytes intravenously. The third purpose of IV therapy is *_____ .

5 to replace current fluid losses

6

In situations when a client is unable to meet nutritional needs through oral intake, total parenteral nutrition (TPN) may be used to meet the client's _____ needs.

6 nutritional

7

There are many clinical situations in which the IV route is preferable for medication administration. This fifth purpose of IV therapy is * _____

_____ .

To meet client needs for blood losses or conditions such as anemia, IV therapy meets another purpose. The last purpose of IV therapy is * _____

_____ .

Laboratory tests used by health professionals to determine the need for IV therapy are the BUN and creatinine levels. The BUN is a serum test used to measure the amount of urea, a by-product of protein metabolism, remaining in the blood that is normally excreted by the kidneys. The normal range for the BUN level is 10–25 mg/dL.

An elevated BUN frequently indicates poor renal function; however, a slightly elevated BUN may also indicate a decrease in the extracellular fluid (ECF) volume.

The normal range for the creatinine-BUN ratio is 1:10–1:20. A ratio of 1:20 or greater is indicative of a decreased extracellular fluid volume deficit. For example, if a client's creatinine-BUN ratio is 0.9:9, the client's creatinine-BUN ratio is within the normal 1:10 ratio. However, if a client's ratio is 1.4:60, this is well beyond the 1:10–1:20 ratio and is considered to be a fluid volume deficit. When the creatinine-BUN ratio increases to the point of extreme imbalance, the client can go into renal failure. For example, a 2.4:40 ratio is indicative of an extreme imbalance as seen in renal failure. The creatinine level is elevated.

8

After the client has been hydrated, the elevated BUN should return to a normal range; if the BUN does not return to normal, it can be an indication of (poor renal function/decrease in body fluids) * _____ .

9

Mary Jones has a creatinine of 0.8 and a BUN of 30. This creatinine-BUN ratio is indicative of * _____ .

Paul Thomas has a ratio of 2.8:50. His creatinine-BUN ratio is indicative of * _____ .

---

7 to provide a mechanism for the administration of medications; to transfuse blood or blood products

8 poor renal function

9 a fluid volume deficit, or dehydration; renal failure

10 hematocrit level, BUN-
     creatinine ratio, and serum
     electrolyte levels

10

A third test in determining the need for IV therapy is the serum electrolyte levels.

Three tests used to determine the necessity of IV therapy are * _____ .

11 excess or significant
     alterations; CONTINUOUS-
     LY on a daily basis; This
     defends the body against
     significant alterations in
     fluid and electrolyte
     balance.

11

Fluids and electrolytes for maintenance therapy should be administered over a period of at least 24 hours and then ordered on a daily basis.

Normally, the administration of IV fluids results in prompt excretion of excess fluid and electrolytes. This response defends the body against * _____ in water and electrolyte balance.

How should fluids and electrolytes for maintenance therapy be scheduled? * _____ Why? * _____

12

If a client receives the full 24-hour maintenance parenteral therapy in 8 hours, two-thirds of the water and electrolytes are in (excess/deficit) _____ of the client's current needs. Normally, a large portion of the excess maintenance fluid is (excreted/retained) _____ .

12 excess; excreted

13

Tolerance for sudden changes in water and electrolytes is limited for very ill clients, clients following major surgery, elderly clients, small children, and infants.

Rapid administration of fluids that exceeds one's physiologic tolerance can cause hyponatremia, pulmonary edema (accumulation of fluid in the lungs), and other complications.

Maintenance parenteral therapy should be administered over a period of * _____ .

Two possible complications of rapid administration of maintenance fluids are * _____ .

13 24 hours; hyponatremia
     and pulmonary edema

▶ IV FLOW RATE

14

Hypertonic IV solutions (those having an osmolality greater than the osmolality of body fluids) should be infused no faster than 2–4 mL/min or as ordered by the health care provider.

14 dextrose 5% in normal saline, dextrose 10% in water, dextrose 10% in normal saline, dextrose 5% in lactated Ringer's solution, hypertonic saline, and multiple electrolyte replacement solutions

List at least five hypertonic solutions to which this might apply. Refer back to Tables 15-1 and 15-2 on pages 277–279 if needed. *_____

_____

_____

_____

Table 17-1 outlines three types of IV therapy. The table includes the desired amount of solution and the recommended rate of flow. The symbol mL (milliliter) has the same equivalence as cc (cubic centimeter). The symbol for drops is gtt.

Today many institutions use IV controllers or pumps to deliver IV fluids, but the health professional still needs to know how to calculate the flow rate and regulate various types of infusion devices.

Take several minutes to study this table carefully. Know the three purposes of therapy and the recommended drip rates. Refer to this table as needed.

15 maintenance therapy, replacement therapy, hydration therapy, nutritional therapy, and a mechanism for the administration of medications and/or blood and blood products

15
The five purposes of IV therapy are *_____ .

16
The type of solution most frequently suggested in hydration therapy is (hyper/hypo/iso) _____ -tonic.

Once urinary output is reestablished, then (maintenance/replacement hydration) _____ therapy is started.

16 isotonic, maintenance

Table 17-1

Rates of IV Administration

Type of Therapy	Amount of Solution Desired (mL)	Rate of Flow
Maintenance therapy	1500–2000	62–83 mL/h or 1–1.5 mL/min if given over 24 h
Replacement with maintenance therapy	2000–3000	83–125 mL/h or 1.5–2 mL/min (depends on individual)
Hydration therapy	1000–3000	60–120 mL/h or 1–2 mL/min

Note: These guidelines may be adapted to individual circumstances. The health care provider orders the 24-h requirements and the health professional computes 1-h requirements from this. The amount of solution to be administered and the rate of flow can vary greatly with the very sick, the elderly, the small child, the infant, and the postsurgical client.

17 a very sick client, an elderly
client, a small child, an
infant, and a postsurgical
client

18 hourly volume; flow rate

17

Identify four types of clients for which the amount of solution to
be administered and the rate of flow can vary greatly.

* _____

_____

18

The physician's order determines the 24-hour fluid requirements,
and the health professional computes the *_____ and
calculates the *_____ .

▶ CALCULATION OF IV INFUSION FLOW RATES

The health care provider's order for IV therapy includes the type
of fluid for infusion and the amount to be administered in a specified period of time. The health professional must compute the
number of milliliters (mL) per hour and then calculate the drops
per minute for the infusion. Volume and pressure infusion pumps
are frequently used to administer IV fluids and are considered essential if the client is receiving continuous heparin, aminophylline,
medications that affect blood pressure and pulse, and infusions
where continuous blood levels are required, as with insulin.

The first step in calculating the drip rate (drops per minute) is
to check the manufacturer's specifications for how many drops
(gtt) per milliliter (mL) are delivered by the infusion set. The number of drops per milliliter varies with each manufacturer and
ranges from 8 to 20 gtt/mL for macrodrip chambers and from 50
to 60 gtt/mL for microdrip chambers.

Example. Order: 3000 mL D$_5$W to run over 24 hours. The
health professional must compute the number of milliliters (mL)
per hour and then calculate the drops per minute. A commonly used formula for this conversion is as follows.

Two-Step Method:

(a) $\dfrac{\text{Total volume}}{\text{Time in hours}} = \text{volume per hour}$

In the above order the formula becomes

$$\frac{3000 \text{ mL}}{24 \text{ h}} = 125 \text{ mL/h}$$

To convert the milliliters per hour (mL/h) to drops per minute (gtt/min), the second part of the formula is

(b) $\dfrac{\text{Volume to be infused (mL/h)} \times \text{gtt/mL (IV set)}}{\text{Time in minutes [e.g., 60 min (1 h)]}} = \text{gtt/min}$

In the above order, if the drip factor is 15 gtt/mL (IV set instruction), the second part of the formula is

$$\frac{125 \text{ mL/h} \times 15 \text{ gtt/mL (IV set)}}{60 \text{ min (1 h)}} = \frac{1875}{60} = 31 \text{ gtt/min}$$

The calculations may be computed in one step using only the second part of the formula if the milliliters per hour is known.

Instead of the two-step formula, a one-step formula may be used:

One-Step Method:

$$\frac{\text{Volume to be infused (mL)} \times \text{gtt/mL (IV set)}}{\text{Hours to administer (h)} \times \text{min/h (60)}}$$

$$= \frac{3000 \text{ mL/24 h} \times 15 \text{ gtt/mL}}{24 \text{ h} \times 60 \text{ min}} = \frac{45,000 \text{ gtt}}{1440 \text{ min}} = 31 \text{ gtt/min}$$

If an IV infusion pump or controller is used, it would only be necessary to calculate the volume per hour (in this case 125 mL) and enter that number on the pump.

Practice the necessary calculations on the following orders for IV therapy.

19

Mr. Dean is ordered 1000 mL of D$_5$/0.9% NS to infuse over 10 hours. The drip factor is 10 gtt/mL. Using the two-step method, how many drops per minute would you regulate the IV?

a. $\dfrac{\text{Volume in mL}}{\text{Time in h}} = \text{mL/h}$ $\underline{\hspace{2cm}} = \underline{\hspace{1cm}} \text{mL/h}$

b. $\dfrac{\text{Volume in mL} \times \text{gtt/mL}}{\text{Time in min}} = \text{gtt/min}$

$\dfrac{\hspace{1cm} \times \hspace{1cm}}{\hspace{2cm}} = \dfrac{}{} = \underline{\hspace{1cm}} \text{gtt/min}$

---

19 a. $\dfrac{1000 \text{ mL}}{10 \text{ h}} = 100 \text{ mL/h}$

b. $\dfrac{100 \text{ mL/h} \times 10 \text{ gtt/mL}}{60 \text{ min/h}}$

$= \dfrac{1000}{60} = 16.6, \text{ or}$

17 gtt/min

20
Mr. Dean is to have a secondary infusion of 50 mL of dextran to run for 1 hour. The drip factor is 20 gtt/mL (IV set instruction). How many drops per minute would you regulate the IV? Remember milliliters per hour is known, so calculating part 1 of the two-step method is not necessary:

$$\frac{\text{Volume in mL} \times \text{gtt/mL}}{\text{Time in min}} = \frac{\times}{\rule{1cm}{0.4pt}} = \underline{\hspace{1cm}} \text{ gtt/min}$$

21
When the dextran infusion is completed on Mr. Dean, he is to receive erythromycin, 1000 g in 250 mL of D_5W to infuse over 1 hour. The drip factor is 15 gtt/mL. How many drops per minute would you give?

$$\frac{\text{Volume in mL} \times \text{gtt/mL}}{\text{Time in min}} = \frac{\times}{\rule{1cm}{0.4pt}} = \underline{\hspace{1cm}} \text{ gtt /min}$$

22
The reason Mrs. Beare had a KVO (keep vein open) infusion was for the intermittent administration of medications and electrolytes. The order reads potassium chloride 40 mEq in 150 mL D_5W to infuse over 3 hours. Drip factor is 15 gtt/mL. How many drops per minute would you give?

$$\frac{\text{Volume in mL} \times \text{gtt/mL}}{\text{Time in min}} = \underline{\hspace{2cm}}$$

23
Instead of using the macrodrip chamber of 15 gtt/mL for Mrs. Beare's potassium chloride, you decide to use a microdrip chamber of 60 gtt/mL. How many drops per minute would you give?

$$\frac{\text{Volume in mL} \times \text{gtt/mL}}{\text{Time in min}} = \underline{\hspace{2cm}}$$

24
Mr. Shirtzer is to receive 1500 mL of $D_5/0.2\%$ NS to infuse over 24 hours. The drip factor is 15 gtt/mL. How many drops per minute would you give?

$$\frac{\text{Volume in mL} \times \text{gtt/mL}}{\text{Time in min}} = \underline{\hspace{2cm}}$$

Sidebar (worked solutions):

20
$$\frac{50 \text{ mL} \times \overset{1}{\cancel{20}} \text{ gtt/mL}}{\underset{3}{\cancel{60} \text{ min}}}$$
$$= \frac{50}{3} = 16.6, \text{ or } 17 \text{ gtt/min}$$

21
$$\frac{250 \text{ mL} \times \overset{1}{\cancel{15}} \text{ gtt/mL}}{\underset{4}{\cancel{60} \text{ min} (1 \text{ h})}}$$
$$= \frac{250}{4} = 62.5, \text{ or } 63 \text{ gtt/min}$$

22
$$\frac{150 \text{ mL} \times 15 \text{ gtt/mL}}{180 \text{ min} (3 \text{ h})}$$
$$= \frac{2250}{180} = 12.5 \text{ gtt/min}$$

23
$$\frac{150 \text{ mL} \times \overset{\overset{1}{\cancel{60}}}{\cancel{60} }\text{gtt/mL}}{\underset{\underset{3}{\cancel{180}}}{\cancel{3} \text{ min} (3\text{h} \times 60 \text{ min})}}$$
$$= \frac{150}{3} = 50 \text{ gtt/min}$$

24
$$\frac{1500 \text{ mL} \times 15 \text{ gtt/mL}}{1440 \text{ min} (24 \text{ h})}$$
$$= \frac{22,500}{1440} = 15.6, \text{ or}$$
16 gtt/min

▶ TYPES OF IV INFUSION DEVICES FOR SHORT-TERM IV THERAPY

There are three common types of infusion devices for routine short-term IV therapy: the butterfly (steel needle), the over-needle-catheter, and the inside-needle-catheter.

The first type is a winged-tip or butterfly set, which consists of a wing-tip needle with a steel cannula, plastic or rubber wings, and a plastic catheter or hub. The needle is $\frac{1}{2}$–$1\frac{1}{2}$ inches long with needle gauges of 16–26. The infusion needle and clear tubing are bonded into a single unit.

A second type of commonly used IV device is the over-needle-catheter (ONC). The bevel of the needle extends beyond the catheter, which is $1\frac{1}{4}$–8 inches in length. The needle is available in gauges of 12–24.

A third type of commonly used IV device is the inside-needle-catheter (INC), which is constructed exactly opposite the ONC. Needle length is $1\frac{1}{2}$–3 inches with a catheter length of 8–25 inches. The catheter is available in gauges of 2–24. The INC set comes with a catheter sleeve guard that must be secured over the needle bevel to prevent severing the catheter.

Catheters used in INCs and ONCs are constructed of silicone, Teflon, polyvinyl chloride, or polyethylene.

25

Three common types of IV infusion devices for short-term IV therapy are *_____ .

Identify three to four types of materials used to make ONC and INC devices. *_____

25 butterfly (wing-tipped), over-needle-catheter (ONC), and inside-needle-catheter (INC); silicone, Teflon, polyvinyl chloride, and polyethylene

Some advantages of the butterfly infusion set are that it is a one-piece apparatus, has a short beveled needle, and is easy to tape securely. The butterfly reduces the risk of secondary puncture and infiltration on puncture. A disadvantage of this IV apparatus is that the butterfly wings prevent manipulation and rotation of the needle in the vein. The butterfly infusion set (only for short-term use of less than 2 hours) is commonly used in children and the elderly, whose veins are likely to be small or fragile.

The ONC with its short large cannula is preferable for rapid IV infusion and is more comfortable for the client.

In INC with its longer narrower catheter is preferred when vein catheterization is necessary for prolonged infusions.

26

Three advantages of the butterfly (winged-tip) infusion device are that it *_____

_____ .

    A disadvantage of the butterfly device is *_____ .
The butterfly is most commonly used for _____ and
_____ whose veins are (large/small) _____ or (fragile/
durable) _____ .

27

Two advantages of the ONC device are *_____ .
    The cannula in the ONC device is (short and large/long and narrow) *_____ .

28

INC devices are preferred for (short/prolonged) _____ infusions.
    The cannula in the INC device is (short and large/long and narrow) *_____ .

Factors to consider in the needle selection for IV therapy include (1) the health professional's preference, (2) the client's condition, and (3) the type or amount of IV solution to be administered.

29

Identify three factors to consider when selecting a needle for an IV infusion. *_____

▶ CENTRAL VENOUS CATHETERS AND LONG-TERM IV THERAPY

Central venous catheters are another type of IV device. These catheters are radiopaque and may have a single, double, or triple lumen. Since the insertion of a central venous catheter presents

---

Sidebar (left margin answers):

26 is a one-piece apparatus, has a short bevel needle, is easy to secure, and has a decreased risk of puncture, (short-term use—less than 2 hours in length); limited manipulation/rotation of needle; children and the elderly; small; fragile

27 good for rapid intravenous infusion of fluids and more comfortable for client; short and large

28 prolonged; long and narrow

29 health professional's preference, client's condition, and type/amount of solution to be infused

critical risks, their insertion is followed by an x-ray to confirm the position and tip placement of the catheter.

30
Central venous catheters are _____ so they may be visualized in x-rays to determine their *_____ . Identify the three types of lumen that may be present in a central venous catheter. *_____

31
Four common reasons for using a central venous catheter are (1) measuring the central venous pressure, (2) infusion of TPN, (3) infusion of multiple IV fluids and/or medications, and (4) infusion of chemotherapeutic or irritating medications.
    Identify four reasons central venous lines are used. *_____
_____
_____
_____
_____

32
Hickman and Groshong are examples of central venous catheters that must be inserted in the operating room. The implantable vascular access device (IVAD) is another example of a central venous line that must be surgically inserted in the operating room.
    Name three types of central venous lines that must be inserted in the operating room. *_____
_____

33
Polyethylene, silicone, and polyvinyl chloride central venous lines can be inserted at the bedside under sterile conditions.
    Name three types of central venous catheters that can be inserted under sterile conditions at the bedside. *_____
_____

34
Veins commonly used to insert central venous lines are the subclavian vein, internal and external jugular veins, femoral vein, and the antecubital vein. A procedure called venous cutdown may be used to insert central venous lines.

30 radiopaque; position and tip placement; single, double, and triple

31 to measure the central venous pressure, to infuse TPN, to infuse multiple IV fluids and/or medications, and to infuse chemotherapeutic or irritating medications

32 Hickman, Groshong, and implantable venous access device (IVAD)

33 polyethylene, silicone, and polyvinyl chloride

34 subclavian, internal and
external jugular veins,
femoral, and antecubital

Name four veins commonly used for access when inserting a central venous catheter. *_____

_____

Peripherally inserted central catheter (PICC) lines are used increasingly in home care settings for clients that require IV therapy (see Figure 17-1). These lines are expected to last from 2 weeks to 1 year and are considered to be convenient and cost effective for long-term therapy. A specifically trained/certified PICC insertion health professional inserts the catheter and an x-ray is taken to confirm accurate placement.

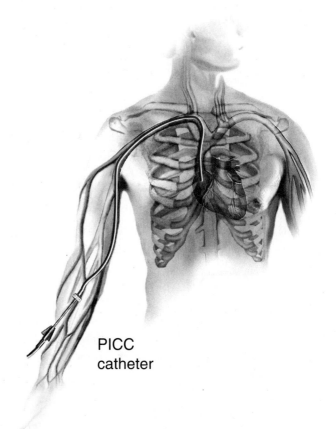

PICC
catheter

Figure 17-1 Peripheral Inserted Central Catheter (PICC) Line for IV Therapy

35

PICC lines may remain in place for _____ weeks to _____ year. They are particularly convenient for use in long-term IV therapy that takes place in the _____ setting.

36

Complications that can occur with insertion of a central venous line into the subclavian and jugular veins are pneumothorax, hemorrhage, air embolism, thrombus dislodgement, and cardiac dysrhythmias. Long-term complications that occur with central venous lines include hemorrhage, phlebitis, air embolism, thrombus formation, infection, dislodgement, cardiac dysrhythmias, and circulatory impairment.

Identify five complications associated with inserting a central venous catheter. *_____

_____

Identify four to five complications associated with the long-term use of central venous catheters. *_____

_____

▶ ASSESSMENT FACTORS IN IV THERAPY

Table 17-2 presents important assessment factors in IV therapy. Once the health care provider orders the IV fluids, the health professional must know and understand the various solutions, needles, catheters, tubings, IV sites, and potential complications in order to accurately assess, initiate, and monitor IV infusions. Table 17-2 provides the assessment, interventions, and rationale related to IV therapy. Study the table carefully and refer to it as needed.

37

When a client receives IV therapy, responsibility begins with assessment of the solutions ordered.

Intravenous solutions with less than 240 mOsm are considered (hypotonic/hypertonic) _____ solutions. Continuous use of this type of solution can cause *_____ . Give an example of a solution that can become hypotonic if its contents are metabolized. *_____

35 2;1; home care

36 pneumothorax, hemorrhage, air embolism, thrombus dislodgement, and cardiac dysrhythmias; hemorrhage, phlebitis, infection, dislodgement, cardiac dysrhythmias, and circulatory impairment

37 hypotonic; water intoxication; 5% dextrose in water

Table 17-2

Assessment Factors in IV Therapy

Assessment	Interventions	Rationale
Types of IV Solutions	Note the types of IV fluid ordered, hypotonic, isotonic, or hypertonic solutions.	An excessive use of hypotonic solutions can cause a fluid volume excess. Excessive use of hypertonic solutions may cause a fluid volume deficit. An isotonic solution has 240–340 mOsm/L; less than 240 is hypo-osmolar, and greater than 340 is hyperosmolar (refer to Chapter 1).
	Report extended use of continuous IVs of dextrose in water.	Dextrose 5% in water administered continuously becomes a hypotonic solution. Dextrose is metabolized rapidly and the remaining water decreases the serum osmolality. Alternate use of D/W with D/NSS (saline) to prevent this complication.
	Observe for signs and symptoms of fluid volume deficit, i.e., dry mucous membranes, poor skin turgor, and increased pulse and respiration rates, when using hyperosmolar solutions. Creatinine/BUN ratio, 1:10/20; hemoconcentration, 1:20 or greater.	Continuous use of hyperosmolar solutions pulls fluid from intracellular compartments to the extracellular compartments. The fluid is excreted by the kidneys. Poor kidney function causes fluid retention, increasing the risk for a fluid volume excess.
Intravenous Tubing and Bag	Inspect IV bags for leaks by gently squeezing.	Microorganisms can enter IV bags through small leak sites, contaminating the fluid.
	Check drop size on the equipment box. Use IV tubing with macrodrip chamber (10–20 gtt/mL) for administering IV fluids at a rate of 50 mL/h or greater.	Use of a microdrip chamber (IV tubing) for fluids that are ordered to run at a rate greater than 50 mL/h is too slow and inaccurate.
	Use microdrip chamber (60 gtt/mL) for administering IV fluids at a rate under 50 mL/h.	Infusion pumps increase the accuracy and decrease the risks associated with IV fluids that are to run for 12–24 h and meet specific client fluid needs.

(continues on the following page)

Table 17-2

(Continued)

Assessment	Interventions	Rationale
	Change IV tubing every 24–48 h at time of new hanging.	Studies have shown that IV tubing left hanging for 48 h is free of bacteria when proper aseptic technique is used.
	New IV containers are hung according to agency policy.	An IV bag should not be used for longer than 24 h. If the order is for KVO (keep vein open), a 250–500-mL container with a microdrip chamber set is suggested.
Needles and IV Catheters (cannulas)	Recognize the types of IV needles and catheters used for IV fluids: Straight needles Scalp vein needles/butterfly (steel) needles Heparin lock Over-needle-catheter (ONC) Inside-needle-catheter (INC)	Needles (straight and scalp vein) are used for short-term IV therapy and for clients with autoimmune problems. Catheters made of silicone and Teflon are less irritating than polyvinylchloride and polyethylene catheters.
	Change IV site every 2–3 days according to agency policy.	Needles and catheters in longer than 72 h increase the risk of phlebitis.
	Check the ONC for placement and function.	There are many types of ONCs, i.e., Angiocath, A-Cath, Vicra Quik-Cath, etc. Catheter length can be 1–3 inches. Care should be taken to avoid severing the catheter with the needle tip.
	Check for fluid leaks at the insertion site after the insertion of an INC.	An INC is used for central venous pressure monitoring, TPN (hyperalimentation), etc. It is frequently inserted in large veins, i.e., subclavian vein, internal jugular or femoral vein. Leaks result from needle punctures that are larger than the catheter.

(continues on the following page)

Table 17-2

Assessment Factors in IV Therapy (Continued)

Assessment	Interventions	Rationale
Injection Site	Insert needle or catheter in the hand or the distal veins of the arm. Use the antecubital fossa (elbow) site last.	The upper extremity is preferred for the infusion site, since the occurrence of phlebitis and thrombosis in the upper extremities is not as prevalent as it is in the lower extremities.
	Avoid using the leg veins if possible.	Circulation in the leg veins is reduced and thrombus formation can occur.
	Avoid using limbs affected by a stroke or mastectomy for IV sites.	Circulation is usually decreased in affected extremities.
	Apply arm board and/or soft restraints to the extremity with the IV when the client is restless or confused.	Prevention of extremity movement with an IV decreases the chance of dislodging the needle and phlebitis.
Flow Rate and Irrigation	Check types of solutions clients are receiving.	Knowledge of tonicity (osmolality) of fluids aids in determining rate of flow. Rate of hypertonic solutions should be slower than isotonic solutions.
	Observe drip chamber and regulate accordingly.	Regulation of IV fluids is important to prevent overhydration, i.e., cough, dyspnea, neck vein engorgement, and chest rales. Do not play "catch-up" with IV fluids.
	Regulate KVO (keep vein open) rate to run 10–20 mL/h or according to agency policy or use an infusion pump.	KVO IVs should run approximately 10–20 mL/h.
	Label IV bag for milliliters (mL) to be received per hour. Check rate of flow every 30 min to 1 h with hypertonic and toxic solutions and every hour with isotonic solutions.	Hypertonic solutions administered rapidly can cause cellular dehydration and, if the kidneys are properly functioning, vascular dehydration.
		Hypertonic fluids act as an osmotic diuretic and can cause diuresis; when administered rapidly, speed shock can occur; and if extravasation occurs, necrotic tissue can result.

(continues on the following page)

Table 17-2

(Continued)

Assessment	Interventions	Rationale
	Restore IV flow if stopped by opening flow clamp, milking the tubing, raising the height of IV bag, or repositioning the extremity.	If IV flow has stopped and does not start by opening clamp, milking tubing, raising the bag, or repositioning extremity, then the IV catheter should be removed. Irrigating IV catheters is prohibited in some institutions and should never be attempted with clotted lines. Forceful irrigation can dislodge clot(s) and cause the movement of an embolus to the lungs.
Position of IV Line	Position and tape IV tubing to prevent kinking.	Kinking of the tubing may cause the IV to be discontinued and to be restarted at a different site.
	Hang IV bag 2½–3 feet above client's infusion site.	The higher the IV bag, the faster the gravity flow rate. If the IV bag is too low, IV fluids may stop due to an insufficient gravity pull.
Infusion Problems and Complications		
1. Infiltration	Observe insertion site for infiltration, i.e., swelling, coolness, and soreness.	Infiltration is accumulation of nonmedicated fluid in the subcutaneous tissue. When infiltration or extravasation occurs, the IV should be discontinued and restarted at a different site. Notify the health care provider if extravasation is observed.
2. Phlebitis	Observe insertion site for phlebitis, i.e., red, swollen, hard, pain, and warm to touch. Apply warm, moist heat to area as ordered.	Phlebitis is an inflammation of the vein that can be caused by irritating substances. Drugs and hyperosmolar solutions may cause phlebitis. Application of moist heat decreases inflammation.

(continues on the following page)

Table 17-2

Assessment Factors in IV Therapy *(Continued)*

Assessment	Interventions	Rationale
3. Systemic infection	Observe for pyrogenic reactions (septicemia), i.e., chills, fever, headache, fast pulse rate. Check vital signs q4h for shocklike symptoms. Utilize aseptic technique when inserting IV catheters and changing IV tubing and IV bag.	Aseptic technique should be used at all times with IV therapy. Prevention of systemic infections is of primary importance.
4. Speed shock	Observe for signs and symptoms of speed shock, i.e., tachycardia, syncope, decreased blood pressure.	Speed shock occurs when solutions with drugs are given rapidly. High drug concentration accumulates rapidly in the body and can cause shocklike symptoms.
5. Air embolism	Remove air from tubing to prevent air embolism.	Air can be removed from tubing by (1) inserting a needle with syringe into side arm of tubing set and withdrawing the air and (2) using a pen or pencil on tubing, distal to the air, and rolling tubing until air is displaced into the drip chamber.
	Observe for signs and symptoms of air embolism. These include pallor, dyspnea, cough, syncope, tachycardia, decreased blood pressure.	Air embolism occurs when air inadvertently enters the vascular system. Injection of more than 50 mL of air can be fatal. It occurs more frequently in the central veins, and symptoms usually appear within 5 min.
	Immediately place client on left side in Trendelenburg position.	Air is trapped in the right atrium, which prevents it from going to the lungs.
6. Pulmonary embolism	Report signs and symptoms of pulmonary embolism, i.e., restlessness, chest pain, cough, dyspnea, tachycardia.	Thrombus originating in the peripheral vein becomes an embolus and can lodge in a pulmonary vessel.

(continues on the following page)

Table 17-2

(Continued)

Assessment	Interventions	Rationale
	Administer oxygen, analgesics, anticoagulants, and IV fluids as ordered.	Preventive measures should be taken, such as *never* forcefully irrigating an IV catheter to reestablish flow and avoiding the use of veins in the lower extremities.
7. Pulmonary edema	Check breath sounds for rales. Check neck veins for engorgement. Decrease IV flow rate.	IV fluids administered too rapidly or in large amounts can cause overhydration. Excess fluids accumulate in the lungs.
8. "Runaway" IV fluids	Monitor IV fluid every hour even if on an electronic infusion pump (EIP).	Control clamp on IV tubing is opened.
	Check EIP flow rate and alarm set.	Alarm was not set properly on EIP.
9. Hematoma	Observe for hematoma with unsuccessful attempts to start IV therapy.	Hematoma (blood tumor) is a raised ecchymosed area.
	Apply ice pack immediately, then warm compresses after 1 hour.	Ice stops bleeding into the tissue. Warm compresses cause vasodilation and improve blood flow and healing.
Additives to IV Fluids	Recognize the untoward reactions of drugs in IV fluids: potassium, Levophed, low-pH drugs, vitamins, antibiotics, antineoplastic drugs.	Potassium, antineoplastic drugs, and Levophed irritate the blood vessels and body tissue. Phlebitis is common with these drugs; and if infiltration occurs, sloughing of tissues may result. Vitamins and antibiotics should not be mixed together. They are incompatible. Always check compatibility charts before adding medications to IV fluids.

(continues on the following page)

Table 17-2

Assessment Factors in IV Therapy *(Continued)*

Assessment	Interventions	Rationale
	Stay with the client 10–15 min when the client is receiving drugs that are classified as a possible cause of anaphylaxis.	Allergic reactions often occur within the first 15 min when drugs are administered by IV.
	Inject drugs into IV container and invert several times before administering.	Equal drug distribution throughout the solution ensures proper dilution. *Do not* add drugs, i.e., potassium, into the IV bag while it is being administered unless the IV is temporarily stopped and the bag is inverted several times to promote equal distribution.
Intake and Output	Check urine output every 4–8 h. If a critically ill client is receiving potassium, urine output should be checked every hour.	If urine output is poor, overhydration can occur when excessive or continuous IV fluids are given. Potassium is excreted by the kidneys; thus, a decreased urine output can result in hyperkalemia.

38

Continuous use of hypertonic solutions can cause which of the following:

( ) a. Overhydration/fluid volume excess

( ) b. Dehydration/fluid volume deficit

( ) c. Water intoxication

It is usually recommended that IV solutions with different osmolality be alternated. Give an example of an appropriate alternating solution. *_____

38 b; 5% D/W, 5% D/NSS, or 5% D/½ NSS (0.45% NaCl)

39

IV containers should be inspected for _____ . If IV fluids are to run for less than 50 mL/h for 12 hours, IV tubing with a (macrodrip/microdrip) _____ chamber should be used.

The macrodrip chamber delivers *_____ gtt (drops) per milliliter. The microdrip chamber delivers _____ gtt/mL/h.

39 leaks or flaws; microdrip; 10 or 20; 60

40

IV tubing should be changed at least every *_____ hours.
KVO means *_____ . An IV container should not hang
longer than _____ hours.

40 24–48; keep vein open; 24

41

Needles or IV catheters should be changed at least every
_____ days. Which of the following needles/catheters are
irritating to the veins and can cause phlebitis?
( ) a. Scalp vein needles
( ) b. Straight needles
( ) c. Polyvinyl chloride catheters
( ) d. Polyethylene catheters
( ) e. Teflon catheters
( ) f. Silicone catheters

41 3; c, d

42

A problem with ONCs is *_____ .
What can happen at the skin site with INCs?
*_____

42 severing the catheter with
the needle tip; A leak can
occur at the infusion
insertion site.

43

Which of the following body areas are preferred for the
insertion of IV devices?
( ) a. Hand veins
( ) b. Distal arm veins
( ) c. Leg veins
What body sites should be avoided? *_____ and *_____
Identify at least two client conditions when an upper extremity
should not be used. *_____

43 a, b; leg veins and affected
limbs resulting from a
stroke or mastectomy;
poor circulation, burns,
scleroderma, and rashes

44

IV fluids running too fast can cause (dehydration/overhydration)
_____ . Give two symptoms of a fluid volume excess.
*_____

44 overhydration; cough and
dyspnea, also neck vein
engorgement and chest
rales

45

KVO should run approximately _____ mL/h. Name two
types of solutions whose flow rate should be checked every
30 minutes to 1 hour.
*_____

45 10–20; hypertonic solutions
and solutions with
potassium or medications
that affect the pulse and
blood pressure (e.g.,
Levophed, epinephrine)

46 opening flow clamp, milking the tubing, raising bag, and repositioning extremity; Irrigation can dislodge clot(s) and cause an embolus (emboli) to travel to the lungs, brain, or heart.

46

Identify two methods of restoring IV fluids that have stopped running. *_____

    Explain the danger of forcefully irrigating the catheter when the IV fluid has stopped dripping. *_____

_____ .

47

Indicate how high an IV bag should hang above the infusion site:

    ( ) a. $2\frac{1}{2}$–3 inches
    ( ) b. $2\frac{1}{2}$–3 feet
    ( ) c. 5–6 feet

47 b

48

Indicate which of the following problems/complications can result from IV therapy:

    ( ) a. Infiltration
    ( ) b. Phlebitis
    ( ) c. Infections (septicemia)
    ( ) d. Bradycardia
    ( ) e. Speed shock
    ( ) f. Air embolus
    ( ) g. Pulmonary embolus
    ( ) h. Hematoma
    ( ) i. Pulmonary edema

48 a, b, c, e, f, g, h, i

49

When an IV infiltrates, the health professional should do which of the following:

    ( ) a. Decrease the flow rate
    ( ) b. Discontinue and restart the IV fluids

    Phlebitis (inflammation of the vein) can result from an IV needle or catheter that has been in the vein too long, solutions with irritating drugs (potassium, Levophed), or hypertonic solutions (25% dextrose) for TPN. Give three symptoms of phlebitis. *_____

_____

49 b; redness, edema (swelling), skin warm to touch, and pain

50
How can pyrogenic reactions (septicemia) be prevented?
*_____
    Give two symptoms of systemic infections. *_____
_____

51
What is speed shock? *_____
What is a hematoma? *_____

52
An air embolus can be fatal if more than _____ mL of air is injected into the vein.
    If an air embolus is expected, what should be done? *_____
_____

53
A pulmonary embolus results when a thrombus in the peripheral veins becomes an embolus and travels to the _____ .
    Identify two ways in which a pulmonary embolus can occur.
*_____
_____

54
Match the symptoms of an air embolus on the left with the pulmonary embolus. Refer to Table 17-2 as needed.
_____ a. Restlessness   1. Air embolus
_____ b. Chest pain   2. Pulmonary embolus
_____ c. Pallor   3. Both 1 and 2
_____ d. Cough
_____ e. Dyspnea
_____ f. Tachycardia

55
Which of the following drug additives in IV solutions can cause phlebitis or, if extravasated, can cause sloughing of the tissue?
( ) a. Potassium
( ) b. Decadron (cortisone)
( ) c. Antineoplastic agents
( ) d. Low-pH drugs (tetracycline)
( ) e. Levophed

---

50 good aseptic technique; chills, fever, headache, and tachycardia

51 Drugs given rapidly in solution. This increases the drug concentration in the body and produces shock-like symptoms.; blood (tumor) or raised ecchymosed area

52 50; Immediately place the client on left side in Trendelenburg position.

53 lungs; forcefully irrigating a clotted IV needle or catheter and IV fluids given in the lower extremities

54 a. 2; b. 2; c. 1; d. 3; e. 3; f. 3

55 a, c, d, e

56 To determine kidney function. Eighty to 90% of body potassium is excreted by the kidney. With kidney impairment or shutdown, hyperkalemia can occur.; If the potassium is not properly distributed in the IV container and its highest concentration is in the lower part of the container, it can be toxic to the myocardium (heart) and irritating to the peripheral veins.

56

In critically ill clients who are receiving potassium in IV solutions, the urine output is monitored hourly. Why? *_____

Explain why potassium should not be injected into an IV bag while it is being administered.

* _____

_____

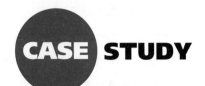

CASE STUDY   REVIEW A

Mr. Deale, age 84, was admitted to the hospital because of malnutrition. His hematocrit and BUN were elevated and his serum electrolytes were decreased. His blood gases were pH of 7.3, $PaCO_2$ of 40, and HCO_3 of 19. Mr. Deale's urine output was decreased. He was to receive 3 liters of fluid for 24 hours, 2000 mL of 5% dextrose in lactated Ringer's, and 1000 mL of 5% dextrose in 0.2% saline with 30 mEq/L of KCl.

ANSWER COLUMN

1. extracellular fluid volume

2. nutrients such as glucose and electrolytes

3. dehydration (fluid volume deficit)

4. renal impairment or failure

1. The first step in treating Mr. Deale's nutritional, fluid, and electrolyte deficits should be the restoration of

* _____

2. Along with the fluid replacement, name two other nutritional replacements that Mr. Deale needs. *_____

_____

3. Mr. Deale's elevated hematocrit and BUN may be indicative of

_____ .

4. After hydration Mr. Deale's BUN does not return to normal. What does the elevated BUN indicate? *_____

_____

5. acidosis (metabolic)

6. pulmonary edema and
   fluid volume excess
7. $1000 \div 8\,h = 125\,mL/h$ *or*

$$\frac{125\,mL/h \times 10\,gtt/mL\,(IV\,set)}{60\,min}$$

$= \dfrac{1250}{60} = 20\text{–}21\,gtt/min$

8. hematocrit; BUN; serum
   electrolytes

9. albumin, plasma or
   Plasmanate, and dextran

10. reduces clotting ability and
    interferes with type and
    cross-matching

5. Mr. Deale's blood gases show a low pH and HCO_3. These findings indicate *_____ .

6. If the IV fluids were administered at a rapid rate, what could happen to Mr. Deale taking into consideration his age and his state of dehydration? *_____
_____

7. Mr. Deale's IV fluid orders were 3000 mL (3 liters) in 24 hours or 1000 mL (1 liter) in 8 hours. Using an IV with a drip factor of 10 gtt/mL, calculate the number of drops per minute. _____

8. The health care provider determines the need for IV therapy by checking on which blood studies? _____, _____, and *_____ .

9. Mr. Deale was ordered to receive a plasma volume expander. Name three solutions that can be used. *_____
_____

10. Identify two potential adverse effects that can occur with dextran. *_____
_____

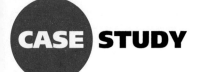 **CASE STUDY**

REVIEW B

Ms. McCann, age 60, has orders to receive 2 liters of 5% dextrose in normal saline (0.9% NaCl) daily. After several days, Ms. McCann's skin turgor was poor and her mucous membranes were dry. Her pulse rate had increased 26 beats per minute.

ANSWER COLUMN

1. hypertonic

2. dehydration, or fluid
   volume deficit; poor skin
   turgor, dry mucous
   membrane, and increased
   heart rate

1. Identify the type of solution osmolality (tonicity) of 5% dextrose in saline. _____

2. What type of fluid imbalance did Ms. McCann have according to her symptoms? *_____ .
   Give three symptoms that were indicative of the fluid imbalance. *_____

3. Needles and catheters should be changed every 3 days (with some exceptions). Check for leaks when using INCs and severing the catheter with ONCs.
4. Change IV tubing every 2 days or according to agency policy.
5. Regulate drip chamber to deliver specified drops per minute with macrodrip or microdrip chambers.
6. Use hands or distal veins in the arm. Avoid using leg veins, antecubital fossa (elbow), or limbs affected with paralysis or impaired circulation.
7. Use aseptic technique when administering and caring for IV therapy.
8. a. Remove air from the IV tubing. b. Do not irrigate an IV that has stopped dripping.
9. Check for infiltration and phlebitis.
10. Monitor urine output every 4–8 hours, every hour when potassium is in the solution.

The health professional has many responsibilities with assessment and monitoring of IV therapy. Describe the nursing interventions related to the following:

3. Needle or catheter: * _____
   _____

4. IV tubing: * _____
   _____

5. Flow rate: * _____
   _____

6. Intravenous insertion site: * _____
   _____

7. Prevention of infection: * _____
   _____

8. Prevention of air and pulmonary emboli:
   a. * _____
   b. * _____

9. Drug additives: * _____
   _____

10. Urine output: * _____
    _____

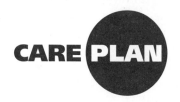

Client Management: Clients Receiving IV Therapy

Assessment Factors

The administration of IV therapy meets five basic purposes: replacement of previous fluid loss, maintenance requirements for fluids and electrolytes, meeting concurrent fluid losses, meeting nutritional needs, and a mechanism for the administration of medications and blood and blood products. An awareness of the specific purpose of the IV therapy is essential to an accurate assessment. Inherent in the administration of IV infusions are numerous procedural responsibilities and implications for the assessment of risk factors created by IV infusions. The assessment factors and diagnoses discussed in this section are limited to the responsibilities and implications for specific risks associated with IV therapy and fluid balance.

Assessment factors related to responsibilities and risk factors associated with IV therapy:

▶ Monitor fluid balance. Knowledge of the specific purpose of the prescribed IV therapy along with a basic understanding of the types of IV solutions is essential in promoting fluid balance with IV therapy. While the health care provider may prescribe the type and amount of IV solution administered, the health professional must coordinate these activities and assess the client for potential risks associated with the prescribed therapy. An accurate record of intake and output, observations for expected and unexpected client responses to IV infusions, close monitoring of laboratory results (electrolytes, hemoglobin and hematocrit, etc.), and keen physical assessment skills focused on the detection of signs and symptoms of dehydration or overhydration are needed to promote early identification of fluid balance problems.

▶ Monitor equipment used in the administration of IV therapy. IV containers and tubing must be closely observed for leaks. IV therapy requires a closed system, and any leaks or openings provide a medium for microorganisms to invade the system and contaminate the solution. Check the drip size on the IV tubing. Drip size can vary from company to company and has implications for accurately meeting fluid requirements of IV therapy (macrodrips vary from 10 to 20 gtt/mL; microdrips generally equal 60 gtt/mL). Macrodrip chambers should be used when administering amounts of fluid greater than 50 mL/h. Microdrip chambers should be used if this amount is to be less than 50 mL/h. Procedures for changing IV tubings and the length of time for their use are usually determined by hospital policy (generally the tubing is changed every 24–48 hours). A single IV container should not be infused over a period longer than 24 hours. Microdrip chambers are suggested to keep the vein open (KVO) with 250–500 mL of fluid running at 10–20 mL/h.

▶ Select and observe infusion sites carefully. The selection of the type of needle or catheter and the infusion site are factors that must be assessed carefully to promote client comfort and reduce risks associated with IV therapy (see Table 17-1 for specifics related to infusion rates). In order to reduce the risks of phlebitis and dislodged thrombus, the upper extremities are preferred infusion sites. Limbs affected by a stroke, mastectomy, or injury should not be used as an infusion site. Soft restraints and arm boards are helpful in preventing dislodgement of the IV needle. Correct positioning of the tubing prevents kinking or obstruction.

▶ Continuously assess the flow rate and patency of the infusion system. Calculating flow rates and the regulation of the IV solution are the responsibility of the health professional. Maintenance of the infusion system and the solution flow rate is necessary to meet the fluid and electrolyte needs of the client. Check the rate every 30 minutes to prevent complications and ensure fluid balance. Patency of the system and regulation of the flow rate can be influenced by various factors other than the tubing clamp (height of the solution, repositioning of the extremity, or milking of the tubing can assist in enhancing the flow rate of sluggish IVs).

▶ Assess for problems and complications of IV infusion. Possible complications of IV infusions include infiltration, extravasation, phlebitis, systemic infections, speed shock, air emboli, pulmonary embolism, pulmonary edema, hematomas, runaway IV fluids, and reactions to additives. Early recognition of the signs and symptoms of these complications is a key responsibility.

Diagnosis 1

Risk for fluid volume excess related to runaway IV or volume infused too great for client's physical condition.

Interventions and Rationale

1. Identify source/reason for excessive fluid intake. Determine whether the fluid overload is accidental in nature or the result of changes in the physiologic status of the client. Report errors in fluid regulation and seek consultation in adjusting fluid volume replacement/maintenance.

2. Assess client's response to fluid overload and risk for medical emergencies (pulmonary edema). Observe for signs and symptoms of fluid overload, frequent vital signs, laboratory studies, etc. Notify health care provider of significant changes in client's condition.

3. Reduce causative factors. Poor regulation of fluid intake and runaway IV infusion are primary causes of a fluid overload

that can be controlled. Accurately calculate flow rate and monitor the rate every 30 minutes to every hour based on client's physical condition.

4. Use electronic infusion pumps as appropriate to regulate IV flow rate. EIPs are preferable if available and mandatory when administering specific medications.

5. Monitor blood values. Electrolytes should be monitored every 4 hours in acutely ill clients and as needed according to the client's physical condition. Creatinine/BUN ratios and the hemoglobin and hematocrit levels should be evaluated every 8 hours until stable.

6. Monitor weight daily. Report sudden weight gains or losses to determine indications of IV fluid changes related to fluid overload or a fluid deficit.

7. Closely assess physiologic responses to fluid load. Monitor vital signs according to physical condition. Auscultate lungs every 2–4 hours for rales, palpate pedal pulses, test for edema in extremities, and monitor for changes in mental status that may result from electrolyte imbalances. Continuous physical assessment of the client's condition is essential to prevent life-threatening conditions that can result from a fluid overload.

Diagnosis 2

Risk for fluid volume deficit related to inadequate fluid intake.

Interventions and Rationale

1. Monitor intake and output. The health professional is responsible for coordinating the factors that control fluid balance for clients. Accurate documentation of intake and output provides essential clues to detecting risks for deficit imbalances. Use an EIP if available. Accurately calculate fluid rate and monitor rate closely (every $\frac{1}{2}$–1 hour observation).

2. Assess for physiologic signs of dehydration. Check mucous membranes for color and dryness, evaluate skin turgor, assess for orthostatic hypotension when checking vital signs, check vital signs every 1–4 hours according to client's physical condition, and check weight daily. Recognize changes in hydration that indicate a change in status and increase risk for fluid volume overload. Confusion is more common in dehydration than in a fluid overload.

3. Monitor lab studies. Electrolyte imbalances are often the first sign of an increased risk for dehydration. Cretinine/BUN ratios and hemoglobin and hematocrit ratios provide evidence of dehydration. Urine specific gravity can be done every 8 hours to assess hydration status. Serum osmolality measurements should be assessed every 24 hours.

Diagnosis 3

Risk for infection related to contaminated IV fluids, contaminated equipment, or a break in aseptic technique.

Interventions and Rationale

1. Use sterile technique. When inserting infusion devices, changing IV tubing, changing site dressings, or changing IV containers, sterile techniques are mandatory. IVs are a closed system, and any break in the system provides the potential for bacterial invasion.

2. Assess IV insertion site. Fluid leakage, pain, redness, swelling, or drainage at the insertion site is abnormal. Examination of the insertion site often provides the first clues to infection potential or inadequate function of the system.

3. Change peripheral IV site every 72 hours or according to agency policy. Procedures for the care of IV sites vary with agency policy. A period of 72 hours is generally considered the maximum time for peripheral infusion sites.

4. Change IV tubing and dressing sites every 24–48 hours according to agency procedure. Dressing changes are essential to the prevention of infections. Confirm expiration dates of IV tubing and fluids before hanging to ensure sterility.

Other Diagnoses to Consider

Risk for tissue perfusion (renal, cardiopulmonary, and peripheral): decreased, related to fluid volume deficit and inadequate fluid replacement. This is a collaborative problem. Interventions are similar to those with a fluid volume deficit with special consideration given to the select systems involved.

Risk for knowledge deficit related to lack of familiarity with IV therapy.

Evaluation/Outcome

1. Evaluate the effects of intravenous (IV) therapy to replace fluid and electrolyte losses, to meet concurrent fluid losses, to maintain fluid balance.

2. Remain free of complications related to IV therapy, phlebitis, infiltration, fluid overload.

3. Continuous assessments of IV flow rate and the tonicity of the prescribed daily IV fluids.

4. Maintain a support system for the client.

UNIT VI

CLINICAL SITUATIONS: FLUID, ELECTROLYTE, AND ACID-BASE IMBALANCES

▶ INTRODUCTION

In clinical and home care settings health professionals provide care for persons experiencing a variety of problems related to fluid and electrolytes. Unit VI addresses clinical situations. The first two chapters focus on the developmental issues related to infants, children, and the aging adult. The remaining chapters focus on trauma and shock, burns, gastrointestinal surgery, renal failure, increased intracranial pressure, oncology and chronic diseases including heart failure, diabetic ketoacidosis, and chronic obstructive pulmonary disease (COPD). In order to assess the client's needs and to provide the appropriate care needed for persons with selected health problems, the health professional must have a working knowledge and understanding of the concepts related to fluid and electrolyte imbalance. Knowledge of these concepts allows the health professional to assess physiologic changes that occur with fluid, electrolyte, and acid-base imbalances and to plan appropriate interventions to assist clients as they adapt to these changes.

In each clinical situation the participant will become acquainted with clients who have fluid and electrolyte imbalances. Clients are presented as part of a clinical situation. Some of the client situations used in this unit have already been presented in earlier case study reviews. The participant in this program will gain an understanding of the physiologic changes involved in each clinical situation.

Fluid Problems of Infants and Children

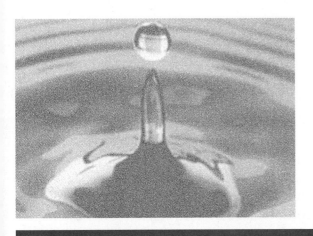

Gail H. Wade, RN, MS

OBJECTIVES

Upon completion of this chapter, the reader should be able to:

- Identify three physiologic factors that influence infants' and children's responses to changes in fluid and electrolyte balance.
- Compare the total body fluid volume in infants and children to the total body fluid volume in the mature adult.
- Identify normal serum electrolyte values for sodium, potassium, and calcium in infants and children.
- Discuss how the electrolyte values for sodium, potassium, and calcium vary in response to fluid balance changes in infants and children.

(continued on next page)

OBJECTIVES (Continued)

● Describe a method to calculate the daily fluid and electrolyte needs of infants and children.

● Describe assessment factors important in determining fluid and electrolyte balance in infants and children.

● Develop diagnoses for infants and children experiencing fluid balance problems.

● Identify interventions specific to selected diagnoses associated with fluid balance problems.

▶ INTRODUCTION

The health professional's understanding of the physiologic differences in infants and children that have implications for fluid and electrolyte balance is essential to providing optimal health care. Since these physiologic differences vary significantly throughout infancy and childhood, important regulatory factors are presented from a developmental perspective. Health professionals need to understand the implications of these developmental characteristics and the potential for fluid balance problems. This chapter addresses those factors as well as normal chemistry values and physiologic factors that influence infants' and children's rapid responses to changes in fluid and electrolyte balance.

▶ PHYSIOLOGIC FACTORS

Physiologic differences in the infant's total body surface area, immaturity of renal structures, high rate of metabolism, and immaturity of the endocrine system in promoting homeostatic control predispose this age group to various fluid and electrolyte imbalances. The proportionately high ratio of extracellular fluid (ECF) to intracellular fluid (ICF) predisposes the infant to rapid losses of body fluid. The infant's limited fluid reserve capacity inhibits adaptation to fluid losses. Additionally the infant's renal structures are not fully developed until the latter half of the second year of life. All of these factors increase the infant's vulnerability to dehydration.

1

The body is composed mostly of water. Body water in the early human embryo represents _____% of body weight, in the newborn infant _____%, and in the adult _____%. (Refer to Chapter 1, question 1.)

The low-birth-weight infant's (premature infant's) body water represents 80–90% of body weight.

1 97; 77; 60

2

Complete the percentage of body weight that is representative of body water in the following:

Early human embryo	_____%
Low-birth-weight infant	_____%
Newborn infant	_____%
Adult	_____%

2 97; 80–90; 77; 60

3

Infants need proportionately more water than adults. The infant's large body surface area and immature kidney limit the infant's ability to retain water. Their kidneys cannot concentrate urine effectively; thus, urine volume is increased. More water is lost through the infant's skin because of the increased body surface area. Since the infant cannot concentrate urine, water is needed to maintain fluid volume lost through the increased urine output and larger body surface area.

Give two reasons why the infant needs a higher percentage of total body water.

*_____

_____

3 a large body surface (greater amounts of water loss through the skin) and inability to concentrate urine (increased urine output due to immature kidneys)

4

Water distribution in the newborn is not the same as in an adult. The ECF in the infant is 50% of body weight. The

percentage of body weight (ECF) in the adult is _____ .
(Refer to Chapter 5.)

The ICF in the infant is 35% of body weight; whereas in the adult it is _____ . (Refer to Chapter 5). The proportionately higher ratio of ECF volume in the infant predisposes the infant to (more, less) _____ rapid losses of fluid volume; consequently, _____ develops more rapidly in infants than adults.

4 20%; 40%; more; dehydration

5

At 1 year, the percentage of the child's total body water is close in amount to the percentage of the adult's (60%) total body water; and, the proportion of ECF (25%) and ICF (40–45%) is also similar to that of the adult.

The extracellular fluid is composed of _____ and _____ fluid. Another name for intracellular fluid is (cellular/vascular) _____ fluid. (Refer to Chapter 1.)

5 interstitial and intravascular; cellular

6

Increased body surface area in the infant causes excess water loss through the _____ . The smaller the infant, the greater the body surface area in proportion to body weight. The infant's kidneys are (mature/immature) _____; thus, the urinary volume is (increased/decreased) _____ .

6 skin; immature; increased

7

It may take 2 years before the child's kidneys are mature.

The infant's immature kidneys decrease the glomerular filtration rate (GFR); thus, the kidney's ability to concentrate urine is (decreased/increased) _____ , while the urine volume is (decreased/increased) _____ .

Giving too much water can cause (dehydration/overhydration) _____ .

7 decreased; increased; overhydration

8

As the child grows, there is muscle growth and cellular growth. More water shifts from the ECF to the ICF compartment.

What do you think is the contributing factor when the child's ICF and ECF proportions become similar to the adults? *_____

8 Increased cellular and muscular growth causes water to shift from the ECF space to the ICF space.

▶ ETIOLOGY

9

The infant has less body fluid reserve than the adult and is more likely to develop a fluid volume deficit.

An infant may lose one-half of ECF daily; however, under normal conditions losses are replaced simultaneously. Adults lose only one-sixth of their ECF in the same length of time.

Name two reasons why an infant may lose one-half of ECF daily. *_____

_____

The infant is likely to develop dehydration more rapidly than adults who lose proportionately similar amounts of water. This increased risk for infants is the result of their (increased/ decreased) _____ fluid reserve.

10

Factors that increase insensible fluid loss are hyperthermia, increased activity, hyperventilation, radiant warmers, and phototherapy.

Keeping an infant covered in a stable cool environment (reduces/increases) _____ insensible fluid loss through the body surface.

11

Serum electrolytes do not vary greatly between infants and adults. The serum sodium level in a newborn fluctuates at birth. It may be low the first 3–6 hours after birth and then rise slightly (2–6 mEq/L increase) during the first 2 days of life.

The infant's normal serum sodium range is 139–146 mEq/L and the child's normal serum range is 135–148 mEq/L. What is the normal adult serum sodium level? *_____

12

A 5-month-old infant who consumes cow's milk and commercially prepared baby food ingests five times more sodium than a breast-fed infant.

The name for an elevated serum sodium level is _____ .

9 large body surface area causing water to be lost through the skin (insensible perspiration) and increased urinary output (immature kidneys cannot concentrate urine); decreased

10 reduces

11 135–146 mEq/L

12 hypernatremia (serum sodium excess)

13

Low-birth-weight infants tend to develop hypernatremia with a normal to low sodium intake. Their body surface area is (greater/lesser) _____ than an average-weight newborn's and their insensible water loss is (increased/decreased) _____ .

Also, low-birth-weight infants' kidneys are more immature than the kidneys of average-weight infants; therefore, more diluted water is excreted. The loss of water is in excess of the loss of solutes. In low-birth-weight infants this increases their risk of developing _____ .

13 greater; increased; hypernatremia

14

Hyponatremia can also occur in infants and children. Another name for hyponatremia is *_____ .
Three causes of hyponatremia are:
 a. Overhydration—water overloading
 b. Continuous administration of oral or parenteral electrolyte-free solutions
 c. Syndrome of inappropriate antidiuretic hormone (SIADH). This results in an excess secretion of ADH causing excess water reabsorption from the distal tubules. Factors attributing to SIADH are CNS injuries or illness (head injuries, meningitis), pneumonia, neoplasm, stress, surgery, and drugs (narcotics, barbiturates).

14 serum sodium deficit

15 overhydration, continuous administration of electrolyte-free solutions, and SIADH

15

Name three causes of hyponatremia. *_____
_____

16

A rapid decrease in the serum sodium, 120 mEq/L or below, can cause CNS changes such as headache, twitching, confusion, and convulsions. In infants, increased irritability or other subtle changes in state and feeding behavior may occur.

Observe for CNS changes when hyponatremia occurs suddenly. Give three CNS symptoms. *_____

16 headache, twitching, and confusion (also convulsions)

17

The normal potassium range for the infant is 3.5–5.0 mEq/L. The top level is slightly higher than the adult's and remains in the upper level for the first few months of the infant's life.

17 cells or ICF (In various institutions, laboratory values may vary slightly.)

Try to recall where the greatest concentration of potassium is found in the body. _____

18

Infants and children may develop hypokalemia (serum potassium deficit) when cellular breakdown occurs from injury, starvation, dehydration, diarrhea, vomiting, diabetic acidosis, and steroids for treating nephrosis. Children do not conserve potassium well. The kidneys continue to excrete body potassium even with little or no potassium intake.

18 dizziness, muscular weakness, abdominal distention, decreased peristalsis, and arrhythmia

Give at least two signs or symptoms of hypokalemia. (Refer to Chapter 6.) *_____

19

Eighty to 90% of body potassium loss is excreted in the urine. When oliguria (decreased urine output) occurs, what type of potassium imbalance results? _____

19 hyperkalemia, or serum potassium excess

20

The infant's normal serum chloride range is 96–116 mEq/L. For the first few months of the infant's life the serum sodium range is *_____ and the serum potassium range is *_____ . The normal range of the child's serum chloride level is 98–111 mEq/L.

20 139–146 mEq/L; 3.5–5.0 mEq/L

21

The serum calcium level in the cord blood is higher than the maternal serum calcium level; however, after birth the infant's serum calcium level decreases to 3.8 mEq/L, or 7.7 mg/dL. In low-birth-weight infants, the serum calcium tends to remain lower for a longer period of time. (A child's normal serum calcium range is 4.5–5.8 mEq/L, or 8–10.8 mg/dL.)

Infants do not have calcium stored in their bones as do adults. If infants are fed cow's milk, their body calcium level may remain low since cow's milk has a high phosphorus content, which lowers the calcium level.

Breast-fed infants receive more calcium and retain it since breast milk contains less phosphorus.

21 the breast-fed infant; Breast milk contains more calcium and less phosphorus, which gives the infant more calcium. Thus, reducing phosphorus allows the infant to retain the calcium.

Which infant retains more body calcium—the infant receiving cow's milk or the breast-fed infant? *_____ . Why? *_____

22

Newborn infants tend to have a low pH, which is indicative of metabolic acidosis. This is the result of increased acid metabolites that result from the infant's increased metabolic rate and physiologic changes during birth. The pH becomes closer to normal after the first few days or weeks of life. In low-birth-weight infants, the pH remains low for several weeks.

The low pH of cow's milk combined with the low serum calcium level in infants (does/does not) _____ result in symptoms of tetany.

23

Ionized calcium levels, important indicators of the child's acid-base balance, are slightly lower than serum calcium levels. The binding of calcium to protein is affected by the pH. When the pH decreases with acidosis, ionized calcium increases and calcium is removed from proteins and is available for chemical reactions. Alkalosis increases the binding of calcium to proteins and decreases the concentration of ionized calcium. Tetany symptoms occur when hypocalcemia (serum calcium deficit) is present in a normal acid-base balance or in an alkalotic state.

Symptoms of tetany are *_____ and *_____ . (Refer to Chapter 8.)

▶ CLINICAL APPLICATIONS

There are several formulas and nomograms for calculating fluid and electrolyte maintenance requirements in infants and children. Table 18-1 suggests a simple method for calculating daily fluid and electrolyte maintenance requirements for infants and children. The formula is based on the assumption that for each 100 calories metabolized, 100 mL of water is required. This method is not used with neonates less than 14 days old or with conditions of abnormal fluid losses.

To calculate the daily fluid and electrolyte needs of infants and children, first calculate the infant's/child's weight in kilograms (kg). Then use this chart to calculate the specific fluid and electrolyte needs according to the body weight in kilograms.

22 does not (Calcium is ionized in an acidotic state regardless of how low it is.)

23 tingling of fingers and twitching around mouth (also, carpopedal spasm)

Table 18-1

Fluid and Electrolyte Maintenance Requirements for Infants and Children According to the Holiday-Segar Method

Body Weight (kg)	Water (mL/kg/day)	Electrolytes (mEq per 100 mL H_2O)
First 10 kg	100	Na^+3
Second 10 kg	50	Cl^-2
Each additional kg	20	K^+2

Source: Adapted from *The Harriet Lane Handbook: A Manual for Pediatric House Officers* (14th ed.), by M. A. Barone (Ed.), 1996, St. Louis: Mosby.

24

Using Table 18-1, calculate which of the following are daily fluid requirements for an infant weighing 6 kg:

( ) a. 300 mL
( ) b. 600 mL
( ) c. 900 mL

24 b

25

Using Table 18-1, calculate the daily fluid requirements of a child weighing 30 kg:

( ) a. 1500 mL
( ) b. 1700 mL
( ) c. 1250 mL

The daily sodium requirement according to the fluid needs of this child is:

( ) d. 17 mEq
( ) e. 45 mEq
( ) f. 51 mEq

The daily potassium and chloride requirements according to the fluid needs for this child are:

( ) g. 34 mEq
( ) h. 17 mEq
( ) i. 30 mEq

25 b; f; g

In situations of minimal fluid and electrolyte imbalances, oral intake of fluids should be encouraged to maintain fluid and electrolyte balance. Table 18-2 contains a list of common fluids and the approximate electrolyte composition.

Table 18-2

Electrolyte Composition of Common Oral Fluids

| Fluid | mEq/liter | | | |
	Na$^+$	K$^+$	Cl$^-$	HCO$_3^-$
Apple juice	0.4	26	—	—
Orange juice	0.2	49	—	50
Grape juice	0.8	29.6	—	—
Gatorade	21	2.5	17	—
Jello (half-strength)	5.5–16.5*	0.1–0.2	—	—
Coca-Cola	4.3	0.1	—	13.4
Pepsi-Cola	0	0	—	—
Ginger Ale	3.5	0.1	—	3.6
Sprite	7.6	0	—	—

*Varies according to flavor. Wild cherry has the highest Na$^+$ and grape and black raspberry the lowest.

Source: Adapted from *Nelson Textbook of Pediatrics* (15th ed.), by R. E. Behrman, 1997, Philadelphia: Saunders; *Whaley & Wong's Nursing Care of Infants and Children* (5th ed.), D. L. Wong, 1995, St. Louis: Mosby.

26

For fluid and electrolyte maintenance in children, decarbonated ginger ale, cola, and full-strength apple juice are not recommended (Wong, 1995). These fluids are high in glucose concentration and thus have a high osmolarity. Therefore, juices diluted with half water are more appropriate. Milk is also not considered a liquid because it forms curds when in contact with stomach renin.

Give two reasons why cola is contraindicated in the maintenance of fluid and electrolyte balance. * _____

_____

26 Cola is high in glucose concentration and osmolality.

27

The encouragement of fluid intake in a child is often a challenge. When possible, the preferences of the child should be considered. Which of the following fluids should be encouraged in a child experiencing anorexia? Refer to Table 18-2 and select all appropriate answers.

( ) a. Full-strength orange juice
( ) b. Half-strength apple juice
( ) c. Half-strength jello
( ) d. Ginger ale

27 b

▶ FLUID VOLUME DEFICITS

Dehydration, a common cause of fluid volume deficit in infants and young children, occurs when the total output of fluid exceeds the total intake. Dehydration associated with diarrhea is the number one cause of fluid and electrolyte imbalances in infants and children. When vomiting occurs with diarrhea, fluid and electrolyte losses are more severe.

28

The most common cause of fluid and electrolyte disturbances in infants and children is:
( ) a. Vomiting
( ) b. Diarrhea
( ) c. SIADH
( ) d. Pyloric stenosis

28 b

The most accurate way to assess fluid volume deficits in infants and children is based on the preillness weight. The following formula can be used to calculate the percent of dehydration. To use this formula, the weight in pounds must be converted to kilograms (kg):

$$\% \text{ Dehydration} = \frac{\text{preillness weight} - \text{illness weight}}{\text{preillness weight}} \times 100\%$$

29

In infants and young children, decreases in body weight of 3–5% are considered mild dehydration; moderate with a weight loss of 6–10%; and severe when the loss is over 10%. In older children, decreases of 3–5% and 6–9% represent moderate and severe dehydration.

Example: Mary weighed 30 pounds, or 13.6 kg, before she became ill. Now she weighs 26 pounds, or 11.8 kg. She has lost 4 pounds, or 1.8 kg.

29 13; severe

The percentage of weight loss is _____%. The degree of dehydration is (mild, moderate, severe) _____ .

30
If a 2-year-old with diarrhea weighed 15 kg prior to the illness and 14 kg when assessed in the clinic, the percent dehydration is _____ and it is classified as _____ dehydration.

30 6-7%; moderate

31
In an older child, this percent of weight loss would be an indicator of _____ dehydration.

31 severe

The degree of body fluid loss can be determined by the weight loss. Body weight loss greater than 1% per day represents loss of body water. For every 1% weight loss, 10 mL/kg of body fluid is lost. Therefore, parents should be encouraged to keep an accurate record of the child's weight. When pre-illness weight is not available, however, clinical observations as described in Table 18-3 can be used. Dehydration is classified as mild, moderate, and severe based on these observations.

32
Indicate which symptoms may be associated with mild dehydration in infants and children.
    ( ) a. Increased heart rate
    ( ) b. Decreased tear production
    ( ) c. Sunken eyeballs
    ( ) d. Confusion
    ( ) e. Increased concentration of urine
32 a, c, e, f
    ( ) f. Elevated specific gravity

33
Indicate which symptoms are typical of moderate to severe dehydration in infants and children.
    ( ) a. Increased heart rate
    ( ) b. Decreased tears
    ( ) c. Sunken fontanels
    ( ) d. Increased specific gravity
    ( ) e. Sunken eyeballs
    ( ) f. Decreased blood pressure
    ( ) g. Decreased skin turgor
33 All of the above.
    ( ) h. Oliguria

Table 18-3

Clinical Assessment of Degree of Dehydration in Infants and Children

% Dehydration (mL/kg)		
Infants	Children	Clinical Assessment
5% (50 mL/kg)	3% (30 mL/kg)	Heart rate (10–15% above baseline) Slightly dry mucous membranes Concentrated urine Sunken eyeballs Alert, restless
10% (100 mL/kg)	6% (60 mL/kg)	Increased severity of above Systolic blood pressure may be low Respirations may be deep and increased Urine reduced and concentrated Decreased skin turgor Sunken anterior fontanel Restless or lethargic Irritable to touch
15% (150 mL/kg)	9% (90 mL/kg)	Marked severity of preceding signs Decreased systolic blood pressure Delayed capillary refill Very deep rapid breathing Significant decrease in urine output Decreased level of consciousness

Source: Adapted from *The Harriet Lane Handbook: A Manual for Pediatric House Officers* (14th ed., p. 218), St. Louis: Mosby. Additional data from Samson & Ouzts (1996), p. 394.

34
With severe dehydration, ECF and ICF are lost. With a slow, progressive fluid loss, the ICF shifts into the ECF compartment (vessels and tissue spaces) to replace the ECF loss. What do you think occurs when dehydration develops rapidly?
*
_____

34 ECF loss is greater than ICF loss. ICF cannot replace ECF loss quickly.

In general, when dehydration occurs in less than 3 days, 80% of the losses are from the ECF and 20% of the losses are from the ICF. If dehydration occurs over a longer period of time, 60% of the losses are from the ECF and 40% of the losses are from the ICF.

35

When a child develops dehydration over a period of 2 days, the percentage of ECF loss may be _____ and the percentage of ICF loss may be _____ .

When dehydration occurs over a period of 1 week, the percentage of ECF loss may be _____ and the percentage of ICF loss may be _____ .

35 80%; 20%; 60%; 40%

▶ TYPES OF DEHYDRATION

36

Dehydration is classified according to the serum concentration of solutes (osmolality). Sodium is the primary contributor to the serum osmolality. Dehydration has three classifications in relation to osmolality and sodium concentration: (a) iso-osmolar dehydration (isonatremic dehydration); (b) hyperosmolar dehydration (hypernatremic dehydration); and (c) hypo-osmolar dehydration (hyponatremic dehydration).

Which type of dehydration has the highest osmolality (concentration)? _____

36 hyperosmolar, or hyper-natremic dehydration

37

All degrees of dehydration are frequently associated with iso-osmolality or isonatremic dehydration. This is the most common type of dehydration, which results in proportionate losses of fluid and sodium.

Hypernatremic dehydration and hyponatremic dehydration indicate involvement of the electrolyte _____ .

37 sodium

Table 18-4 lists the three types of dehydration: isonatremic, hypernatremic, and hyponatremic. For each of the dehydrations, the water and sodium loss, serum sodium level, ECF and ICF loss, causes, symptoms, and treatments are described. Study the table carefully and refer to it as needed.

38

With isonatremic dehydration, there is a proportionate loss of the ions _____ and _____ . The serum sodium level is between _____ and _____ . The ECF volume is (increased/decreased) _____ .

38 sodium; water; 130 mEq/L; 150 mEq/L; decreased

Table 18-4

Types of Dehydration: Isonatremic, Hypernatremic, and Hyponatremic

Types of Dehydration	Water and Sodium Loss	Serum Sodium Level	ECF and ICF Loss	Causes	Symptoms	Treatment
Isonatremic dehydration (iso-osmolar or isotonic dehydration)	Proportionately equal loss of water and sodium	130–150 mEq/L	Extracellular fluid volume is markedly decreased (severe hypovolemia). Since sodium and water loss are approximately the same, there is no osmotic pull from ICF to ECF. The plasma volume is significantly reduced and shock occurs from decreased circulating blood volume. ICF volume remains virtually constant.	Diarrhea, vomiting, and malnutrition (decreases in fluid and food intake) are the most common causes.	With severe fluid loss, symptoms are characteristic of hypovolemic shock: rapid pulse rate, rapid respiration; and later, a decreasing systolic blood pressure. Other symptoms are weight loss, irritability, lethargy, pale or gray skin color, dry mucous membranes, reduced skin turgor, sunken eyeballs, sunken fontanels, absence of tearing and salivation, and decreased urine output.	Fluid should be restored rapidly to correct hypovolemic shock. Iso-osmolar solutions, i.e., Ringer's lactate and 5% dextrose in 0.2% NaCl or 0.3% NaCl, are some of the choices. Replacement should be calculated over 24 h; if dehydration is severe, half of the amount of solution should be given over the first 8 h and the remaining half over the next 16 h.
Hypernatremic dehydration (hyperosmolar or hypertonic dehydration) (second leading type of dehydration in children)	Water loss is greater than sodium loss; sodium excess	↑ 150 mEq/L	ECF and ICF volumes are both decreased. Increased ECF osmolality (solutes) results in a shift of fluid from the ICF to the ECF causing severe cellular dehydration. ECF depletion may not be as severe as ICF depletion. Loss of hypo-osmolar fluid raises the osmolality of ECF.	Severe diarrhea (water is lost in excess to solutes) and high solute intake with decreased water intake are the two most common causes. Others include fever, poor renal function, rapid breathing, or any combination of these conditions.	Shock is less apparent since ECF loss is not as severe. Symptoms include weight loss, avid thirst, confusion, convulsions, tremors, thickened and firm skin turgor, sunken eyeballs and fontanels, absence of tearing, moderately rapid pulse, moderately rapid respirations, frequently normal blood pressure, normal to decreased urine output, and intracranial hemorrhage.	The goal is to increase the ICF and ECF volumes without causing water intoxication. Giving excessive hypo-osmolar solutions or only 5% dextrose in water would dilute ECF, causing water to shift to the ICF and water intoxication (ICF volume excess) to occur. A gradual reduction over 48 h of solution is safest. Dextrose 5% with 0.2% NaCl may be ordered and later lactated Ringer's solution. With normal urinary flow, potassium can be added to the solution (2–3 mEq/kg).

(continues on the following page)

Table 18-4

Types of Dehydration: Isonatremic, Hypernatremic, and Hyponatremic (Continued)

Types of Dehydration	Water and Sodium Loss	Serum Sodium Level	ECF and ICF Loss	Causes	Symptoms	Treatment
Hyponatremic dehydration (hypo-osmolar or hypotonic dehydration)	Sodium loss is greater than water loss; excess water	↓ 130 mEq/L	ECF is severely decreased, and ICF is increased. The osmolality of ECF is lower than the osmolality of ICF. Water shifts from the ECF to the ICF (lesser to the greater concentration). The cerebral cells are frequently affected first as the excess water interferes with brain cell activity.	Severe diarrhea (sodium is lost in excess of water), excessive water intake, electrolyte-free fluid infusions (5% dextrose in water), sodium-losing nephropathy, and diuretic therapy.	Thirst, weight loss, lethargy, comatose, poor skin turgor, clammy skin, sunken and soft eyeballs, absence of tearing, shock symptoms (rapid pulse rate, rapid respirations, and low systolic blood pressure), and decreased urine output.	Ringer's lactate or 5% dextrose in 0.45% NaCl (1/2 NSS) can help to correct the serum sodium level (125–135 mEq/L). For serum sodium of 15 mEq/L, normal saline can be used. For serum sodium of 15 mEq/L or less, 3% saline may be indicated. Rapid fluid correction with electrolytes can cause an excessive shift of cellular fluid into the plasma. The result can be overhydration and congestive heart failure.

39 diarrhea and vomiting, also malnutrition; rapid pulse rate, rapid respiration, and decreasing systolic blood pressure (others could be gray skin color, lethargy)

39

Two common causes of isonatremic dehydration are * _____

_____ .

   With severe dehydration, shock symptoms are common. Give three shock symptoms. * _____

_____

40

With hypernatremic dehydration, which is lost to a greater degree: (water/sodium)? _____ The serum sodium level is _____ mEq/L. ECF and ICF volumes are decreased. Which body fluid compartment has the largest fluid loss: (ECF/ICF)?

_____

40 water; 150 ↑; ICF

41

Give two causes of hypernatremic dehydration. * _____

_____

   Shock symptoms (are/are not) _____ common with this type of dehydration.

   Check the symptoms found with hypernatremic dehydration:

( ) a. Avid thirst   ( ) d. Skin turgor firm and thickened

( ) b. Convulsions   ( ) e. Absence of tearing

( ) c. Tremors   ( ) f. Excess urine output

41 severe diarrhea and high solute intake; are not; a, b, c, d, e

42

With hyponatremic dehydration, the loss of _____ is greater than the loss of _____ . The serum sodium level is _____ mEq/L. ECF is (increased/decreased) _____ and ICF is (increased/decreased) _____ .

42 sodium; water; 130; decreased; increased

43

Give three causes of hyponatremic dehydration. * _____

_____

   Check the symptoms found with hyponatremic dehydration:

( ) a. Thirst   ( ) e. Sunken, soft eyeballs

( ) b. Weight gain   ( ) f. Rapid pulse rate

( ) c. Poor skin turgor ( ) g. Rapid respiration

( ) d. Clammy skin   ( ) h. Low systolic blood pressure

43 severe diarrhea, excessive water intake, and electrolyte-free fluid infusions (others are sodium-losing nephropathy and diuretic therapy); a, c, d, e, f, g, h

▶ TREATMENT OPTIONS

44

44 restore fluid; electrolyte
balance and prevent
hypovolemic shock

Regardless of the type of dehydration, immediate treatment of infants and children is needed to prevent hypovolemic shock. Oral rehydration is the treatment of choice for children with mild to moderate dehydration. The primary goal of rehydration therapy is to *_____ and *_____.

For mild dehydration, parents should be urged to give the child any kind of oral fluid that the child tolerates and to continue feeding. Formula can be given to infants. If these approaches are unsuccessful, then oral electrolyte solutions should be given.

Table 18-5 contains a list of oral electrolyte solutions that are used for rehydration and maintenance. Generic brands of the solution that are similar to Pedialyte are also available. When purchasing generic brands, however, it is important to select the appropriate solution for the type of rehydration or maintenance therapy needed.

45

The two major types of oral electrolyte fluids are those for rehydration and those used for maintenance. Rehydration solutions contain more sodium than do maintenance solutions. Oral Electrolyte solutions that may be used for rehydration are _____ and _____ .

45 Rehydralyte; ORS (WHO)

Table 18-5

Oral Electrolyte Solutions

Product	Na (mEq/L)	K (mEq/L)	Cl (mEq/L)	Base (mEq/L)	Glucose (g/L)
Infalyte	50	25	45	30	30
Naturalyte	45	20	35	48	25
Pedialyte	45	20	35	30	25
Ricelyte	50	25	45	34	30
Rehydralyte	75	20	65	30	25
ORS (WHO)	90	20	80	30	20

Source: Adapted from *Seminars in Pediatric Infectious Disease* (5th ed., p. 231), by J. Snyder, 1994.

Nausea and mild vomiting are not contraindications of oral rehydration therapy. Oral rehydration solutions are given in small amounts of 5–10 mL every 5–10 minutes and increased as tolerated. Administering the solution with a teaspoon or an oral syringe may help to monitor the amounts more accurately. Rehydration therapy for mild dehydration is 50 mL/kg given over 4 hours. For moderate dehydration, 100 mL/kg should be given over 4 hours.

46

For a child weighing 20 kg with mild dehydration, how much rehydration fluid should be given over 4 hours? *_____ In the first hour? *_____

46 1000 mL; 250 mL

Once rehydration is accomplished, the child should be encouraged to resume a normal diet. Some physicians prescribe diluted or lactose-free formulas for infants while others believe that full-strength formula can be given. Breast-fed infants may supplement their feedings with an electrolyte solution (usually 100 mL/kg is recommended). Any ongoing losses (through stool or emesis) should also be replaced. For each loss through diarrhea stools, 10 mL/kg of child's body weight should be replaced with an electrolyte solution.

47

Breast-fed infants on maintenance therapy are sometimes given *_____ of an oral electrolyte solution to supplement breast feedings. Formula fed infants may be given *_____ or *_____ formulas.

47 100 mL/kg; lactose free; half-strength regular

48

For a child weighing 15 kg that has two diarrhea stools, how much replacement solution should be given? *_____

48 300 mL

With the resumption of a normal diet, physicians may prescribe 100 mL/kg of oral electrolyte solution to supplement the diet. Diets that are low in simple carbohydrates and contain easily digestible foods such as cereal, yogurt, cooked vegetables, and soups can be given to older children. Toddlers may tolerate soft or pureed foods. The BRAT diet (bananas, rice, apples, and toast or tea) is no longer recommended because of its limited nutritional value. Also, the diet is high in carbohydrates and low in electrolytes. Other foods to avoid are fried foods, soda, or jello water.

49

A child who is recovering from dehydration should receive a _____ diet that is low in _____ and contains easily digestible foods such as *_____

_____ .

49 regular (normal); carbohydrates; cooked vegetables, yogurt, cereal, soups

50

Name three oral electrolyte solutions that might be used in the maintenance phase of rehydration therapy. *_____

_____

These solutions contain similar concentrations of glucose and important electrolytes such as _____ , _____ , _____ , and _____ .

50 Infalyte, Naturalyte, and Pedialyte; sodium; chloride; potassium; calcium

Oral rehydration therapy is replaced with parenteral therapy in infants and children with severe vomiting, gastric distention, and severe dehydration.

51

Emergency treatment of unstable children with severe dehydration is needed to prevent or correct *_____ . In emergency situations, fluids should be restored (slowly, rapidly) _____ .

51 hypovolemic shock; rapidly

Overhydration can lead to cerebral edema with neurologic symptoms such as seizures. Therefore, careful consideration of parameters for rehydrating children is essential. Initial expansion of ECF volume to treat or prevent shock is usually accomplished with 20 mL/kg of Ringer's lactate (isotonic fluid). Once the type of dehydration is diagnosed, specific IV solutions are used. Maintenance requirements are usually calculated for a 24-hour period and focus on definitive fluid and electrolyte replacement.

52

The amount of fluid replaced is based on the calculated loss and fluid maintenance requirements. Refer to pages 346 and 347 for calculation of fluid maintenance needs. The formula for determining the fluid loss is

Percentage of dehydration (fluid loss in mL/kg)
× child's body weight in kilograms (kg)

A child who weighs 20 kg and has an estimated dehydration level of 10% has lost 10% of body weight, or 100 mL/kg. Based on this formula, *_____ is the amount of fluid lost.

52 2000 mL

53
For the first 8 hours of rehydration, half of the fluid lost plus the required maintenance fluid is replaced. In the preceding example, how much fluid should be replaced during the first 8 hours of rehydration? *_____ for body fluid loss plus *_____ for maintenance fluids, making a total of _____ mL of fluid to be administered over 8 hours or _____ mL each hour.

53 1000 mL; 500mL; 1500; 188

54
The second half of the required fluids is replaced over the next 16 hours. If a child requires 2000 mL of deficit fluids and 1500 mL of maintenance fluids over a 24-hour period, how many milliliters should be administered in the last 16 hours of daily rehydration therapy? _____
How much should be administered hourly? *_____

54 1750; 110 mL

Continued replacement over the next 48–72 hours is based on the calculated maintenance plus the estimated fluid deficit over that period.
The type of IV fluid administered is determined by the type of dehydration.

55
With hyponatremic dehydration, fluids are usually replaced and maintained with *_____ (refer to Table 18–4). For rehydration therapy when isonatremic dehydration is suspected, *_____ may be used. If serum sodium is below 115 mEq/L, what type of IV fluid may be indicated? *_____

55 5% dextrose with 0.45 normal saline; 5% dextrose with 0.2 or 0.3% normal saline; 3% saline

56
The severity of hypernatremic dehydration is often difficult to assess because fluid shifting between the intercellular and extracellular spaces preserves the circulating volume. Therefore,

56 too much

the potential of giving (too much, too little) *_____ fluid is present.

57

The goal for correcting hypernatremic dehydration is to avoid causing what major type of fluid imbalance? *_____

What electrolytes should be replaced when correcting hypernatremic dehydration? _____ and _____

57 water intoxication; calcium; later potassium with normal kidney function

58

Serum Na correction in hypernatremia should not occur any more rapidly than 0.5–1.0 mEq/L/h. To ensure that serum Na levels do not decrease too rapidly or too slowly, serum Na levels should be monitored every 2–4 hours and the fluid rate adjusted accordingly. Too rapid administration of fluid may lead to *_____ . When serum sodium reaches 120–125 mEq/L, fluid restrictions should be initiated.

58 cerebral edema

59

While severe dehydration is treated with *_____ , after the fluid and electrolyte imbalances have stabilized, *_____ is initiated.

59 intravenous therapy; oral rehydration therapy

Table 18-6 lists the assessments with rationales for determining fluid and electrolyte imbalance in infants and children. The table can be utilized as an assessment tool in the hospital, community agency, or home. In the assessment column, check or fill in the blanks. The rationales should be eliminated when used as a tool. Study the table and complete the related questions. Refer back to the table as needed.

60

The signs and symptoms of fluid balance deficits may vary with the age of the child. In the hospital, children should be assessed at least every 8 hours. Infants should be assessed more frequently. The infant or child with an existing imbalance should be assessed at least every hour.

The fluid status of a child in fluid and electrolyte imbalance should be closely monitored every _____ .

60 hour

Table 18-6

Head-to-Toe Assessment of Fluid and Electrolyte Imbalance in Infants and Children

Observation	Assessment	Rationale
Behavior and Appearance	Irritable/restless Anorexia Purposeless movement Unusual cry Lethargic Lethargy with hyperirritability on stimulation Unresponsive (comatose)	Early symptoms of fluid volume deficit are irritability, purposeless movements, and an unusual or high-pitched cry in infants. Young children may experience thirst with restlessness. As dehydration continues, lethargy and unconsciousness may occur.
Skin	Color _____ Temperature _____ Feel _____ Turgor _____	Skin color may be pale (mild), gray (moderate), or mottled (severe) depending on the degree of dehydration. Temperature is usually cold except with hypertonic dehydration where the temperature may be hot or cold. Skin feels dry with isotonic dehydration; clammy with hypotonic dehydration; and thickened and doughy with hypertonic dehydration. Turgor is measured by pinching the skin on the abdomen, chest wall or, medial aspect of the thigh and assessing the rate of skin retraction (elasticity). As dehydration progresses, elasticity decreases from fair to very poor. With hypertonic dehydration, turgor may remain fair. Skin turgor on obese infants or children may appear normal even with a deficit. Undernourishment can cause poor tissue turgor with fluid balance.
Mucous Membranes	Dryness in oral cavity (cheeks and gums) _____ Dry tongue with longitudinal wrinkles _____	The mucous membranes and tongue are dry with a fluid deficit. Sodium deficit causes the tongue to appear sticky, rough, and red. A dry tongue may also indicate mouth breathing. Some medications and vitamin deficiencies cause dryness of mucous membranes. Dryness in the oral cavity membranes (cheeks and gums) is a better indicator of fluid loss.

(continues on the following page)

Table 18-6

Head-to-Toe Assessment of Fluid and Electrolyte Imbalance in Infants and Children (Continued)

Observation	Assessment	Rationale
Eyes	Sunken _____ Tears _____ Soft eyeballs_____	Sunken eyes and dark skin around them may indicate a severe fluid volume deficit. Tears are absent with moderate to severe dehydration. (Tearing is not present until approximately 4 months of age.) Soft eyeballs may indicate isonatremic or hyponatremic dehydration.
Fontanel	Sunken _____ Bulging _____	Depression of the anterior fontanel is often an indicator of fluid volume deficit. A fluid excess results in bulging fontanel.

Vital Signs
Temperature
	Admission
	Temperature_____
	    Time _____(1)_____
	    Time _____(2)_____
		Body temperature can be subnormal or elevated. Fever increases insensible water loss. The child's extremities may feel cold because of hypovolemia (fluid volume deficit), which decreases peripheral circulation. A subnormal temperature may be due to reduced energy output.

Pulse	Admission pulse _____
	Pulse rate
	    Time _____ (1)_____
	    Time _____ (2)_____
	    Pattern _____
		A weak and rapid pulse rate (over 160 for infant and over 120 for child) may indicate a fluid volume deficit (hypovolemia) and the possibility of shock. A full, bounding, not easily obliterated pulse may indicate a fluid volume excess. An irregular pulse can be due to hypokalemia. A weak, irregular rapid pulse may indicate hypokalemia, while a weak slow pulse may indicate hypernatremia.

Respiration	Admission rate _____ Respiration Time _____ (1)_____ Time _____ (2)_____ Pattern _____	Note the rate depth and pattern of the infant's breathing. Dyspnea and moist rales usually indicate fluid volume excess. Rapid breathing increases insensible fluid loss from the lungs. Rapid, deep, vigorous breathing (Kussmaul breathing) frequently indicates metabolic acidosis. Acidosis can be due to poor hydrogen excretion by the kidneys, diarrhea, salicylate poisoning, or diabetes mellitus. Shallow, irregular breathing can be due to respiratory alkalosis.

(continues on the following page)

Table 18-6

(Continued)

Observation	Assessment	Rationale

Blood Pressure	Admission BP _____
	Blood pressure
	  Time _____ (1)_____
	  Time _____ (2)_____
		Elasticity of young blood vessels may keep blood pressure stable even when a fluid volume deficit is present. Increased blood pressure may indicate fluid volume excess. Decreased blood pressure may indicate severe fluid volume deficit, extracellular shift from the plasma to the interstitial space, or sodium deficit.

Neurological Signs	Abdominal distention _____
	Diminished reflexes
	  (hypotonia) _____
	Weakness/paralysis _____
	Tetany tremors
	  (hypertonia) _____
	Twitching, cramps _____
	Sensorium
	  Confusion _____
	  Comatose _____
	  Other _____
		Abdominal distention and weakness may indicate a potassium deficit. Tetany symptoms can indicate a calcium and/or magnesium deficit. Serum calcium deficits occur easily in children, since their bones do not readily replace calcium to the blood. Confusion can be due to a potassium deficit and/or fluid volume deficit.

Neurovascular Signs	Capillary filling time _____	A measure of systemic perfusion. Moderate to severe dehydration is often accompanied by delayed capillary filling time of >2–3 s.
Weight	Preillness weight _____ Current weight _____	Weight loss can indicate the degree of dehydration (fluid loss): *Mild*—2–5% in infants and young children *Moderate*—5–10% in infants and young children; 3–6% in older children. *Severe*—10–15% in infants and young children; 6–9% in older children. Fluid loss can also be estimated by considering that 1 g of weight loss equals 1 mL of fluid loss. Edema and ascites can occur with fluid imbalances. Fluid overloads can result in hepatomegaly (enlarged liver). Weights should be taken on the same scale, at the same time each day, and with the same covering.

(continues on the following page)

Table 18-6

Head-to-Toe Assessment of Fluid and Electrolyte Imbalance in Infants and Children (Continued)

Observation	Assessment	Rationale

Urine	Number of voidings in 8 h _____
	 Amt mL/8 h _____
	 Amt mL/h _____
	 Urine color _____
	 Specific gravity _____
	 Urine pH _____
		Accurate measurements of intake and output from all sources is essential. Normal output ranges are:
		   Infants: 2–3 mL/kg/h
		   Young children: 2 mL/kg/h
		   Older children: 1–2 mL/kg/h
		 By subtracting the weight of a saturated urine diaper from a dry diaper, output in infants and toddlers can be determined (1 g wet diaper = 1 mL urine). Because of evaporative losses, diapers must be weighed within 30 min of the void to be accurate. Specific gravity can be obtained by refractometer or dipstick. Accurate assessment can be made within 2 h of the void. Oliguria (decrease in urine output) with very concentrated urine (dark yellow color) and increased specific gravity (>1.030) can indicate a moderate to severe fluid volume deficit, plasma to interstitial fluid shift, sodium deficit or severe sodium excess, potassium excess, or renal insufficiency. An elevated specific gravity is also indicative of glycosuria and proteinuria. With severe fluid deficit the infant may not void for 16–24 h and not show evidence of abdominal distention. Polyuria (increased urine output) with low specific gravity (<1.010) can indicate fluid excess, renal disease, a sodium deficit, or extracellular shift from interstitial fluid to plasma or decreased antidiuretic hormone (ADH). An acidic pH may indicate metabolic or respiratory acidosis, alkalosis with severe potassium deficit, or a fluid deficit. Alkaline urine may result from metabolic or respiratory alkalosis, hyperaldosteronism, acidosis with chronic kidney infection and tubular dysfunction, or diuretic therapy.

(continues on the following page)

Table 18-6

(Continued)

Observation	Assessment	Rationale
Stools	Number _____ Consistency _____ Color _____ Amount _____	The consistency, color, and amount of each stool should be noted. If the stool is liquid, it should be measured. Frequent liquid stools can lead to fluid volume deficit, potassium and sodium deficit, and bicarbonate deficit (acidosis).
Vomitus	Number _____ Consistency _____ Color _____ Amount _____	Vomitus needs to be described according to consistency, color and amount. Frequent vomiting of large quantity leads to fluid loss, potassium and sodium loss, as well as hydrogen and chloride loss (alkalosis).

Other Fluid Loss	GI suction
	  Amount _____
	Drainage tube
	  Amount _____
	Fistula
	  Color _____
	  Amount _____
	Other
	  Amount _____
		Fluid loss from all sources should be measured. Fluid loss from GI suctioning, drainage tubes, and fistula can contribute to severe fluid and electrolyte imbalance.

Blood Chemistry and Hematology	Electrolytes
	Time _____ Time _____
	K _____ _____
	Na _____ _____
	Cl _____ _____
	Ca _____ _____
	Mg _____ _____
	BUN _____ _____
	Creatinine
	  _____ _____
	Hgb _____ _____
	Hct _____ _____
		One set of blood chemistry is not sufficient for assessment. Electrolytes should be frequently monitored when they are not in normal range.
		Norms are:
		K:
		  Newborn 3.0–6.0 mEq/L
		  Infant & older 3.5–5.0 mEq/L
		Na:
		  Newborn 136–146 mEq/L
		  Infant 139–146 mEq/L
		  Child 135–148 mEq/L
		Cl:
		  Newborn 97–110 mEq/L
		  Child 98–111 mEq/L
		Ca:
		  Newborn 7–12 mg/dL
		  Child 8–10.8 mg/dL

(continues on the following page)

Table 18-6

Head-to-Toe Assessment of Fluid and Electrolyte Imbalance in Infants and Children (Continued)

Observation	Assessment	Rationale
		Mg:
		All ages 1.3–2.0 mEq/L
		BUN:
		Newborn 4–18 mg/dL
		Child 5–18 mg/dL
		Creatinine:
		Newborn 0.3–1.0 mg/dL
		Infant 0.2–0.4 mg/dL
		Child 0.3–0.7 mg/dL
		Hgb:
		Newborn 14.5–22.5 g/dL
		Infant 9–14 g/dL
		Child 11.5–15.5 g/dL
		Hct:
		Newborn 44–72%
		Infant 28–42%
		Child 35–45%
		An elevated BUN can indicate fluid volume deficit or kidney insufficiency.
		Elevated creatinine frequently indicates kidney damage.
		Elevated hemoglobin and hematocrit may indicate hemoconcentration caused by fluid volume deficit. If anemia is present, the hemoglobin and hematocrit may appear falsely normal.

	Blood gases
	  pH _____
	  PaCO$_2$ _____
	  PaO$_2$ _____
	  HCO$_3$ _____
	  BE _____
		After the first day of life, normal range for pH is 7.35–7.45. A pH of 7.35 or less indicates acidosis. A pH of 7.45 or higher indicates alkalosis.
		Newborns and infants have PaCO$_2$ levels that range between 27 and 41 mm Hg. After infancy, PaCO$_2$ levels range from 35 to 48 mm Hg in males and from 32 to 45 mm Hg in females. Lower values indicate respiratory alkalosis or compensation (overbreathing, hyperventilating). Higher values mean respiratory acidosis.

(continues on the following page)

Table 18-6

(Continued)

Observation	Assessment	Rationale
		Normal range for HCO_3 in all ages is 21–28 mEq/L. BE (base excess) varies with age. Normal BE ranges are: Newborn (-10)–(-2) mEq/L Infant (-7)–(-1) mEq/L Child (-4)–$(+2)$ mEq/L HCO_3 below 21 and BE less than the normal value for age indicates metabolic alkalosis. HCO_3 above 28 and BE higher than the normal value for age indicates metabolic acidosis.

61

Neurologic changes may indicate a fluid and electrolyte imbalance. Match the neurologic assessment on the left with the probable imbalance. (Refer to Chapters 6 and 8 on potassium and calcium and Chapter 2 on dehydration and edema.) Some answers may be used more than once.

_____ 1. Abdominal distention   a. Potassium deficit
_____ 2. Confusion   b. Calcium deficit
_____ 3. Muscle weakness   c. Fluid volume excess
_____ 4. Tetany symptoms   d. Fluid volume deficit

61 1. a; 2. a, c, d; 3. a; 4. b

62

A weight loss of 12% is comparable to which of the following degrees of dehydration (fluid loss)?

( ) a. Mild dehydration
( ) b. Moderate dehydration
( ) c. Severe dehydration

62 c

63 Subcutaneous fat can give the appearance of normal skin turgor, or abdominal distention may mask poor skin turgor in heavy infants and toddlers.

63

Tissue (skin) turgor can be misleading as an indicator of fluid volume loss. Explain why. *_____
_____

64

Indicate in which areas of the body skin turgor should be checked.

( ) a. Face   ( ) d. Top of thighs

( ) b. Chest wall   ( ) e. Medial aspect of thighs

( ) c. Abdomen

64 b, c, e

65

To determine dryness of the mucous membrane, which part of the mouth should be assessed?

( ) a. Cheeks and gums of the oral cavity

( ) b. Teeth

65 a

66

Sunken eyeballs and fontanels frequently do not occur in infants until there is a 10% body weight loss (as fluid loss). Give the type of fluid imbalance that would be present with a 10% fluid loss. *_____

66 moderate to severe dehydration, or the upper range
of moderate dehydration

67

Delayed capillary refill time of greater than 3 seconds is most likely indicative of fluid volume _____ .

67 deficit

68

Normal specific gravity for a young infant is 1.002–1.010 and for a child is 1.005–1.030. If the child's urinary output is decreased and the specific gravity exceeds 1.030, the fluid imbalance is *_____ .

68 fluid volume deficit, or
hypovolemia

69

Hyperkalemia (serum potassium excess) can result from (polyuria/oliguria) _____ .

69 oliguria (↓ urine output)

70

Frequent and increased quantities of vomitus and stools can lead to which of the following:

( ) a. Hypokalemia

( ) b. Hyperkalemia

( ) c. Hyponatremia

( ) d. Hypernatremia

( ) e. Acidosis

( ) f. Alkalosis

( ) g. Dehydration

70 a, c, e (↑ stools due to loss
of HCO_3), f (↑ vomitus due
to loss of HCl), g

71

Vital signs should be monitored every *_____ minutes for seriously ill infants or children. Check which of the following vital signs can indicate a fluid volume loss/deficit.

( ) a. Subnormal temperature
( ) b. Rapid, weak pulse
( ) c. Rapid respiration (Kussmaul)
( ) d. Fever
( ) e. Shallow breathing
( ) f. Systolic pressure below 80

72

An irregular pulse (dysrhythmia) can be caused by a (potassium deficit/potassium excess) *_____ .

A full bounding pulse can mean *_____ .

Why are blood pressure readings in infants and young children a poor indicator of fluid imbalance? *_____

_____

73

An elevated BUN (blood urea nitrogen) can indicate *_____

_____ ,

whereas an elevated serum creatinine indicates *_____ .

74

Arterial blood gases (ABGs) are used to assess acid-base balance. In the child:

a. pH of 7.27 indicates *_____
b. pH of 7.48 indicates *_____
c. $PaCO_2$ of 28 indicates *_____
d. $PaCO_2$ of 60 indicates *_____
e. HCO_3 of 34 and BE of +8 indicates *_____
f. HCO_3 of 18 and BE of −6 indicates *_____

75

The fluid imbalance that can result from gastrointestinal suction and from secretions from drainage tubes and fistula is

_____ .

Name the two important electrolytes that are lost from gastrointestinal suctioning. *_____

_____

71 15–30; a (in some cases can indicate loss), b, c, d, f

72 potassium deficit; fluid volume excess; Firm elasticity of young blood vessels keeps blood pressure stable.

73 dehydration (fluid volume deficit) or kidney insufficiency (renal damage); kidney damage

74 a. acidosis; b. alkalosis; c. hyperventilation due to respiratory alkalosis or compensation for metabolic acidosis; d. respiratory acidosis; e. metabolic alkalosis; f. metabolic acidosis

75 dehydration (fluid volume deficit); potassium and sodium (important electrolytes), also hydrogen, chloride, bicarbonate, and magnesium

76

From the following list of observations and nursing assessments, check the ones that indicate fluid volume deficit (hypovolemia or dehydration).

( ) a. BUN elevated
( ) b. Hemoglobin and hematocrit elevated
( ) c. Increased secretions from GI suction
( ) d. Increased blood pressure
( ) e. Irritability, high-pitched cry
( ) f. Confusion, disorientation
( ) g. Weight gain
( ) h. Decreased, concentrated urine
( ) i. Avid thirst
( ) j. Poor skin turgor
( ) k. Absence of tearing and salivation
( ) l. Sunken eyeballs and anterior fontanel
( ) m. Increased number and quantity of vomitus and stools
( ) n. Temperature 98.2°F or 36.8°C
( ) o. Rapid, weak pulse
( ) p. Rapid breathing

76 a, b, c, e, f, h, i, j, k, l, m, o, p

CASE STUDY REVIEW

Tonya, age 4, has had diarrhea and anorexia for 3 days. She has taken only sips of fruit juices for the last 3 days. She weighed 38 pounds, or 17.3 kg, preillness and now weighs 35 pounds, or 15.9 kg. Her cheeks and gums are dry and her skin turgor is reduced. She is irritable. Tonya has voided once in the last 24 hours. Vital signs: temperature 99°F, or 37.2°C, pulse rate 110, respirations 32, BP 90/60. Results of the BUN and creatinine are pending.

1. Because of diarrhea, anorexia, decreased fluid intake, and weight loss, the health professional would assume the fluid imbalance to be which of the following:
   ( ) a. Intracellular fluid volume excess (water intoxication)
   ( ) b. Extracellular fluid volume excess (edema or overhydration)
   ( ) c. Extracellular fluid volume deficit (dehydration)

1. c

2. In kilograms, Tonya has lost _____ kg. What degree of dehydration is present? _____ (Refer to Table 18-3 if needed.) The severity of her dehydration is (mild/moderate/severe) _____ .

2. 1.4; 8%; moderate

3. The onset of fluid loss (dehydration) has been _____ days. The percentage of fluid loss from the ECF is _____ and from the ICF is _____ .

3. 3; 60%; 40%

4. cheeks and gums dry, reduced skin turgor, irritable, voided once (decreased urine output), and pulse rate and respiration increased

4. List Tonya's signs and symptoms of dehydration from the health assessment. *_____
   _____
   _____

5. No; Blood pressure for that age group is normal; however, a baseline blood pressure from an office visit would be helpful.

5. Is Tonya's blood pressure indicative of shock? _____ Explain. *_____

6. The ranges of serum electrolytes for a child of this age are:
   a. K*_____
   b. Na*_____
   c. Cl*_____
   d. Ca*_____
   (Refer to Table 18-6.)

6. a. 3.5–5.0 mEq/L; b. 135–148 mEq/L; c. 98–111 mEq/L; d. 8–10 mg/dL

7. One would expect Tonya's serum potassium to be (increased/decreased) _____ , serum sodium to be (increased/decreased) _____ , serum chloride to be (increased/decreased) _____ , and serum calcium to be (increased/decreased) _____ .

7. decreased; decreased; decreased; decreased

8. dizziness, soft muscles, abdominal distention, decreased peristalsis, dysrhythmia, and decreased BP

8. Give some signs and symptoms of hypokalemia. *_____
   _____

9. tetany; tingling of fingers and twitching of mouth (others—tremors and carpopedal spasms)
10. increased; dehydration; With a decreased urine output, there is an increase in serum solutes such as urea (due to hemoconcentration).

11. 1365; 40.8, or 41; 27.2, or 27

12. isonatremic; The serum sodium level for isonatremic dehydration is 130–150 mEq/L.

13. rapidly
14. rapid pulse rate, rapid respiration, and decreasing blood pressure (others—clammy skin, pale or gray color)
15. P 130 (rapid pulse rate) and R 35 (rapid respirations). Baseline vital signs are helpful.

16. oliguria or decreased; decreased; 1.030 (or more)

9. With a serum calcium level of 7.4 mg/dL, one should observe for symptoms of _____ . Give two of the symptoms.
   * _____

10. Tonya's BUN should be (increased/decreased) _____ . The most likely cause of her BUN is _____ . Explain.
    * _____

11. Tonya's preillness weight is 38 pounds, or 17.3 kg. Calculate Tonya's daily fluid maintenance requirements. _____ mL per 24 hours (Refer to Table 18-1 if needed).
    Her daily sodium requirement is _____ mEq/L and her daily potassium requirement is _____ mEq/L. (Refer to Table 18-1 as needed.)

12. Tonya's type of dehydration according to her serum sodium level is (isonatremic/hypernatremic/hyponatremic) _____ . Why? * _____
    _____

13. For the type of dehydration in question 12, fluids should be replaced (slowly/rapidly) _____ .

14. Name three shock symptoms that can occur. * _____
    _____

15. Identify Tonya's vital signs that are indicative of impending shock due to hypovolemia (fluid volume loss). * _____ and * _____

16. With moderate dehydration, the changes in the urine output and concentration are (refer to Table 18-3 if needed):
    Urine volume _____
    Urine osmolality _____
    Urine specific gravity _____

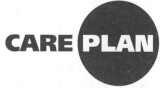

Client Management

Assessment Factors

▶ Early detection of pertinent symptoms and prompt therapeutic management of fluid and electrolyte disturbances are critical in the care of infants and children. Fluid balance is so precarious that life-threatening changes can occur rapidly with little symptomatic warning. Conditions that promote fluid imbalances in infants and children include vomiting, diarrhea, sweating, fever, burns, injury, and diseases such as diabetes and renal and cardiac anomalies. A thorough assessment integrates the health history obtained from the parents with data from the physical examination and laboratory tests.

▶ Knowledge requirements and basic assessment techniques vary for infants and children. Understanding the implications of variations in laboratory studies, total body fluid volume, and developmental differences that influence the responses of infants and children to fluid problems provides a basis for data comparison. Assessment begins with observations of the infant's/child's general appearance and behavioral changes. Knowing baseline data from the infant's/child's health history is important to the assessment and interpretation of the findings.

▶ Monitor vital signs according to the severity of the illness. A baseline reading of the infant's or child's vital signs is important to the interpretation of changes. Seriously ill infants and children need their vital signs monitored every 15 minutes. An elevated temperature can occur with early fluid depletion and can indicate a fluid deficit. An elevated or a subnormal temperature can indicate dehydration. Blood pressure is not a reliable sign of fluid imbalance in young children. A rapid, weak, thready pulse is a symptom of shock. A bounding, not easily obliterated pulse occurs with fluid volume excess when the interstitial fluid shifts to the plasma. A bounding, easily obliterated pulse may indicate an impending circulatory collapse and a sodium deficit. The overall cardiac status reflects changes in levels of important electrolytes. A potassium imbalance is life threatening in a child.

▶ Dyspnea and moist rales can occur with a fluid volume excess. Respiratory stridor may indicate a calcium deficit. Assess skin and mucous membranes; the skin is usually pale during a fluid deficit and flushed during a fluid excess. The extremities often become cold and mottled with the presence of a fever and a severe fluid volume deficit. Skin elasticity can be assessed by pinching the skin on the abdomen or inner thigh (dent test). In fluid depletion the skin remains raised for several seconds. The skin may feel dry or cold and clammy in sodium deficits (hypotonic dehydration). Fluid deficits cause the mucous membranes of the mouth to become dry. The tongue is observed to have longitudinal wrinkles. A sodium excess (hyperosmolar dehydration) causes a sticky, rough, red, dry tongue.

▶ Tears and salivation are decreased to absent in fluid volume deficits of infants and children. Fluid volume deficits cause the fontanels and eyeballs to appear soft and sunken. Conversely, in fluid excess the fontanels bulge and feel taut.

▶ Tingling fingers and toes, abdominal cramps, muscle cramps, lightheadedness, nausea, and thirst are important symptoms of electrolyte imbalances in infants and children. Other sensory and neurologic signs may include hypotonia and flaccid paralysis indicative of a potassium deficit. Hypertonia is evidenced as a positive Chvostek sign, tremors, cramps, or tetany, which are indicative of a calcium deficit. A magnesium deficit causes twitching.

▶ Knowing the variations in serum electrolyte ranges for infants and children can help prevent complications of electrolyte imbalances of sodium, potassium, chloride, calcium, and magnesium (see Table 18-1 for serum electrolyte norms).

▶ Even small weight changes are crucial in fluid balance problems of infants and children. Rapid loss or gain in weight indicates fluid deficits and fluid excesses in the fluid regulation process. Although baseline data on normal output is important, normal output varies with the age of the child. Normal output ranges for an infant are 2–3 mL/kg/h and for young children it is 2 mL/kg/h. Immature kidneys limit the child's ability to concentrate urine. Urine should be monitored for specific gravity and acidity. A specific gravity of less than 1.010 is low and indicates a fluid excess. A specific gravity of 1.030 is high and may indicate a fluid deficit with a sodium excess. An elevated specific gravity is usually accompanied by glycosuria and proteinuria. The specific gravity of infants and children can be used to monitor their hydration level. Fixed low specific gravity readings indicate renal disease.

Diagnosis 1

Fluid volume deficit related to decreased fluid reserve.

Interventions and Rationale

1. Identify source of fluid deficit. Fluid deficits result from a decreased fluid intake or an abnormal fluid loss in conditions such as diabetes insipidus, adrenocortical insufficiency, vomiting, diarrhea, hemorrhage, burns, and diabetes mellitus. Fluid deficits in infants and children are accentuated by three factors associated with their immaturity: (a) their pro-

portionately high body surface area; (b) their high rate of metabolism; and (c) their immature renal structures. All of these factors limit the infant's ability to conserve fluid and compensate for fluid deficits.

2. Monitor laboratory values for selected electrolytes (Na, Cl, K, Ca). Recognize differences between the normal values of infants and children and the normal values of adults. Report even small changes in laboratory values. The increased vulnerability of infants and children to fluid deficits are not easily detected in observable signs and symptoms. Be able to recognize specific symptoms of electrolyte imbalance.

3. Closely assess changes in general appearance and neurologic and behavioral signs. Lethargy with hyperirritability on stimulation is an early sign of fluid volume deficit (see Table 18-6). Dry mucous membranes are often the first symptom of fluid deficits. Sunken fontanels are an indication of a fluid volume deficit in an infant.

4. Monitor weight daily. Amount of weight loss is a key assessment factor for determining the severity of the fluid imbalance. Knowledge of weight in kilograms is essential to determine the degree of dehydration and calculate the fluid replacement needs (see Table 18-1) of infants and children.

5. Monitor vital signs. A baseline value of the infant or child's normal vital signs is important in determining the degree of the fluid deficit and assessing for hypovolemic shock (see Table 18-2). Check physician's records or ask the parents for the normal values of the child or infant.

6. Measure intake and output. The immature development of the renal structures in infants and children limits the kidney's ability to concentrate urine and increases the infant's risk for dehydration. A balance in intake and output is important in restoring fluid balance.

7. Integrate observations to determine the type (iso-osmolar, hypo-osmolar, or hyperosmolar) and degree of dehydration (mild, moderate, or severe). Knowledge of the type and degree of dehydration assists in identifying the ratio of ICF volume and ECF volume. This information is important in the proper selection of fluids and the regulation of the rate and volume of fluid replacement.

Diagnosis 2

Fluid volume excess related to inadequate excretion of fluid or alteration of fluid volume regulation.

Interventions and Rationale

1. Although fluid volume excess is less common than are deficits, it is important to first identify the source of the fluid volume excess. Fluid overload can be caused by rapid infusions of IV or dialysis fluid, tap water enemas, or with rapid reduction of glucose levels in diabetic ketoacidosis. Other causes that may occur in the home setting are diluted formula and water intoxication associated with swallowing pool water during swimming activities. Regulatory mechanisms in infants are not as developed as in the older child. Therefore, they are often unable to excrete a fluid overload effectively.

2. Monitor intake and output as well as laboratory values. The ingestion or infusion of excessive amounts of fluids can result in reduced sodium levels and CNS symptoms. Specific gravity measurements are used to assess urine concentration. The kidney's reduced ability to concentrate urine results in an excessive, diluted urine output. Urine output should be at least 1–2 mL/kg/h (refer to Table 18-6).

3. Assess neurologic symptoms. Neurologic symptoms of a fluid overload include lethargy, irritability, headache, and/or generalized seizures. These symptoms result because water moves into the brain more rapidly than sodium moves out.

4. Assess for edema. Immaturity of the kidneys and inadequate hormone production may predispose infants and young children to fluid imbalances that result in edema. Infants and young children who look well hydrated may have edema. Early recognition of edema as a consequence of fluid overload is essential. Edema may be localized to a specific body area or generalized. Common areas for assessing edema are the extremities, face, perineum, and torso.

Diagnosis 3

Diarrhea related to irritable bowel.

Interventions and Rationale

1. Identify causative factors. Compare and contrast dietary patterns 24 hours prior to the onset of diarrhea with normal dietary patterns. Assess for the possibility of allergies, contaminated foods, dietary indiscretions, bacterial or viral infections, antibiotic usage, exposure to other children in day

care settings, or malabsorption problems. Rotavirus, the most common pathogen associated with diarrhea in hospitalized infants and children, can be identified through a stool culture. Frequent use of antibiotics may deplete the normal intestinal flora leading to colonization and toxin production by *Clostridium difficile* resulting in diarrhea and pseudomembranous colitis. Diarrhea may also be associated with upper respiratory and urinary tract infections. Although the cause may be unknown, whenever possible, causative factors should be eliminated.

2. Monitor vital signs, weight changes, and laboratory values. Determine the extent of fluid and electrolyte imbalance based on changes in these assessment factors.

3. Assess stools for frequency, consistency, blood pH, and carbohydrate malabsorption. Liquid/diarrhealike stools contain significant fluid content and must be measured in infants and children to determine their fluid balance status. Compare frequency and consistency of bowel movements to the infant's normal pattern.

4. If mild to moderate dehydration is suspected, oral rehydration therapy should be initiated. Oral rehydration solutions (ORSs) can be used to treat most types of dehydration in the home setting. To determine the appropriate amount of maintenance fluid requirements, refer to Table 18-1. Stool losses should be replaced with equal volumes of ORSs. Clear liquids such as fruit juices, soft drinks, and gelatin should be discouraged. These fluids are high in carbohydrates and may exacerbate the diarrhea. Caffeinated beverages act as a mild diuretic and may increase fluid and sodium losses.

5. Severe dehydration requires IV fluid replacement. Once the child is stabilized, oral rehydration therapy should be introduced.

6. A regular diet that contains easily digestible foods such as cereal, yogurt, cooked vegetables, and soups should be given. Avoid high-fiber foods as they often cause the bowel to expand and stimulate peristalsis. A BRAT (bananas, rice, applesauce, toast or tea) is no longer recommended. Formula (either half strength or lactose free) and breast feeding can be continued. Initially, there may be a higher output of stool. The benefits of a nutritionally sound diet, however, outweigh the problems with stool output. Losses are replaced with oral rehydration solutions.

7. Parental education is an important aspect of treatment. They should be taught how to recognize signs and symptoms of fluid imbalance. In addition, techniques for providing oral rehydration therapy should be discussed as well as fluids and foods to encourage and avoid. Oral rehydration therapy is very labor intensive. Small amounts of fluids (1–2 teaspoons) can provide up to 300 mL of fluid per hour.

Diagnosis 4

Altered nutrition: less than body requirements, related to anorexia secondary to (altered level of consciousness, vomiting, diarrhea, and nausea).

Interventions and Rationale

1. Identify cause of nutritional deficit. Diarrhea and vomiting are the most common causes of fluid and electrolyte problems in infants and children. These conditions prevent the absorption of adequate nutrients and threaten the precarious fluid balance of infants and young children.

2. Initiate a regular diet as soon as possible (see 6 in Diagnosis 3). Knowledge of the nutritional requirements of various age groups is essential to adequate nutritional replacement. Changes in metabolic needs are affected by the child's physical status and pathophysiologic conditions. The health professional can help the parents plan a diet that is nutritionally sound, developmentally appropriate, and pleasing to the child.

3. Monitor weight. Weight gains or losses are indicative of nutritional status and fluid balance. Small gains or losses are significant in infants and children.

Diagnosis 5

Impaired tissue integrity related to the effects of chemical destruction or tissue deficits, secondary to fluid and electrolyte imbalances (diarrhea, edema).

Interventions and Rationale

1. Identify risk factors for threats to tissue integrity. Tissue destruction can occur from chemical irritants or mechanical destruction. Conditions such as diarrhea, excessive or unusual secretions, urinary incontinence, and edema increase

the tissue's vulnerability to destruction. Proper identification and treatment of risk factors reduce the infant's vulnerability to these risks. Since maturity factors in infants and children reduce their ability to adapt, early identification and treatment of risk factors can prevent major complications.

2. Eliminate or reduce causative factors. Diarrhea and edema are symptoms that require early interventions to reduce the risk of tissue destruction.

3. Assess nutritional status. Nutritional status affects the tissue's vulnerability to breakdown. Inadequate protein consumption reduces healing power and increases tissue vulnerability. Vitamins and minerals are also important to the health of body tissues. In fluid imbalance conditions, one's nutritional state is often compromised.

4. Promote mobility as tolerated. Many fluid imbalance problems promote lethargy and immobility. Since adequate circulation is essential to tissue nutrition and oxygenation, frequent position changes and movement promote circulation and reduce the risk of tissue breakdown. Reposition infants carefully to reduce risks related to mechanical destruction of tissues.

5. Keep the skin clean and dry. Cleanse with a mild soap and pat dry. If the skin is irritated, a hair dryer placed on the "cool" setting can be used to dry the skin. When possible, the skin should be left open to the air. Protective ointments such as zinc oxide may be applied. Most importantly, diapers should be changed frequently and the skin assessed. With diarrhea stools, skin breakdown can occur very rapidly.

Other Diagnoses and Interventions to Consider

1. Altered oral mucous membranes related to fluid deficit (dehydration):

   ▶ Apply a thin layer of a water-soluble ointment to the lips to prevent cracking (glycerin and lemon swabs have a drying effect and should be avoided).

   ▶ Rinse mouth with water or warm saline (do not allow swallowing if oral fluids are restricted).

   ▶ Clean teeth and gums with a soft sponge. Dryness may cause inflammation, bleeding, or lesions that need interventions to promote comfort and reduce complications.

▶ Instruct parents to provide these interventions in situations when child is too young or unable to care for self. Maintenance of moist, adequately perfused mucous membranes is important in fluid balance problems.

2. Altered urinary elimination related to kidney function:

▶ Monitor intake and output. Toilet-trained children and independent older children may not understand the importance of measuring intake and urinary output. This independence may pose a threat to accurate monitoring of intake and output. Altered urine output may indicate dysfunctions such as inadequate blood volume regulatory mechanisms of aldosterone and ADH, excessive fluid intake, or marked fluid loss (hemorrhage, GI bleeding). Monitor urine for presence of protein or glucose and measure its pH level. The preferred method of measuring urine output in diapered infants and children is simply to compare the dry and wet weight of the diaper. (Weight in grams corresponds to volume voided.) Urine can be aspirated from cloth diapers to obtain urine for specific gravity measurements.

▶ Urine can be aspirated from diapers or a dipstick used to obtain specific gravity readings. In children with superabsorbent diapers, the diaper should be weighed within 30 minutes of voiding to ensure accurate measurement.

▶ Monitor kidney function for early signs of renal insufficiency. The specific gravity of urine, sufficient amounts of output (30 mL/h), BUN, serum creatinine, potassium, phosphorus, ammonia, and creatinine clearance times are important in the diagnosis of renal insufficiency (Refer to Table 18-6 for normal values).

3. Sensory-perceptual alterations related to metabolic changes secondary to fluid and electrolyte imbalance (acidosis):

▶ Identify sensory-perceptual alterations. Children can experience different sensory-perceptual alterations depending upon the type of fluid and electrolyte imbalance. Fluid deficits promote irritability and lethargy while fluid shifts that cause cerebral edema may cause irritability and restlessness. Complaints of headaches and nausea with episodes of vomiting are not uncommon. Severe cerebral edema can cause convulsions. Selected electrolyte imbalances result in dizziness, muscle cramping or twitching, and tingling of the fingers and toes.

- ◗ Monitor laboratory values. An elevated BUN or serum creatinine can alter sensory-perceptual experiences.

- ◗ Maintain a cool, quiet environment. To reduce unnecessary stimulation, interventions should be organized in a manner that allows for uninterrupted rest periods. Unnecessary interruptions should be prevented during these quiet times.

- ◗ Provide developmentally appropriate diversional activities. Asking the child and parent what activities the child enjoys during quiet times is helpful.

4. Knowledge deficit (parental) related to detection, care, and treatment of fluid and electrolyte imbalance:

- ◗ Teach parents basic fluid balance principles. Knowledge of basic principles of fluid and electrolyte balance can alert parents to symptoms of fluid overload and fluid deficits for early detection of potential complications.

- ◗ Involve parents in the infant's/child's care as much as possible. Promoting trust by involving parents enhances treatment and reduces unnecessary anxiety of parents during the infant's/child's illness.

- ◗ Teach basic fluid replacement strategies. Many hospitalizations or complications from fluid problems can be prevented by early detection and appropriate fluid replacement strategies initiated at home by alert parents.

Evaluation/Outcome

1. Evaluate that the cause of the ECFV problem has been eliminated or controlled (disease state identified, vomiting and/or diarrhea controlled, hemorrhage, etc., and the electrolyte imbalance and/or fluid intake adjusted appropriately).

2. Evaluate effectiveness of interventions through selected electrolyte studies (Na, Cl, K, Ca) return to normal range.

3. Document daily weight (in kilograms for infant and young children) for return to stable baseline weight (consult parents if necessary).

4. Evaluate general appearance for improvement in signs and symptoms of fluid imbalance (lethargy, hyperirritability, sunken or bulging fontanels in infants, edema, weak/shrill cry, seizures, etc.).

5. Monitor for fluid balance through intake and output measures. Document parental understanding of teaching related to the sign and symptoms of dehydration in children.

6. Evaluate hydration status (return of moist pink mucous membranes, good skin turgor, etc.) of infant or child.

7. Monitor weight frequently (small gains or losses are significant in infants and children).

Fluid Problems of the Aging Adult

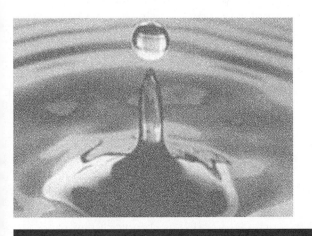

OBJECTIVES

Upon completion of this chapter, the reader should be able to:

- Describe structural and functional changes that occur with normal aging of the respiratory, renal, cardiac, integumentary, and gastrointestinal systems.
- Discuss the effects of normal aging (on the respiratory, renal, cardiac, integumentary, and gastrointestinal systems) that have implications for fluid and electrolyte balance.
- List risk factors, especially chronic diseases, that may cause fluid and electrolyte problems for the older adult.
- Identify common body fluid problems experienced by the aging adult.

(continued on next page)

OBJECTIVES (Continued)

● **Assess normal physiologic changes in the aging client as they relate to the signs and symptoms of fluid problems in the aging adult.**

● **Identify appropriate interventions for aging clients experiencing fluid and electrolyte imbalances.**

▶ INTRODUCTION

The normal aging process has a wide range of effects on the structure and function of various body systems. Changes in respiratory, cardiac, renal, gastrointestinal, and integumentary systems can present fluid and electrolyte problems for the older adult.

This chapter looks at the normal physiologic changes and the effects of chronic illness as they relate to the signs and symptoms of fluid and electrolyte imbalance in the aging adult.

▶ PHYSIOLOGIC CHANGES

Structural and functional changes that occur as a result of the aging process are usually measured in terms of the body's ability to adapt. Additional risk factors such as chronic diseases increase the debilitating effects of normal functional changes in all of the body's systems and further inhibit the aging client's ability to maintain fluid and electrolyte balance.

Assessments provide information about age-related changes and factors that may place older adults at risk for fluid and electrolyte imbalances. Miller (1990) proposed the Functional Consequences Model of Gerontological Nursing (Figure 19-1) to show how age-related changes and risk factors such as stress and disease may combine to cause negative functional consequences. Appropriate interventions, however, can foster positive functional consequences and decrease the debilitating effects of risk factors.

Table 19-1 lists (a) age-related structural and functional changes in five major body systems, (b) risk factors for fluid and electrolyte imbalance, (c) age-related changes and potential risk factors, and (d) interventions to foster positive functional outcomes. Study the table and practice stating the specific changes, risk factors, and interventions to enhance positive functional outcomes in each system.

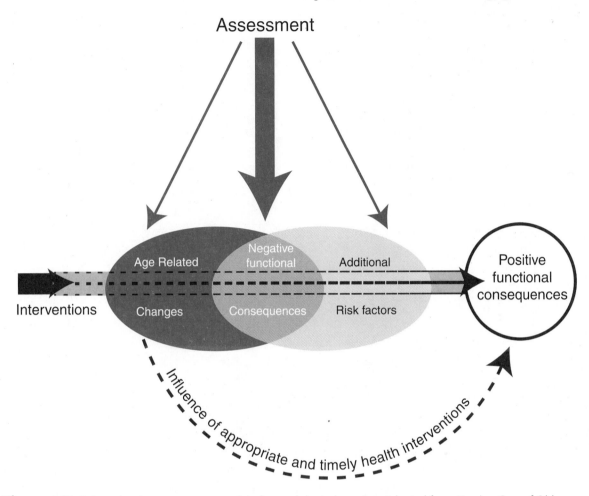

Figure 19-1 Functional consequences model of gerontological nursing. Adapted from *Nursing Care of Older Adults* (p. 53), by C. Miller, 1990, Philadelphia: Lippincott. Adapted with permission.

Table 19-1

Major Structural Changes, Risk Factors, and Functional Outcomes in Aging Adults

Body System	Structural Changes	Risk Factors	Functional Outcomes	Nursing Interventions
Pulmonary function decreased	Loss of elasticity of parenchymal lung tissue with 20% decrease in weight Increased rigidity of chest wall Fewer alveoli Decreased strength of expiratory muscles	Chronic diseases Emphysema Asthma Chronic bronchitis Bronchiectasis Injuries smoking Longer sleeping hours Exposure to air pollutants Occupational exposure to toxic substances Infection Decreased immune system response	Defective alveolar ventilation Accumulation of bronchial secretions Increased CO_2 retention Increased difficulty in regulating pH Decreased tolerance for exercise Decreased vital capacity response Increased residual volume	Increase breathing capacity to enhance the elimination of CO_2 by: 1. Breathing exercises with prolonged expiration 2. Coughing after a few deep breaths 3. Frequent position changes 4. Chest clapping 5. Intermittent positive pressure breathing (IPPB)
Renal function decreased	Arteriosclerotic changes in large renal vessels Decrease in number of functioning nephrons (begins by age 40) 30–50% less by age 70 Decrease in size and weight of the kidneys Increase interstitial tissue Decrease in number glomeruli Thickening of glomeruli and tubular membranes Increased potential for development of diverticuli	Medications (e.g., diuretics) Genitourinary diseases (e.g., infections, obstructions)	Reduced glomerular filtration Decreased renal blood flow Impaired ability to excrete water and solutes causing: 1. A decrease in H^+ excretion; thus metabolic acidosis can occur 2. Reduced ability to concentrate urine 3. Increased accumulation of waste products in body 4. Decreased ability to excrete drugs Decline in urine creatinine clearance Overall decrease in adaptive capacity of the kidneys to stress	Assess adaptive capacity and maintain optimal renal function by: 1. Checking fluid intake and output balance 2. Encouraging fluid intake as appropriate 3. Checking acid-base balance according to serum CO_2 or HCO_3 4. Testing specific gravity to determine kidneys' ability to concentrate urine 5. Noting drugs that may be toxic to renal function 6. Observing for side effects from drug accumulation 7. Observing for desired effects of drugs

Circulation and cardiac function decreased	Increased rigidity and decreased elasticity of arterial walls (arteriosclerosis) Decreased elasticity of blood vessels Thickening of cardiac vessels and valves Decrease in number of conductive cells	Obesity Smoking Dietary habits that contribute to risk factors: Hyperlipidemia, excess salt and calories Inactivity Low potassium intake Diuretic therapy Excessive alcohol consumption Stress Air pollution Hormone changes	Potential increase in blood pressure Stasis of blood causing back pressure on capillaries, which in turn causes fluid to move into tissue areas causing edema Decreased cardiac output and decreased blood flow Decreased cardiac reserve (capacity of heart to respond to increased burden) slows the adaptive functions as evidenced by: 1. Heart rate same as young adults except under stress takes longer to return to normal 2. Increased incidence of edema and congestive heart failure Diminished strength of cardiac contractions Decreased cardiac output and stroke volume Decreased compensatory responses to blood pressure changes	Assess adaptive capacity of heart and maintain circulation and cardiac function by: 1. Checking blood pressure for elevations resulting from arteriosclerotic changes 2. Determining blood flow by checking peripheral pulses 3. Checking lungs and dependent extremities for edema from increased capillary pressure 4. Checking pulse rates (apical and radial) and character to determine heart contraction, cardiac output, and pulse deficit 5. Noting changes in heart rate following activity 6. Assessing chest sounds for moist rales

(continues on the following page)

Table 19-1

Major Structural Changes, Risk Factors, and Functional Outcomes in Aging Adults (Continued)

Body System	Structural Changes	Risk Factors	Functional Outcomes	Nursing Interventions
Gastrointestinal function decreased	Atrophy of gastric mucosa Muscular atrophy and loss of supportive structures in small intestines	Alcohol or medications Psychosocial factors (e.g., isolation, depression) Factors that interfere with ability to obtain, prepare, consume, or enjoy food and fluids (e.g., immobility, mental impairment) Extraintestinal disorders (diabetes, vascular disorders, and neurologic changes)	Decrease in gastric secretions, especially HCl Metabolic alkalosis related to decreased HCl Atrophic gastritis due to decreased HCl Weakened intestinal wall causing diverticuli Decreased motility (peristalsis) of gastrointestinal tract (may cause constipation) Decreased calcium absorption Decreased solubility and absorption of some drugs	Assess for adaptive changes and maintain gastrointestinal function by: 1. Discussing client preferences for foods 2. Suggesting dietary alterations according to physiologic changes, individual preferences, and nutritional needs; may need increased calcium and vitamin D 3. Encouraging fluid intake 4. Checking frequency, consistency, and stool color in bowel elimination 5. Assessing bowel sounds and level of peristalsis
Liver function and endocrine gland function decreased	Liver cell decrease in size and character Hormonal cells decrease in size and character, and outputs dwindle	Liver or endocrine diseases Medications (e.g., steroids, cardiac medications, antibiotics) Alcohol consumption	Liver: 1. Decreased hepatic capacity to detoxify drugs 2. Decreased synthesis of cholesterol and enzyme activity Hormonal: 1. Decreased overall metabolic capacity 2. Decreased endocrine gland function to react to adverse drug action	Assess adaptive liver and endocrine gland functioning by: 1. Noting drugs client is taking that may be toxic to liver 2. Observing for toxic effects of drug buildup 3. Observing for desired effects of drugs 4. Assessing alcohol consumption and teaching accordingly 5. Assessing for jaundice

| Skin function decreased | Epidermis—thinner
Dermis—thinning and loss of elasticity and strength
Blood flow—decreased
Sebaceous gland—decreased production
Sweat gland—decreased production
Decrease in number of nerve endings | Exposure to ultraviolet rays (sunlight)
Adverse medication effects
Personal hygiene habits (e.g., too frequent bathing)
Immobility
Friction
Chemical
Mechanical injury
Temperature—too high or low
Pressure
Gene influence | Dryer, coarser skin
Increased threshold level to pain and temperature sensitivity
Decreased ability to produce sweat
Impaired ability to maintain body temperature | Maintain skin integrity and function by:
1. Maintaining hydration
2. Maintaining optimal skin temperature
3. Maintaining mobility to enhance circulation
4. Turning patient and elevating extremities when necessary to minimize edema and skin breakdown
5. Educating elderly about decreased sensitivity to pain and temperature
6. Providing special mattress or sheepskins for those at risk |

ANSWER COLUMN

1

The aged person adapts more slowly and thus has more difficulty maintaining homeostasis necessary for fluid and electrolyte balance. This factor is complicated by diminished efficiency of pulmonary, renal, cardiac, gastrointestinal, and integumentary functions.

The changes occurring in the aged are _____ and

_____ .

1 functional; structural; fluid; electrolyte imbalances

With diminished pulmonary, renal, cardiac, integumentary, and gastrointestinal functions, the aged person is prone to _____ and * _____ .

2

2 decreases; loss of elasticity of the parenchymal lung tissue; increased rigidity of the chest wall (also fewer alveoli)

The aging process (increases/decreases) _____ the effectiveness of pulmonary ventilation and gas exchange.

The maximal breathing capacity is reduced due to * _____ and * _____ .

3

Environmental toxins and/or progressive subclinical exhaustion of internal respiratory reserve and repair mechanisms in the elderly contribute to poor diffusion of respiratory gases, which results in * _____ and * _____ .

Reduced ventilation can cause which of the following:

( ) a. CO_2 retention
( ) b. CO_2 excretion
( ) c. respiratory alkalosis
( ) d. respiratory acidosis

Name four clinical diseases that cause a decrease in breathing capacity, poor diffusion, and reduced ventilation. * _____

_____

3 defective alveolar ventilation; accumulation of bronchial secretions; a, d; emphysema, asthma, chronic bronchitis, and bronchiectasis

4 breathing exercises with prolonged expiration, coughing and deep breathing, changing positions, chest clapping, and intermittent positive-pressure breathing (IPPB) treatments

4

Name five research-supported interventions that can increase breathing capacity and facilitate the elimination of CO_2.

* _____

_____

5

The renal function in the aged is (increased/decreased)

_____ .

    The persistent renal vasoconstriction and decreased numbers of functioning nephrons resulting from arteriosclerotic changes cause *_____ and *_____ .

6

Aged kidneys show evidence of a reduction in their ability to *_____ water and solutes.

    The kidneys' ability to excrete hydrogen (increases/decreases) _____ with age. The resulting acid-base imbalance is *_____ .

7

The aged kidneys' ability to concentrate urine is _____ , resulting in *_____ .

8

Decreased renal function may result in (decreased/increased) _____ drug excretion and (increased/decreased) _____ accumulation of the drug in the body.

9

Name at least four interventions for assessing and maintaining renal functions. *_____

_____

10

In the aging process, circulation and cardiac function are (increased/decreased) _____ .

    The increased rigidity and decrease in elasticity of the arterial walls due to arteriosclerotic changes can cause *_____ and *_____ .

11

Stasis of blood in the veins can cause back pressure on the capillaries, increasing *_____ . The result of increased capillary pressure is _____ .

---

5 decreased; a reduced glomerular filtration rate; impaired ability to excrete water and solutes

6 retain or excrete; decreases; metabolic acidosis

7 reduced/decreased; a buildup (accumulation) of waste products in the body

8 decreased; increased
9 checking fluid intake and output, encouraging fluid intake, testing urine specific gravity, and noting drugs that may be toxic to renal function; also, observing lab results for signs of acid-base imbalance (according to the serum CO_2 or HCO_3)

10 decreased; an increased blood pressure; stasis of the blood

11 capillary pressure/permeability; edema

12

12 cardiac output; blood flow

The diminished strength of heart contractions can cause a decrease in *_____ and *_____ .

13

13 the capacity of the heart to respond to increased burden; quickly returns to normal; takes longer to return to normal

The aged person has a decrease in cardiac reserve. Cardiac reserve is *_____

_____ .

   Under stress, the heart rate increases both in the young adult and in the elderly. After stress, what happens to the heart rate in the young adult? *_____ In the elderly? *_____

14

14 checking blood pressure for elevation or hypertension, determining blood flow in lower extremities by checking pulses (peripheral), checking for edema, checking apical and radial pulse rates for pulse deficit, and noting changes in heart rate following activities, also, assessing chest sounds for moist rales

Name at least five interventions for assessing and maintaining circulation and cardiac function. *_____

_____

_____

_____

15

15 slowed; HCl; metabolic alkalosis

Gastrointestinal functions are (increased/slowed) _____ in the aged.

   Atrophy of the gastric mucosa occurs with aging, causing a reduction in the important gastric secretion of _____ .

   The resulting acid-base imbalance is *_____ .

16

16 decrease

The muscular atrophy in the small intestine that occurs in aging can (increase/decrease) _____ gastrointestinal motility (peristalsis) when stressed.

17

17 constipation

The aging adult frequently has a reduced ability to detect stimulation and/or decreased propulsion force to stimulate a bowel movement. This type of bowel problem can result in _____ .

18

18 weakened; outpouches in the intestinal wall due to a weakened structural area

The supportive structures in the intestinal wall (villae) are (strengthened/weakened) _____ and can cause diverticuli as a result of normal aging. Describe diverticuli. *_____

_____

19 discuss food preferences, suggest a diet to meet individual nutritional needs and preferences, encourage fluid intake, note color and consistency of bowel movements, and check frequency of bowel elimination and activity.

19

Name at least five interventions for assessing and maintaining gastrointestinal function. *_____

_____

_____

_____

20

Aging skin is (more/less) _____ prone to injury and (slower/faster) _____ to heal. This occurs because of the skin's tendency toward (thinning/thickening) _____ of the epidermis and a (thinning/thickening) _____ of the dermis in the aging adult. These changes result in (decreased/increased) _____ elasticity and strength of the skin, which may be tested in fluid and electrolyte imbalances that cause either _____ or _____ which makes the skin more vulnerable to injury.

20 more; slower; thickening; thinning; decreased; overhydration; edema

21

Fluid imbalances causing dehydration promote drying of the skin and make it more fragile to handle. Fluid imbalances causing overhydration and edema stretch the skin and make it thinner and more vulnerable to injury. Identify five factors that the health professional should consider to decrease the client's risk for skin injury. *_____

_____

21 friction, chemical injury, mechanical injury, temperature, and pressure

22 maintain hydration, maintain optimal skin temperature, increase mobility (turn frequently), elevate edematous extremities, and encourage use of loose or nonrestrictive clothing

22

Identify four to five interventions aimed at maintaining optimal skin integrity. *_____

_____

▶ ASSESSMENT FACTORS

The normal structural and functional losses that occur as a result of the aging process have important implications for assessments. The physiologic changes that alter the structure and function of the respiratory, renal, cardiac, gastrointestinal, and integumentary systems reduce the aging client's ability to adapt to changes that affect fluid and electrolyte balance. Many of these age-related changes predispose clients to chronic diseases, that further decrease the client's ability to adapt to fluid and electrolyte changes.

By recognizing the changes due to normal aging and additional risk factors such as chronic diseases, fluid and electrolyte problems can often be prevented or detected before major complications have occurred. A critical assessment in clients at risk for fluid imbalances requires accurate measurement of fluid intake and output. The magnitude of fluid problems in older adults is often evidenced by discrepancies between their fluid intake and output. Laboratory determinations of electrolytes and clinical assessments such as skin turgor, edema, and chest sounds provide additional information for planning and implementing care.

23

The total body water in the healthy adult is _____ %. In normal aging the total body water decreases to approximately 54% (percentages vary for males and females). Changes include a slight (increase/decrease) _____ in extracellular fluid and a(n) (increase/decrease) _____ in intracellular fluid.

23 60; increase; decrease

24

Hypokalemia is a common deficit experienced by the aged. Potassium is not conserved well at any age. Many aged people receive diuretics (potassium wasting) and steroids, which tend to (increase/decrease) _____ the serum potassium level. (Review Chapter 6, potassium with drug relationship, if needed.)

24 decrease

25

The aged person's ECF is (increased/decreased) *_____ , and the ICF is (increased/decreased) _____ because of the drop in the number of body cells (an approximate 30% decrease).

The total body water in the aged is approximately _____ %.

Total body water measurements in the aged are consistent with cell (mass/number) _____ , not cell (mass/number) _____ .

25 slightly increased; decreased; 54; mass; number

The six potential body fluid problems commonly experienced by the aged include dehydration, edema, water intoxications, constipation, diarrhea, and diaphoresis. Table 19-2 lists these six fluid problems with their related causes and suggested interventions.

Table 19-2

Body Fluid Problems in the Aged

Problems	Etiology	Interventions
Fluid Volume Deficit: Dehydration	1. Insufficient water intake 2. Increased urinary output 3. Decreased thirst mechanism 4. Diminished response to ADH (antidiuretic hormone) 5. Reduced ability to concentrate urine	1. Measure fluid intake and output to assess fluid balance 2. Encourage adequate oral fluid intake 3. Assess osmolality of IV fluid intake 4. Assess for clinical signs and symptoms of hypovolemia (dehydration) 5. Monitor other types of fluid therapy, e.g., IV clysis and tube feeding. Adjust rate of IV fluid according to age and physiologic state
Fluid Volume Excess Edema	1. Slightly elevated ECF 2. Overhydration from IV therapy 3. Increased capillary pressure 4. Cardiac insufficiency	1. Measure fluid intake and output to assess fluid balance 2. Adjust IV flow rate to prevent overhydration 3. Assess for peripheral edema in morning 4. Assess chest sounds for moist rales 5. Observe for signs and symptoms of hypervolemia—overhydration
Water intoxication	1. Hypo-osmolar solutions with copious amounts of drinking water	1. Assess types of IV fluids, e.g., 5% dextrose in water replacement to prevent complications 2. Observe for signs and symptoms of water intoxication 3. Check laboratory results for osmolar effects (Hgb, Hct, electrolytes, BUN)
Alternate Bowel Elimination: Constipation	1. Decrease in water intake 2. Muscular atrophy of small and large intestines with decrease in GI motility 3. Perceptual loss of bowel stimulation	1. Encourage fluid intake 2. Assess bowel sounds for peristalsis 3. Administer mild laxative, and teach dangers of abuse 4. Have patient eat at regular times 5. Offer bedside commode 6. Increase roughage in diet as tolerated 7. Observe color, consistency, and frequency of stools

(continues on the following page)

Table 19-2

Body Fluid Problems in the Aged *(Continued)*

Problems	Etiology	Interventions
Alternate Bowel Elimination: Diarrhea	1. Tube feedings with too much carbohydrate 2. Constipation—with small amount of liquid stools 3. Partially digested nutrients 4. Viral or bacterial infection	1. Assess for problem causing diarrhea 2. Administer drug(s), e.g., Lomotil, Kaopectate, to decrease motility of bowel 3. Observe color, frequency, and consistency of stool

Diaphoresis	1. Excessive perspiration
	  a. Fever
	  b. High environmental temperature and/or humidity
		1. Identify cause of problem

26 decreased; insufficient water intake and increased urinary output

27 measure fluid intake and output for balance, encourage taking fluids orally, assess signs and symptoms of dehydration (hypovolemia), and assess intravenous fluid (type and rate), also, adjust replacement fluid rate according to age and condition of the client

28 pulmonary edema from overhydration

26

The thirst mechanism in the elderly is frequently (decreased/ increased) _____ , resulting in a decreased fluid intake.

Name two factors that can result in dehydration for the elderly. *_____

_____

27

Name four interventions to correct dehydration in the older person. *_____

_____

_____

28

Overloading the vascular system with fluids (hypervolemia) can result in congestive heart failure (CHF). The type of edema occurring in CHF is *_____ .

29

Peripheral edema can result from dependent or refractory edema. When the feet and ankles are edematous in the

29 refractory; cardiac-renal impairment or insufficiency with little to no diuretic effect; nondependent (since edema is present in the morning and is not necessarily due to gravity)

30 a. X; b. X; c. —, in the morning; d. —, chest sounds; e. —, of hypervolemia (overhydration)

31 Dextrose 5% in water (D₅W) is an iso-osmolar solution; however, if it is given without other solutes, the dextrose is metabolized by the body, leaving only water; it becomes a hypo-osmolar solution.

32 a. X; b. X; c. —, mild laxatives or stool softeners; d. X; e. X

33 tube feedings with too much carbohydrate, constipation with small liquid stools, partially digested nutrients, and viral or bacterial infections; identification of the problem causing diarrhea

morning, the type of edema present is called _____ edema. This type of edema results from *_____ and may also be called (dependent/nondependent/independent) _____ edema.

30
Identify selected interventions for correcting edema in the aged by selecting the correct answers and adjusting the incorrect answers.
( ) a. Measure fluid intake and output to assess fluid balance.
( ) b. Adjust intravenous flow rate according to age and patient condition.
( ) c. Assess for peripheral edema in the evening for refractory or nondependent edema.
( ) d. Assess bowel sounds.
( ) e. Observe for signs and symptoms of hypovolemia.

31
Explain why 5% dextrose in water might be considered a hypo-osmolar solution. *_____
_____
_____

32
Identify appropriate interventions related to constipation and adjust the incorrect answers:
( ) a. Encourage fluid intake.
( ) b. Assess bowel sounds for peristalsis.
( ) c. Administer harsh cathartics.
( ) d. Offer bedside commode.
( ) e. Have meals at regular times.

33
Name four causes of diarrhea in the aged. *_____
_____
 What is the most important intervention for correcting diarrhea? *_____
_____

34 diaphoresis; fever and high environmental temperature and high humidity

34

The sixth fluid problem occurring with the aged is _____ , or excessive perspiration. Two causes of excessive perspiration are *_____ .

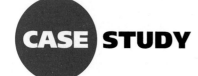

REVIEW A

Mrs. Palmer, age 89, is a resident in a nursing home. She has been hypoventilating and says that she has some difficulty with breathing. An assessment further reveals an elevated blood pressure (168/100), an increased pulse rate (104), edema in the extremities, a urinary output of 500 mL/day, and a recent weight gain of 10 pounds.

ANSWER COLUMN

1. pulmonary; renal; cardiac; gastrointestinal; integumentary; endocrine
2. a. loss of elasticity of the parenchymal lung tissue; b. increased rigidity of the chest wall

3. CO_2; respiratory acidosis
4. breathing exercise with prolonged expiration, coughing after a few deep breaths, and changing positions, also, chest clapping
5. increased rigidity of the arterial walls due to arteriosclerotic changes
6. increased capillary pressure forcing fluid into the tissues (nondependent edema)

1. As an aged person, Mrs. Palmer's body systems most prone to changes are _____ , _____ , _____ , _____ , _____ , and _____ .

2. Mrs. Palmer's reduced breathing capacity may be due to
   a. *_____
   b. *_____

3. Hypoventilation can result in _____ retention, which may cause an acid-base imbalance called *_____ .

4. Identify at least three interventions that can improve Mrs. Palmer's pulmonary function. *_____
   _____

5. Mrs. Palmer's blood pressure is elevated due to *_____
   _____
   _____

6. The physiologic reason for edema in her lower extremities is
   *_____
   _____ .

7. Identify three interventions regarding Mrs. Palmer's blood pressure and edema.

7. a. check blood pressure;
   b. determine blood flow in lower extremities by checking pulses; c. check for edema in the morning to determine if it is dependent or nondependent edema

8. 25; 600; inadequate;
   a. inadequate fluid intake;
   b. kidneys unable to excrete water and solute (you could have answered: reduced glomerular filtration rate and decrease in number of functioning nephrons)

9. check intake and output, encourage fluid intake, and check acid-base balance, also, test specific gravity

10. reduced motility of the gastrointestinal tract and loss of perception for bowel elimination

11. suggest diet (foods) to meet nutritional needs and maintain bowel function and encourage fluid intake; also, check frequency of bowel elimination and determine the presence of peristalsis (bowel sounds)

a. *_____ .
b. *_____ .
c. *_____ .

8. Urine output should be _____ mL/h or _____ mL/24 h to maintain adequate renal function. Mrs. Palmer's urine output was 500 mL in 24 hours, which is (adequate/inadequate) _____ . Identify two possible reasons for her poor urinary output.
   a. *_____
   b. *_____

9. Identify at least three interventions in regard to Mrs. Palmer's renal function. *_____
   _____

10. What two physiologic factors can cause Mrs. Palmer's constipation? *_____
    _____

11. Two interventions aimed at alleviating constipation are
    *_____

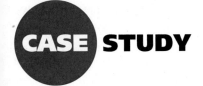

CASE STUDY   REVIEW B

Tom Fellows is a 67-year-old single man who until recently lived alone in his own house. He now lives in an intermediate-care unit of a continuing care facility where his meals are provided. He is independent in activities of daily living but requires help with shopping and money management. He was a financial analyst who led an active social life that included almost nightly "happy hours" with work associates until his retirement 5 years ago. After his retirement he started to drink alone. He quit going to the dining room for his meals and gradually stopped drinking fluids other than his beer and wine. The day shift recorded his vital signs as temperature 99°F, pulse 104, and respirations 28. His laboratory studies revealed an elevated hemoglobin and hematocrit. Other laboratory studies revealed serum potassium, 3.4 mEq/L; serum Na, 147; and Cl, 105 mEq/L (review Chapters 6–10 for normal electrolyte ranges). His skin and mucous membranes were very dry. He complained of constipation.

ANSWER COLUMN

1. dehydration, edema, and constipation

2. insufficient water intake (you might have answered that a decreased thirst mechanism was present)

3. a. vital signs: temperature slightly elevated, pulse and respirations elevated; b. Hgb, Hct, and BUN elevated; c. serum sodium elevated; d. skin and mucous membranes very dry

4. Yes. Frequently a person can have edema and be dehydrated due to hypovolemia in the vascular system with increased fluids in the interstitial space.

5. assess the IV fluid according to the type ordered and its osmolality and adjust the rate of IV fluids according to client's age and physiologic state. The nurse should also assess fluid intake and output balance.

6. water intoxication, or ICFVE

7. hypervolemia or overhydration (pulmonary edema) constant irritating cough, engorged veins (neck and hand), and dyspnea

1. From this history, identify three fluid problems. *_____
   _____

2. What is the clinical source of Mr. Fellows' dehydration?
   *_____
   _____

3. Identify four clinical signs and symptoms of dehydration experienced by Mr. Fellows.
   a. *_____
   b. *_____
   c. *_____
   d. *_____

4. Is it possible to have dehydration and edema at the same time? _____ Explain why. *_____
   _____

Mr. Fellows was given IV fluids for several days and then later given tube feedings daily.

5. While Mr. Fellows was receiving IV fluids, identify at least two interventions aimed at maintaining an appropriate fluid balance for clients receiving IV fluids. *_____
   _____

6. If Mr. Fellows receives continuous IV replacements with 5% dextrose in water, what type of fluid problem might result?
   *_____ .

7. If the intravenous fluids were administered too rapidly, what type of fluid imbalance is Mr. Fellows most likely to develop?
   *_____ Identify three symptoms of this imbalance.
   *_____

8. diarrhea

9. poorly conserved; deficit; hypokalemia

10. increased

8. Tube feedings high in carbohydrate can cause what type of a fluid problem? _____ .

9. The normal potassium level in the aged is *_____ , and therefore fluid balances often result in a potassium (deficit/excess) _____ called _____ .

10. Fluid imbalances can cause Mr. Fellows to be at an (increased/ decreased) _____ risk for skin breakdown.

Diagnoses and Related Interventions and Rationale

The purpose of assessing clients such as Mrs. Palmer and Mr. Fellows is to form diagnoses based on the assessment data. Interventions are selected to foster positive functional outcomes. Review the Functional Consequences Model of Gerontological Nursing in Figure 19-1 to review age-related changes and additional risk factors to be considered when forming diagnoses and planning interventions for older adults. Then answer the following study questions for Mrs. Palmer and Mr. Fellows:

1. What are the major body systems affected by the client's health problems?

2. What are the client's age-related structural changes related to fluid and electrolyte balance?

3. What are the client's additional risk factors for fluid and electrolyte imbalances?

4. What are the functional changes related to the client's structural changes and additional risk factors?

5. What are the most important diagnoses related to fluid and electrolyte balance for these clients?

6. What negative functional consequences can be prevented?

7. What interventions can help these clients prevent negative functional consequences?

Use Table 19-3 to organize your replies to the study questions about Mrs. Palmer and Table 19-4 for those about Mr. Fellows. Refer to Tables 19-1 and 19-2 as needed.

Diagnoses

Refer to Table 19-3.

Interventions and Rationale

Refer to Table 19-3.

Table 19-3

Mrs. Palmer

Body System Affected	Structural Changes	Risk Factors	Functional Changes	Diagnoses	Interventions	Rationale
Cardiac	Arteriosclerosis Increased capillary pressure Decreased effectiveness of cardiac contractions	Recent weight gain of 10 pounds Low protein intake	High blood pressure Edema Decreased cardiac output Increased heart rate	Fluid volume excess: edema, related to decreased cardiac output as evidenced by taut, shiny skin	1. Monitor intake and output, body weight, vital signs, and neck veins for distension 2. Monitor hemoglobin and hematocrit 3. Administer diuretics as ordered by physician 4. If on diuretics, monitor K$^+$	Checking for overhydration is important to measure the effectiveness of medical treatment and interventions Hemoglobin and hematocrit concentration are important to assess fluid balance changes A↓ Hgb and Hct levels can indicate fluid overload Diuretics increase fluid loss and decrease edema. Many diuretics cause potassium loss
Respiratory	Loss of elasticity of the parenchymal lung tissue Increased rigidity of the chest wall	Immobility Exertion Hypoventilation	CO_2 retention Respiratory acidosis *and* Reduced breathing capacity	Risk for respiratory insufficiency Impaired gas exchange Ineffective breathing patterns	1. Monitor chest for adventitious sounds 2. Observe for cough, which may indicate pulmonary edema 3. Breathing exercises—prolonged expiration	To assess for fluid overload Cough is an early sign of fluid overload Assists clients to remove excess CO_2

System	Physiologic changes	Contributing factors	Alteration	Nursing diagnosis	Interventions	Rationale
					4. Coughing after a few deep breaths	To enhance gas exchange ($O_2 + CO_2$)
					5. Change position frequently	Assist in lung expansion
					6. Chest clapping	Loosens mucus
Renal	Persistent renal vasoconstriction from arteriosclerotic changes and decreased numbers of functioning nephrons	Medications Genitourinary obstructions	Reduced glomerular filtration rate and ability to excrete water and solute	Fluid volume deficit related to decreased fluid intake	1. Assess intake and output	To determine amount of excess fluid loss
					2. Encourage oral fluids as tolerated	Assist with fluid replacement
					3. Assess acid-base balance	To observe for metabolic changes
					4. Assess urine specific gravity (SG)	Increased urine SG indicates inadequate fluid intake or decreased renal function
Gastrointestinal	Atrophy of gastric mucosa Loss of supportive structure of small and large bowel	Immobility Medications	Decreased mobility of GI tract Loss of perception of signs for bowel elimination	Risk for constipation related to decreased fluid volume, age-related changes, and immobility	1. Encourage fluids as tolerated	To assist with proper bowel elimination
					2. Increase mobility as tolerated	Physical mobility enhances GI mobility
					3. Encourage proper diet to ensure elimination	A balanced diet with fiber enhances bowel elimination
					4. Assess bowel sounds	To determine functional status of the GI system
					5. Check frequency of bowel elimination and consistency of stools	To determine risk of bowel complications

(continues on the following page)

Table 19-3

Mrs. Palmer (Continued)

Body System Affected	Structural Changes	Risk Factors	Functional Changes	Diagnoses	Interventions	Rationale
Liver* Integumentary	Loss of elasticity and strength of skin Decreased blood flow, sebaceous and sweat gland production	Edema Immobility	Taut, shiny skin reduces protective function	Impaired skin integrity related to edema and immobility	1. Avoid friction, prolonged pressure, chemical irritation, mechanical injury, excessive temperature variations	To reduce possible skin breakdown due to edema and/or immobility
					2. Encourage mobility to enhance circulation	Good circulation improves skin repair
					3. Raise extremities	To improve circulation and reduce edema
					4. Implement interventions for fluid volume excess and pulmonary congestion (PC) respiratory insufficiency	Fluid balance reduces risks to integumentary system

*Not applicable.

Table 19-4

Mr. Fellows

Body System Affected	Structural Changes	Risk Factors	Functional Changes	Diagnoses	Interventions	Rationale
Cardiac* Respiratory* Renal	Persistent renal vasoconstriction Decreased number of functioning nephrons	Obstructions Disease Medications	Decreased thirst mechanism Reduced glomerular filtration rate Decreased ability to excrete water and solute	Fluid volume deficit related to decreased desire to drink fluids secondary to high alcohol intake and social isolation, as evidenced by dry lips, furrowed tongue, and decreased skin turgor	1. Observe for decreased skin turgor, decreased urine output 2. Measure intake and output 3. Check specific gravity of urine 4. Observe lab results for increased red blood cell count, hematocrit, and hemoglobin	Decreased skin turgor is a sign of dehydration. Decreased urine output may be due to dehydration or renal dysfunction To determine fluid balance To assess renal function Provide clues to extent of fluid deficit
Gastrointestinal	Muscular atrophy and loss of supportive structure of small and large intestine Atrophy of gastric mucosa	Alcohol intake Poor diet Immobility Decreased motivation to drink fluids other than alcohol Social isolation	Decreased GI secretions Decreased motility Constipation	Potential complication: gastrointestinal bleeding Colonic constipation related to inadequate intake of food and fluids and lack of exercise, as evidenced by infrequent bowel movements, small, hard stools	1. Increase fluid intake of water and fluids 2. Assess fluid balance 3. Encourage a balanced diet with increased roughage 4. Assess bowel sounds 5. Observe color and consistency of stools 6. Hemoccult stools	To enhance bowel elimination and soften stools Fluid balance reduces risk for constipation Balanced diet with fiber stimulates bowel elimination To assess for constipation and/or bleeding Observe for GI bleeding to assess GI motility
Liver	Atrophy of liver cells	Heavy alcohol use Aspirin Social isolation		Potential complication: gastrointestinal bleeding	1. Observe for accumulation of fluids in third spaces	Liver damage can cause fluid shift, e.g., ascites
Integumentary*						

*Not applicable.

Evaluation/Outcome

1. Evaluate intake and output for fluid balance.
2. Evaluate effectiveness of medications and fluid replacement in treatment.
3. Monitor nutritional intake to ensure fluid balance.
4. Evaluate body weight and vital signs for return to normal client values.
5. Evaluate skin turgor, sensitivity, circulation, temperature, and moisture to reduce effects of risk factors.
6. Monitor lab results for Hgb, Hct, Na, Cl, K, and Ca until findings are within normal range.
7. Monitor reduction of signs and symptoms related to fluid imbalance.
8. Maintain a support system.

Trauma and Shock

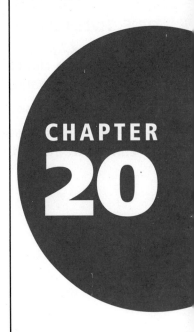

CHAPTER

20

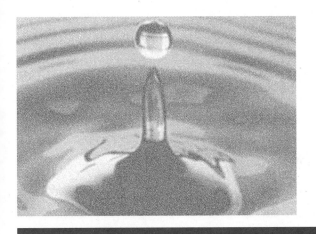

OBJECTIVES

Upon completion of this chapter, the reader should be able to:

- Discuss the physiologic changes in fluids and electrolytes that occur as a result of traumatic injuries and shock.
- Describe the clinical manifestations associated with traumatic injuries and shock.
- Discuss the assessment guidelines for fluid, electrolyte, and acid-base imbalances in the traumatically injured client.
- Identify the four types of shock and the physiologic basis for specific clinical symptoms.

(continued on next page)

OBJECTIVES (Continued)

● Discuss the clinical management of traumatic injuries as they relate to the four types of shock.

● Identify the assessment factors for evaluating shock and trauma clients.

● Develop diagnoses and interventions with rationales appropriate in the clinical treatment of trauma and shock clients.

▶ INTRODUCTION

There are numerous physiologic changes in fluids and electrolyte imbalances that occur as a result of traumatic injuries and shock. Swift and accurate assessment and intervention are necessary to protect the life of the injured client. This chapter is divided into two sections relating to fluid and electrolyte changes, trauma and shock.

▶ TRAUMA

Fluid, electrolyte, and acid-base changes occur rapidly in the acutely traumatized client. Quick assessments and actions are needed for the best chance of survival.

In trauma (acute injury), the sodium shifts into cells, potassium shifts out, and the fluid shifts from the vascular to the interstitial spaces and cells. These shifts can result in severe fluid and electrolyte imbalances.

ANSWER COLUMN

1 potassium and sodium;
Fluid shifts from the
vascular to the interstitial
spaces and cells.

1

The two electrolytes that change spaces during trauma are
*_____ .

Explain the fluid shifts during trauma. *_____
_____

Pathophysiology

Following a severe traumatic injury, there is cellular breakdown due to cell damage and hypoxia. The physiologic changes that occur during trauma are described in Table 20-1. Be familiar with these physiologic changes and their causative factors. The information in this table will help you to accurately assess traumatic injuries.

2
Explain what happens to the following electrolytes and water:
  a. Potassium *_____
  b. Sodium *_____
  c. Chloride *_____
  d. Water *_____

3
The sodium pump is necessary for cellular activity (see Chapter 7).
  Explain the sodium pump action. *_____
_____

4
During and after an acute injury, fluids shift to _____ and
*_____ .
  Do you know what is meant by fluids shifting to the third space? *_____
_____ .

5
With vascular fluid deficit (loss), the serum osmolality is (increased/decreased) _____ .
  What happens to the permeability of capillaries as a result of injury? *_____ .

6
Explain how ADH and aldosterone restore water balance.
ADH *_____
Aldosterone *_____

---

2 a. potassium is lost from the cells; b. sodium shifts into the cells; c. chloride shifts into the cells; d. water shifts into the cells

3 To maintain cellular activity, sodium shifts into the cells and potassium shifts out of the cells. Or, sodium shifts into the cell and depolarization occurs, and then potassium shifts back into the cell and repolarization occurs.

4 cells and injured site(s) or cells and interstitial (third) space; Fluids shift to the interstitial space at the injured site. Fluid in the third space is considered physiologically useless or nonfunctional fluid.

5 increased; it increases

6 ADH promotes water absorption from the distal tubules of the kidneys due to hypovolemia and/or the increased serum osmolality.; Aldosterone causes sodium to be reabsorbed from the distal tubules of the kidney when hyponatremia or stress is present.

Table 20-1

Physiologic Changes Associated with Trauma

Physiologic Changes	Causative Factors
Potassium, sodium, chloride, bicarbonate	Potassium is lost from cells due to catabolism (cellular breakdown). As potassium leaves, sodium and chloride with water shift into the cells. The sodium pump does not function properly (see Chapter 7).
Fluid changes	Fluids along with sodium shift into cells and to the third space (interstitial space—at the injured site). The increased cellular and third-space fluids cause a vascular fluid deficit (dehydration) and hyponatremia. Serum osmolality may be normal or increased due to the fluid deficit and excess solutes other than sodium, such as potassium and urea. Remember, sodium influences the osmolality of plasma. (see Chapter 1). The volume and composition of extracellular fluid (ECF) fluctuates depending on the number of cells injured and the body's ability to restore balance. Two to three days following injury, fluid shifts from the third space at the injured site back into the vascular space.
Protein changes	Trauma results in nitrogen loss due to increased protein catabolism, decreased protein anabolism, and/or a protein shift with water to the interstitial space. The colloid osmotic pressure is decreased in the vascular fluid and increased in the interstitial fluid (tissues), which causes fluid volume deficit (vascular) and edema.
Capillary permeability	Increased capillary permeability causes water to flow into and out of the cells and into tissue spaces. This contributes to hypovolemia (fluid volume deficit).
Hormonal influence	ADH and aldosterone help to restore the ECF. A vascular fluid deficit and/or increased serum osmolality stimulates ADH secretion, which causes water reabsorption from the distal tubules of the kidneys. In certain traumatic situations (surgery, trauma, pain), SIADH (syndrome of inappropriate ADH) occurs and causes excess water reabsorption from the kidneys. Aldosterone is secreted from the adrenal cortex due to hyponatremia and stress. Aldosterone promotes sodium reabsorption from the renal tubules and is reabsorbed with water. Potassium is excreted.
Kidney influence	Kidney activity is altered during and after a severe traumatic injury. Sodium, chloride, and water shift to the injured site, which causes hypovolemia. Decreased circulatory flow can decrease renal arterial flow, which can cause temporary or permanent kidney damage. Decreased kidney function results in hyperkalemia.

(continues on the following page)

Table 20-1

(Continued)

Physiologic Changes	Causative Factors
Acid-base changes	With cellular breakdown and hypoxia from decreased perfusion, nonvolatile acids (acid metabolites), e.g., lactic acid, increase in the vascular fluid, causing metabolic acidosis.
	Kidneys conserve or excrete the hydrogen ion to maintain the acid-base balance. Decreased kidney function can cause hydrogen retention and acidosis.
	The lungs try to compensate for the acidotic state by blowing off excess CO_2—hyperventilation. Blowing off CO_2 decreases the formation of carbonic acid.

7

The syndrome of inappropriate antidiuretic hormone secretions (SIADH) frequently occurs following surgery, trauma, stress, pain, and CNS depressants (narcotics). The water reabsorption can be continuous for several days.

The nurse should assess for what type of fluid imbalance:

( ) a. Overhydration (hypervolemia)

( ) b. Dehydration (hypovolemia)

7　a

8

Kidneys are the chief regulators of sodium and water balance. Kidneys conserve sodium when there is a sodium deficit. The hormone that is responsible for sodium reabsorption is

_____ . This hormone also causes potassium (excretion/ retention) _____ .

8　aldosterone; excretion

9

A decrease in circulation from trauma, stress, or shock can cause a decrease in renal arterial blood flow. What effect does this have on the kidney? *_____

_____

For circulating blood to perfuse the kidneys, the systolic blood pressure should be _____ mm Hg or greater. (Refer to Chapter 2, ECFV deficit.)

9　temporary or permanent kidney damage; 70

10

Severe trauma resulting in inadequate tissue perfusion with hypoxia releases nonvolatile acids (acid metabolites), such as lactic acid, from cells. What type of acid-base imbalance can occur? * _____ .

How do the lungs compensate for this imbalance?

* _____ .

10 metabolic acidosis; by blowing off CO_2 (reducing carbonic acid)

11

From the following list of fluid, electrolyte, and acid-base changes, check those that are affected by trauma, and correct the incorrect responses.

( ) a. Cellular loss of potassium
( ) b. Sodium shifts into cells
( ) c. Hypervolemia or overhydration
( ) d. Fluid shifts to the cells and injured site(s)
( ) e. Protein loss
( ) f. Decreased capillary permeability
( ) g. ADH secretion promoting reabsorption of water from the kidneys

11 a, b, d, e, g; Corrections: c. hypovolemia or dehydration; f. increased capillary permeability

Clinical Manifestations

The health care professional assesses injured sites, orders fluid replacements, and performs medical or surgical interventions as needed.

Responsibility for care is ongoing assessment and monitoring of fluid electrolyte and acid-base imbalances as they occur.

12

The three imbalances that the health professional should assess are * _____

12 fluids, electrolytes, and acid-base

The clinical manifestations that frequently occur in traumatic injuries depend upon the type of imbalance (fluid, electrolyte, or acid-base) and include changes in vital signs, behavioral changes, cardiac conduction changes, venous changes, renal changes, neuromuscular changes, integumentary changes, and laboratory findings. Table 20-2 lists the signs and symptoms that may occur as the result of trauma. For further clarification of these changes and rationale, refer to Table 20-3 on assessment.

Table 20-2

Clinical Manifestations Related to Trauma

Clinical Manifestations	Signs and Symptoms
Vital Signs Pulse	Increased pulse rate (tachycardia) Irregular pulse rate Full-bounding pulse
Blood Pressure	Blood pressure decreases when severe fluid loss occurs Pulse pressure narrows
Respiration	Increased breathing (tachypnea) Dyspnea Deep, vigorous breathing (Kussmaul breathing)
Temperature	Hypothermia commonly associated with shock
Behavioral Changes	Irritability, restlessness, and confusion
Cardiac Conduction Changes	ECG: T-wave changes (inverted or peaked), ST-segment changes, and cardiac dysrythmias
Venous Changes	Neck and hand vein engorgement No vein engorgement with fluid loss
Renal Changes	Hourly urine output decreases
Neuromuscular Changes	Muscular weakness
Integumentary Changes	Poor skin turgor Dry mucous membrane Edema Diaphoresis Draining wound, exudate
Laboratory Findings Electrolytes ↓ or ↑	Serum potassium, sodium, magnesium, chloride may be decreased or increased
Serum CO_2	Decreased CO_2 indicates metabolic acidosis; increased CO_2 indicates metabolic alkalosis or respiratory alkalosis
BUN ↑	Increased BUN: fluid loss or decreased renal function
Serum creatinine ↑	Increased serum creatinine indicates decreased renal function
Arterial blood gases: pH, $PaCO_2$, HCO_3	Decreased pH and HCO_3 indicate metabolic acidosis

13 a. tachycardia, irregular pulse rate, or full-bounding pulse; b. decreased blood pressure, narrow pulse pressure with severe fluid loss; c. tachypnea, dyspnea, or deep vigorous breathing; d. hypothermia is commonly associated with shock

13

Indicate the typical effects of trauma on the vital signs:
   a. Pulse *_____
   b. Blood pressure *_____
   c. Respiration *_____
   d. Temperature *_____

14

Behavioral changes are frequently observed with fluid and electrolyte imbalances.
   Name two behavioral changes that can occur following severe trauma. *_____

14 irritability and confusion (also restlessness, disorientation)

15

Trauma usually results in loss of body fluid. When elevated above the heart level the neck veins become (engorged/flat) _____ .

15 flat

16

Urine output following trauma may be _____ .
   Following trauma, urine output should be checked (every hour/every 8 hours/once a day) _____ .

16 decreased; every hour

17

Integumentary changes may not be noted immediately following severe trauma with fluid losses. However, after several hours or a day, the skin turgor can be affected and mucous membranes become (dry/wet) _____ .
   These signs indicate (hypovolemia/hypervolemia) _____ .

17 dry; hypovolemia

18

Many abnormal laboratory results occur in severe trauma.
   Cellular breakdown and poor urine output (increase/decrease) _____ the serum potassium level.
   Poor renal function causes the BUN and serum creatinine to (increase/decrease) _____ .
   Frequently, metabolic acidosis results following severe trauma due to cellular breakdown and poor tissue perfusion. Which arterial blood gas changes are indicative of metabolic acidosis?
   ( ) a. pH decreased
   ( ) b. $PaCO_2$ increased
   ( ) c. HCO_3 decreased

18 increase; increase; a, c

Clinical Applications

Accurate assessment is vitally important when planning and implementing care. Table 20-3 is a guide that may be used when assessing the client for fluid, electrolyte, and acid-base imbalances. The table includes key observations, assessment factors, and rationale. To understand the significance of the assessment, the rationale helps to identify the type of imbalance that is present. Use this table in clinical assessments.

19

Vital signs should be constantly monitored following an acute injury. Tachycardia or pulse rate greater than 120 can indicate _____ and should be reported.

19 hypovolemia or fluid volume deficit

20

Blood pressure does not immediately fall after an injury. With a fluid volume deficit, the pulse rate increases first, and later the blood pressure drops if fluid loss is not replaced.
    A pulse pressure of less than 20 can indicate _____ .

20 shock

21

A respiratory rate greater than 32 can indicate _____ .
    Deep, rapid, vigorous breathing occurring after cellular damage or shock due to acute injury can indicate (metabolic acidosis/metabolic alkalosis) *_____ . Why?
    *_____

21 hypovolemia or fluid volume deficit; metabolic acidosis; Acid metabolites, such as lactic acid, are released from cells due to anaerobic metabolism from inadequate perfusion.

22

Temperature changes frequently do not occur immediately after injury. When there is a slight temperature elevation, this can indicate _____ .
    If a high temperature elevation occurs 2–5 days after the injury, what might it indicate? _____ .

22 hypovolemia or a fluid volume deficit or dehydration; infection

23

Irritability, apprehension, restlessness, and confusion are usually the result of hypoxia and of fluid and electrolyte imbalances. Name two fluid and one electrolyte imbalance associated with the stated behavioral changes.
Fluid imbalances: *_____
Electrolyte imbalance: _____

23 hypovolemia or fluid volume deficit and water intoxication; hypokalemia

Table 20-3

Assessment of Fluid, Electrolyte, and Acid-Base Imbalances in the Traumatically Injured Client

Observation	Assessment		Rationale
1. Vital signs: Pulse	Pulse rate Volume Pattern	_____ _____ _____	Changes in vital signs (VS) are indicators of client's physiologic status. Several VS should be taken and the first reading acts as the baseline for comparison. Pulse rate and pattern should be monitored frequently. Pulse rate >120 may indicate hypovolemia and the possibility of shock. Full, bounding pulse can mean hypervolemia and an irregular pulse can mean hypokalemia.
Blood pressure	Admission BP Time Time	_____ _____	Decrease in BP (systolic and diastolic) may not occur until severe fluid loss has occurred. Several BP readings should be taken, and the first BP reading acts as the baseline and for comparison. A drop in systolic pressure can indicate hypovolemia. Pulse pressure (systolic minus diastolic) of <20 can indicate shock.
Respiration	Respiration Pattern	_____ _____	Note changes in rate, depth, and pattern. A rate >32 can indicate hypovolemia. Deep, rapid, vigorous breathing can indicate acidosis as a result of cellular damage and shock. Hyperventilating (fast, shallow breathing) can be due to anxiety or hypoxia. Head injury can produce a wide variety of respiratory patterns.
Temperature	Temperature on admission	_____	Hypothermia is a common finding in shock; an elevated temperature can indicate infection.
2. Behavioral changes	Irritable Apprehensive Restless Confused Delirious Lethargic	_____ _____ _____ _____ _____ _____	Irritability, apprehension, restlessness, and confusion are indicators of hypoxia and later of fluid and electrolyte imbalances (hypovolemia, water intoxication, and potassium imbalance).
3. Neurologic and neuromuscular signs	Sensorium Confused Semiconscious Comatose Muscle weakness Pupil dilation Tetany Tremors Twitching Others	_____ _____ _____ _____ _____ _____ _____ _____	Changes in sensorium can be indicative of fluid imbalance. Tetany can indicate a calcium and magnesium deficit. Hypercalcemia can occur with multiple transfusions of banked blood.

(continues on the following page)

Table 20-3

(Continued)

Observation	Assessment		Rationale
4. Fluid loss	Wound(s)	_____	Note the presence of an open draining wound. Kidneys regulate fluids and electrolytes. Monitoring the urine output hourly is most important. Oliguria can indicate a lack of fluid intake or renal insufficiency due to decreased circulation/circulatory collapse or hypovolemia.
	Urine		
	Number of voidings	_____	
	Amount	_____	
	mL/h	_____	
	mL/8 h	_____	
	mL/24 h	_____	
	Color	_____	
	Specific gravity	_____	
	Vomitus		Frequent vomiting in large quantities leads to fluid, electrolyte (potassium, sodium, chloride), and hydrogen losses. Metabolic alkalosis can occur.
	Number	_____	
	Consistency	_____	
	Amount	_____	
	Nasogastric tube		Gastrointestinal secretions should be measured. Large quantity losses of GI secretions can cause hypovolemia.
	Amount—mL/8h	_____	
	Amount—mL/24 h	_____	
	Drain(s)		Excess drainage could contribute to fluid loss and should be measured if possible.
	Number	_____	
	Amount	_____	
5. Skin and mucous membrane	Skin color		Pale and/or gray-colored skin can indicate hypovolemia or shock. Flushed skin can be due to hypernatremia, metabolic acidosis, or early septic shock.
	Pale	_____	
	Gray	_____	
	Flushed	_____	
	Skin turgor		Poor skin turgor can result from hypovolemia/dehydration. This may not occur until 1–3 days after the injury.
	Normal	_____	
	Poor	_____	
	Edema—pitting peripheral		Edema indicates sodium and water retention. Sodium, chloride, and water shift into the cells and to the injury site(s) (interstitial or third space).
	Feet	_____	
	Legs	_____	
	Dry mucous membranes	_____	Dry, tenacious (sticky) secretions and dry membranes are indicative of dehydration or fluid loss. This may not occur until 1–3 days after the injury.
	Sticky secretions	_____	
	Diaphoresis	_____	Increased insensible fluid loss can result from diaphoresis (excess perspiration). Amount of fluid loss from skin can double.
6. Chest sounds and vein engorgement	Chest rales	_____	The chest should be checked for rales due to overhydration (pulmonary edema) following fluid administration/resuscitation.

(continues on the following page)

Table 20-3

Assessment of Fluid, Electrolyte, and Acid-Base Imbalances in the Traumatically Injured Client (*Continued*)

Observation	Assessment		Rationale
	Neck vein engorgement	_____	Neck and hand vein engorgement are indicators of fluid excess. Rales and vein engorgement can occur from excess IV fluids or rapid IV administration.
	Hand vein engorgement	_____	
7. ECG (EKG)	T wave		Flat or inverted T waves indicate cardiac ischemia and/or a potassium deficit. Peaked T waves indicate a potassium excess.
	Flat	_____	
	Inverted	_____	
	Peaked	_____	
8. Fluid intake	Oral fluid intake		Oral fluids should not be given until the injury(s) can be assessed. If surgery is indicated, the client should be NPO.
	Amount		
	mL/8 h	_____	
	mL/24 h	_____	
	Types of IV fluids		Crystalloids, i.e., normal saline, lactated Ringer's, are normally ordered first to restore fluid loss, correct shocklike symptoms, restore or increase urine output, and serve as a lifeline to administer IV drugs.
	Crystalloids	_____	
	Colloids	_____	
	Blood	_____	
	Amount		Five percent dextrose in water can cause water intoxication (ICF volume excess) and is contraindicated as a resuscitation fluid in shock states.
	mL/8 h	_____	
	mL/24 h	_____	
	mL/h	_____	
9. Previous drug regimen	Diuretics	_____	A drug history should be taken and reported to the physician. Potassium-wasting diuretics taken with a digitalis preparation can cause digitalis toxicity in the presence of hypokalemia. Steroids cause sodium retention and potassium excretion.
	Digitalis	_____	
	Steroids	_____	
	Beta blockers	_____	
	Calcium channel blockers	_____	
			Long-term steroid use can impair adrenal function in shock states and impair the client's ability to mount a stress response. A steroid bolus or "stress dose" is indicated for steroid-dependent clients. Beta blockers and calcium channel blockers block the effects of the sympathetic nervous system. They may block the compensatory mechanisms for shock.

(continues on the following page)

Table 20-3

(Continued)

Observation	Assessment		Rationale
10. Chemistry, hematology, and arterial blood gas changes	Electrolytes *Serum* K _____ Na _____ Cl _____ Ca _____ Mg _____	*Urine/24 h* K _____ Na _____ Cl _____	Electrolytes should be drawn immediately after a severe injury and used as a baseline for future electrolyte results. (See Chapter 6 for normal values.) Urine electrolytes are compared to serum electrolytes. Normal range for urine electrolytes are: K 25–120 mEq/24 h Na 40–220 mEq/24 h Cl 150–250 mEq/24 h
	Serum CO_2	_____	Serum CO_2 >32 mEq/L indicates metabolic alkalosis and <22 mEq/L indicates metabolic acidosis.

	Osmolality
	  Serum
	  Urine
		_____
		_____
			Serum osmolality >295 mOsm/kg indicates hypovolemia/dehydration and <280 mOsm/kg indicates hypervolemia. Urine osmolality can be 100–1200 mOsm/kg with a normal range of 200–600 mOsm/kg.

	BUN Creatinine	_____ _____	An elevated BUN can indicate fluid volume deficit or kidney insufficiency. Elevated creatinine indicates kidney damage. Normal range: BUN 10–25 mg/dL Creatinine 0.7–1.4 mg/dL
	Blood glucose	_____	Blood sugar increases during stress (up to 180 mg/dL, or higher in diabetics).
	Hbg _____	Hct _____	Elevated hemoglobin and hematocrit can indicate hemoconcentration caused by fluid volume deficit (hypovolemia).

(continues on the following page)

Table 20-3

Assessment of Fluid, Electrolyte, and Acid-Base Imbalances in the Traumatically Injured Client *(Continued)*

Observation	Assessment	Rationale

	Arterial blood gases (ABGs)
	pH
	PaCO$_2$
	HCO$_3$
	BE
		pH: <7.35 indicates acidosis and >7.45 indicates alkalosis.
		
		PaCO$_2$ (respiratory component):
		  Norms 35–45 mm Hg
		Respiratory acidosis (↓ pH, ↑ PaCO$_2$) may occur due to inadequate gas exchange. A ↑ pH and ↓ PaCO$_2$ indicate respiratory alkalosis from hyperventilation.
		
		HCO$_3$ (renal component):
		  Norms 24–28 mEq/L
		A ↓ HCO$_3$ and ↓ pH means metabolic acidosis, which is the most common acid-base imbalance following injury from inadequate perfusion and lactic acid production. (See Table 20-1).
		A ↑ HCO$_3$ and ↑ pH means metabolic alkalosis.
		
		BE (base excess)
		  Norms +2 to −2. Same as bicarbonate.
		A base excess of <−2 (also termed base deficit) is an indication of poor perfusion/inadequate resuscitation.

24

Match the neurologic and neuromuscular signs on the left with fluid and electrolyte imbalances on the right:

_____ 1. Decreased sensorium   a. Hypokalemia

_____ 2. Muscle weakness   b. Hypovolemia

_____ 3. Tetany—tremors   c. Hypocalcemia
 and twitching

24 1. b; 2. a; 3. c

25

Oliguria is not uncommon following an acute injury. Decreased urine output can be due to *_____ .

 Do you recall what elevated specific gravity (>1.030) indicates? *_____ .

25 hypovolemia, or a lack of fluid intake; dehydration/hypovolemia, or lack of fluid intake

26

Vomitus, nasogastric tubes, and diarrhea can cause what type of fluid imbalance? _____ .

Indicate which acid-base imbalance listed on the right occurs with the causes of fluid loss listed on the left:

_____ 1. Vomiting a. Metabolic alkalosis
_____ 2. Nasogastric tubes (loss b. Metabolic acidosis
    of stomach secretions)
_____ 3. Diarrhea

26 hypovolemia; 1. a; 2. a; 3. b

27

Pale or gray-colored skin can indicate _____ .

Poor skin turgor, dry mucous membranes, and tenacious or sticky mucous secretions are indicative of _____ .

27 hypovolemia or shock; dehydration or fluid loss

28

When the client is receiving IV therapy at an increased flow rate to correct fluid loss, the client should be assessed for potential signs of overhydration.

Excess and/or rapidly administered IV fluids can cause what type of fluid imbalance? _____

Name two symptoms associated with this imbalance. (Refer to Chapter 3, section on ECFVE.) *_____

28 overhydration, or ECFV excess (extracellular cellular fluid volume excess); chest rales and neck or hand vein engorgement (also constant irritating cough or dyspnea)

29

A flat or inverted T wave can indicate _____ , and a peaked T wave can indicate _____ .

29 hypokalemia or potassium deficit or cardiac ischemia; hyperkalemia or potassium excess

30

Immediately after an acute injury, oral fluids (should/should not) _____ be given. Why? *_____
_____ .

30 should not; The client may need surgery and would be NPO (nothing by mouth).

31

Indicate which of the following are crystalloids used in IV therapy for shock states:

( ) a. Dextrose 5% in water (D_5W)
( ) b. Dextran 40, 6%
( ) c. Plasmanate
( ) d. Normal saline (0.9% NaCl)
( ) e. Lactated Ringer's

31 d, e;

to restore fluid loss and correct shocklike symptoms (correction may be temporary) (also, increase urine output); Water intoxication (ICFV excess). In early shock/trauma massive infusions of D_5W can also cause hyperglycemia. Dextrose 5% in water should never be used as a replacement fluid in shock states.

32 c, d, e

33 increase (release of potassium from severe tissue damage; if urine output is poor, serum K can also increase).; decrease

34 hypovolemia; hypervolemia; It is caused from overhydration or hemodilution (excess water in proportion to solutes).

35 fluid volume deficit or renal insufficiency; renal insufficiency; hypovolemia or fluid volume deficit

36 metabolic acidosis

Give two reasons for using crystalloids. *_____
_____ .
What type of fluid imbalance occurs when using 5% dextrose in water as a resuscitation fluid? *_____

32
Identify the drugs that cause sodium retention.
( ) a. Diuretics
( ) b. Digitalis
( ) c. Cortisone
Which of the following drugs cause potassium excretion?
( ) d. Diuretics (potassium wasting)
( ) e. Digitalis
( ) f. Cortisone

33
After severe tissue injury, serum potassium levels _____ . If lactic acid is released from the cells due to a cellular breakdown, the serum CO_2 would (increase/decrease) _____ . Serum CO_2 is a bicarbonate determinant.

34
A serum osmolality greater than 295 mOsm/kg indicates (hypovolemia/hypervolemia) _____ .
A serum osmolality less than 280 mOsm/kg indicates (hypovolemia/hypervolemia) _____ . Why? *_____
_____

35
An elevated BUN can indicate *_____ or *_____ .
After hydration, if the BUN does not return to normal, the elevated BUN indicates *_____ .
An elevated hemoglobin and hematocrit level can indicate hemoconcentration caused by _____ .

36
What type of acid-base imbalance is present if the client's arterial blood gases are: pH 7.25; $PaCO_2$ 35 mm Hg; and HCO_3 18 mEq/L? *_____

37

From the following list of observations and assessments, mark the ones that indicate fluid volume deficit (hypovolemia).

( ) a. Pulse 76
( ) b. Blood pressure 86/68
( ) c. Irritability, restlessness, confusion
( ) d. Specific gravity 1.034
( ) e. Excess GI drainage (>2 liters)
( ) f. Dry mucous membrane and dry, tenacious mucous secretions
( ) g. Chest rales
( ) h. Peaked T waves
( ) i. Elevated BUN and Hgb

37 b, c, d, e, f, i

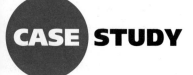

CASE STUDY REVIEW

Marjorie Rockland, age 58, was in a motor vehicle crash and was taken by ambulance to the emergency department of a large medical center. Her vital signs on admission are blood pressure 134/88, pulse rate 106, respiration 30, and temperature 98.8°F (37.1°C). She complained of pain in her abdomen and leg. A liter of 0.9% normal saline solution (NSS) is started. Blood chemistry, x-rays (leg), and CT scan (abdomen) are ordered. Abdominal area appears distended, and there are diminished bowel sounds. A nasogastric tube is inserted and attached to intermittent suction.

ANSWER COLUMN

1. fluid loss or hypovolemia or impending shock
2. normal; heart rate (pulse) was compensating for fluid loss and in response to injury. Later, if heart rate does not compensate, blood pressure will fall.
3. crystalloids. This group of solutions increases fluid volume and acts as a lifeline for emergency IV drugs.

1. Ms. Rockland's pulse rate indicates tachycardia (mild to moderate) and can be indicative of *_____ .

2. Her blood pressure is (normal/high/low) _____ and may mean *_____ .

3. Name the solution category for NSS. *_____

4. Intraabdominal injury (most likely a traumatized or injured area)
5. to remove accumulated stomach and intestinal fluid (secretions) that resulted from an abdominal injury; gastric decompression

6. a. tachycardia from fluid volume deficit (hypovolemia); b. drop in BP and pulse pressure 20 indicate hypovolemia and shock (impending); c. tachypnea from hypovolemia and stress

7. a. N; b. L; c. N; d. N
8. to monitor urine output (common practice following a traumatic injury); adequate
9. GI injury or abdominal injury

10. hypovolemia and/or hypoxemia

11. hypovolemia (severe) and shock
12. Fluid shifts from the vascular fluid to the cells and to the injured sites (third spaces—abdominal area and injured leg tissue area). Fluids are also lost from GI suction and from diaphoresis.

4. A distended abdomen and decreased peristalsis can indicate
   *_____ .

5. The purpose for the nasogastric tube connected to suction would be *_____ .

   The x-rays showed a fractured right femur and the CT scan of the abdomen revealed possible abdominal fluid. Vital signs 1 hour later were blood pressure 106/86, pulse rate 128, respiration 34. Ms. Rockland was apprehensive and restless and had periods of confusion. Blood chemistry results were K 3.7 mEq/L, Na 134 mEq/L, Cl 99 mEq/L, serum CO_2 24 mEq/L. A Foley catheter was inserted, and 350 mL of urine was obtained. The secretions from GI suction were "bloody."

6. Changes in the vital signs indicate:
   a. Pulse *_____
   b. Blood Pressure *_____
   c. Respiration *_____

7. Indicate whether the results from the blood chemistry are normal (N), low (L), or high (H).
   (   ) a. Potassium
   (   ) b. Sodium
   (   ) c. Chloride
   (   ) d. Serum CO_2

8. Why is a Foley catheter inserted? *_____
   Was the amount of urine obtained (adequate/inadequate)?
   _____.

9. Bloody GI secretions can indicate *_____ .

10. Ms. Rockland's apprehension, restlessness, and bouts of confusion can indicate _____ .

    Two hours after admission, Ms. Rockland's vital signs are blood pressure 84/66, pulse rate 136, respiration 36. Her skin color is gray and she is diaphoretic. Urine output is averaging 15–20 mL/h. Blood chemistry, type, and cross-match and blood gases are ordered. A second liter of NSS to run wide open is ordered.

11. Vital signs are indicative of *_____ .

12. Explain why there is a fluid volume deficit. *_____
    _____

13. No. It is less than 25 mL/h.

14. No. Dextrose 5% in water (D_5W) is not an appropriate solution and can cause water intoxication if used in large quantities.

15. a. normal; b. hyponatremia; c. hypochloremia; d. metabolic acidosis; e. stress; f. hypovolemia/ dehydration; g. acidosis; h. low normal; i. metabolic acidosis

13. Is the hourly urine output adequate? _____ Why? *_____

14. Is 5% dextrose in water an appropriate IV solution to be used in this case? _____ Why? *_____
_____

She is immediately scheduled for the OR. The second laboratory results are K 5.0 mEq/L, Na 130 mEq/L, Cl 94 mEq/L, serum CO_2 18 mEq/L, blood sugar 166 mg/dL, BUN 32 mg/dL, ABG—pH 7.32, $PaCO_2$ 35 mm Hg, HCO_3 19 mEq/L.

15. Her lab results indicate:
    a. Potassium _____
    b. Sodium _____
    c. Chloride _____
    d. Serum CO_2 *_____
    e. Blood sugar _____
    f. BUN _____
    g. pH _____
    h. $PaCO_2$ _____
    i. HCO_3 *_____

▶ SHOCK

The state of inadequate perfusion, known as *shock,* occurs when the hemostatic circulatory mechanism, which regulates circulation, fails to maintain adequate circulation. With shock, the cardiac output is insufficient to provide vital organs and tissues with blood. There are four categories of shock: (1) hypovolemic, which includes hematogenic from hemorrhage; (2) cardiogenic; (3) septic; and (4) neurogenic. Most shock-induced conditions are associated with trauma.

38 inadequate perfusion; maintain adequate circulation or provide adequate blood to vital organs and tissues

38
Shock is a state of *_____ .
    Shock occurs when the hemostatic circulatory mechanism fails to *_____ .

39
A common feature of shock, regardless of the cause, is a low circulating blood volume in relation to the vascular capacity.

There is a loss of blood, not necessarily from hemorrhaging, but from "pooling" in body areas so that adequate blood does not circulate. This causes inadequate tissue perfusion.

A low blood volume is known as _____ .

A disproportion between the volume of blood and the capacity (size) of the vascular chamber is the essential feature of

_____ .

39 hypovolemia; shock

40

A common feature of shock is * _____ .

With shock, is hypovolemia always due to hemorrhaging?

_____

Explain. * _____

40 a low circulating blood volume or loss of blood; No! It can be due to pooling of blood in body areas.

Pathophysiology

The physiologic changes resulting from shock include a decrease in blood pressure, an increase in vasoconstriction of the blood vessels, an increase in heart rate, a decrease in metabolism (inadequate oxygenation of the blood, electrolyte changes, metabolic acidosis, and a decline in liver glycogen), and a decrease in renal function. Table 20-4 describes these physiologic changes. Study the table, noting if there is an increase or decrease in action or function. Refer to the table as needed as you proceed to the questions.

41

Place I for increase and D for decrease beside the physiologic factors as they occur with shock.

_____ a. Arterial blood pressure

_____ b. Kidney function

_____ c. Heart rate

_____ d. Anaerobic metabolism

_____ e. Vasoconstriction

41 a. D; b. D; c. I; d. I; e. I

42

When there is a low blood pressure, the pressoreceptors in the carotid sinus and aortic arch cause an increase in the systemic vasomotor activity that leads to what two activities in order to maintain homeostasis? * _____

Increased systematic vasomotor activity occurs in order to maintain _____ .

42 vasoconstriction and cardiac acceleration; homeostasis

Table 20-4

Physiologic Changes Resulting from Shock

Physiologic Changes	Rationale
Arterial blood pressure: decreased	Reduced venous return to heart decreases cardiac output and arterial blood pressure (BP).
	Decrease in BP is sensed by pressoreceptors in carotid sinus and aortic arch, which leads to immediate reflex increase in systemic vasomotor activity. (This center is found in medulla.) Cardiac acceleration and vasoconstriction occur in order to maintain homeostasis with respect to blood pressure. This may be sufficient for early or impending shock.
Vasoconstriction of blood vessels: increased	Increased sympathetic nervous system activity causes vasoconstriction. Vasoconstriction tends to maintain blood pressure and reduce discrepancy between blood volume and vascular capacity (size). Vasoconstriction is greatest in skin, kidneys, and skeletal muscles and not as significant in cerebral vessels. Coronary arteries actually dilate with a decrease in blood volume. This is a compensatory mechanism to provide sufficient blood to the heart muscle (myocardium) for heart function.
Heart rate: increased	Heart rate is increased to overcome poor cardiac output and to increase circulation. Rapid, thready pulse is often one of first identifiable signs of shock.
Metabolism: decreased	Fall in plasma hydrostatic pressure reduces urinary filtration. Unopposed plasma colloid osmotic pressure draws interstitial fluid into vascular bed. Blood loss results in loss of serum potassium, phosphate, and bicarbonate. Inadequate oxygenation of cells prevents their normal metabolism and leads to anaerobic metabolism and the formation of nonvolatile acids (acid metabolites), thus lowering serum pH values. With a fall in serum pH and a decrease in HCO_3, metabolic acidosis results. A rise in blood sugar is first seen due to release of epinephrine; later, blood sugar falls due to a decline in liver glycogen.
Kidney function: decreased	Low blood pressure causes inadequate circulation of blood to the kidneys. Renal ischemia is the result of a lack of O_2 to the kidneys. Renal insufficiency follows prolonged hypotension. Systolic blood pressure must be 70 mm Hg and above to maintain kidney function.
	One of the body's compensatory mechanisms in shock is to shunt blood around kidney to maintain intravascular fluid. Deficient blood supply makes tubule cells of kidneys more susceptible to injury.
	Urine output of less than 25 mL/h may be indicative of shock and/or decrease in renal function.

43

Increased sympathetic activity results in (vasoconstriction/vasodilation) _____ .

   Vasoconstriction is greatest in what three parts of the body?
*
_____ .

   The coronary arteries (dilate/constrict) _____ with a decrease in blood volume.

44

Heart rate in shock is (increased/decreased) _____ to overcome poor cardiac output and to increase circulation.

   The pulse rate is _____ and _____ .

   A person with a pulse rate above 120 has (bradycardia/tachycardia) _____ .

45

The following metabolic changes occur with shock:

   Fluid is drawn from the interstitial space into the vascular space due to what kind of pressure? *_____

   Inadequate oxygenation of cells leads to the formation of nonvolatile acids (acid metabolites), causing the pH to (rise/fall)
_____ .

   A fall in pH and HCO_3 leads to (metabolic acidosis/metabolic alkalosis) *_____ .

   In shock, there is a release of epinephrine, which causes the blood sugar to (rise/fall) _____ . Later, there is a (rise/fall)
_____ in blood sugar due to a decline in liver glycogen.

46

In shock, the compensatory mechanisms shunt the blood around the kidney in order to maintain the volume of
*_____ . This results in a lack of oxygen in the kidneys known as *_____ , causing a decrease in kidney function.

   The systolic blood pressure for kidney function must be at least *_____ .

   An indication of shock related to kidney dysfunction is a urine output of less than *_____ .

47

Extracellular fluid volume shifts occur during shock. In *early* shock, fluid is shifted from the interstitial space to the intravascular space to compensate for the fluid deficit in the

---

43 vasoconstriction; skin, kidneys, and skeletal muscles; dilate

44 increased; rapid and thready; tachycardia

45 colloid osmotic pressure; fall; metabolic acidosis; rise; fall

46 intravascular fluid; renal ischemia; 70 mm Hg; 25 mL/h

vascular system. More fluid in the vascular system increases the venous return to the heart; thus it increases cardiac output.

As the interstitial fluid becomes depleted, tissue (dehydration/edema) _____ occurs.

47 dehydration

48

In *late* shock, fluid is forced from the intravascular space (blood vessels) back into the interstitial space (tissues).

In early shock, fluid is shifted from the * _____ to the * _____ . Why? * _____

48 interstitial space; intravascular space; This shift compensates for fluid deficit in the vascular system.

Etiology

The clinical symptoms and related physiologic basis for each of the four types of shock—hypovolemic, cardiogenic, septic (also known as endotoxic or vasogenic), and neurogenic—are presented. Table 20-5 describes the four types of shock, the clinical causes, and the rationale and physiologic changes that occur with each type.

Study the table carefully, noting the causes (etiology) for each type of shock. Refer to the glossary for unfamiliar terms and refer to the table as needed.

49

The four types of shock are * _____

_____ .

49 hypovolemic, cardiogenic, septic, and neurogenic

50

Match the following types of shock with the appropriate clinical causes.

a. Hypovolemic shock
b. Cardiogenic shock
c. Septic shock
d. Neurogenic shock

___ 1. High spinal anesthesia, emotional factors, or trauma from an extensive operative procedure
___ 2. Hemorrhaging from surgery or injury, burns, or GI bleeding
___ 3. Severe bacterial infection, immunosuppressant therapy
___ 4. Myocardial infarction, cardiac failure, and cardiac tamponade

50 1. d; 2. a; 3. c; 4. b

Table 20-5

Types and Clinical Causes of Shock

Type of Shock	Clinical Causes	Rationale and Physiologic Results
Hypovolemic: Hematogenic (from hemorrhage)	Severe vomiting or diarrhea—acute dehydration Burns, intestinal obstruction, fluid shift to third space Hemorrhage that results from internal or external blood loss	Blood, plasma, and fluid loss from decreased circulating blood volume *Physiologic Results* 1. Decreased circulation 2. Decreased venous return 3. Reduced cardiac output 4. Increased afterload 5. Decreased preload 6. Decreased tissue perfusion
Cardiogenic	Myocardial infarction Severe arrhythmias Congestive heart failure Cardiac tamponade Pulmonary embolism Blunt cardiac injury (formerly "cardiac contusion")	Because of these clinical problems, the pumping action of the heart is inadequate to maintain circulation. (Pump failure of myocardium.) *Physiologic Results* 1. Decreased circulation 2. Decreased stroke volume 3. Decreased cardiac output 4. Increased preload 5. Increased afterload 6. Increased venous pressure 7. Decreased venous return 8. Decreased tissue perfusion
Septic: Endotoxic Vasogenic	Severe systemic infections Septic abortion Peritonitis Debilitated conditions Immunosuppressant therapy	Septic shock is characterized by increased capillary permeability that permits blood, plasma, and fluid to pass into surrounding tissue. Often caused by a gram-negative organism. *Physiologic Results* 1. Vasodilatation and peripheral pooling of blood 2. Decreased circulation 3. Decreased preload, early shock and increased preload, late shock 4. Decreased afterload, early shock and increased afterload, late shock. 5. Decreased tissue perfusion

(continues on the following page)

Table 20-5

(Continued)

Type of Shock	Clinical Causes	Rationale and Physiologic Results

Neurogenic	Mild to moderate neurogenic shock:
	  Emotional stress
	  Acute pain
	  Drugs: narcotics, barbiturates,
	    phenothiazines
	  High spinal anesthesia
	  Acute gastric dilation
	Severe neurogenic shock:
	  Spinal cord injury
	Trauma:
	  Extensive operative procedure
		Neurogenic shock is caused by loss of vascular tone.
		Physiologic Results
		1. Decreased circulation
		2. Vasodilatation and peripheral pooling of blood
		3. Decreased cardiac output
		4. Decreased venous return
		5. Decreased tissue perfusion

51

Match the following types of shock with the appropriate rationale.

  a. Hypovolemic shock
  b. Cardiogenic shock
  c. Septic shock
  d. Neurogenic shock

  ___ 1. Failure of the myocardium causes a decrease in the circulating blood volume
  ___ 2. Loss of vascular tone with vasodilation
  ___ 3. Decrease in blood volume due to loss of blood and plasma
  ___ 4. Increase in capillary permeability resulting from an infection

51 1. b; 2. d; 3. a; 4. c

52

Match the following types of shock with the physiologic results. Your response may be used more than once.

a. Hypovolemic shock
b. Cardiogenic shock
c. Septic shock
d. Neurogenic shock

____ , ____ , ____ , ____   1. Decreased circulation
____ , ____ , ____   2. Decreased cardiac output
____ , ____   3. Vasodilatation
____ , ____ , ____   4. Decreased venous return
____ , ____ , ____ , ____   5. Decreased tissue perfusion

52 1. a, b, c, d; 2. a, b, d; 3. c, d; 4. a, b, d; 5. a, b, c, d

Clinical Manifestations

The clinical manifestations of shock are listed in Table 20-6 with the types of shock and rationale that are related to the signs and symptoms. Immediate medical action needs to be taken when shock occurs so that it can be reversed. Therefore, the health professional should frequently check for signs and symptoms of shock when impending shock is suspected.

Study the table carefully and be able to explain the signs and symptoms that frequently occur in shock.

Table 20-6

Clinical Manifestations of Shock

Signs and Symptoms	Types of Shock	Rationale
Skin: pale and/or cold and moist (except when caused by a spinal cord injury)	Hypovolemic Cardiogenic Neurogenic Septic (late)	Pale, cold, and/or moist skin results from increased sympathetic action. Peripheral vasoconstriction occurs and blood is shunted to vital organs. Skin is warm and flushed in early septic shock. Skin is warm and dry in neurogenic shock due to spinal cord injury.
Tachycardia (pulse fast and thready)	Hypovolemic Cardiogenic Septic	Increased pulse rate is frequently one of the early signs, except in neurogenic shock, in which the pulse is often slower than normal. Norepinephrine and epinephrine, released by the adrenal medulla, increase the cardiac rate and myocardial contractibility. Tachycardia, pulse >100, generally occurs before arterial blood pressure falls.

(continues on the following page)

Table 20-6

(Continued)

Signs and Symptoms	Types of Shock	Rationale
Apprehension, restlessness	Hypovolemic Cardiogenic Septic Neurogenic	Apprehension and restlessness, early signs of shock, result from cerebral hypoxia. As the state of shock progresses, disorientation and confusion occur.
Muscle weakness, fatigue	Hypovolemic Cardiogenic Septic Neurogenic	Muscle weakness and fatigue, which occur early in shock, are the result of inadequate tissue perfusion.
Arterial blood pressure: early, a rise in or normal BP; late, a fall in BP	Hypovolemic Cardiogenic Septic Neurogenic	In early shock blood pressure rises or is normal as a result of increased heart rate. As shock progresses, blood pressure falls because of a lack of cardiac and peripheral vasoconstriction compensation.
Pulse pressure: narrowed, <20 mm Hg		Narrowing of pulse rate occurs because the systolic BP falls more rapidly than the diastolic BP.
Pressures: CVP, PAP, PCWP—decreased in hypovolemic, septic, neurogenic; increased in cardiogenic	Hypovolemic Cardiogenic Septic Neurogenic	Normal values: 1. Central venous pressure (CVP): 5–12 cm H_2O. With decreased blood volume CVP <5 cm H_2O. 2. Pulmonary artery pressure (PAP): 20–30 mm Hg systolic, 10–15 mm Hg diastolic. With blood volume depletion or pooling of blood PAP in hypovolemic <10 mm Hg, septic <10 mm Hg, neurogenic <10 mm Hg. In cardiogenic shock PAP >30 mm Hg. 3. Pulmonary capillary wedge pressure (PCWP): 4–12 mm Hg. With blood volume depletion or peripheral pooling the PCWP in hypovolemic, septic, and neurogenic <10 mm Hg and in cardiogenic >20 mm Hg.
Respiration: increased rate and depth (tachypnea)	Hypovolemic Cardiogenic Septic Neurogenic	Increased hydrogen ion concentration in the body stimulates the respiratory centers in the medulla, thus increasing the respiratory rate. Acid metabolites, e.g., lactic acid from anaerobic metabolism increases the rate and depth of respiration. Rapid respiration acts as a compensatory mechanism to decrease metabolic acidosis.
Temperature: subnormal	Hypovolemic Cardiogenic Neurogenic	Body temperature is subnormal in shock because of decreased circulation and decreased cellular function. In septic shock the temperature is elevated.
Urinary output: decreased	Hypovolemic Cardiogenic Septic Neurogenic	Oliguria (decreased urine output) occurs in shock because of decreased renal blood flow caused by renal vasoconstriction. Blood is shunted to the heart and brain. Urine output should be >25 mL/h.

53 apprehension and
restlessness; cerebral
hypoxia

53

Two early mental changes occurring in shock are *_____

_____ .

  They generally result from *_____ .

54

The central venous pressure (CVP), pulmonary artery pressure
(PAP), and pulmonary capillary wedge pressure (PCWP) are
decreased in which types of shock?
  ( ) a. Hypovolemic
  ( ) b. Cardiogenic
  ( ) c. Septic
  ( ) d. Neurogenic

54 a, c, d
55 Increased hydrogen ion
concentration stimulates
the respiratory center in
the medulla; OR nonvolatile
acids (acid metabolites)
from anaerobic metabo-
lism increase respiratory
rate and depth.; Note: The
purpose of increased rate
and depth of respiration is
to decrease the acidotic
state.
56 Decreased urinary output
is the result of decreased
renal blood flow caused by
renal vasoconstriction.

55

Increased rate and depth of respirations are present in shock.
Why? *_____

_____

56

Frequently the urinary output is decreased in all types of shock.
Why? *_____

_____

57

In shock, tachycardia is frequently seen before the arterial blood
pressure begins to fall.
  The heart beats faster to (increase/decrease) _____ the
circulating blood volume. This is an early compensatory
mechanism to overcome shock.
  With shock, what happens to the arterial blood pressure?
*_____ .

57 increase; it will first rise
and then fall

58

Some signs and symptoms follow. Check the ones that are true
about shock. Correct the false ones.

58 a. Arterial blood pressure
rises, then falls; b. Tachycardia occurs in neurogenic
shock and is common in
other forms of shock.;
c. Fast and deep; d. X; e. Not
in early septic shock;
f. Decreased output; g. It is
low in hypovolemic (hema-
togenic) shock; h. Pale or
cold and moist, or both

(   ) a. Arterial blood pressure low
(   ) b. Bradycardia
(   ) c. Respiration slow and deep
(   ) d. Apprehension, restlessness
(   ) e. Temperature low in all types of shock
(   ) f. Urine output increased
(   ) g. Central venous pressure high in cardiac shock and in
              hypovolemic shock
(   ) h. Skin pale and hot

Clinical Applications

59

Normal blood pressure is the usual level of blood pressure in a
person and varies to some extent from person to person.

    A systolic blood pressure of less than 90 mm Hg is significant
for shock in most people.

    A systolic pressure of 70 mm Hg is necessary to maintain the
coronary circulation and renal function (urinary output). A
person with a systolic pressure of 50–60 mm Hg is said to be in

59 shock

          _____ .

60

A low pulse pressure, which is the difference between the
systolic and diastolic pressures, is indicative of shock. The systolic
blood pressure usually decreases before the diastolic.

    To maintain coronary circulation and renal function, the
systolic pressure should be at least *_____ .

60 70 mm Hg; shock

    A pulse pressure of 20 mm Hg is indicative of _____ .

61

Blood supply to the organs most susceptible to acute anoxia
(absence or lack of oxygen), i.e., the brain and the heart, is
maintained as long as possible at the expense of the less vital
organs and tissues.

    The two organs most susceptible to anoxia are the *_____

61 heart and brain

_____ .

    The brain can survive 4 minutes in an anoxic state before
cerebral damage occurs.

62

Which of the following physiologic symptoms indicate shock?

( ) a. Arterial blood pressure less than 90

( ) b. Pulse pressure of 55 mm Hg

( ) c. Pulse pressure of 20 mm Hg

Which two organs are most susceptible to acute anoxia?

( ) a. Heart

( ) b. Brain

( ) c. Intestines

The organ that cannot survive anoxia longer than 4–6 minutes without permanent damage is the _____ .

62 a, c; a, b; brain

Clinical Management

To maintain body fluid volume and particularly the intravascular fluid, fluid resuscitation must begin immediately for clients who are in shock or impending shock. Improvement of blood volume is needed to maintain tissue perfusion and oxygen delivery. The types of solutions for fluid replacement include crystalloids or balanced salt solutions and colloid solutions.

Crystalloids

Crystalloids expand the volume of the ECF (intravascular and interstitial spaces). The two common types of crystalloids used for fluid replacement are normal saline solution (0.9% sodium chloride) and lactated Ringer's solution. Lactated Ringer's solution contains the electrolytes sodium, potassium, calcium, and chloride with their milliequivalents, which are similar to the plasma values.

Table 20-7 lists examples of crystalloids that can be used for fluid replacement.

Table 20-7

Crystalloids for Fluid Replacement

Crystalloids	mEq/L						
	Na	K	Ca	Mg	Cl	Lactate	Gluconate
0.9% NaCl (NSS)	154	—	—	—	154	—	—
Lactated Ringer's	130	4	3	—	109	28	—

63 0.9% NaCl (normal saline solution) and lactated Ringer's solution

63
Name two commonly prescribed crystalloids that are used for fluid resuscitation. *_____

64
Normal saline solution (0.9% NaCl) is a popular IV solution used for fluid resuscitation because it is iso-osmolar (approximately the same milliosomoles as plasma). Excess use of normal saline can increase the serum sodium level and can cause (hypochloremia/hyperchloremia) _____ .
  If metabolic acidosis is present, the chloride level can (increase/decrease) _____ the acidotic state.

64 hyperchloremia; increase

65
The lactate of the lactated Ringer's solution acts as a buffer to increase the pH, thus decreasing the acidotic state. Large quantities of lactated Ringer's solution might cause metabolic (acidosis/alkalosis) _____ .

65 alkalosis

66
If the client has a liver disorder, the lactate is not metabolized into bicarbonate; therefore lactic acid can result.
  If large quantities of lactated Ringer's solution are administered to a client with a liver disorder, the metabolic acidotic state can be (intensified/lessened) _____ .
  Alternating the crystalloid solutions, such as normal saline solution and lactated Ringer's solution, usually (maintains/disturbs) _____ the electrolyte and acid-base balance.

66 intensified; maintains

67
Intravenous solutions containing calcium should NOT be administered with blood transfusions. The calcium in the solution precipitates when it comes in contact with blood.
  Indicate which of the following solutions can be administered through the same IV line with blood.
  ( ) a. 0.9% NaCl (normal saline solution)
  ( ) b. Lactated Ringer's solution
  ( ) c. D₅W
  ( ) d. D₅0.45 NSS

67 a

68 hypo-osmolar; The dextrose is rapidly metabolized, leaving water, a hypo-osmolar solution. Use of D_5W can lead to intracellular fluid volume excess (water intoxication) or cellular swelling.

69 more; less

68

The crystalloid 5% dextrose in water (D_5W) should never be ordered for total fluid replacement during shock. Dextrose 5% in water is an iso-osmolar solution, but if it is used in large volumes, it becomes a (hypo-osmolar/hyperosmolar) _____ solution. Why? * _____

_____

Colloids

Colloids are substances that have a higher molecular weight than crystalloids and therefore cannot pass through the vascular membrane. Colloids increase the intravascular fluid volume. When colloid therapy is used, less fluid is needed to reestablish the fluid volume in the vascular space.

Table 20-8 lists the colloids that may be used for fluid replacement.

69

In comparison with crystalloids, colloids are (more/less) _____ expensive. Colloid therapy requires (more/less) _____ solution replacement than needed with crystalloid solutions for fluid replacement.

Table 20-8

Colloids

Colloids*	Brand Names	Comments
Blood products	Packed RBCs Whole blood	Used to replace blood loss.
Albumin, 5% or 25%	Albuminar Plasbumin	Not used in acute shock; 1–4 mL/min.
Plasma protein fraction, 5%	Plasmanate	Rapid infusion rate can decrease blood pressure.
Hetastarch	Hespan	Synthetic starch similar to human glycogen. Very expensive.
Dextran 40	Dextran	Low-molecular-weight dextran 40 may prolong bleeding time.

70

Colloid solutions are useful in replacing fluid losses from which of the following:

( ) a. Intravascular space (blood vessels)
( ) b. Interstitial space (tissue area)
( ) c. Cellular space (cells)

70 a

71

Prior to a blood transfusion, what two crystalloid solutions can be used to manage shock? *_____

71 lactated Ringer's and
   normal saline solution

72

Which crystalloid solution is the only one compatible to infuse in the same line as blood? *_____

72 0.9% normal saline solution
   (NSS)

73

The colloids albumin 5%, plasma protein fraction (Plasmanate), and hetastarch increase the vascular volume to approximately the same amount that is infused. With the low-molecular-weight dextran (40), the vascular fluid is expanded by one to two times the amount that is infused. With albumin 25%, the vascular volume is expanded four times the amount that is infused.

To increase the vascular volume more than the amount of colloid that is infused, which of the following colloid solutions might be used?

( ) a. Albumin 5%
( ) b. Albumin 25%
( ) c. Plasmanate
( ) d. Dextran 40
( ) e. Hetastarch

73 b, d

Crystalloids are the first choice for treating hypovolemic shock. Crystalloids can restore fluid volume in the vascular and interstitial spaces and improve renal function; however large quantities of crystalloids are needed. Excessive infusions of crystalloids might cause fluid overload in clients who are elderly or who have heart disease. Frequently, a combination of crystalloids and colloids is used for fluid replacement. If severe blood loss occurs, blood transfusion may be necessary after infusion of 1–2 liters of crystalloids. Each fluid replacement situation differs and each individual situation must be evaluated separately.

There are many suggested formulas for restoring fluid loss, especially for clients in hypovolemic shock who have lost massive amounts of blood and/or body fluid. The simplest formula for fluid replacement is the 3:1 rule: for every 1 mL of blood lost, 3 mL of crystalloid solution is necessary to restore fluid volume (to a point that if hypotension persists despite 2 liters of crystalloid solution replacement, a blood transfusion should be considered). Table 20-9 outlines the calculation of blood loss and fluid replacement for three states of hypovolemic shock from hemorrhage.

74

If a client is in Class I shock due to hemorrhage, blood volume loss is *_____ and systolic blood pressure is probably _____ . The replacement fluid for this blood volume loss is _____ . This shock state is considered _____ .

74 up to 750 mL (up to 15% BV); normal; crystalloid; mild

75

If a client is in Class II hypovolemic shock, blood volume loss is *_____ , and systolic blood pressure is probably _____ . The replacement fluid for this blood volume loss is _____ . The heart rate is probably _____ .

75 750–1500 mL (15–30% BV); normal; crystalloid; <100

Table 20-9

Calculation of Blood Loss and Fluid Replacement for Four States of Hypovolemic Shock from Hemorrhage

	Class I	Class II	Class III	Class IV
Blood loss (mL)	Up to 750 mL	750–1500 mL	1500–2000 mL	2000 mL or more
Blood loss (%BV)	Up to 15%	15%–30%	30%–40%	40% or more
Heart rate	<100	>100	>120	>140
Blood pressure	Normal	Normal	Decreased	Decreased
Fluid replacement (3:1 rule)	Crystalloid	Crystalloid	Crystalloid and blood	Crystalloid and blood
	Mild Shock State	Moderate Shock State	Severe Shock State	Severe Shock State

76

If a client is in Class III or IV hypovolemic shock, the shock state is considered _____ . Blood volume loss is *_____;
systolic blood pressure is _____; heart rate is *_____ .
Replacement fluid will consist of _____ and _____ .

Table 20-10 outlines the clinical management for alleviating four types of clinical shock: hypovolemic, cardiogenic, septic, and neurogenic. Many years ago the first and foremost treatment of shock was to administer a vasopressor drug. The drug constricts the dilated blood vessels that occur with shock and raises the blood pressure. Vasopressors act as a temporary treatment for shock, and the shock continues to increase if the cause is not alleviated or removed. Today vasopressors are only used for severe shock and types of shock nonresponsive to treatment. Note that vasopressors are *not* effective in the treatment of hypovolemic shock, since constricting blood vessels does not aid in the circulation of blood when the cause is most obvious—a lack of blood, causing hypovolemia. Replacing blood volume loss should correct this type of shock. Remember, removal of the cause is first and foremost in alleviating various types of shock.

Study this table carefully and be able to explain the treatments for each type of shock.

77

What is shock? *_____
     What is a common feature of shock? *_____

_____

78

The clinical management for *hypovolemic shock* may consist of which of the following:
     ( ) a. Blood Products
     ( ) b. Digitalization
     ( ) c. Vasopressors
     ( ) d. Oxygen
     ( ) e. Lactated Ringer's solution
     ( ) f. Normal saline
     ( ) g. Electrolyte replacement
     ( ) h. Lidocaine

---

76 severe; 1500–2000 mL or more (30%–40% BV or more); decreased; <120–140; crystalloid and blood

77 a state of inadequate perfusion; low circulating blood volume or hypovolemia. This can be due to loss of blood from the body or "pooling" of blood in selected areas.

78 a, e, f, g

Table 20-10

Clinical Management for Various Types of Shock States

Hypovolemic Shock	Cardiogenic Shock	Septic Shock	Neurogenic Shock
1. O_2	1. O_2	1. O_2	1. O_2

2. IV fluids, such as
  a. Lactated Ringer's
  b. Normal saline
  c. Blood products
3. No vasopressors
4. Electrolyte replacement
	2. IV therapy is limited when pulmonary congestion is present and venous pressure is elevated. Close monitoring CVP and PCWP
	3. Vasopressors, if necessary
	4. Antiarrythmics Sodium nitroprusside/ Nipride nitroglycerin/NTG; (decrease preload and decrease afterload). Intropic drugs (e.g., dobutamine/Dobutrex, amrinone/Inocor) Sedatives Diuretics
		2. IV therapy crystalloids
		3. Vasopressors for nonresponsiveness
		4. Blood cultures
		5. IV antibiotics
			2. IV therapy
			3. Vasopressors, if necessary
			4. Atropine for symptomatic bradycardia

Note: Examples of vasopressors are (1) levarterenol bitartrate/Levophed, (2) dopamine hydrochloride/Intropin, (3) Epinephrine Infusion.

79

When administering crystalloids, such as normal saline or lactated Ringer's solution, for hypovolemic shock, these IV solutions may be given rapidly at first to decrease the symptoms of shock and prevent fluid shift into the interstitial space at the injured site. Later, the flow rate should be slowed.

What type of fluid imbalance can occur if massive quantities of crystalloids are rapidly administered intravenously?

79 overhydration (hypervolemia). This occurs most likely with the older adult, child, or debilitated person.

80

Clinical management for *cardiogenic shock* may consist of which of the following:

( ) a. IV therapy
( ) b. No vasopressors
( ) c. Antibiotics
( ) d. Oxygen
( ) e. Intropic drugs
( ) f. Sedation
( ) g. Sodium nitroprusside/Nipride

80 a, d, e, f, g

81

Clinical management for *septic shock* may consist of which of the following:
( ) a. Blood culture
( ) b. Antibiotics in IV fluids
( ) c. Vasopressors
( ) d. Digitalization
( ) e. Massive IV therapy with whole blood

81 a, b, c

82

Antibiotics and pain medications should be given intravenously if the client is in shock. Since circulation is poor, medications given intramuscularly (IM) are not fully absorbed. If given IM, after circulation is restored, the accumulated drug in the tissue spaces can be toxic.

Do you think the same dosage prescribed for IM should be given intravenously? *_____

82 Not always. Please check with the health care provider. Frequently, large doses are given diluted in 50–100 mL of IV solution. IV morphine is given slowly (approximately 5 minutes). In some cases, one-half of the IM dose is given IV.

83

Clinical management for *neurogenic shock* may consist of which of the following:
( ) a. Blood culture
( ) b. Vasopressors
( ) c. IV therapy as needed
( ) d. Massive IV therapy

83 b, c

84

Explain the action of vasopressors (see introduction to Table 20-10, if necessary). *_____

_____

The three vasopressors listed at the bottom of Table 20-10 are *_____

_____ .

84 Vasopressors constrict blood vessels in hopes of improving circulation.; levarterenol bitartrate/ Levophed, dopamine HCl/Intropin, and epinephrine

85

Vasopressors should be used with care; however, they are helpful at the right time and with the right clinical problem.

When vasopressors are used, cardiac dysrhythmias may occur.

Levophed (levarterenol bitartrate), a strong vasopressor, is norepinephrine, which increases blood pressure and cardiac output by constricting blood vessels. Epinephrine works in the same manner.

Maintaining the blood pressure higher than 90 mm Hg with Levophed and epinephrine infusions can cause * _____ .

85 cardiac dysrhythmias

86

Levophed and epinephrine are (strong/weak) _____ vasopressors and can cause cardiac dysrhythmias.

Vasopressors are titrated according to the blood pressure and should be checked every 2–5 minutes.

86 strong

87

Dopamine HCl (Intropin) is a catecholamine precursor of norepinephrine. It increases blood pressure and cardiac output. It also dilates renal vessels at low dose (<5 mcg/kg/min), thus increasing renal blood flow and the glomerular filtration rate.

Levophed causes vasoconstriction, which affects the renal arteries and can decrease kidney function. The vasopressor that increases blood pressure, cardiac output, and urinary output is * _____ .

87 dopamine HCl

88

Dopamine is helpful in the treatment of cardiogenic shock but is limited when severe hypotension exists.

What two vasopressors can be used in severe shock? * _____

88 Levophed and epinephrine

89

Dobutamine/Dobutrex is an adrenergic drug that increases blood pressure moderately by raising the heart rate and cardiac output. Dobutamine is effective in increasing myocardial contractility. It is frequently used with sodium nitroprusside.

Explain why dobutamine is not used to treat severe hypotension. * _____

89 Dobutamine has only a
    moderate effect on
    increasing blood pressure.

90

Identify the treatments listed below that may be used in various types of shock by placing:

H for hypovolemic shock
C for cardiogenic shock
S for septic shock
N for neurogenic shock

   Some treatments may be used for more than one type of shock.

_____ a. IV therapy: lactated Ringer's, normal saline
_____ b. Digitalis products
_____ c. Electrolyte replacement
_____ d. Sedatives
_____ , _____ , _____ e. Vasopressors
_____ f. Oxygen
_____ , _____ g. Limited IV therapy
_____ h. IV Antibiotics
_____ i. Lidocaine

90 a. H; b. C; c. H; d. C; e. C, S, N; f. C; g. C, N; h. S; i. C

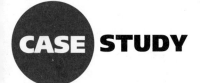 **CASE STUDY**

REVIEW

Mr. Martz, age 58, had diverticulitis. The diverticulum ruptured, causing peritonitis and systemic septicemia. His vital signs are temperature 104°F (40°C), pulse 126 rapid and thready, respirations 32, and blood pressure 65/45. His urinary output is 25 mL/h. His skin is warm and dry. He is markedly apprehensive and restless. He is diagnosed as being in septic shock.

ANSWER COLUMN

1. circulation or blood volume

2. capillary permeability, permitting blood and plasma to pass into the surrounding tissues

1. Shock occurs when the hemostatic circulatory mechanism fails to maintain adequate *_____ .

2. Septic shock is characterized by *_____
_____ .

3. pulse 126, respiration 32, blood pressure 65/45 and low pulse pressure, and apprehension and restlessness
4. septicemia (bacterial infection)

5. shock

6. 600; kidney dysfunction or insufficiency
7. decreased renal function and output. It can lead to renal failure if prolonged.
8. pulse rate increases; heart beats faster to maintain circulating blood volume. Increased pulse rate is an early compensatory mechanism to overcome shock.

9. severe
10. oxygen, crystalloids, blood culture, IV antibiotics, vasopressors as needed

11. dopamine or Levophed
12. It dilates the renal arteries and increases blood flow and urine output in low doses (<5 mcg/kg/min).

3. Identify four of Mr. Martz's clinical signs and symptoms of shock.* _____
_____
_____ .

4. Mr. Martz's temperature was elevated due to _____ .

5. His pulse pressure was 20 mm Hg (65 minus 45), which is indicative of _____ .

6. His urine output is _____ mL for 24 hours, which is in the low "normal" range. If his urine output goes below 25 mL/h, what may this indicate?* _____

7. Since Mr. Martz's systolic blood pressure dropped below 70 mm Hg, what can occur to his renal function?* _____

8. In shock, which frequently occurs first, does blood pressure decrease or does pulse rate increase?* _____
_____
Why?* _____ .

9. Based on Mr. Martz's blood pressure, the state of shock is (mild/moderate/severe) _____ .

10. Name the four methods for managing septic shock.* _____
_____

11. If vasopressors were used for Mr. Martz, which two would be indicated? _____ or _____

12. What advantage does dopamine hydrochloride have on kidney function that other vasopressors do not have?* _____
_____

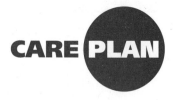

Client Management
Assessment Factors

▶ Check vital signs and report signs and symptoms that may indicate hypovolemia and shock: tachycardia, narrowing of the pulse pressure [difference between systolic and diastolic (less than 20 mm Hg is an indicator of shock)], tachypnea (rapid breathing), and skin cool and clammy.

▶ Obtain a drug history of the injured client. Report if the client is regularly taking insulin, potassium-wasting diuretics, digitalis, steroid preparations, beta blockers or calcium channel blockers.

▶ Relate acute clinical problem with the signs and symptoms of hypovolemia and shock.

▶ Assess the behavioral and neurologic status of the injured client and/or the client in shock. Irritability, apprehension, restlessness, and confusion are symptoms of fluid volume deficit. Apprehension and restlessness are early symptoms of shock.

▶ Check urinary output. Less than 25 mL/h or 200 mL/8 h can indicate fluid volume deficit or renal insufficiency. In severe shock, severe oliguria or anuria might occur.

▶ Check laboratory results, especially ABGs, hemoglobin, hematocrit, serum electrolytes, BUN, and serum creatinine. Report abnormal laboratory results immediately.

Diagnosis 1

Fluid volume deficit related to traumatic injury and/or shock.

Interventions and Rationale

1. Monitor vital signs. Compare the vital signs with those taken on admission, and report abnormalities immediately. Significant vital sign changes that could be due to fluid loss or shock include rapid, thready pulse rate, drop in blood pressure, and narrowing of the pulse pressure (<20 mm Hg).

2. Check skin color and turgor. Note changes. Pallor, gray, cold, clammy skin, and poor skin turgor are symptoms of shock and fluid volume deficit.

3. Record amounts of vomitus, diarrhea, stools, secretions from nasogastric suction, and drains that contribute to fluid losses.

4. Check the mucous membranes for dryness. Observe for dry tenacious secretions.

5. Monitor IV therapy. Crystalloids are usually rapidly administered initially to hydrate the client and to increase urine output. Normal saline solution and/or lactated Ringer's solution are the choice crystalloids for fluid replacement. Colloids may be used in combination with crystalloids for the aged client with cardiac problem (fluid excess should be avoided).

6. Monitor central venous pressure (CVP) and pulmonary capillary (arterial) wedge pressure (PCWP) that is needed to adjust fluid balance. Norm for CVP is 5–12 cm/H_2O and for PCWP it is 4–12 mm Hg. Keeping PCWP between 12 and 15 mm Hg in shock conditions provides the filling pressure required for adequate stroke volume and cardiac output. If PCWP drops below 10 mm Hg, administration of fluids is usually needed. If PCWP is greater than 18 mm Hg, fluid restriction may be necessary.

7. Draw blood chemistry, hematology, and arterial blood gases as ordered. Report abnormal findings immediately to the physician.

8. Monitor laboratory results, especially the serum electrolytes. The serum potassium (K) levels can vary after trauma. The low K serum level can be due to excess urine output. The serum K level may be normal even though there is a cellular potassium deficit. Hyperkalemia can occur due to excessive cellular breakdown and oliguria (decreased urine output). The serum potassium level should be known before administering potassium in IV fluids.

9. Monitor ECG readings and report arrhythmias, ST-T changes, potassium imbalance, or cardiac ischemia.

Diagnosis 2

Fluid volume excess related to massive infusions of crystalloids.

Interventions and Rationale

1. Monitor IV fluid therapy. Regulate flow rate to prevent overhydration (hypervolemia).

2. Auscultate the lungs for rales. Overhydration from excess fluids and rapid administration of IV fluids can cause pulmonary edema. Heart failure can be another result.

3. Instruct the client to cough and breathe deeply to expand and provide effective ventilation and/or obtain an order for an incentive spirometer.

4. Check for neck vein engorgement when overhydration is suspected. Check jugular vein at a 45° angle.

5. Check for pitting edema in the feet and legs. Weigh client daily to determine if there is fluid retention.

Diagnosis 3

Urinary retention related to fluid volume deficit and shock.

Interventions and Rationale

1. Monitor urine output. Hourly urine should be measured and, if less than 25 mL/h, the IV fluid rate should be increased as ordered. Don't forget to check for overhydration when pushing fluids—IV or orally. Renal artery vasoconstriction occurs in shock, which causes a decrease in kidney perfusion.

2. Report systolic blood pressure of 80 mm Hg or *less* immediately. Kidney damage can occur due to hypotension if SBP is less than 70 mm Hg.

3. Check the BUN and creatinine. If both are highly elevated, it could be due to renal insufficiency. If they are slightly elevated and return to normal when the patient is hydrated, it could be due to the fluid volume deficit.

Diagnosis 4

Altered tissue perfusion: renal, cardiopulmonary, cerebral, and peripheral, related to decreased blood volume and circulation secondary to hypovolemia and shock.

Interventions and Rationale

1. Monitor blood pressure continuously when administering vasopressors. Monitor for cardiac dysrhythmias. If urine output is poor, low-dose dopamine may be added to the therapeutic regime.

2. Monitor arterial blood gases (ABGs). Metabolic acidosis frequently results from cellular damage due to severe hypovolemia and shock. In acidosis, the pH is below 7.35, HCO_3 is below 24 mEq/L, and base excess (BE) is less than -2. Signs of Kussmaul breathing (rapid, vigorous breathing) may be present. Respiratory acidosis may also result due to the lungs' inability to excrete carbon dioxide. The ABGs that indicate respiratory acidosis include pH <7.35 and $PaCO_2$ >45 mm Hg. Dyspnea may be present.

Evaluation/Outcome

1. Skin warm and dry, mucous membranes moist, pulse and blood pressure within normal range, urine volume and specific gravity within normal range.

2. Weight stable, patient has no rales or rhonchi, breathing pattern and rate are normal; peripheral pulses are present, no venous neck engorgement, CVP and PCWP are within client's normal baseline.

3. BUN, creatinine arterial blood gases, hemoglobin, and hematocrit stable and within normal limits.

4. Client alert and oriented to person and place, not restless, and there is no peripheral edema.

5. Electrocardiogram ST segment and T wave are within normal limits.

6. Nail beds, oral mucous membranes, and conjunctiva show good oxygenation.

Burns and Burn Shock

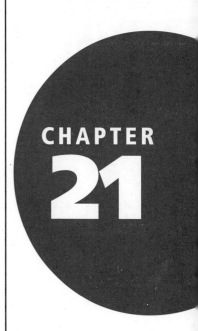

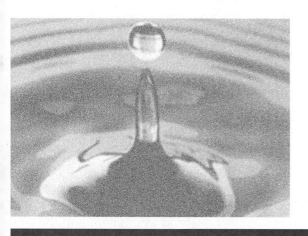

Larry Purnell, RN, PhD

OBJECTIVES

Upon completion of this chapter, the reader should be able to:

- Explain the physiologic changes and fluid and electrolyte imbalances resulting from burns and burn shock.
- Describe the classifications of burn severity and the degrees of burns.
- Explain one method for determining the percentage of total body surface burns (TBSB).
- State treatment priorities in the clinical management of burns and burn shock.
- Apply selected principles of fluid balance in the assessment and care of burned patients in two clinical situations.
- Describe assessment factors, diagnoses, and interventions commonly associated with burns and burn shock.

▶ INTRODUCTION

Burns vary in severity depending upon the depth of tissue involvement and the percentage of burned surface area of the body. An extracellular fluid volume shift occurs soon after the burn and results in a fluid imbalance. An assessment concerning the burn areas, tissue involvement, and signs and symptoms of fluid imbalance should be performed immediately. Monitoring vital signs, hourly urine output, and fluid replacement are a few of the prioritized responsibilities required during the first 5–7 days after a moderate to severe burn.

This chapter discusses thermal burns caused by exposure to or contact with flames, hot liquids, hot objects, or steam. It includes the pathophysiologic changes resulting from burns, classification systems used to assess tissue depth of the burns and the degrees of burns, methods used to determine percentage of total body surface burned, the three classifications of burns (mild, moderate, and critical), and important factors to consider in the clinical management of burns. Two clinical situations of burned cases are presented. In the first situation, the focus is on fluid replacement during the first 48 hours. The focus in the second situation is on the assessment of burned areas by percent and laboratory studies as they relate to assessment and the clinical management of fluid and electrolyte imbalances of burned clients. The health professional assesses the burn areas, the significance of the laboratory test results, and fluid replacement as it relates to interventions. A case study review related to the second situation is provided. Assessment factors, diagnoses, and interventions with rationales are listed following the second case study.

▶ PHYSIOLOGIC CHANGES

Table 21-1 describes the physiologic changes associated with burns. There is an increased capillary permeability, increased serum osmolality, increased circulatory resistance, decreased cardiac output, decreased renal function, increased hemolysis, electrolyte imbalances, acidosis, an increased hematocrit, and a decreased protein serum level.

Table 21-1

Physiologic Changes Associated with Burns and Burn Shock

Physiologic Factors	Rationale
Capillary permeability: increased	There is a rapid shift of fluid and protein from the intravascular space (vessels) to the burned site. If more than 15–25% of the total body surface is burned, fluid (edema) accumulates in burned and unburned tissue spaces. Fluid shift to the burned site and tissue spaces is referred to as *fluid shift to the third space*. This fluid is nonfunctional, which causes a vascular fluid deficit (hypovolemia). This is referred to as *burn shock*. Most of the fluid shift occurs during the first 18 hours but can persist for 48 hours postburn. Approximately 40–50% of vascular fluid can be lost to burned site and tissue spaces within the first 18 hours.
Serum osmolality: increased	Hemoconcentration results from loss of vascular fluid. The serum osmolality exceeds 295 mOsm/L since the proportion of solutes is greater than water.
Electrolyte imbalances: decreased Serum Sodium (hyponatremia)	Sodium enters the edema fluid in the burned area, lowering the sodium content of the vascular fluid. Hyponatremia may continue for days to several weeks because of sodium loss to edema fluid, sodium shifting into cells, and later, diuresis. After 48 hours, fluid shifts from the burned and interstitial spaces to the vascular space. Sodium and excess fluid are excreted by the kidneys.
Cellular potassium: decreased	Potassium is lost from the cells.
Serum potassium: increased (hyperkalemia)	Potassium leaves the cells as sodium shifts into the cells. Hyperkalemia can occur if urine output is decreased. Serum potassium values may vary from normal to a deficit or an excess depending on the urine output and the length of time after the initial burn.
Serum calcium: decreased (hypocalcemia)	Hypocalcemia occurs because of calcium loss to edema fluid at the burned site (third-space fluid). Multiple infusions of citrated blood decreases the serum calcium level.
Serum protein: decreased	Protein is lost to the burned site due to increased capillary permeability. Serum protein levels remain low until healing occurs.
Hematocrit: increased	Hematocrit level is elevated due to hemoconcentration from hypovolemia. Anemia is present postburn due to blood loss at burned site and hemolysis, but it is not assessed until the client is adequately hydrated.
Hemolysis: increased (destruction of cells)	Hemolysis causes a liberation of hemoglobin (free hemoglobin) which can cause renal damage.

(continues on the following page)

Table 21-1

Physiologic Changes Associated with Burns and Burn Shock *(Continued)*

Physiologic Factors	Rationale
Cardiac output decreased	With more than 40% of the total body surface area burned, cardiac output can be decreased 50% or more due to hypovolemia. Cardiac output = stroke volume × heart rate. Tachycardia is a compensatory response. Beta receptors in the myocardium increase heart rate.
Circulatory resistance: increased	Hypovolemia and decreased blood pressure are sensed by pressoreceptors in the aorta and carotid bodies and in the sympathetic nervous system to cause vasoconstriction in order to increase blood flow to the vital organs, i.e., heart, brain, and lungs.
Renal function: decreased	Severe decreased blood volume (hypovolemia) causes a fall in blood pressure and oliguria or anuria. Systolic blood pressure below 60 mm Hg can cause renal insufficiency. Excess ADH (SIADH) is secreted during the first 48 hours, which causes water to be reabsorbed from the renal tubules and urine output to be decreased. Free hemoglobin from hemolysis is excreted by the kidneys as red-color urine and can cause renal damage.
Metabolic acidosis: increased	Burns cause cellular breakdown, and the cells release acid metabolites (lactic acid). Bicarbonate loss accompanies loss of sodium.

ANSWER COLUMN

▶ PATHOPHYSIOLOGY

1

Following a burn, there is an extracellular fluid volume shift in which fluid and electrolytes shift from the intravascular space (plasma) to the interstitial spaces of the burned area. (See Chapter 4 on ECF shift, if necessary.) This results in a(n) (increase/decrease) _____ of circulating plasma volume.

1   decrease

2

With a decrease in circulating plasma volume, burn shock occurs. It is characterized by restlessness, confusion, tachycardia, decreased blood pressure, decreased urine output, metabolic acidosis, and a paralytic ileus.

Burn shock results from *_____ .

2 a decrease in circulating plasma volume

3

Capillary permeability is (increased/decreased) _____ during the first 48 hours postburn. If less than 25% of the total body surface is burned, fluid accumulates in which of the following:

( ) a. Burned site
( ) b. Unburned tissue spaces
( ) c. Both of the above

3 increased; a. If more than 25% of body surface area is burned, fluid shifts to the burned site and to unburned tissue spaces.

4

What is meant by fluid shift to the third space? *_____
_____ .

Most of the fluid shift occurs during the first _____ hours, but may persist for _____ hours postburn. If 50% of the vascular fluid is lost to burned and unburned tissue spaces, severe (hypervolemia/hypovolemia) _____ occurs.

4 Fluid shifts from the vascular to the tissue (burned or unburned) spaces.; 18; 48; hypovolemia

5

Hemoconcentration is present in early burns. Explain why. *_____
_____
When this occurs, the serum osmolality is (increased/decreased) _____ and the hematocrit is (increased/decreased) _____ .

5 Fluid leaves the vascular (intravascular) space, causing hypovolemia or dehydration.; increased; increased

6

Electrolyte imbalances occur postburn. Hyponatremia is common because of which of the following:

( ) a. Sodium is lost to edema fluid at the burned site.
( ) b. Sodium shifts into cells.
( ) c. Diuresis occurs 48 hours postburn.

6 a, b, c

7

Intracellular potassium is lost from the cells and is replaced by sodium. Decreased urine output (oliguria) usually occurs in the early postburn period. With oliguria, the serum potassium level (increases/decreases) _____ . Why? *_____
_____

7 increases. Kidneys excrete 80–90% of potassium loss.

8 calcium loss to edema fluid at the burned site; hypocalcemia

9 decreased. Protein leaks from the vascular system to the burned site because of increased capillary permeability.

10 renal; b

11 increased; decreased

12 before

13 b, c, d

14 a, b

8

A serum calcium deficit may result from *_____ .
Multiple infusions of citrated blood can cause (hypocalcemia/ hypercalcemia) _____ .

9

Serum protein is (increased/decreased) _____ . Why?
*_____

10

Erythrocytes or red blood cells are destroyed by hemolysis (destruction of red blood cells). The free hemoglobin released from the red blood cells may cause damage to the _____ system.
   Erythrocytes are destroyed as a result of which of the following:
   ( ) a. Increased plasma protein
   ( ) b. Hemolysis

11

As a result of burn shock, there is (increased/decreased) _____ circulatory resistance and (increased/decreased) _____ cardiac output.

12

Once vascular fluid volume is reestablished, the diminished number of red blood cells (erythrocytes) becomes apparent; thus anemia results. Hemoconcentration is present (after/before) _____ rehydration.

13

Renal function decreases as a result of which of the following:
   ( ) a. Hypervolemia
   ( ) b. Hypovolemia
   ( ) c. Systolic BP <60 mm Hg
   ( ) d. SIADH (syndrome of inappropriate antidiuretic hormone secretion)

14

Metabolic acidosis results from which of the following:
   ( ) a. Loss of serum bicarbonate
   ( ) b. Increase in acid metabolites
   ( ) c. Excess vascular fluid

15

Indicate which of the following may occur as the result of burns. Correct the wrong statements.

( ) a. Increased capillary permeability
( ) b. Elevated serum osmolality in early postburn
( ) c. Hypovolemia
( ) d. Hemolysis
( ) e. Hemoconcentration before hydration
( ) f. Metabolic alkalosis
( ) g. Increased serum protein
( ) h. Hyperkalemia with oliguria
( ) i. Hyponatremia
( ) j. Hypercalcemia

15 a. X; b. X; c. X; d. X; e. X; f.—(metabolic acidosis); g.—(decreased serum protein); h. X; i. X; j.—(hypocalcemia)

▶ CLINICAL MANIFESTATIONS

Degree and Depth of Burns

The degrees of burn are rated by two different classification methods. The older method, in which burns are classified as first-, second-, or third-degree burns, is still commonly used. The newer method classifies burns as (1) superficial, (2) partial thickness superficial, (3) partial thickness deep, and (4) full thickness. Because both classification methods are used in clinical practice, it is necessary to learn both methods. Burns involve the three layers of skin: the *epidermis,* which is the outer layer of skin; the *dermis,* known as the true skin; and *subcutaneous tissues,* called the fatty tissues. Additionally, the underlying muscle and bone can be involved and some authors describe this as fourth-degree burns.

Depth of burn injury is described as superficial epidermal, partial thickness, and full thickness. These relate to first-, second-, and third-degree burns. Carefully study Table 21-2 and proceed to the frames that follow.

16

Define the following terms:

a. Epidermis *_____
b. Dermis *_____
c. Subcutaneous tissue *_____

16 a. the outer layer of skin; b. true skin; c. fatty tissue

Table 21-2

Degree and Depth of Burns and Their Characteristics

Type and Degree	Depth	Characteristics	Pain	Course of Healing
Superficial epidermal (first degree)	Epidermis	Erythema, dry, blanches with pressure	Painful, hyperesthetic (very sensitive)	2–3 days
Partial thickness (first to second degree)	Epidermis Upper dermis	Pink to deep red blisters, moist blanches with pressure	Very painful to touch and air currents	Heals in 3 weeks
Deep (second degree)	Epidermis Deep dermis	Mottled, moist, or dry blisters	Extremely painful to touch and air currents	Varies with burn depth and presence or absence of infection
Full thickness (third degree)	Epidermis Dermis Subcutaneous	Dry, pearly white to charred, inelastic, and leathery	No pain or sensation	
Fourth degree	Muscle and bone	Color variable		Amputation of extremities likely; grafting required for healing

Note: From "Burn Trauma: The Emergent Phase of Care. Contemporary Perspectives in Trauma Nursing (An Independent Home Study Continuing Education Course)," by K.K. Bryant, 1991, Forum Medicum, Inc., 4. Copyright 1991 by Forum Medicum. Adapted with permission.

---

17 superficial epidermal; partial thickness; deep; full thickness; or first degree; second degree; third degree; fourth degree

18 epidermis

19 erythema, dry and blanching; are

17

Type or degree of burn injury is classified as * _____ , * _____ , * _____ , or * _____ .

18

Superficial epidermal burns involve which layer of skin? _____

19

Superficial epidermal burns are characterized by * _____ .
Superficial epidermal burns (are/are not) _____ painful.

20
What two skin layers are involved in partial-thickness superficial burns? *_____

21
Partial-thickness superficial burns are described as *_____
_____ .
   Partial-thickness superficial burns are (tender/very painful)
*_____ .

22
Which two skin layers are involved in partial-thickness deep burns? *_____

23
Partial-thickness deep burns are described as *_____ .
Partial-thickness deep burns are (slightly painful/extremely painful) _____ .

24
Which three skin layers are involved in full-thickness burns?
  *_____
_____

25
Full-thickness burns are described as *_____ .
Full-thickness burns are (very painful/not painful) _____ .

26
Fourth-degree burns involve *_____ , (do/do not)
_____ involve pain, and are described as *_____ .

27
Superficial first-degree burns heal within *_____ .
  Partial-thickness burns (first to second degree) heal within
*_____ .
  Deep burns (second degree) heal according to *_____ .
  Full-thickness burns (third and fourth degree) require
*_____ for healing.

---

20 epidermis and upper dermis

21 pink to deep red, blisters, and moist blanches; very painful

22 epidermis and deep dermis

23 mottled, moist, or dry blisters; extremely painful

24 epidermis, dermis, and subcutaneous tissue

25 dry, pearly white, inelastic, and leathery; not painful

26 muscle and bone; do not; having variable color

27 2-3 days; 3 weeks; burn depth and presence/absence of infection; skin grafting

28

Place SE for superficial epidermal, PT for partial thickness; and FT for full thickness according to the depth, characteristics, and pain of burns.

_____ a. Epidermis and upper dermis burned

_____ b. Slightly painful

_____ c. Epidermis, dermis, and subcutaneous tissues burned

_____ d. Very painful

_____ e. Epidermis only

_____ f. Extremely painful

_____ g. Dry and blanches

_____ h. No pain

_____ i. Epidermis and deep dermis burned

_____ j. Moist or dry with blisters

_____ k. Pearly white and leathery

28 a. PT; b. SE; c. FT; d. PT; e. SE; f. PT; g. PT; h. FT; i. PT; j. PT; k. FT

Methods Used to Determine Percentage of Total Body Surface Burns

29

There are several methods used for determining the percentage of total body surface burned. The Berkow formula determines the percentage according to age and 19 predetermined surface body areas. Another method is the Lund and Browder chart, which estimates the body surface areas in small proportions, i.e., upper arm 2%, forearm $1\frac{1}{2}$%, and hand $1\frac{1}{2}$%. The rule of nines is frequently used as a quick method of estimation because it can be easily recalled. The three methods used to determine the percentage of total body surface area that has been burned are
* _____ .

29 the Berkow formula, Lund and Browder chart, and rule of nines

Figure 21-1 explains the rule of nines used to estimate the total body surface area burned. The rule of nines uses 9% or multiples thereof in calculating the burned body surface. The five main regions in the estimation of burned surface are in italics. Be sure to know the five regions and the percentages of each.

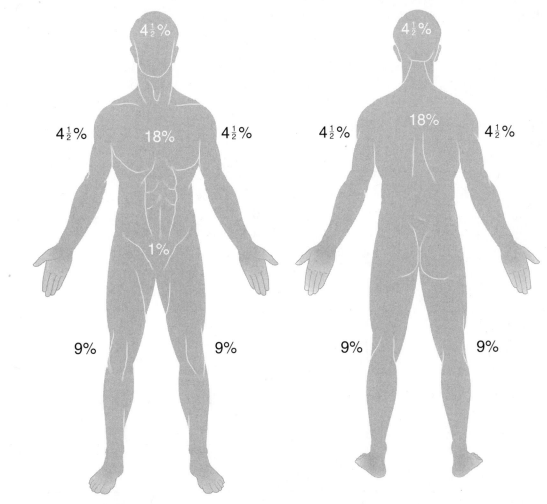

Figure 21-1 Rules of nines for estimation of body surface.

Region	Percentage of Body Surface (%)
Head and neck	9
1. Anterior head and neck (4.5%)	
2. Posterior head and neck (4.5%)	
Upper extremities	18
3. Right arm—anterior (4.5%) and posterior (4.5%)	
4. Left arm—anterior (4.5%) and posterior (4.5%)	
Trunk and buttocks	36
5. Anterior surface (18%)	
6. Posterior surface (18%)	
Lower extremities	36
7. Right leg and thigh—anterior (9%) and posterior (9%)	
8. Left leg and thigh—anterior (9%) and posterior (9%)	
9. *Perineum and genitalia* (1%)	1

30 head and neck, upper extremities, trunk and buttocks, lower extremities, and perineum and genitalia

31 rule of nines; depth of burned tissue (also burned surface area); 9; 9

32 18; 18

33 a. $4\frac{1}{2}$; b. 9; c. 36; d. 9; e. 1; f. $4\frac{1}{2}$; g. 18; h. 36

30

The rule of nines and the depth of burned tissue are used in planning parenteral therapy for burned persons.

What are the five main regions of the body used in the rule of nines? *_____

_____

31

In planning parenteral therapy for burns, the *_____ and *_____ are used.

The estimated percentage used for the anterior and posterior surfaces of each arm is _____%.

The estimated percentage used for the anterior and posterior surfaces of the head and neck is _____%.

32

The estimated percentage used for the anterior surface of the trunk is _____%.

The estimated percentage used for the anterior and posterior surfaces of each thigh and leg is _____%.

33

Complete the percentages on the following chart:

Region		Percentage of Body Surface (%)
Anterior head and neck	a.	_____
Left anterior and posterior arm	b.	_____
Anterior and posterior surfaces of trunk and buttocks	c.	_____
Anterior surface of right thigh and leg	d.	_____
Perineum and genitalia	e.	_____
Anterior right arm	f.	_____
Posterior trunk and buttocks	g.	_____
Anterior and posterior surfaces of lower extremities	h.	_____

Classifications of Burns

Table 21-3 differentiates between minor, moderate, and critical burns according to the degrees and percentage of burns. Know the three classifications or burns, the degrees, and the percentages. It is important to note that this classification is for the adult person. Infants, children, the elderly, and individuals with chronic illnesses may need to be classified differently than the healthy adult.

34

The three classifications of burns are *_____

_____ .

34 minor burns, moderate burns, and major burns

35

To be classified as minor burns, the skin surface involved must be first degree or second degree of less than _____% of body surface or third degree of less than _____% of body surface.

35 15; 2

36

To be classified as moderate burns, the skin surface involved must be second degree of _____ to _____% of body surface or third degree of less than _____% of body

36 15; 25; 10

Table 21-3

Classification of Burns: American Burn Association

Minor Thermal Burns	Moderate Thermal Burns	Major Thermal Burns
Second-degree burn <15% of TBSA in adults or <10% in children	Second-degree burns 15–25% of TBSA in adults or 10–20% in children	Second-degree burns >25% of TBSA in adults or >20% in children
Third-degree burn <2% of TBSA (not involving face, hands, feet, perineum)	Third-degree burns of <10% of TBSA (not involving hands, face, feet, perineum)	Third-degree burns >10% of TBSA. All burns involving hands, face, feet, and perineum.
		All poor risk clients

surface, provided that the hands, face, feet, eyes, ears, or genitalia are not burned.

37

To be classified as major burns, the skin surface involved must be second degree of over _____% of body surface or third degree of more than _____% of body surface or the burn must be of the hands, face, eyes, ears, _____ , or _____ .

37 25; 10; feet or genitalia

38

Place the word *minor* for minor burns, *moderate* for moderate burns, or *critical* for critical burns beside the following statements:

a. _____ Burns of the hands, face, feet, or genitalia

b. _____ Third-degree burns of less than 10% of body surface

c. _____ Third-degree burns of more than 10% of body surface

d. _____ Second-degree burns of 15–25% of body surface

e. _____ Second-degree burns of over 25% of body surface

f. _____ Second-degree burns of less than 15% of body surface

g. _____ Third-degree burns of less than 2% of body surface

38 a. major; b. moderate; c. major; d. moderate; e. major; f. minor; g. minor

▶ CLINICAL MANAGEMENT

39

Minor burns are generally treated in the health care provider's office or emergency room, and the person seldom needs hospitalization.

Moderate burns and burns (first and second-degree) greater than 15% of total body area should receive intravenous fluids.

Minor burns and burns less than 15% of total body surface area frequently (do/do not) _____ need intravenous fluids unless the person is a child, elderly, or in poor health. People

39 do not

with burns greater than 10% of total body surface area may need intravenous fluids.

40

Persons with burns involving >15% of body surface require careful, planned intravenous replacement therapy for survival.

In those with over 50% of the body surface involved, the mortality rate is high regardless of careful, planned intravenous therapy.

Individuals with 15–50% of body surface burns, having received fluid replacement, have a (good/poor) _____ prognosis, whereas those with 50% or more have a (good/poor) _____ prognosis.

40 good; poor

41

Various formulas have been devised and used as a basis for initiating therapy in the treatment of burns.

Accurately measured hourly urine flow is an important index for the determination of adequate intravenous therapy. For all severely burned persons, an indwelling catheter is advisable to obtain *_____ .

41 accurate hourly urine outputs

42

The desired rate of urine flow is 30–50 mL (cc) per hour. Less than 25 mL of urine output per hour for an adult indicates insufficient fluid intake or kidney dysfunction.

After 48–72 hours, the urine output can increase to 100 mL or more per hour from diuresis due to a fluid shift into the intravascular space (vessels). For a burned person, the desired urine output per hour is *_____ . Less than 25 mL/h indicates which of the following:

( ) a. Too much fluids
( ) b. Not enough fluids
( ) c. Kidney dysfunction

42 30–50 mL; b, c

43

During the first 48 hours, fluid replacement should be at least three times the urine output because of the fluid shift to the burned and unburned tissue areas.

When the intravenous flow rate is increased to correct hypovolemia and to increase urine output, the health care

43 overhydration; constant, irritating cough, dyspnea, and neck vein engorgement (also chest rales)

44 renal damage

45 a, c

46 a fluid volume deficit or hemoconcentration; b

47 b

professional should observe for what type of fluid imbalance?_____
Give three symptoms of overhydration. *_____
_____

44
To determine whether poor urine output is due to renal damage or inadequate fluid intake, a Fluid Challenge Test can be used. This test consists of giving 500–1000 mL of fluid in $\frac{1}{2}$ hour.
    A failure to increase urine output indicates *_____ .

45
High-protein liquids, between meals or at mealtime, are helpful for cell reconstruction. Which of the following liquids are high in protein?
    (   ) a. Eggnog
    (   ) b. Ginger ale
    (   ) c. Milkshake
    (   ) d. Coca-Cola

46
A very high hematocrit reading indicates *_____ .
    Many health care providers prefer to maintain the hematocrit (Hct) at 45 or above for the first 48 hours after the burn, thus during rehydration, the hematocrit will:
    (   ) a. Drop very low
    (   ) b. Return to a normal range
    (   ) c. Show a marked increase

47
The greatest fluid shift occurs during the first 18 hours after a burn and reaches its peak in 48 hours. Therefore, the critical period for fluid and electrolyte replacement is which of the following:
    (   ) a. The first 36 hours
    (   ) b. The first 48 hours
    (   ) c. The first 72 hours

48
A major hazard in burn cases is infection. This frequently delays the reabsorption of edema fluid from the site of the burn.

Surgical aseptic (sterile) techniques are employed to reduce the possibility of _____ .

Infection causes the edematous fluid to be reabsorbed (more slowly/more quickly) *_____ .

48 infection; more slowly

49

After 48 hours, capillary permeability lessens, fluid reabsorption begins, and edema starts to subside. This is the *stage of diuresis,* which generally begins after 2 days. However, it may take as long as 2 weeks before this stage develops, depending upon the severity of the burns. Explain what happens when the stage of diuresis begins:

    a. Capillary permeability (increases/decreases) _____ .

    b. Fluid (reabsorption/excretion) _____ begins.

    c. Edema starts to (increase/subside) _____ .

49 a. decreases; b. reabsorption; c. subside

50

Extracellular fluid volume shift from the interstitial space to the intravascular space occurs during the stage of diuresis. This most likely occurs _____ hours after the burn. A delay in the stage of diuresis varies with *_____ .

50 48; the severity of the burn

51

After 48 hours, IV therapy is frequently restricted or decreased, providing the serum sodium and potassium levels are near normal.

Continuous IV therapy may result in overhydration. This can be hazardous because it can overload the circulation, causing pulmonary edema and cardiac failure.

After 48 hours, IV fluid administration is (increased/decreased) _____ .

Overloading the circulation can result in which of the following:

    ( ) a. Pulmonary edema

    ( ) b. Gastritis

    ( ) c. Cardiac failure

    ( ) d. Pancreatitis

51 decreased; a, c

Fluid Correction Formulas

There are many formulas for calculating fluid replacement during the first 48 hours after burns. Table 21-4 gives three types of formulas. Brooke and Evans are similar except for the amount of colloid and electrolyte replacement. Parkland's formula does not call for colloid and free water during the first 24 hours. Parkland supporters believe that early colloid replacement shifts to the burned site, thus, by giving lactated Ringer's infusions, cardiac output increases and cell function is restored. Refer to Table 21-4 as needed.

52

The three formulas used for fluid replacement during the first 48 hours postburn are * _____ .

52 the Brooke Army Hospital, Evans, and Parkland

53

Four solutions used for colloid replacement are * _____
_____ .

Two electrolyte solutions used are * _____ .

53 blood, dextran, plasma, and albumin; lactated Ringer's and normal saline

Table 21-4

Formulas for Fluid Replacement During First 48 Hours for Burn Shock

Name	First 24 Hours	Second 24 Hours
Brooke Army Hospital	Colloid*: 0.5 mL/kg × % of burned area Electrolyte†: 1.5 mL/kg × % of burned area Water: 2000 mL D_5W	One-half ($\frac{1}{2}$) amount of colloid and electrolyte of the first 24 hours Water: 2000 mL D_5W
Evans	Colloid: 1 mL/kg × % of burned area Electrolyte: 1 mL/kg × % of burned area Water: 2000 mL D_5W	One-half ($\frac{1}{2}$) amount of colloid and electrolyte of the first 24 hours Water: 2000 mL D_5W
Parkland	Colloid: none Electrolyte: 4 mL/kg × % of burned area Water: none	Colloid: 20–60% of calculated plasma volume Water: 2000 mL D_5W

Note: Over 50% of body surface burns are calculated at 50% burns for fluid replacement purposes. 1 kg = 2.2 pounds.

*Colloid used: blood, dextran, plasma, albumin.

†Electrolyte used: lactated Ringer's or normal saline.

▶ CLINICAL APPLICATIONS

54

Mr. Greene, weighs 154 pounds, or _____ kg, and has 30% of his body surface burned.

To estimate his fluid needs for the first 24 hours, calculate his fluid needs according to the Brooke's formula as:

a. 0.5 mL colloid × 70 (kg of body weight) × 30 (% of burned body surface) = _____ mL of colloid to be given. (*Note:* When multiplying by 30, do not use the decimal point.)

b. 1.5 mL electrolyte × 70 (kg of body weight) × 30 (% of burned body surface) = _____ mL of lactated Ringer's to be given.

c. Plus 2000 mL of dextrose in water.

The total amount of parenteral fluid that Mr. Greene should receive in the first 24 hours following his burns is _____ mL.

54 70; a. 1050; b. 3150; 6200

55

For the second 24 hours, according to Brooke's formula, Mr. Greene should receive:

a. _____ mL of colloid

b. _____ mL of lactated Ringer's

c. _____ mL of dextrose in water

The total amount of parenteral fluid for the second 24 hours would be

d. _____ mL.

55 a. 525; b. 1575; c. 2000; d. 4100

56

After 48 hours of parenteral therapy, Mr. Greene should receive (more/less) _____ intravenous fluid.

After 48 hours, fluid shifts from the burned and unburned tissue spaces to the vascular area, and if the same quantity of IV fluids is given, what type of fluid imbalance can occur?

_____

56 less; overhydration, hypervolemia, or fluid volume excess

57

Over 50% of body surface burns are calculated as _____% burns for fluid replacement purposes.

57 50

58

During the first 24 hours, one-half of the fluids is given in the first 8 hours and the other half is given in the remaining 16 hours.

Mr. Greene should receive _____ mL of intravenous fluids in the first 8 hours and _____ mL in the remaining 16 hours of the first day.

Mrs. Silver, age 35, received 25% of second- and third-degree body surface burns when her farmhouse caught fire.

The following areas of her body were burned:

Face, 5%
Right arm and hand, 9%
Left arm, 5%
Back and upper chest, 6%

59

The total body surface area burned of Mrs. Silver is _____%.

60

Since the face, hand, and upper chest were burned, Mrs. Silver would be considered to have which of the following:

( ) a. Minor burns
( ) b. Moderate burns
( ) c. Major burns

Mrs. Silver's laboratory studies were:

Hemoglobin   13.5 g
Hematocrit   44%
White blood count   20,300 cells/mm^3
Polymorphonuclear cells (polys)   65%

A venous section (cutdown) was performed. In the emergency room she received:

Two injections of morphine sulfate: 1. 10 mg (gr $\frac{1}{6}$) (IM)
                                     2. later 10 mg (gr $\frac{1}{6}$) (IV)
1000 mL normal saline with 2 million units of aq. penicillin IV
1000 mL normal saline with 5 million units of aq. penicillin IV
Tetanus toxoid: 0.5 mL

58 3100; 3100

59 25

60 c

Mrs. Silver received tetanus toxoid because she was subject to infection by anaerobic microbes, such as *Clostridium tetani*.

61

She received morphine sulfate for *_____ . She received aqueous penicillin because of which of the following:
( ) a. Her hemoglobin was elevated.
( ) b. Her hematocrit was elevated.
( ) c. Her WBC was elevated.

Mrs. Silver's laboratory studies in Table 21-5 show her results at the time of her injury.

62

Mrs. Silver's serum chloride, sodium, and potassium (are/are not) _____ in the normal range.
Due to her low serum CO_2 on admission, she is in a state of metabolic _____ .

61 relief of pain; c

62 are; acidosis

Table 21-5

Laboratory Studies for Mrs. Silver

Laboratory Tests	On Admission	Day 1	Day 2	Day 3	Day 4	Day 5	Day 6	Day 7
Hematology Hemoglobin (12.9–17.0 g)	13.5	17.6						
Hematocrit (40–46%)	44	49 54	56 52 61	64	55	51	46 36	35
WBC (white blood count) (5000–10,000/mm³)	23,000	11,685						
Biochemistry BUN (blood urea nitrogen) (10–25 mg/dL)*	11	14						
Plasma/serum† CO_2 50–70 vol % / 22–32 mEq/L	30/14	44/20	44/20		57/26		57/26	
Plasma/serum chloride (95–108 mEq/L)	105	105	105		97		103	
Plasma/serum sodium (135–146 mEq/L)	141	137	137		134		141	
Plasma/serum potassium (3.5–5.3 mEq/L)	4.3	4.8	4.8		4.2		4.4	

*mg/100 mL = mg/dL.
†*Plasma* and *serum* are used interchangeably.

63

63 a. Cl, 95–108 mEq/L; b. Na, 135–146 mEq/L; c. K, 3.5–5.3 mEq/L

In the preceding question you noted that Mrs. Silver's serum electrolytes were within normal range. Can you recall the normal range for the following electrolytes without referring to Table 21-5?

  a. Plasma chloride. *_____

  b. Plasma sodium. *_____

  c. Plasma potassium. *_____

64

64 elevated; fluid volume deficit (You may have answered hemoconcentration. O.K.)

Her hematocrit in relation to her hemoglobin during the first 48 hours following admission is *_____ and is an indication of *_____ .

65

Her elevated WBC indicates which of the following:

  ( ) a. An increased number of white blood cells

  ( ) b. Infection

  ( ) c. Head cold

65 a, b, d

  ( ) d. Inflammatory stress response

66

Mrs. Silver weighed 65 kg and had a total of 25% body burns. Calculate the following fluid replacement needs using the Brooke Army Hospital formula:

  a. $0.5 \times 65 \times 25 =$ _____ mL colloid

  b. $1.5 \times 65 \times 25 =$ _____ mL electrolyte

                plus ___2000___ mL dextrose/water

  c.   Total _____ mL for first 24 hours

During the first 8 hours, Mrs. Silver should receive one half of the intravenous fluid.

  d. This amount is _____ mL. Intravenous fluids ordered for the first 8 hours are:

          812.5 mL colloid

          2437.5 mL electrolyte

          2000   mL dextrose in water

          5250   total for 24 hours

          2625   mL for first 8 hours

Note: Lactated Ringer's is not ordered because her electrolytes are not low. In the clinical setting, numbers may be rounded off.

Orders for the second 8 hours include:

> 500 mL colloid
> 250 mL electrolyte
> <u>400</u> mL 5% dextrose in water
> 1150 mL for the second 8 hours

Later she received 1500 mL D$_5$W for the third 8 hours.
e. The total amount of colloid ordered is _____ mL.
f. The total amount of electrolyte ordered is _____ mL.
g. The total amount of dextrose in water ordered is
   _____ mL.

67
Calculate the amount of fluids that she should receive during the second 24 hours according to the Brooke formula.
a. _____ mL colloid
b. _____ mL electrolytes
c. _____ mL D$_5$W

68
In Mrs. Silver's case, urine output was measured hourly and tested for specific gravity.

After the first 8 hours, Mrs. Silver's urine output was 250 mL/h; thus the IV flow rate was decreased.

During the third 8 hours, her urine output fell to 5–10–15 mL/h for 3 consecutive hours.

The fluid flow rate should be (increased/decreased) _____ .

Which of these intravenous fluids should be given to correct Mrs. Silver's decrease in urine output:

( ) a. Blood
( ) b. Normal saline
( ) c. 5% dextrose in water
( ) d. 10% dextrose in saline

69
Mrs. Silver's urine specific gravity ranged from 1.005 to 1.017. The specific gravity of urine is the weight (waste products) in relationship to water, 1.000. The specific gravity norm for urine is (1.010–1.030).

66 a. 812.5; b. 2437.5; c. 5250;
   d. 2625; e. 812.5 (800–825);
   f. 2437.5 (2450–2500); g. 2000

67 a. 406 (400–425); b. 1218
   (1200–1225); c. 1000

68 increased; b, c

Mrs. Silver's urine specific gravity of 1.005 and 1.008 indicates there are (more/less) _____ waste products in her urine than normal. These waste products are more concentrated in her (urine/plasma) _____ .

69 less; plasma

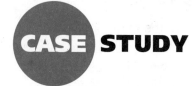

REVIEW

Mrs. Silver, age 35, received 25% second- and third-degree body surface burns. Using the rule of nines, her face received 5%, right arm and hand 9%, left arm 5%, and back and upper chest 6%. On admission, her hematocrit was 44%; on the first day it rose to 49 and 54%. By the second day, it was 56–64%. Her serum CO_2 on admission was 14 mEq/L, and on the second and third days it was 20 mEq/L. Her serum electrolytes were in normal range.

ANSWER COLUMN

1. intravascular; interstitial
2. Elevated; Hemoconcentration was present due to ECF volume shift to the interstitial space (burned area), or you could answer dehydration due to ECF volume shift.
3. Metabolic acidosis; Due to a loss of serum bicarbonate and an increase in body acid metabolites (cellular breakdown).
4. infection

5. rule of nines, Lund and Browder's, and Berkow

6. Critical; Mrs. Silver had burns to the hand and face plus a total of 25% second- and third-degree burns.

1. After a burn, there is an extracellular fluid volume shift from the _____ to the _____ space.

2. Mrs. Silver's hematocrit was _____ the first and second days following the burn. Explain why. *_____
_____

3. What type of acid-base imbalance did Mrs. Silver have the first 3 days? *_____ Explain the reason for this imbalance. *_____
_____

4. Besides fluid and electrolyte imbalance, another hazard in burn cases is _____ .

5. Name three methods used to estimate body burn surface.
*_____

6. Mrs. Silver's burns were classified as (minor/moderate/critical) _____ . Explain why. *_____
_____

Mrs. Silver's fluid replacement was based on the Brooke Army Hospital formula. Review the Brooke formula and Mrs. Silver's fluid replacement the first 24 hours.

7. Brooke; Evans and Parkland

8. measured hourly urine output

9. 30; 50; insufficient fluid intake; kidney dysfunction

10. plasma; blood; albumin and dextran

11. normal saline and lactated Ringer's solution

12. Normal saline.; Mrs. Silver's serum electrolytes were in normal range, so saline was given. Also, saline (NaCl) replaces the sodium loss to the burn area and to diuresis.

13. interstitial spaces; the intravascular space

14. irritating cough, dyspnea, engorged neck and hand veins, and moist rales

7. In planning Mrs. Silver's parenteral therapy, the _____ formula was used based on the rule of nines. Name two other formulas for determining fluid needs. *_____ _____

8. An important index for the determination of adequate parenteral therapy is an accurate record of *_____ .

9. Urine output should be maintained between _____ and _____ mL/h. Less than 25 mL of urine output can indicate *_____ or *_____ .

10. Mrs. Silver's colloid replacement solutions were _____ and _____ . What two other colloids can be used? *_____

11. Name two types of electrolyte solutions used in parenteral therapy for burns. *_____

12. Give the type of electrolyte solution that Mrs. Silver received _____ Why? *_____ _____

13. After 2 days or, at the longest, 2 weeks, the stage of diuresis occurs. This is when the extracellular fluid volume shifts from *_____ to *_____ .

14. Overhydration or hypervolemia is a hazard when large quantities of intravenous fluids are administered for fluid replacement and for increasing urinary output. Give four symptoms of overhydration. *_____ _____

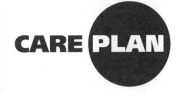

Client Management

Assessment Factors

▶ Assess: blood pressure, temperature, pulse, and respiration. An increase in pulse rate with a decrease in blood pressure (even slightly) and an increase in respiration can be indicative of shocklike symptoms due to hypovolemia resulting from the fluid shift to the burned site. A pulse pressure of less than 20 mm Hg can indicate severe hypovolemia. An elevated temperature can indicate an infection. A lower than normal temperature can indicate heat loss due to loss of skin.

▶ Assess burns, including the surface area and status of burned tissue. Burns are assessed according to the depth of tissue involvement, i.e., superficial, partial, partial-deep, and full thickness or by the degree of the burns. The classification method used for burns, either by depth or degree, is determined by institutional preference.

▶ Record the skin surfaces involved indicating the color of the burn and the intensity of pain related at each burn site.

▶ A quick estimation of the percentage of total burned body surface areas can be accomplished using the rule of nines.

▶ Urine output is a key factor in fluid and electrolyte balance for burned clients. Insufficient urine output, <30 mL per hour or <250 mL per 8 hours, can indicate a change in body fluid loss resulting from a fluid shift to the burned areas and surrounding tissues (third-space fluid).

▶ Assess for presence of bowel sounds. Hypokalemia can cause a paralytic ileus.

Diagnosis 1

Fluid volume deficit related to fluid shift to the burned site.

Interventions and Rationale

1. Monitor vital signs: every hour to every 4 hours depending on the severity of the burns and burn shock. A pulse rate greater than 100 may indicate impending or the presence of shock. Check strength of peripheral pulses. If systolic pressure is below 90 mm Hg, shock is probable.

2. Monitor urine output. Measure urine output and specific gravity at specified times such as ordered by the doctor or according to unit policy.

3. Check laboratory test results. Electrolytes, BUN, creatinine, protein, arterial blood gases, and CBC (hematocrit, hemoglobin, WBC) have implications for care. Altered test results may be the result of hemodilution. Report significant changes.

4. Monitor fluid intake (oral and intravenous). The fluid intake can be as high as three times the amount of urine output depending upon the severity of the burns. IV therapy is usually not indicated if the percentage of burn is less than 15% of the body surface area for an adult and less than 10% of the body

surface area for a child, elderly client, or a client with a debilitating preexisting illness.

5. Calculate the flow rate of IVs. During the first 24 hours, one half of the daily IV fluid order is usually administered in the first 8 hours and the second one half in the next 16 hours.

6. Monitor potassium replacement. When the client is receiving intravenous fluids with potassium, the serum potassium level is elevated because of hypovolemia in conjunction with a decreased urine output. Notify the physician, as a change in the IV order is indicated. Intravenous fluids without potassium should be run rapidly to improve renal function and to decrease the potassium level.

Diagnosis 2

Risk for fluid volume excess related to fluid shift from burned site to the vascular system and the administration of a large volume of IV fluids.

Interventions and Rationale

1. Monitor vital signs: blood pressure, pulse, respirations, and invasive hemodynamic parameters (e.g., CVP, PAP/PCWP) as appropriate.

2. Monitor fluid intake (oral and intravenous). Intravenous fluid is usually decreased after 3–5 days postburn as a result of the fluid shift back into the vascular system (blood vessels). If massive fluid replacement is continued as fluid shifts back into circulation, hypervolemia or overhydration results.

3. Observe the vascular system: vein engorgement, jugular vein distention, and hand vein engorgement can occur several days postburn and may indicate impending hypervolemia.

4. Monitor breath sounds. Report the presence of chest rales. Respiratory changes may occur due to hypervolemia (fluid overload).

5. Check laboratory test results: Electrolytes, protein, BUN, creatinine, hematocrit, and hemoglobin have implications for care. The test results may be altered due to hemodilution. Report significant changes.

6. Weigh client daily or as indicated. Weight changes may indicate changes in fluid or nutritional status.

7. Monitor urine output. Urine output may be greatly increased (two to three times the normal volume) when the vascular system is overloaded. Insufficient urine output during the fluid shift to the vascular space may be indicative of renal impairment from burn shock or cardiac insufficiency.

Diagnosis 3

Altered urinary elimination; decreased, related to hypovolemia.

Interventions and Rationale

1. Monitor fluid intake and urine output. Fluid intake requirements during the first several days following major burns is greatly increased due to fluid loss from the burns and the fluid shift to the burned site (third space). The administration of IV fluids must be decreased during the period in which body fluids shift back into circulation. If urine output remains low with the second phase of the fluid shift (back into circulation), renal insufficiency should be suspected. Urine output should be closely monitored during the first week postburn.

2. Check laboratory test results. Elevated BUN and serum creatinine are usually indicative of renal dysfunction.

3. Monitor respiratory status. Auscultate lung fields for rales every 2–4 hours. Renal insufficiency resulting in hypervolemia frequently accompanies fluid retention in the lungs.

Diagnosis 4

Risk for ineffective airway clearance and risk for ineffective breathing pattern related to inhalation injury, tracheal edema, and/or hypervolemia.

Interventions and Rationale

1. Maintain client airway. Check for symptoms of inhalation injury: singed facial/nasal hairs, wheezing, stridor, hoarseness, and chest rales. Swelling and inflammation from inhalation injury obstruct air exchange.

2. Monitor respiratory status. Check respirations frequently and assess chest sounds to evaluate quality of air exchange and respiratory status.

3. Administer oxygen per order (usually by nonrebreather face mask) to reduce effects of reduced air exchange.

4. Maintain airway equipment at bedside (airway, ambubag, tracheotomy tray) for respiratory emergency.

5. Suction oropharyngeal and tracheal secretions prn to reduce the effects of obstruction of airway from increased burn secretions.

6. Turn position every 2 hours if not contraindicated to enhance full expansion of the lungs, enhance movement of fluid, and reduce respiratory complications.

7. Maintain head of bed 30°–45°, if permitted. This facilitates breathing by decreasing pressure on the diaphragm.

Diagnosis 5

Altered tissue perfusion: related to hypervolemia

Interventions and Rationale

1. Assess skin: color, temperature, quality, healing of lesions. Elevate edematous extremities. Keep warm and dry. Evaluate for signs of infection.

2. Turn every 2 hours to prevent pressure sites and skin breakdown.

3. Check peripheral pulses and assess chest sounds for pulmonary congestion.

4. Monitor Hgb, Hct, electrolytes, BUN. Electrolytes, BUN, hematocrit, and hemoglobin may be elevated due to a decrease in vascular fluid.

5. Monitor weight. Weigh daily to determine loss or gain of fluid.

6. Monitor renal function, fluid balance. Check urine output and specific gravity to assess effectiveness of treatment regime.

7. Assess mental status for orientation. Changes in mental status may indicate inadequate tissue oxygenation.

Diagnosis 6

Risk for body image disturbance related to physical appearance from burn injury.

Interventions and Rationale

1. Assess causative factors. Have client describe self and encourage verbalization of feelings. Respond realistically, support positive perceptions, and note denial behaviors or overuse of defense mechanisms.

2. Assist client and significant others' acceptance of body changes. Establish therapeutic relationship, discuss fears and conflicts, and encourage client to acknowledge and accept feelings. Provide accurate information. Encourage client to look at and touch affected body parts.

3. Promote wellness. Begin counseling as soon as possible. Provide positive feedback. Complete teaching exercises in small time frames. Refer to appropriate support groups.

Evaluation/Outcome

1. Evaluate that fluid volume is maintained at a functional level: skin has good turgor; blood pressure and pulse are in normal ranges; urine specific gravity and volume are within normal range; mucous membranes are moist; and potassium, BUN creatinine, hemoglobin, and hematocrit are within normal ranges.

2. Weight is stable, there are no pulmonary rales or rhonchi and no venous engorgement, and CVP and PAP/PCWP are within normal baseline for that client's cardiorespiratory status. Intake equals output, including insensible fluid loss.

3. Respirations are within normal range without use of accessory muscles of breathing. Client able to handle respiratory secretions without suctioning.

4. Client is alert and oriented to person and place, peripheral pulses are within client's normal range, and arterial blood gases are within normal range.

5. Nail beds, oral mucous membranes, and conjunctiva show good oxygenation.

Gastrointestinal Surgery with Fluid and Electrolyte Imbalances

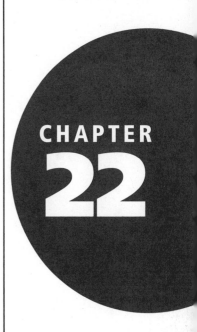

CHAPTER

22

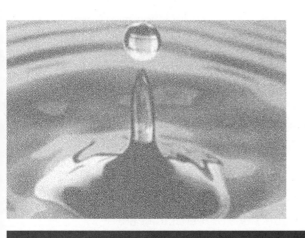

OBJECTIVES

Upon completion of this chapter, the reader should be able to:

- Identify five major electrolytes that may be affected by gastrointestinal (GI) surgery.
- Discuss the physiologic implications of sodium, potassium, and chloride imbalances associated with major GI surgery.
- Discuss the effects of gastric intubation on fluid and electrolyte balance.
- Describe the physiologic implications of hydrogen and bicarbonate balance with alterations in the GI system.
- Identify important assessment factors associated with fluid and electrolyte balance that may occur with major GI surgery.
- Identify selected diagnoses and interventions related to fluid and electrolyte balance associated with major GI surgery.

▶ INTRODUCTION

The main functions of the gastrointestinal (GI) tract are the ingestion, absorption, and transportation of fluids and nutrients. Diseases and illnesses that interrupt these daily functions place the client at risk for developing fluid and electrolyte imbalances. Diagnostic testing and preparation for gastrointestinal surgery may further increase the client's risk for fluid and electrolyte imbalance. Postoperatively, the client may be NPO, have gastrointestinal drainage tubes, and delayed peristalsis. Preexisting cardiopulmonary, endocrine, and renal conditions in conjunction with diuretics, glucocorticoids, mineralocorticoids, and insulin requirements place the client undergoing major surgery at risk for fluid and electrolyte imbalances. Alterations in fluid volume status can occur rapidly; astute assessment skills and timely interventions may prevent or decrease potential complications.

ANSWER COLUMN

1 ingestion, absorption, and transportation

2 fluid; electrolyte

3 NPO; drainage tubes; decreased peristalsis

4 a. cardiopulmonary disorders (congestive heart failure); b. endocrine disorders (diabetes mellitus), glucocorticoid disorders (Cushing's disease), mineralocorticoid disorders (Addison's disease); c. renal disease (renal impairment or kidney failure). You may have included other conditions as well as the ones mentioned.

1

Three of the main functions of the GI tract are *_____ _____ of fluids and electrolytes.

2

Diseases and illnesses that interrupt the normal functions of the GI tract place the client at risk for _____ and _____ imbalances.

3

Postoperative treatment modalities that increase the client's risk for fluid and electrolyte imbalance include _____ , *_____ , and *_____.

4

Name at least three preexisting conditions that increase the surgical client's risk for fluid and electrolyte imbalances.

a. *_____

b. *_____

c. *_____

▶ FLUID AND ELECTROLYTE ALTERATIONS

5

Clients undergoing minor surgery usually experience little or no fluid and electrolyte alterations.

In major surgery, sodium and water may be retained and potassium may be lost. Before potassium is administered, it is necessary to make certain that:

( ) a. The person can tolerate food
( ) b. Renal function is adequate

6

After major surgery, there is a tendency for sodium _____ , water _____ , and potassium _____.

7

Many clients undergoing gastrointestinal surgery experience fluid and electrolyte imbalances prior to surgery. Treatment of these imbalances must be considered prior to surgery in conjunction with concurrent fluid losses. Replacement of fluid losses is necessary before, during, and following surgery.

Frequently, these clients have a fluid deficit and will need additional fluids to reestablish renal function. Which type of intravenous solution is indicated to reestablish renal function:

( ) a. Hydrating solutions
( ) b. Plasma expanders
( ) c. Replacement solutions with potassium replacement

8

Some clients undergoing gastrointestinal surgery may require fluid and electrolyte replacement therapy for which of the following:

( ) a. Before surgery
( ) b. During surgery
( ) c. After surgery

9

Gastric or intestinal intubation (tube passed into the stomach or intestines) for suctioning purposes may be inserted before surgery. This alleviates vomiting due to an obstruction in the

5　b

6　retention; retention; loss

7　a

8　a, b, c

gastrointestinal tract or decompresses the stomach or bowel, or both, before and after an operation.

For gastric intubation, a Levine tube or Salem sump is inserted via the nose into the stomach. For an intestinal intubation, a Miller-Abbott tube or Cantor tube is inserted via the nose and stomach into the intestines. The intestinal tubes are longer than the gastric tube and they contain a small balloon filled with air or mercury on the end which helps the tube pass into the lower intestines. A gastric or an intestinal tube is frequently used following abdominal surgery in order to remove secretions until peristalsis returns and to relieve abdominal distention.

Gastric or intestinal intubation before abdominal surgery is used to *_____

_____ .

Gastric or intestinal intubation after abdominal surgery is used to *_____

_____

and to *_____ .

9 alleviate vomiting and decompress the bowel or stomach; remove secretions until peristalsis returns; relieve abdominal distention

Table 22-1 lists the electrolytes that are in the stomach and intestines. Note which electrolytes are more concentrated in gastric and intestinal fluids. The client experiencing vomiting, diarrhea, or intubation (gastric or intestinal) loses fluid and electrolytes. Study the table and be able to state which electrolytes are lost.

10 potassium, chloride, and hydrogen; sodium and bicarbonate (chloride is in high concentration in the stomach and the intestines)

10

Identify three highly concentrated electrolytes that are lost with vomiting and gastric intubation. *_____

Name two other electrolytes that are lost from the stomach.

*_____

Table 22-1

Concentration of Electrolytes in the Stomach and Intestine (mEq/L)

Area	Body Fluid	Na^+	K^+	Cl^-	HCO_3^-	
Stomach	Gastric juice	60.4	9.2	100*	0–14	H^+*
Small intestine	Intestinal juice	111.3*	20*	104.2*	31*	

*Electrolytes that are highly concentrated in these areas.

11 sodium, potassium, and bicarbonate

12 intestines; intestines

13 intestines; metabolic acidosis

14 stomach; metabolic alkalosis

15 hypokalemia alkalosis

11
What are the three major electrolytes lost by clients with diarrhea or intestinal intubation? *_____
Another electrolyte lost from the intestines is _____.

12
Sodium ions are more plentiful in the (stomach/intestines) _____.

Potassium ions are more plentiful in the (stomach/intestines) _____.

13
Bicarbonate ions are more plentiful in the (stomach/intestines) _____.

What type of acid-base imbalance results when a large amount of bicarbonate is lost? *_____

14
Hydrogen is more plentiful in the (stomach/intestines) _____ .

What type of acid-base imbalance results when hydrogen is lost? *_____

15
Name the electrolyte-acid-base imbalances that can occur if potassium, chloride, and hydrogen are lost from the stomach.
*_____

▶ CLINICAL APPLICATIONS

Mr. Drum was admitted to the hospital complaining of severe, persistent hiccups and abdominal pain. The client noticed a mass in the lower left quadrant of his abdomen for approximately 5–6 days before admission. Mr. Drum experienced several episodes of this left groin mass that could be reduced manually.

Mr. Drum stated he had not had a bowel movement for the past 3 days and he was not able to "keep anything down" over the past 3 days. His skin was warm and dry with poor turgor. He was very weak.

16

Which of the following signs and symptoms might indicate that Mr. Drum had a fluid volume deficit:

( ) a. Vomiting—unable to retain food for 3 days
( ) b. Skin warm, dry, and lacking elasticity
( ) c. Not having a bowel movement for 3 days
( ) d. Weakness
( ) e. Hernia could be manually reduced
( ) f. Severe abdominal pain in left lower quadrant

16 a, b, d

Table 22-2 gives the laboratory studies for Mr. Drum and shows how his results changed from the norm at the time of his illness.

Table 22-2

Laboratory Studies of Mr. Drum

Laboratory Tests	On Admission	First Day	Second Day	Third Day	Fourth Day
Hematology					
Hemoglobin (12.9–17.0 g)	21.2	18.4	13.1	13.2	
Hematocrit (40–54%)	58	54	38	39	
WBC (white blood count) (5000–10,000/mm^3)	10,700				
Biochemistry					
BUN (blood urea nitrogen) (10–25 mg/dL)*	85	68	68	19	19
Plasma/serum[†] CO$_2$					
50–70 vol%	52	61	—	72	50
22–32 mEq/L	24	28	—	38	22
Plasma/serum chloride (98–108 mEq/L)	73	78	73	91	97
Plasma/serum sodium (135–146 mEq/L)	122	128	122	132	145
Plasma/serum potassium (3.5–5.3 mEq/L)	5.2	4.0	4.0	4.2	4.1

*mg/100 mL = mg/dL.

[†]*Plasma* and *serum* are used interchangeably.

Memorize the "normal" laboratory ranges as given in Table 22-2 in the left-hand column. Use the values throughout the chapter. Refer to Table 22-2 as needed.

17

The "normal" ranges from hemoglobin, hematocrit, and white blood count are *_____ , *_____ , and *_____ , respectively.

17 12.9–17.0 g; 40–54%; 5000–10,000/mm³

18

BUN is the abbreviation for blood urea nitrogen. Explain how urea is formed. *_____

How is it excreted? *_____

What is the "normal" BUN range? _____

18 by-product of protein metabolism; through the kidney; 10–25 mg/dL

19

The "normal" serum CO_2 range is _____ vol %, or _____ mEq/L.

Would a client with a serum CO_2 of 38 mEq/L be in metabolic (acidosis/alkalosis)? _____. Refer to Chapter 12 for further clarification.

19 50–70; 22–32; alkalosis

20

The "normal" range of the serum chloride is 95–108 mEq/L. Identify the "normal" range of the serum potassium and serum sodium: serum potassium: *_____ mEq/L; serum sodium: *_____ mEq/L. Refer to Chapters 6–7 for further clarification.

20 K, 3.5–5.3; Na, 135–146

21

Which of Mr. Drum's admission laboratory results indicate a fluid and electrolyte imbalance:

( ) a. Hemoglobin 21.2 g
( ) b. Hematocrit 58%
( ) c. Serum CO_2 52%
( ) d. Serum CO_2 24 mEq/L
( ) e. Serum chloride 73 mEq/L
( ) f. Serum sodium 122 mEq/L
( ) g. Serum potassium 5.2 mEq/L

21 a, b, e, f

488 ● Unit VI Clinical Situations: Fluid, Electrolyte, and Acid-Base Imbalances

22 fluid volume deficit (If you
answered hemoconcentra-
tion or dehydration, OK.)

23 b

24 a, d

25 a. O; b. D; c. K, D; d. O; e. O; f. E;
g. M; h. O; i. E

22
Mr. Drum's elevated hemoglobin and hematocrit on admission
and the first day postoperatively indicate *_____.

23
A high BUN is indicative of renal impairment or dehydration or
both. Mr. Drum's elevated BUN indicates which of the following:
( ) a. An increased urine output
( ) b. A retention of urea, the by-product of protein
metabolism, in the circulating blood
( ) c. An abnormal excretion of urea, the by-product of
protein metabolism

24
The third day postoperatively, Mr. Drum's plasma CO_2 increased.
This indicates which of the following:
( ) a. An increased bicarbonate ion in the plasma
( ) b. A decreased bicarbonate ion in the plasma
( ) c. Metabolic acidosis
( ) d. Metabolic alkalosis

25
Below are some of Mr. Drum's laboratory results. Use the
following symbols to label the imbalance that they might indicate:

D for dehydration
K for kidney dysfunction
E for electrolyte imbalance
M for metabolic alkalosis
O for normal range or for those that do not pertain to the
above four

Some results may be associated with more than one imbalance.
_____ a. Hematocrit 40%
_____ b. Hemoglobin 21.2 g
_____ c. BUN 68 mEq/L
_____ d. BUN 19 mEq/L
_____ e. Serum potassium 4.0 mEq/L
_____ f. Serum sodium 122 mEq/L
_____ g. Serum CO_2 38 mEq/L
_____ h. Serum CO_2 28 mEq/L
_____ i. Serum chloride 73 mEq/L

◗ CLINICAL MANAGEMENT

Preoperative

The preoperative management for Mr. Drum should include:

1. Hydrate rapidly utilizing 4–5 liters over the next 6–8 hours.

2. Insert a Levine tube and connect to low intermittent suction.

3. Prepare for OR for a left inguinal herniorrhaphy as soon as he is hydrated.

4. Monitor renal function—urine output.

Solution for hydration: 4500 cc 5% D/$\frac{1}{2}$ NS (dextrose in $\frac{1}{2}$ normal saline or 0.45%)

26

Which of the following conditions resulted from Mr. Drum's vomiting?

( ) a. Severe fluid volume deficit
( ) b. Water intoxication
( ) c. A loss of sodium and chloride
( ) d. A low serum bicarbonate level
( ) e. A low serum potassium level

26 a, c

27

He was hydrated (before/after) _____ the herniorrhaphy. A gastric tube was inserted to do which of the following:

( ) a. Relieve distention
( ) b. Remove secretions from the stomach
( ) c. Lessen vomiting
( ) d. Provide nutrition

27 before. On admission his potassium was high normal, probably because of the severe fluid volume deficit that caused hemoconcentration.; a, b, c

Postoperative

28

The postoperative fluid and electrolyte management for Mr. Drum should include the following:

1. Connect gastric tube to low suction and check drainage hourly.

2. Administer and monitor parenteral therapy to run at 125 mL/h.

1000 cc 5% D/$\frac{1}{2}$ NS
1000 cc 5% D/NS
1000 cc 5% lactated Ringer's

3. Ranitidine (Zantac) 50 mg in 100 mL/D$_5$W; infuse 15–20 minutes every 6–8 hours.

4. Check urine output hourly and test for specific gravity and pH.

5. Assess serum electrolyte findings.

6. Administer antibiotic as prescribed for febrile condition.

7. Encourage client to cough and deep breathe every 30 minutes for the first 4 hours.

Mr. Drum received gastric intubation following surgery to
*_____ and *_____ .

29

Gastrointestinal secretions contain solid particles that may accumulate and obstruct the tube. Irrigating the tube will assure patency and proper drainage.

Frequent irrigations, using large amounts of water, should be avoided to prevent electrolyte washout.

Irrigation of Mr. Drum's tube will assure *_____ .
Name the "major" electrolytes lost through frequent gastric irrigation with large quantities of water. _____ ,
_____ , and _____

30

The gastric tube should be irrigated at specific intervals with small amounts of normal saline to keep it patent.

A change in the client's position helps to alleviate tube obstruction.

The use of small amounts of air to check the patency of the tube may be ordered instead of irrigating the tube to help prevent the loss of fluids and electrolytes. Listen with the stethoscope over the stomach for a "whoosh" sound when air is injected into the tube.

Three methods to maintain the patency of Mr. Drum's gastric tube are *_____
_____ .

---

28 relieve abdominal distention; remove gastric secretions

29 patency for proper drainage; potassium; hydrogen; chloride

30 irrigate at specific intervals with small amounts of saline, change the client's position, and introduce small amounts of air and listen with a stethoscope for a "whoosh" sound

31 The electrolytes in the stomach would be diluted, and suction would remove them. H2 receptor antagonists (cimetidine, famotidine, ranitidine) are commonly administered to clients via the gastric tube. These drugs suppress HCl production, thus minimizing the amount of HCl removed by suction.

32 is not; a feeling of fullness, vomiting, abdominal distention, and diminished bowel sounds

33 has not; a small amount of fluid return indicates peristalsis has returned

31

Mr. Drum was allowed sips of water to alleviate the dryness in his mouth and lessen irritation in his throat.

Special attention should be taken to limit the amount of water by mouth, because water dilutes the electrolytes in the stomach and the suction then removes them.

What might happen to Mr. Drum's electrolytes if he drinks a lot of water during gastric intubation? *_____

_____

32

After Mr. Drum's gastric tube is removed, the nurse should observe for:

1. A feeling of fullness

2. Vomiting

3. Abdominal distention

4. Diminished bowel sounds

These symptoms indicate that Mr. Drum's gastrointestinal tract (is/is not) _____ functioning.

The four signs and symptoms that indicate Mr. Drum's peristalsis has not returned to normal are *_____

_____ .

33

Frequently, the tube is clamped for a period of time and then unclamped. The amount of residual gastric fluid is measured. A large residual of gastric fluid released when the tube is unclamped indicates that peristalsis has not returned.

A feeling of fullness, vomiting, and abdominal distention are signs and symptoms that indicate that peristalsis (has/has not) _____ returned.

Using the clamping and unclamping method, how would one know if peristalsis has returned? *_____ .

34

Since suction removes fluids and electrolytes, oral fluid intake is restricted and parenteral therapy is initiated.

Mr. Drum received intravenous fluids containing dextrose, saline, and lactated Ringer's to do which of the following:

( ) a. Replace sodium and chloride loss
( ) b. Maintain nutritional needs
( ) c. Maintain electrolyte balance
( ) d. Replace and maintain the fluid volume

34 a, b, c, d

35

If Mr. Drum received 3–4 (or more) liters of 5% dextrose in water (D_5W) with no other solutes, what type of fluid imbalance could occur?

( ) a. Dehydration
( ) b. Overhydration
( ) c. Water intoxication

Why? *_____

_____

35 b (maybe), c; The diluted fluid in the vessels (vascular) shifts to the cells due to the process of osmosis.; Osmosis causes fluid to diffuse from the lesser to the greater concentration.

36

Mr. Drum received an ampule of sodium bicarbonate IV push. This would do which of the following:

( ) a. Increase the plasma CO_2 or bicarbonate
( ) b. Decrease the plasma CO_2 or bicarbonate
( ) c. Reduce his metabolic acidotic state
( ) d. Reduce his metabolic alkalotic state

36 a, c

37

Mr. Drum should be encouraged to cough and deep breathe to help keep the lungs inflated and promote effective gas exchange. Inadequate ventilation due to pain, narcotics, and anesthesia causes alveolar collapse and eventually leads to CO_2 retention (respiratory acidosis).

In respiratory acidosis, Mr. Drum would (hypoventilate/hyperventilate) _____ .

Indicate the type of breathing associated with alveolar collapse and CO_2 retention (respiratory acidosis). (Refer to Chapter 14 if needed.)

( ) a. Deep, rapid, vigorous breathing
( ) b. Dyspnea—difficult or labored breathing
( ) c. Overbreathing

37 hypoventilate; b

CASE STUDY

REVIEW

Preoperatively, Mr. Drum's fluid and electrolyte status and kidney function should be assessed. All laboratory findings should be checked to assess the fluid balance.

ANSWER COLUMN

1. dehydration

2. dehydration; renal impairment

3. With dehydration, potassium is lost from cells and accumulates in ECF. If urine volume is low, the serum potassium level could increase.

4. serum potassium level decreased, with hydration

5. metabolic alkalosis

6. hypervolemia or overhydration

7. water intoxication. Dextrose is metabolized rapidly by the body, leaving water or hypo-osmolar, fluid which passes into cells.

1. Mr. Drum's elevated hemoglobin and hematocrit on admission and the first day postoperatively is indicative of _____ .

2. His elevated BUN is also indicative of _____ and possibly of *_____ .

3. Mr. Drum's serum sodium and chloride were low due to fluid loss. His serum potassium was 5.2 mEq/L on admission. Explain why Mr. Drum's serum potassium is a high normal with vomiting and dehydration. *_____
_____
_____

4. What happened to Mr. Drum's serum potassium level when he was hydrated? *_____
_____

5. Mr. Drum's increased serum CO_2 may indicate *_____
_____ .

6. What type of fluid imbalance may occur when rapidly hydrating a debilitated individual with 4–5 liters of fluid intravenously? *_____
_____

7. If Mr. Drum were hydrated with 4–5 liters of 5% dextrose in water, what type of fluid imbalance might occur? *_____

Explain why. *_____
_____

8. a. sodium; chloride;
   b. nutritional; c. electrolyte;
   d. fluid volume
9. depletion of electrolytes in the GI tract
10. irrigating with small amounts of saline, changing the client's position, and introducing a small amount of air and listening with a stethoscope for a "whoosh" sound
11. to determine kidney function. Also, it can be an indication of overhydration. When fluids—orally and parenterally—are being pushed and urine output is low, overhydration can occur.
12. to inflate the lungs and promote effective gas (O_2 and CO_2 exchange

8. Mr. Drum received intravenous fluids containing dextrose, saline, and lactated Ringer's for:
   a. Replacing _____ and _____ loss
   b. Maintaining _____ needs
   c. Maintaining _____ balance
   d. Replacing and maintaining * _____

9. Frequent irrigations of the gastric tube with a large quantity of water might have what effect? * _____
   _____

10. The three methods used to maintain the patency of Mr. Drum's gastric tube are * _____
    _____

11. Why is it important to assess Mr. Drum's urine output pre- and postoperatively? * _____
    _____
    _____

12. Why is it important for Mr. Drum to cough and deep breathe after surgery? _____
    * _____

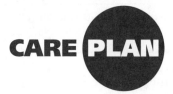

Client Management

Assessment Factors

▶ Clients undergoing gastrointestinal surgery are at an increased risk for fluid and electrolyte disturbances. Preexisting health status and medications further increase the potential risk for fluid and electrolyte disturbances. Clients with preexisting cardiac, pulmonary, endocrine, and renal disease who have gastrointestinal surgery add further challenges. Uncorrected preoperative hypovolemia and anemia may increase the risk of fluid and electrolyte disturbances postoperatively.

▶ Astute assessments and early interventions improve the client's recovery rate and decrease postoperative complications. Fluid and electrolyte imbalances may have deleterious effects on cardiac conductivity, contractility, and rhythm. Pulmonary gas exchange and renal tissue perfusion are also affected by fluid and electrolyte imbalances. Gastrointestinal intubation tubes are used postoperatively to decompress the stomach and intestines to prevent abdominal distension and prevent or relieve nausea and vomiting. The amount of GI drainage must be considered when assessing fluid and electrolyte balance.

▶ To reduce the client's risk for postoperative complications, assess vital signs with close attention to blood pressure and pulse rate, rhythm, and volume. Decreased fluid volume causes hypotension, orthostatic hypotension, decreased pulse pressure, and reflex tachycardia. Potassium disturbances may cause cardiac conduction and rhythm disturbances. Assess peripheral pulses for presence and quality. Hypovolemic states may decrease peripheral pulse quality and may ultimately lead to peripheral thrombosis in extreme states.

▶ Auscultate cardiac sounds for presence or worsening of an S_4, which may indicate an overstretched myocardium from a fluid volume excess. Check respirations every 2 hours or more frequently if indicated. Hypoventilation may occur as a result of the decreased rate and depth of respirations due to pain from the abdominal incision and the side effects of anesthesia and pain medications. Ausculate lungs for rales or crackles, which indicate retention of fluid in the alveoli. Frequent coughing and deep breathing will expand the lung alveoli, help prevent the occurrence and buildup of pulmonary secretions, and prevent atelectasis.

▶ Measure intake and output hourly in the acute stage and every 8 hours for clients who have stabilized. Careful monitoring of intake and output is essential to ascertain the client's ongoing fluid volume status. Daily weights are essential for monitoring the overall fluid volume status. Urinary output relative to specific gravity also helps determine the adequacy of the client's renal perfusion.

▶ Assess skin turgor at least every 8 hours: Hot, dry, scaly skin with poor turgor indicates a fluid volume deficit. Sacral and/or peripheral edema may indicate a fluid volume excess. Assess serum electrolytes daily and more frequently according to the client's overall health status. Low potassium (hypokalemia) levels may indicate excess diuresis, inadequate replacement, or postoperative excess antidiuretic hormone release. High potassium levels (hyperkalemia) may indicate excess potassium administration or impaired renal tubule function even when the total output is adequate in volume. Monitor creatinine/BUN and hemoglobin-hematocrit ratios as an indicator of fluid volume status as well as impaired renal functioning. Creatinine/ BUN ratios greater than 1:20 indicate a fluid volume deficit.

Hemoglobin-hematocrit ratios greater than 1:3 also indicate a fluid volume deficit.

▶ Ascertain current and preoperative medication regimes. Potassium-wasting diuretics such as HydroDiuril may further aggravate low potassium levels. Potassium-sparing diuretics such as aldactone may precipitate or further aggravate high potassium levels. Clients receiving steroids also need close monitoring of potassium. Steroids may cause or aggravate hypokalemia and hypernatremia as well as increase fluid retention.

▶ Assess client's bowel sounds. Oral fluids and foods are not introduced postoperatively until bowel sounds have returned. Be sure to turn off the suction to GI intubation tubes before auscultation of the abdomen.

▶ Maintain patency of GI tubes to ensure proper functioning. Irrigating GI tubes with normal saline or air every 2 hours will help ensure their patency. Proper location of gastric tubes may be determined by auscultating the stomach for a "whoosh" sound while injecting air into the tube. Changing the client's position frequently helps to prevent the tube lumen from lodging against the gastric mucosa.

▶ Assess the client's mental status pre- and postoperatively. Changes in mental status reflecting irritability and confusion may be a primary indicator of a fluid volume excess or deficit. Left untreated, the client's condition may deteriorate to the point of seizures or coma.

▶ Assess blood glucose for clients with preexisting hyperadrenal secretions and diabetes mellitus. Uncontrolled hyperglycemia will cause osmotic diuresis and fluid volume deficit.

Diagnosis 1

Ineffective airway clearance related to pain, ineffective coughing, deep breathing, and viscous mucous secretions.

Interventions and Rationale

1. Elevate head of bed 45°–90° and change every 2 hours to promote lung expansion and take advantage of gravity decreasing diaphragmatic pressure.

2. Encourage coughing and deep breathing hourly while awake, and wake every 2–4 hours during sleeping hours, to improve alveolar expansion, mobilize secretions, and prevent atelectasis.

3. Splint abdominal incision to decrease pain and maximize effects of coughing and deep breathing exercises. (Administer pain medication as often as needed.)

4. Suction orally and/or nasotracheally to clear airway.

5. Auscultate lung fields for rales (crackles) and respiratory movement.

6. Observe for signs of respiratory distress—tachypnea, restlessness, anxiety, moistness of mucous membranes, and use of accessory muscles of breathing.

7. Maintain adequate hydration to liquify and mobilize pulmonary secretions.

8. Provide opportunities for rest to prevent fatigue and facilitate coughing and deep breathing.

Diagnosis 2

Fluid volume deficit related to GI loss, decreased fluid intake, and fluid volume shift.

Interventions and Rationale

1. Monitor intake and output at least every 8 hours and weigh daily to determine changes in fluid volume. In normovolemic clients, intake should be approximately 500 mL more than output in a 24-hour period. For hypovolemic clients intake should be greater than 500 mL for the total output in 24 hours. Hypervolemic clients should have an output equal to or greater than their intake.

2. Take blood pressure and pulse (include orthostatics) every 4 hours or more frequently if client is unstable. Hypovolemic clients will have reflex tachycardia and hypotension. A blood pressure decrease of more than 20 mm Hg systolic or a pulse increase of more than 10 beats per minute with position changes indicate hypovolemia.

3. Check mucous membranes and skin turgor. Poor skin turgor with dry scaly skin and dry mucous membranes indicates a fluid volume deficit.

4. Check temperature every 4 hours. Body water acts as a coolant and temperature increases as body water decreases.

5. Monitor for peripheral and sacral edema to determine fluid shifts from ECF to ICF volume.

6. Palpate peripheral pulses every 4 hours for presence and volume. Hypovolemia decreases the volume of peripheral pulses.

7. Assess creatinine/BUN and Hgb-Hct ratios for hemoconcentration which indicates hypovolemia versus renal failure.

8. Assess serum potassium and sodium to determine changes. Hyperkalemia and hypernatremia may be early indicators of decreased body waters.

9. Measure urine specific gravity every 8 hours as the fluid volume decreases, unless there is renal failure.

10. Note medications that can alter fluid status and electrolyte alterations such as diuretics, insulin, and steroids.

Diagnosis 3

Pain related to trauma of abdominal surgery, decreased or absent bowel sounds, and decreased GI motility.

Interventions and Rationale

1. Ascertain cause of pain and treat accordingly. Medicate for surgical wound pain. Ascertain and maintain the correct functioning of GI tubes to decrease distention, nausea, and vomiting.

2. Evaluate client's response and attitude to pain. Determine pain characteristics and degree of pain; use a 0–10 scale. Observe verbal and nonverbal cues. Explore cultural aspects of pain and methods of control.

3. Medicate for pain to enhance effectiveness of ambulation, coughing, and deep breathing exercises.

4. Use diversional activities to increase pain threshold, e.g., visitors, television, calm environment, relaxation exercises, and reading.

Evaluation/Outcome

1. Evaluate that the source of the ECFV problem has been eliminated or controlled.

2. Evaluate the effectiveness of interventions (fluid replacement therapy, medications, pain control measures, etc.) in balancing fluid needs and promoting comfort.

3. Monitor intake and output for effective regulation of fluid and electrolyte replacement.

4. Monitor vital signs (particularly BP and pulse) for stability or indications of a fluid imbalance.

5. Evaluate mucous membranes and skin turgor for appropriate oxygenation and return to normal pink status.

6. Monitor creatinine/BUN and Hbg-Hct ratios for return to normal range.

7. Monitor electrolyte (Na, Cl, K, Ca) and blood gas levels to confirm fluid and electrolyte balance.

8. Monitor urine specific gravity to detect potential renal problems.

9. Evaluate effectiveness of medications (diuretics, insulin, steroids, etc.) in maintaining fluid balance.

CHAPTER
23

Renal Failure: Hemodialysis, Peritoneal Dialysis, and Continuous Renal Replacement Therapy

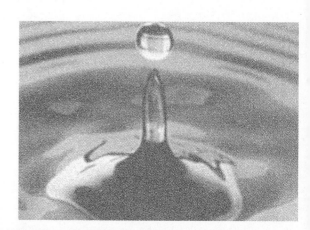

OBJECTIVES

Upon completion of this chapter, the reader should be able to:

- Discuss the physiologic changes related to acute and chronic renal failure.
- Identify the etiologic factors associated with acute and chronic renal failure.
- Discuss common fluid, electrolyte, and acid-base imbalances in renal failure.
- Define the three types of clinical management for renal failure.
- Discuss the purposes for continuous renal replacement therapy (CRRT), hemodialysis, and peritoneal dialysis.
- Discuss the important assessment factors associated with the clinical management of renal failure.

(continued on next page)

OBJECTIVES (Continued)

● **Describe selected complications associated with the clinical management of renal failure.**

● **List selected diagnoses and interventions with rationales for clients with renal failure.**

▶ INTRODUCTION

Renal failure is the inability of the kidneys to excrete the by-products of cell metabolism and normal amounts of body water. Renal failure is classified as acute or chronic. *Acute renal failure (ARF)* results from an acute insult, primarily ischemia, toxicity, or obstruction. *Chronic renal failure (CRF)* frequently results from a disease process that affects the renal parenchyma and eventually causes cessation of renal function.

ANSWER COLUMN

1 renal failure

1

The term that describes the kidneys' inability to excrete waste products and the normal amounts of body water is

* _____ .

▶ PATHOPHYSIOLOGY

Acute renal failure (ARF) may progress through four phases: initial, oliguric, diuretic, and recovery. The characteristics of these four phases are described in Table 23-1.

2

2 oliguric; diuretic; dehydration (if you answered electrolyte loss, true, but the greatest risk is ECFV deficit or dehydration)

When the urinary volume is less than 400 mL/day and azotemia is present, the client is in the _____ phase.

If a sudden increase in urine output occurs (1.5 liters or more per day), the client is in the _____ phase. In the diuretic phase the greatest risk is _____ .

Table 23-1

Phases of ARF

Phases	Characteristics
Initial	This phase begins when the insult occurs and continues until signs of azotemia and/or oliguria appear.
Oliguric	Urine output is less than 400 mL/day. BUN and creatinine are markedly elevated. Dialysis is initiated in this phase.
Diuretic	It starts with a sudden increase in urine output, 1.5 liters (1500 mL) or more per day. Nephrons do not concentrate urine sufficiently to conserve electrolytes and water. Risk of dehydration and death are high. This phase can continue for days to weeks.
Recovery	This phase is noted by a decrease in azotemia with kidneys showing an ability to concentrate urine. It may last from weeks to months.

3 recovery phase

3

The phase of ARF in which the kidneys can concentrate urine and azotemia is less apparent is called the *_____ .

    Chronic renal failure (CRF) is defined as insidious, progressive loss of renal function that is irreversible. The three stages of CRF are (1) decreased renal reserve, (2) renal insufficiency, and (3) end-stage renal disease (ESRD). Table 23-2 lists the three stages and the pathophysiologic factors associated with these stages.

4 decreased renal reserve, renal insufficiency, and end-stage renal disease

4

The three stages of chronic renal failure are *_____

_____

5

In stage I, renal function is _____ % of normal; in stage II, renal function is _____ % of normal; and in stage III, renal function is _____ % of normal.

5 40-70; 20-40; <15

6

Indicate the blood urea nitrogen (BUN) and serum creatinine response to the three stages of CRF:
    a. Stage I: BUN _____ , creatinine _____
    b. Stage II: BUN _____ , creatinine _____
    c. Stage III: BUN *_____ , creatinine *_____

6
  a. normal; normal;
  b. increased; increased;
  c. markedly elevated;
  markedly elevated

Table 23-2

Stages of CRF

Stages	Pathophysiologic Factors
Stage I: decreased renal reserve	Residual renal function is 40–70% of the normal kidney function. Excretory and regulatory renal functions are intact. Renal laboratory studies are asymptomatic (BUN and serum creatinine are normal). At least a 50–60% loss of renal function is required before signs of renal failure are evident. No symptoms are evident until there is a loss of at least 80% renal function.
Stage II: renal insufficiency	Residual renal function is 20–40% of the normal kidney function. There is a decrease in the glomerular filtration rate (GFR), solute clearance, ability to concentrate urine, and hormone secretion. Renal laboratory studies reveal a rising BUN and serum creatinine, mild azotemia, polyuria, nocturia, and anemia. Signs and symptoms become more severe if the kidneys are stressed, i.e., fluid volume depletion or exposure to a nephrotic substance.
Stage III: end-stage renal disease (ESRD)	Residual renal function is <15% of the normal kidney function. Excretory, regulatory, and hormonal renal functions are severely impaired and unable to maintain homeostasis. Renal laboratory studies and physical symptoms reveal markedly elevated BUN and serum creatinine levels. Anemia, hyperphosphatemia, hypocalcemia, metabolic acidosis, hyperuricemia, hyperkalemia, fluid overload, usually oliguric, and urine osmolality similar to serum osmolality. A uremic syndrome develops and all body systems are affected by renal failure. Mortality rate is 100% if peritoneal dialysis, hemodialysis, or renal transplant is not implemented.

7

Hyperkalemia, hyperphosphatemia, hypocalcemia, and metabolic acidosis occur frequently with which stage of CRF?

_____

7   stage III

) ETIOLOGY

The causes of ARF are listed in three categories: ischemia, toxicity, and obstruction. Table 23-3 lists examples of the causes, with contributing problems.

Table 23-3

Causes of ARF

Ischemia	Toxicity	Obstruction

Dehydration
Shock:
  Distributive/sepsis
  Hypovolemic/hemorrhagic
  Cardiogenic
	Antibiotics:
	  Aminoglycosides
	  Penicillins
	  Cephalosporins
	Nonsteroidal anti-inflammatory drugs
	Organic compounds:
	  Carbon tetrachloride
	  Methyl alcohol
	Miscellaneous:
	  Myoglobin, transfusion reactions
		Prerenal:
		  Arterial emboli
		  Aneurysm
		Postrenal:
		  Ureteral obstruction
		  Bladder obstruction
		  Catheter obstruction

8 ischemia, toxicity, and
   obstruction

8
Acute renal failure usually results from insult to the kidney causing a rapid deterioration of renal function. The three major categories of the causes of ARF are *_____ .

9 shock; antibiotics, e.g.,
   aminoglycosides; arterial
   emboli (prerenal) or
   ureteral obstruction
   (postrenal)

9
Give examples of the following major causes of ARF:
Ischemia: _____
Toxicity: _____
Obstruction: *_____

Causes of CRF are listed in Table 23-4.

10 pyelonephritis;
    glomerulonephritis

10
An example of an infectious disease causing CRF is _____ .
A major cause of end-stage renal failure (ESRF) is _____ .

11 diabetes mellitus
12 diabetes mellitus, diabetes
    insipidus, hepatorenal
    syndrome, hypertensive
    nephropathy, and systemic
    lupus erythematosus
    (others: scleroderma,
    amyloidosis)

11
Approximately 25% of the clients with ESRD have the systemic chronic disease *_____ .

12
Name five systemic diseases that can lead to ESRD. *_____

Table 23-4

Causes of CRF

Etiology	Examples
Congenital/developmental disorders	Bilateral renal hypoplasia Fused kidney Ectopic or displaced kidney Bilateral renal dysplasia
Cystic disorders	Polycystic kidney disease Medullary cystic kidney disease
Tubular disorders	Renal tubular acidosis (RTA) Fanconi's syndrome
Glomerular disorder	Glomerulonephritis (major cause of ESRD)
Neoplasms	Benign tumor Malignant tumor Wilm's tumor
Infectious diseases	Pyelonephritis Renal tuberculosis
Obstructive disorders	Nephrolithiasis Retroperitoneal fibrosis
Systemic diseases	Diabetes mellitus (DM): approximately 25% of ESRD clients with DM. Approximately 50% of Type I DM (juvenile onset) develop ESRD within 20 years of onset of DM. Diabetes insipidus Systemic lupus erythematosus (SLE) Hepatorenal syndrome Hypertensive nephropathy Amyloidosis Scleroderma Primary hyperparathyroidism Goodpasture's syndrome Henoch-Schoenlein purpura

13

Urine output in renal failure varies. No urine output is labeled *anuria*. In ARF the cause of anuria may be prerenal or postrenal obstruction. In CRF anuria indicates total loss of parenchymal function.

13 acute renal failure; chronic
renal failure; no urine
output; prerenal or
postrenal obstruction;
total loss of parenchymal
function

ARF means *_____ .

CRF means *_____ .

Anuria, which is *_____ , differs in ARF and CRF. In ARF anuria may be the result of *_____ ,

_____ and in CRF anuria may cause

*_____ .

14

Normal urine output exceeds 30 mL/h. Urine output of less than 400–500 mL per 24 hours is *oliguria*. No urine output is called

_____ .

14 anuria

In ARF ischemia and nephrotoxicity are the causes of oliguria, whereas in CRF oliguria indicates a decline in parenchymal function.

15

Symptoms of ARF and CRF appear when renal function decreases to at least 20%. When renal function decreases to less than 15%, death results if dialysis treatment is not initiated.

Indicate which of the following problems contribute to acute and chronic renal failure by using ARF for acute renal failure and CRF for chronic renal failure.

_____ a. Severe dehydration (hypovolemia)
_____ b. Diabetes mellitus
_____ c. Bladder obstruction
_____ d. Glomerulonephritis
_____ e. Hypertension nephropathy
_____ f. Severe fluid volume deficit
_____ g. Systemic lupus erythematosus
_____ h. Aminoglycoside therapy
_____ i. Pyelonephritis
_____ j. Nephrosclerosis
_____ k. Carbon tetrachloride
_____ l. Sepsis

15 a. ARF; b. CRF; c. ARF; d. CRF;
e. CRF; f. ARF; g. CRF; h. ARF;
i. CRF; j. CRF; k. ARF; l. ARF

▶ CLINICAL MANIFESTATIONS

16

Two measurements of nitrogenous waste products, by-products of protein metabolism, are BUN and creatinine. A rise in the level of BUN and creatinine is known as azotemia.

The two by-products of protein metabolism or nitrogenous waste products are *_____ . Azotemia occurs when *_____ .

16 BUN and creatinine; BUN and creatinine levels rise

17

In ARF, the earliest sign after the insult is a rise in the BUN and serum creatinine accompanied by oliguria or nonoliguria.

The two renal laboratory results that can indicate an early sign of ARF are *_____ .

17 increased BUN and increased serum creatinine

The earliest manifestations of the disease that may lead to CRF are hematuria and proteinuria. At least 50–60% loss of renal tissue is required before signs are evident. If undetected, renal disease progresses, renal function degenerates, and azotemia ensues. No symptoms are evident until loss of renal tissue is at least 80%.

18

In ARF oliguria is usually caused by _____ and _____ . In CRF oliguria indicates *_____ .

In CRF two early manifestations of renal disease are

_____ .

18 ischemia and nephrotoxicity; a decline in parenchymal function; hematuria and proteinuria

Fluid, Electrolyte, and Acid-Base Imbalances

Table 23-5 outlines the fluid, electrolyte, and acid-base changes that occur in renal failure and lists the rationale for the signs and symptoms. Study the table carefully, noting the changes that occur.

19

In renal failure fluid overload can occur from the following pathologic response:

a. *_____
b. *_____
c. *_____

19 a. decreased urine output; b. sodium retention; c. reduced oncotic pressure

20 elevated jugular venous pressure, pitting edema, weight gain, increased blood pressure, dyspnea, and increased central venous pressure (others: moist rales, pulmonary edema, elevated pulmonary artery, and wedge pressures)

20

Name six symptoms of fluid overload (noninvasive and invasive).

*_____

_____

Table 23-5

Fluid, Electrolyte, and Acid-Base Imbalances in Renal Failure

Imbalances	Rationale	Signs and Symptoms
Fluid Overload Decreased urine output	Inability of the kidneys to concentrate, dilute, and excrete urine with normal or excessive intake of fluid. When creatinine clearance is less than 4–5 mL/min, volume overload is usually the major problem.	Noninvasive: elevated jugular venous pressure Pitting edema: preorbital, hands, feet, sacral, anasarca
Sodium retention	Increased tubular reabsorption of sodium due to reduced renal perfusion and/or increased renin-angiotensin-aldosterone secretion. Occurs in ischemia and malignant hypertension.	Increased blood pressure Weight gain Moist rales Dyspnea Pulmonary edema
Reduced oncotic pressure	Loss of intravascular protein through damaged glomeruli leads to decreased intravascular volume. ADH secretion increases water retention to maintain intravascular volume. Continued protein loss decreases oncotic pressure in capillaries and causes water to move into the interstitial space. Seen in nephrotic syndrome, glomerular diseases, and liver ascites.	Invasive: increased central venous pressure Elevated pulmonary artery and wedge pressure
Potassium Excess Potassium retention	*Hyperkalemia* Inability of the kidneys to excrete potassium in severe oliguric and anuric states.	Noninvasive: weakness, parathesia Nausea, vomiting ECG: elevated T wave Tachycardia Cardiac arrest
Cellular injury	Massive tissue injury, acidosis, and protein catabolism cause potassium to leave cells.	Invasive: serum K >5.3mEq/L Decreased pH (arterial blood) Decreased serum CO_2 and arterial HCO_3

(continues on the following page)

Table 23-5

(Continued)

Imbalances	Rationale	Signs and Symptoms
Potassium Deficit Potassium loss	*Hypokalemia* Excessive loss of GI secretions or excessive loss in dialysis.	Noninvasive: muscle weakness Abdominal distention Arrhythmia
Diuretic phase of ARF	Excessive loss of electrolytes and water due to the kidneys' inability to concentrate urine.	Anorexia, N/V ECG: flat or inverted T wave, prominent U wave, and AV block
Renal tubular acidosis	Nonoliguric azotemia causes excretion of K^+. Present in Fanconi's syndrome, nephrotic syndrome, multiple myeloma, cirrhosis, and some drug toxicities.	Invasive: serum K <3.5 mEq/L
Sodium Excess Increased tubular sodium absorption	*Hypernatremia* With decreased intravascular volume, aldosterone secretion increases sodium retention to improve intravascular volume. May be seen in nephrotic syndrome and liver ascites.	Noninvasive: edema Dry tongue Tachycardia Thirst Weight gain Increased BP
Dietary sodium ingestion	Increased dietary ingestion of sodium, especially in anuric states.	Invasive: serum Na >146 mEq/L
Sodium Deficit Sodium loss	*Hyponatremia* Excessive loss of gastrointestinal secretion through suction, vomiting, and diarrhea.	Noninvasive: decreased skin turgor Decreased BP
Diuretic phase of ARF	Excessive loss of electrolytes and water because of the kidneys' inability to concentrate urine.	Rapid pulse Dry mucous membrane Muscle weakness Invasive: serum Na <130 mEq/L
Excessive fluid intake	Increased fluid intake with oliguria or anuria present dilutes the serum sodium level.	
Metabolic acidosis	Sodium shifts into cells as potassium shifts to plasma during acidosis.	

(continues on the following page)

Table 23-5

Fluid, Electrolyte, and Acid-Base Imbalances in Renal Failure *(Continued)*

Imbalances	Rationale	Signs and Symptoms
Phosphorus Excess Phosphorus (phosphate) retention	*Hyperphosphatemia* Occurs because of decreased renal phosphate excretion, which increases metabolic acidosis. Phosphorus affects serum calcium level by altering the balance of their reciprocal relationships. Parathyroid hormone (PTH) (parathormone) enhances phosphorus or phosphate excretion in the urine.	Noninvasive: nausea and diarrhea Tachycardia Tetany with low Ca Hyperreflexia Muscle weakness Flaccid paralysis Invasive: serum P >4.5 mg/dL or >2.6 mEq/L
Calcium Deficit Increased phosphorus retention	*Hypocalcemia* Decreases the balance between calcium and phosphorus. PTH demineralizes the bone to increase serum calcium. Untreated hypocalcemia and hyperphosphatemia lead to renal osteodystrophy and metastatic calcification (deposits of calcium phosphate crystals in soft tissues). The goal is to maintain serum Ca-P product of approximately 40 mg/mL.	Noninvasive: tetany Muscle twitching Tingling Carpopedal spasm Laryngeal spasm Abdominal cramps Muscle cramps Decreased clotting Cardiac dysrhythmias Positive Chvostek sign Positive Trousseau sign
Decreased absorption of calcium from intestines	Impaired vitamin D activity from renal impairment causes reduced calcium absorption.	Invasive: serum Ca <9 mg/dL or <4.5 mEq/L PTH >375 mEq/mL Ca-P product >70 mg/dL
Metabolic Acidosis Hydrogen ion retention	Inability of kidneys to excrete daily hydrogen ion load.	Noninvasive: weakness Lassitude; Increased respiration (rate and depth)
Reduced buffering mechanisms in tubules	Refer to Chapter 11, on renal regulatory mechanisms.	Restlessness Flushed skin

(continues on the following page)

Table 23-5

(Continued)

Imbalances	Rationale	Signs and Symptoms
Ammonia	Reduced nephron function inhibits conversion of ammonia and HCl to NH_4Cl for excretion.	Invasive: pH <7.35 HCO_3 <24 mEq/L Anion gap >16 mEq/L
Phosphate salts	Reduced nephron function inhibits the combination of hydrogen ion with $NaHPO_4$ to form NaH_2PO_4 for excretion.	
Bicarbonate (HCO_3)	With damaged nephrons, less HCO_3 is regenerated and reabsorbed in the tubules.	
Retention of metabolic acids	Inability of the kidneys to excrete uric, sulfuric, phosphate, and other acids of metabolism.	
Lactic acid formation	Occurs from tissue hypoxemia from an ischemic insult.	
Increased fat breakdown	Malnutrition from decreased nutritional intake causes accumulation of ketone acids.	
Urine Sodium and Osmolality		
Urine sodium	Ischemic state increases ADH and aldosterone secretions. Renal efforts to conserve sodium show fewer Na ions in urine, <20 mEq. However, damaged nephrons cannot filter sufficiently; therefore it is possible that urine sodium level >20 mEq.	
Urine osmolality	Ischemic state increases renal filtration; thus urine osmolality >500 mOsm/kg/H_2O. Injured nephrons with impaired filtration have urine osmolality similar to plasma, 290 mOsm/kg/H_2O.	

21 severe oligura and anuria; ventricular tachycardia and cardiac arrest

22 a. loss of GI secretions or from dialysis; b. diuretic phase of ARF; c. renal tubular acidosis

23 a. increased tubular absorption; b. dietary ingestion

24 a. loss of GI secretions; b. diuretic phase of ARF; c. excessive fluid intake; d. metabolic acidosis

25 decreased excretion of phosphate; hypocalcemia or calcium loss (deficit)

26 muscle twitching, tingling, and laryngeal spasms (also carpopedal spasm and positive Chvostek and Trousseau's signs); metabolic acidosis

27 cardiac muscle irritability

21

A potassium excess occurs primarily with which urinary symptoms? *_____ .

A potassium excess can cause cardiac muscle to exhibit which two symptoms? *_____

22

Name the conditions that may cause potassium deficits.

a. *_____

b. *_____

c. *_____

23

Name the conditions that may cause sodium excess.

a. *_____

b. *_____

24

Name the conditions that may cause sodium deficits.

a. *_____

b. *_____

c. *_____

d. *_____

25

An excess serum phosphorus/phosphate level in renal failure is caused by *_____ . The retention of phosphorus/phosphate alters the balance between calcium and phosphorus. The result of the calcium imbalance is _____ .

26

Calcium deficit results in symptoms of tetany, three of which are

*_____

In which acid-base imbalance are the symptoms of tetany decreased? *_____ .

27

Calcium deficits enhance the toxic effect of a high serum potassium by increasing cardiac muscle irritability.

When a low serum calcium exists, the serum potassium must be monitored to prevent *_____ .

28
Name the metabolic changes associated with renal failure that cause metabolic acidosis.

a. *_____ ⎯ _____

b. *_____

c. *_____

d. *_____

e. *_____

28 a. hydrogen ion retention; b. reduction of buffering mechanisms; c. retention of metabolic acids; d. lactic acid formation; e. increased breakdown of fats

29
What respiratory symptom occurs in metabolic acidosis? *_____

29 an increased respiratory rate and depth or Kussmaul breathing

30
Two urinary tests for assessing damaged nephrons are
*_____ .

30 urine sodium and urine osmolality

31
A low urine sodium indicates increased ADH and aldosterone secretions. Nephrons damaged by ischemia or toxins cannot filter sufficiently and the urine sodium can be _____ .

31 increased

32
The urine osmolality measures the kidneys' ability to dilute and concentrate urine. Damaged nephrons impair filtration and decrease the kidneys' ability to concentrate urine. As a result of damaged nephrons, the urine is (diluted/concentrated) _____ .

32 diluted

Table 23-6 explains the effects of renal failure on body systems. Refer to the table as needed to answer the following frames.

33
Which of the following body systems are affected by renal failure?

( ) a. Cardiovascular

( ) b. Respiratory

( ) c. Eye

( ) d. Neurologic

( ) e. Gastrointestinal

( ) f. Integumentary

( ) g. Musculoskeletal

( ) h. Endocrine

( ) i. Hematologic

33 a, b, d, e, f, g, h, i

Table 23-6

Systemic Effects of Renal Failure

Body Systems	Rationale
Neurologic	Uremic waste products cause slow neural conduction. Changes in personality, thought processes, levels of consciousness, and seizures can occur.
Cardiovascular	Fluid retention causes fluid overload, hypertension, and cardiac hypertrophy. Electrolyte imbalance causes arrhythmias. Uremic waste products can irritate the pericardium and lead to pericarditis and cardiac tamponade.
Respiratory	Fluid retention causes pulmonary edema. Thick bronchial secretions and impaired immune response increase susceptibility to bacterial infections.
Gastrointestinal	Ulcerations can develop anywhere in the mucosa of the GI tract from the breakdown of urea to ammonia. Metallic taste in mouth, hiccups, indigestion, nausea, and urine smell to breath from buildup of uremic waste products are added effects.
Hematologic	Failure of the kidneys to secrete erythropoietin results in decreased red cell production and anemia. Platelet survival is diminished and bleeding tendencies are increased. Immune deficiency develops from uremic waste products.
Musculoskeletal	Brittle bones and metastatic calcification result from bone demineralization in response to phosphorus and calcium imbalance.
Endocrine	Secondary hyperparathyroidism can develop from phosphorus and calcium imbalances. Sexual and menstrual dysfunctions are the result. Growth and mental retardation occur in children and carbohydrate and lipoprotein metabolism are altered.
Integumentary	Uremic waste products cause pruritis and dryness. Retained pigments and anemia give the skin a bronze cast.

❚ CLINICAL MANAGEMENT: DIALYSIS

Dialysis is the process of filtrating uremic waste products and excess body fluid through a semipermeable membrane to restore body homeostasis.

Diffusion is the movement of molecules/solutes in a solution. In diffusion the rate of movement across the permeable membrane is greater from the areas of higher concentration to the areas of lower concentration.

Osmosis is the movement of water molecules across a semipermeable membrane from an area of higher water concentration to an area of lower water concentration.

Ultrafiltration is the pressure gradient that enhances the movement of water molecules across the semipermeable membrane.

34

The movement of molecules across a semipermeable membrane from an area of higher concentration to an area of lower concentration is _____ .

The pressure gradient that enhances the movement of water molecules is called _____ .

The movement of water molecules across a semipermeable membrane from an area of higher water concentration to one of lower water concentration is called _____ .

34 diffusion; ultrafiltration; osmosis

35

Types of dialysis therapy are continuous renal replacement therapy (CRRT), hemodialysis, and peritoneal dialysis.

The objectives for all these types are to restore electrolyte balance, to remove uremic waste products, and to restore the patient's dry weight. *Dry weight* is normal body weight without excess fluid.

Name two goals of dialysis. *_____

35 to restore electrolyte balance and to remove uremic waste products (also to restore client's dry weight)

Continuous Renal Replacement Therapy

36

The type of dialysis most effective in the treatment of ARF is continuous renal replacement therapy (CRRT). In CRRT, an extracorporeal circuit is created with arterial to venous blood flow using the client's mean arterial pressure (MAP) as the primary driving force. This acute treatment is administered in the ICU setting.

For CRRT, the client's *_____ is used as the primary driving force for creating the arterial to venous blood flow.

36 mean arterial pressure (MAP)

37

CRRT uses a hemofilter which is a very porous blood filter with a semipermeable membrane that is positioned in an extracorporeal circuit with arterial outflow to venous return access.

A very porous blood filter with a semipermeable membrane used in CRRT is called a _____ .

37 hemofilter

38

Unlike hemodialysis, CRRT requires cannulation of both an artery and a vein for extracorporeal blood flow.

Types of CRRT are (1) slow continuous ultrafiltration (SCUF), (2) continuous arteriovenous hemofiltration (CAVH), and (3) continuous arteriovenous hemodialysis (CAVHD).

CRRT requires cannulation in both an _____ and a _____ .

38 artery; vein

39 slow continuous ultrafiltration, continuous arteriovenous hemofiltration, and continuous arteriovenous hemodialysis

39

The three types of CRRT are *_____

_____ .

Indications for CRRT in the ICU setting include:

1. Clients with CRF with a preexisting vascular access who are clinically unable to tolerate routine hemodialysis procedures, such as with acute pulmonary edema, CHF, recent gastrointestinal bleeding, and/or cardiogenic shock.

2. Clients with ARF who are too hemodynamically unstable for aggressive hemodialysis and for whom peritoneal dialysis is contraindicated. Examples include postoperative cardiac bypass surgery, recent myocardial infarction, sepsis, ARDS, and postoperative vascular bypass surgery.

3. Clients with ARF who are very catabolic and require daily clearance of uremic toxins and electrolyte and bicarbonate replacements.

4. Clients with oliguria who require large quantities of IV fluids either as medication or hyperalimentation.

40

Indicate which clients with the following clinical health problems might be candidates for CRRT:

( ) a. Has CRF and cardiogenic shock occurs
( ) b. Has ARF and has an acute myocardial infarction
( ) c. Has an early stage of pyelonephritis
( ) d. Has ARF and has blood uremic toxins
( ) e. Has oliguria and requires large amounts IV therapy
( ) f. Has polyuria and does not receive sufficient fluids

40 a, b, d, e

41

Hemodialysis and peritoneal dialysis are similar in the following ways: Both use dialysate, which is a solution that contains electrolytes approximating normal plasma, and both use a semipermeable membrane.

List two ways in which hemodialysis and peritoneal dialysis are similar. *_____

Hemodialysis

42

In hemodialysis the artificial kidney (AK) is a semipermeable membrane made of a cellophanelike material through which only molecules of a particular size can diffuse.

The semipermeable membrane of the artificial kidney is a membrane through which only molecules of a *_____

_____ .

43

The dialysate solution is prepared in the delivery system, where it is mixed to the correct concentration, heated, and pumped into the artificial kidney.

List the functions of the delivery system:

a. *_____
b. *_____
c. *_____

44

Dialysate for hemodialysis contains five basic components: calcium chloride, magnesium chloride, potassium chloride, sodium chloride, and sodium acetate or bicarbonate. The concentration of these iso-osmolar/isotonic components resembles low plasma concentrations, but it can be prepared to correct an electrolyte or acid-base imbalance.

If a client has a potassium excess, the dialysate can be prepared with low potassium. If a client has metabolic acidosis, acetate or bicarbonate in dialysate can be used.

Dialysate can be individualized for correcting imbalances of _____ and _____ .

---

41 They both use dialysate similar in composition to normal plasma, and they both use a semipermeable membrane.

42 particular size can diffuse

43 a. mixes dialysate in the correct concentration; b. heats dialysate; c. pumps dialysate

44 electrolytes or potassium; acid-base or acidosis

45

There are no uremic waste products in the dialysate. Therefore urea, creatinine, and other metabolic waste products diffuse rapidly from the blood across the membrane into the dialysate.

Uremic waste products rapidly diffuse from the _____ into the _____ .

45 blood; dialysate

46

Vascular access to the client's bloodstream must be obtained to initiate hemodialysis. This access is surgically created or obtained by catheterizing a large vein.

To initiate hemodialysis, vascular access to the _____ must be obtained.

46 bloodstream

47

During hemodialysis blood is pumped through tubing to the membranes of the AK. Two common types of AK design are the flat plate and hollow fiber. The flat plate is a stack of plastic plates with two membranes between each plate. Blood flows between these membranes. The hollow fiber has thousands of tiny hairlike fibers through which blood flows.

By using the flat-plate AK blood flows *_____ .
With the hollow-fiber AK blood flows *_____ .

47 between the membranes; through the tiny hairlike fibers

48

A complication of hemodialysis is blood clotting in the blood lines and AK. This can be prevented by administering heparin, an anticoagulant, during the procedure.

Heparin administered during hemodialysis prevents _____ .

48 clotting

49

The delivery system pumps dialysate through the AK and around membranes. A negative pressure gradient, created by the delivery system, pulls excess water from the blood across the semipermeable membrane. A positive pressure gradient that pushes excess water across the membrane can occur. Ultrafiltration results and excess fluid is removed from the client's bloodstream.

A negative pressure gradient results from *_____

_____ .

Excess fluid is removed from the client by _____ .

49 the pull of water across the semipermeable membrane; ultrafiltration

50

the normal body weight without excess fluid; cardiovascular

50

The goal of ultrafiltration is to obtain the client's dry weight and prevent cardiovascular complications such as hypertension, pulmonary edema, and ventricular hypertrophy.

    Dry weight is *_____ .

Maintaining the client's dry weight prevents _____ complications.

51

uremic waste products; electrolyte balance; excess fluid

51

Hemodialysis treatment takes 3–4 hours to complete. The results should be the removal of *_____ , restoration of *_____ , and removal of *_____ .

    Hemodialysis is done on a constant basis for client with CRF and intermittently for those in ARF until renal function improves.

Peritoneal Dialysis

52

peritoneum

52

In peritoneal dialysis the peritoneum that surrounds the abdominal cavity is used as the semipermeable membrane.

    The semipermeable membrane used in peritoneal dialysis is the _____ .

53

plasma; sterile

53

The dialysate for peritoneal dialysis is a sterile solution that contains similar levels of sodium, magnesium, calcium, and chloride as the plasma.

    The dialysate electrolyte levels of sodium, magnesium, calcium, and chloride are similar to _____ .

    The dialysate solution is _____ .

54

The client's potassium level may be high. Adding too much potassium to the solution could increase the hyperkalemic state OR similar answer.

54

Potassium is not included in peritoneal dialysate solutions. The health care provider prescribes the amount of potassium that can be added to the dialysate according to the client's serum potassium level.

    Why do you think potassium is not added to the solution? *_____ .

55

Acid-base balance is corrected in peritoneal dialysis by adding acetate, a bicarbonate precursor, to the dialysate solution. This buffers metabolic acids.

　　Acetate can be added to peritoneal dialysate to correct what acid-base disorder? *_____

55 metabolic acidosis

56

Ultrafiltration is accomplished in peritoneal dialysis by creating an osmotic pressure gradient with glucose. The glucose concentration in the dialysate creates a hyperosmolar solution that pulls water across the peritoneal membrane.

　　Glucose in peritoneal dialysate creates an *_____ gradient. The dialysate solution in peritoneal dialysate is

_____ .

56 osmotic pressure;
　　hyperosmolar

57

Peritoneal dialysate has four concentrations of glucose: 1.5, 2.5, 3.5, and 4.5%. The physician prescribes the concentration needed on the basis of the client's state of fluid overload. The higher the glucose concentration, the more hyperosmolar the solution. The result is more ultrafiltration.

　　More ultrafiltration occurs in peritoneal dialysis when the dialysate has a *_____ .

57 high glucose concentration

58

Peritoneal dialysis begins by inserting a catheter into the peritoneal cavity. Capillary beds within the layers of peritoneum provide an indirect access to the bloodstream for the dialysate.

　　Access for peritoneal dialysis is obtained by a _____ .

58 catheter

59

A serious complication of peritoneal dialysis is peritonitis, the result of an infection caused by the peritoneal catheter, e.g., contamination.

　　Peritonitis is a serious complication of *_____ . It is caused by an *_____ .

59 peritoneal dialysis;
　　infection associated with
　　the catheter

60

Two liters of dialysate is usually infused by gravity into the peritoneal cavity where it remains (dwells) for a prescribed time.

Infusion of fluid by gravity takes approximately 10 minutes for a 2-liter volume. The dwell or equilibration period provides time for diffusion and osmosis to occur. A typical dwell or equilibration time for acute peritoneal dialysis is 30–60 minutes; in chronic peritoneal dialysis, the dwell time is 4–6 hours. The excess fluid, electrolytes, and uremic waste products (ultrafiltrate) move through the peritoneal membrane into the dialysate. The solution is then drained from the abdomen by gravity. The drainage of 2 liters of dialysate and ultrafiltrate takes approximately 10 minutes providing that the catheter is patent.

Dialysate solution is infused by gravity into the *_____ .

How is the dialysate removed from the abdomen? *_____

61

The approximate time for infusion or inflow of solution by gravity is _____ minutes.

The time for the dialysate to dwell (equilibrate) in the peritoneal cavity for acute conditions is _____ minutes.

The approximate time for the return of dialysate and ultrafiltrate (excess fluid, electrolytes, and uremic waste products) is _____ minutes.

62

Each infusion of fresh dialysate is referred to as an exchange. The treatment plan prescribed by the nephrologist includes the dialysis regimen, combined with the method of peritoneal dialysis, dialysis solution concentration, the frequency of exchanges, and the infusion volume and prescribed dwell time.

When ordering peritoneal dialysis, four of the treatment plans that the nephrologist must prescribe are *_____

_____ .

63

When a peritoneal catheter is first inserted, heparin is added to the dialysate to maintain catheter patency by preventing the obstruction of the peritoneal catheter with fibrin and/or blood.

The purpose of heparin in the dialysate is to *_____ .

64

The amount of dialysate returned by gravity determines the amount of fluid loss from the body. The return must be

---

60 peritoneal cavity; by gravity

61 10; 30–60; 10

62 dialysis regimen, method of peritoneal dialysis, dialysis solution concentration, and frequency of exchanges (others: infusion volume and dwell or equilibration time)

63 maintain catheter patency (prevent fibrin and clot formation)

accurately measured to maintain fluid balance. If the dialysate return is more than the amount of the infusion fluid being removed, there is a fluid imbalance.

The process by which this exchange occurs is called

_____ .

64 ultrafiltration; retained

When the amount of dialysate returned is less than the amount infused, fluid is being (retained/excreted) _____ . An accurate record of these differences must be maintained.

65

If 2000 mL of dialysate is infused and 2500 mL is returned, an excess of 500 mL is being _____ .

65 ultrafiltrated or excreted; retained

If 2000 mL of dialysate is infused and 1500 mL is returned, 500 mL is being _____ .

66

Retained dialysate can be reabsorbed and can lead to a fluid overload. Symptoms of fluid overload or overhydration are increased blood pressure, dyspnea, constant irritating cough, neck vein engorgement, chest rales, and edema.

66 retention of dialysate fluid; increased blood pressure, dyspnea, neck vein engorgement, and chest rales (also edema and irritated cough)

One cause of fluid overload during peritoneal dialysis is the

* _____ .

Name four symptoms associated with fluid overload. * _____

_____

67

Excessive ultrafiltration can result in dehydration. Solutions such as 2.5% (398 mOsm/L) and 4.5% glucose dialysate (486 mOsm) or excessive exchanges can result in dehydration if not properly monitored. Symptoms of dehydration are decreased blood pressure, poor tissue turgor, tachycardia, dry mucous membranes, and hypernatremia.

67 4.5% glucose dialysate; excessive exchanges; decreased blood pressure, poor tissue turgor, and tachycardia (also dry mucous membranes)

Dehydration can result from * _____ or * _____ .

Name three symptoms of dehydration and fluid loss. * _____

_____

Table 23-7 compares the three types of dialysis treatment for renal failure. Unlike hemodialysis, CRRT is a continuous form of therapy which achieves a more stable maintenance of the volume and composition of body fluids. Rapid intercompartmental fluid shifts observed in hemodialysis are avoided and blood pressure

Table 23-7

Comparison of Hemodialysis, Peritoneal Dialysis, and CRRT

Hemodialysis	Peritoneal	CRRT
Rapid removal of fluid	Fluid removed slowly	Rapid removal of fluid
Potassium lowered quickly	Potassium lowered slowly	Allows for removal or addition of electrolytes independent of changes in total body water
Waste products removed quickly	Waste products removed at a slower rate	
Rapid removal of poisonous drugs	Inefficient for removal of poisonous drugs	
Treatment time 3–4 hours	Usual treatment process includes three to four exchanges per day	A continuous treatment process
Requires complex equipment and specialized training	Uses less complex equipment and less specialized personnel	Requires the use of a simple filter and ICU personnel
Requires vascular access	Requires no direct access to the bloodstream; causes no blood loss; used for clients with poor vascular access, i.e., children and the elderly	Requires vascular access
Requires large doses of heparin	Requires none or very small amounts of heparin	Requires the use of heparin and close monitoring for clotting in both the filter and tubing
Poorly tolerated by clients with cardiovascular disease	Minimal stress to clients with cardiovascular disease	Minimal stress for patients with cardiovascular disease
Contraindicated for clients in shock or hypotension	Can be used for clients with unstable cardiovascular status	Can be used for clients with unstable cardiovascular status
Can be used for clients with abdominal trauma	Contraindicated for clients with a colostomy, abdominal adhesions, ruptured diaphragm, or recent surgery	Can be used for clients with abdominal trauma or who are hemodynamically unstable
Cost is high	Cost effective	Cost effective
Risk of clotting increased with vascular access	Risk for peritonitis increased	Risk of clotting access increased; Risk of dehydration from inappropriate fluid replacement increased
Treatment prescribed for chronic or acute conditions	Treatment prescribed for chronic or acute conditions	Treatment is prescribed only for acute conditions and is provided only in ICU setting

instability is prevented. The solute concentration changes observed in intermittent therapy are often avoided; thus the health care provider is able to remove or add electrolytes independent of changes in total body water. CRRT is used only as an acute therapy. This treatment takes place in an ICU (intensive care unit) for a limited period of time until there is a recovery in the client's kidney function or either peritoneal dialysis or hemodialysis is instituted.

68

Enter HD for hemodialysis, PD for peritoneal dialysis, and CRRT for continuous renal replacement therapy for the effect of the appropriate dialysis procedure:

_____ a. Removes fluid rapidly

_____ b. Removes excess potassium slowly

_____ c. Removes waste products quickly

_____ d. Needs no direct access to the bloodstream

_____ e. Is used in the ICU setting as an acute treatment

_____ f. Requires complex equipment and specialized training

_____ g. Can be used for hemodynamically unstable clients

_____ h. Is poorly tolerated by clients with cardiovascular disease

_____ i. Has high cost

_____ j. Risk of peritonitis

_____ k. Requires small amounts of heparin

68 a. HD; b. PD; c. HD; d. PD; e. CRRT; f. HD; g. CRRT; h. HD; i. HD; j. PD; k. PD

▌ CLINICAL APPLICATIONS

Mr. Tom Smith, age 36, sustained critical injuries in a motor vehicle accident. Assessment in the emergency room indicated that he suffered from blunt trauma to the chest and abdomen and two fractured femurs. He was also in shock. He went to surgery immediately for an exploratory laparotomy in which a splenectomy, aspiration of a large retroperitoneal hematoma, and repair of a ruptured diaphragm were performed. It was noted that he had bilateral contusion of both kidneys. An open reduction of his fractures was done and he was placed in balanced traction.

His urine after surgery was grossly bloody and the output ranged from 10 to 20 mL/h. Mr. Smith experienced hypotension after his injury and surgery. He was transfused with eight units of whole blood. Postoperatively, Mr. Smith was sent to the SICU on ventilatory support with a subclavian line for fluids, nutritional support, and hemodynamic monitoring. Laboratory studies were done daily.

69

Because Mr. Smith was hemodynamically acutely unstable due to an abdominal injury, the choice of treatment can be either _____ or _____ .

69 hemodialysis; CRRT

70

The intravascular fluid volume lost from Mr. Smith's injuries can cause increased ADH and aldosterone secretion.

Two days after his accident Mr. Smith's serum sodium increased. Which hormone prevents excretion of sodium?

_____

70 aldosterone

Table 23-8 lists the lab results, urine output, weight, and urinary sodium for Mr. Smith during admission, surgery, and the first four days of hospitalization. Refer to the table as you respond to the questions.

71

Which factors in Mr. Smith's history contributed to the development of the initial phase of ARF? _____ and * _____

71 hypotension; hemorrhagic shock

72

A rise in serum potassium is noted the day after surgery. An increase in potassium in this situation is caused by * _____ .

72 massive tissue damage

73

Mr. Smith shows signs of oliguric azotemia on the second and third days. What are the two clinical indicators of decreased renal function? * _____

_____

73 urine output less than 400 mL in 24 hours and elevated BUN and creatinine

Table 23-8

Laboratory Studies I: Tom Smith

Tests	Admission	Surgery	Day 1	Day 2	Day 3	Day 4
Potassium (serum) (3.5–5.3 mEq/L)	3.6	4.2	6.5	5.1	5.9	6.8
Sodium (serum) (135–146 mEq/L)	138	142	144	143	144	143
Chloride (serum) (95–108 mEq/L)	110	110	110	108	103	104
CO_2 (serum) (22–32 mEq/L)	17	24	27	29	25	21
BUN (10–25 mg/dL)			30	34	57	84
Creatinine (serum) (0.6–1.2 mg/dL)			1.6	4.7	7.2	10.2
Urine output (mL/24 h)			580	440	320	290
Weight (lb)		185	189	191	196	198
Urine sodium (mEq/L)						93

74 ischemia and toxicity

74
The nephrologist who cared for Mr. Smith diagnosed his renal problem as acute renal failure secondary to shock and myoglobinuria. Shock and myoglobinuria are listed under which two causes of renal failure? *_____

75 hyperkalemia

75
On the fourth day Mr. Smith's serum potassium measures 6.8 mEq/L. His ECG showed peaked T waves and signs of cardiac irritability. These are symptoms of (hypokalemia/ hyperkalemia) _____ .

76
Hyperkalemia can be treated temporarily by methods that decrease serum potassium. (Refer to Chapter 6 on potassium if needed.)

List four methods used in the treatment of hyperkalemia:

a. * _____

b. * _____

c. * _____

d. * _____

76 a. Kayexalate and sorbitol;
b. IV sodium bicarbonate;
c. 10% calcium gluconate;
d. insulin and glucose

77

ECG changes indicate a need to rapidly lower Mr. Smith's serum potassium level. Name two methods that can be used to shift potassium back into the cells. * _____

77 sodium bicarbonate and glucose and insulin

78

Another treatment prescribed for Mr. Smith was a Kayexalate retention enema. Kayexalate, a cation exchange resin, is mixed with sorbitol and given orally or rectally to induce an "osmotic diarrhea." The sodium in Kayexalate is exchanged with potassium in the intestines to lower the serum potassium level.

The resin used in excreting potassium from the intestine is

_____ .

78 Kayexalate

79

It is noted that Mr. Smith had had a 13-pound weight increase since admission. Edema is evident in his hands, feet, and face. His blood pressure is 160/80 and his central venous pressure (CVP) and pulmonary artery wedge pressure (PAWP) are elevated. Auscultation of lung fields revealed coarse rales bilaterally. These symptoms indicate what type of fluid imbalance? * _____

79 fluid overload OR overhydration

80

Mr. Smith's electrolytes for day 4 show a serum Na 143, Cl 104, and CO_2 21. He has an anion gap of 18. An anion gap greater than 16 mEq/L is indicative of what condition? _____ (Refer to Chapter 12 on anion gap if necessary.)

80 acidosis. If you answered metabolic acidosis—OK.

81

Once the urine is clear of blood, a random urine sodium test is ordered. The result of 93 mEq/L means that the kidneys are unable to concentrate urine. What does this test indicate about the nephrons? * _____

81 they are damaged

82 Mr. Smith is hemodynamically unstable and has abdominal trauma. Peritoneal dialysis is contraindicated after abdominal surgery. CRRT prevents the rapid intercompartmental fluid shifts which occur in hemodialysis, and is poorly tolerated in a hemodynamically unstable client.

83 vascular access

84 ultrafiltration; the use of a low-potassium dialysate

85 rapid shift of fluids and electrolytes during hemodialysis

86 agitation; twitching; seizures

87 acidosis, hyperkalemia, and fluid overload

82
The decision is made to prescribe CRRT until Mr. Smith regains kidney function or becomes stable enough to tolerate hemodialysis. Explain why CRRT is selected over peritoneal dialysis or hemodialysis. *_____

_____

_____

83
Several days later, a decision was made for Mr. Smith to have hemodialysis for 3 hours every day. What type of access is needed for hemodialysis? *_____

84
During hemodialysis what method is used to remove excess fluid? _____
     What can be done in hemodialysis to lower the serum potassium? *_____

85
In hemodialysis the rapid shift of fluids and electrolytes can cause central nervous system disturbances such as agitation, twitching, and seizures. This is known as the *disequilibrium syndrome.*
     This condition is caused by a *_____ .

86
Observe for signs of the disequilibrium syndrome that include _____ , _____ , and _____ .

     Table 23-9 lists Mr. Smith's test results on days 6, 14, 35, 37, 40, and 47. He is given hemodialysis until day 49. Refer to the table as needed.

87
On day 14 Mr. Smith became anuric. He also developed a severe infection that caused catabolism and increased his BUN, creatinine, and WBC count. Hemodialysis time is increased to 5 hours per day. From Table 23-9 what three problems are controlled with dialysis on day 14? *_____

_____

Table 23-9

Laboratory Studies II: Mr. Smith

Tests	Day 6	Day 14	Day 35	Day 37	Day 40	Day 47
WBCs (5000–10,000 mm³)		38,000				
Potassium (serum) (3.5–5.3 mEq/L)	5.3	5.2	3.8	3.9	3.8	4.8
Sodium (serum) (135–146 mEq/L)	142	135	134	128	133	147
Calcium (serum) (9–11 mg/dL)		8.5		8.6		
Chloride (serum) (95–108 mEq/L)	102	93	99	90	97	112
Phosphorus (serum) (2.5–4.5 mg/dL)		9.7		4.2		
CO_2 (serum) (22–32 mEq/L)	25	25	21	21	22	17
BUN (10–25 mg/dL)	71	110	86	89	86	140
Creatinine (serum) (0.6–1.2 mg/dL)	9.2	11.1	7.1	6.5	5.8	4.3
Weight (lb)	193	180	171	169	165	164
Intake (mL/24 h)	600	600	600	600	3000	4955
Output (mL/24 h)	170	0	250	550	3000	4650

88 metastatic calcification

88
Mr. Smith's serum phosphorus is very high (9.7 mg/dL). When the serum calcium and phosphate are multiplied, the Ca × P product is 83.1. This is an indication of *_____ .

89
The nephrologist ordered a phosphate binding agent to lower the serum phosphorus. This agent contains aluminum, which

89 a phosphate binding agent
OR an agent that contains
aluminum, e.g., Amphojel
or Basaljel

attracts and binds phosphorus compounds in the intestines for excretion in the stool.

The drug/agent that lowers serum phosphate is *_____
_____ .

90

On day 35 Mr. Smith's urine output returned and hemodialysis was decreased to 4 hours per day. By day 37 his urine output increased further and dialysis times were reduced.

Note: Electrolytes stabilize to low normal levels in daily dialysis therapy.

His intake and output were about the _____ . His serum phosphorus was within high normal limits because of the *_____ prescribed.

90 same; phosphate binding
agent (phosphate binders)

91

On day 40 Mr. Smith's urinary output increased to 3000 mL/24 h. This indicates that he is in the _____ phase of ARF. Identify a potential serious complication of this phase? _____

91 diuretic; dehydration

92

By day 47 Mr. Smith's urine output continues to be high, but his serum sodium and BUN are also high. Skin turgor is poor, mucous membranes are dry, and he complains of thirst. His blood pressure is 120/60 and his pulse is 92. These symptoms are indicators of what type of fluid imbalance? _____

92 dehydration

93

By day 55 Mr. Smith is no longer azotemic and his urine output and electrolytes are in normal range. This phase of ARF is _____ .

93 recovery

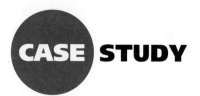

REVIEW

Mrs. Alice Grady, age 68, has a 3-year history of renal insufficiency from glomerulonephritis and a history of several myocardial infarctions. Mrs. Grady is admitted to the hospital for shortness of breath with no dyspnea. Her laboratory results on admission are Hgb 6.1 g/dL, Hct 19%, BUN 78 mg/dL, creatinine 5.2 mg/dL, serum CO_2 13 mEq/L, serum potassium 5.6 mEq/L, serum sodium 124 mEq/L, serum calcium 8.4 mg/dL, and serum phosphorus 5.2 mg/dL. Physical assessment reveals edema of her face, hands, and lower legs. Lung sounds indicate bilateral coarse rales but no frothy sputum. Blood pressure is 170/98 and her jugular venous pressure is elevated. She notes a weight gain of 5 pounds in the preceding 3 days and her urine output is approximately 500 mL per day. Mrs. Grady complains of thirst.

ANSWER COLUMN

1. periods of time; nephrons

2. glomerulonephritis

3. Anemia. Kidneys are not producing erythropoietin to stimulate the bone marrow to build red blood cells.

4. elevated; azotemia

5. decreased; acidosis

6. 3.5–5.3 mEq/L; potassium retention due to oliguria and massive tissue destruction

7. decreased; excessive fluid intake, and metabolic acidosis

8. It causes minimal stress to clients with cardiovascular disease; it is frequently used for clients with unstable cardiovascular disease.

9. weight gain, edema, increased blood pressure, and bilateral rales (also elevated jugular venous pressure)

1. Chronic renal failure usually develops over *_____ . A progressive loss of _____ is the result.

2. What is the cause of Mrs. Grady's chronic renal failure? _____

3. Mrs. Grady's low hemoglobin and hematocrit indicate what clinical condition? _____ Explain why? *_____ _____

4. Her BUN and serum creatinine are (elevated/decreased) _____ , which is indicative of _____ .

5. Mrs. Grady's serum CO_2 is (elevated/decreased) _____ , which is indicative of _____ .

6. Her serum potassium is 5.6 mEq/L. The normal range of potassium is *_____ . Identify two reasons why hyperkalemia occurs in renal failure. *_____ _____

7. Her serum sodium is (elevated/decreased) _____ . Identify two reasons for her hyponatremia. *_____ _____

8. Peritoneal dialysis is chosen to treat Mrs. Grady's uremia. Why is peritoneal dialysis the best choice for her? *_____ _____

9. What four symptoms indicate signs of fluid overload? *_____ _____

10. After trocar insertion, the first exchange of peritoneal dialysate is a 4.25% dextrose dialysate with no potassium.

10. hyperosmolar; ultrafiltration; diffusion of potassium into the dialysate

The 4.25% dextrose dialysate is _____ . It is used for _____ . Dialysate without potassium increases *_____ _____ .

11. When dialysate infuses into the peritoneum, it can push the diaphragm upward. One must assess the client for signs of *_____ _____ .

11. respiratory distress

12. dehydration

12. Excessive use of 4.25% dextrose dialysate can lead to _____ .

13. Strict measurement of dialysate from each exchange

13. An essential intervention during peritoneal dialysis to maintain fluid balance is *_____ .

14. Retention of dialysate during exchanges can lead to *_____ _____ .

14. fluid overload

15. On the second day of peritoneal dialysis Mrs. Grady's potassium is 2.8 mEq/L, which indicates _____ . Potassium must be added to the _____ .

15. hypokalemia; dialysate

16. phosphate binding agents, e.g., Amphojel

16. Mrs. Grady's phosphorus is slightly elevated. The drug given to decrease her serum phosphorus is *_____ .

17. To prevent fluid overload in the future, it is important to determine Mrs. Grady's *_____ .

17. dry weight

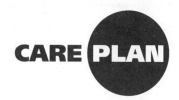

Client Management

Assessment Factors

▶ Obtain a client history concerning frequency and amounts of urination, fluid intake, and history of any past renal health problems.

▶ Obtain baseline vital signs for abnormal findings and for comparison with future vital signs. Obtain client's weight.

▶ Record the amount of urine output for 8 hours. Report if the urine output amount is not within the desired range (>30 mL/h).

▶ Check admitting laboratory results, especially the BUN, serum creatinine, serum electrolytes, and complete blood count (CBC).

▶ Assess for signs and symptoms that relate to the client's abnormal laboratory values.

◗ Assess for edema in the extremities. A decrease in urine output in conjunction with edema in the lower extremities can indicate a renal disorder.

Diagnosis 1

Fluid volume excess related to fluid retention secondary to renal failure.

Interventions and Rationale

1. Monitor fluid intake and output. Report a decrease in urine output of less than 30 mL per hour.

2. Monitor vital signs. Report abnormal vital signs, such as an increase in pulse rate, an increase or decrease in blood pressure, and difficulty breathing.

3. Check for signs of hypervolemia, i.e., constant irritating cough, neck and hand vein engorgements, dyspnea, and chest rales.

4. Check weights daily before breakfast. Weigh the client with the same clothes and on the same scale. An increase in weight may indicate fluid retention. One liter of fluid weighs approximately 2.2 pounds.

5. Check for edema in the lower extremities early in the morning before the client rises. The presence of feet, ankle, and/or leg edema in the morning frequently indicates a renal or cardiac dysfunction.

6. Check abdominal girth. Monitor for fluid shifts by noting rigidity or girth changes in the abdomen.

7. Encourage clients to follow a restricted sodium diet and fluid limitation as ordered by the health care provider.

Diagnosis 2

Fluid volume deficit related to excess ultrafiltration or diuresis.

Interventions and Rationale

1. Monitor vital signs, especially the pulse rate and blood pressure. An increased pulse rate with a decreased blood pressure may be indicative of a fluid volume deficit.

2. Monitor fluid balance associated with dialysis procedures. Excessive ultrafiltration during hemodialysis causes hypotension. If blood pressure postdialysis is low, it may cause

decreased blood flow through the vascular access and result in clotting. Excessive ultrafiltration from peritoneal dialysis can produce hypovolemia and hypernatremia because of the rapid movement of water across the peritoneum.

3. Monitor urinary output in the diuretic phase of ARF. Excessive urine output can deplete the intravascular volume and cause severe dehydration.

4. Replace fluid loss rapidly as prescribed to increase blood pressure and perfusion to vital organs when hypovolemia is due to the dialysis procedure.

Diagnosis 3

Altered tissue perfusion: renal, cardiopulmonary, cerebral, related to hypovolemia and decrease in cardiac output secondary to dialysis.

Interventions and Rationale

1. Monitor vital signs and ECG. Report abnormal findings that may indicate poor tissue perfusion.

2. Check for signs of edema. Edema decreases tissue perfusion.

3. Monitor CVP and PAWP for early signs of decreased cardiac output and decreased perfusion.

4. Check specific gravity (SG) to detect changes in the concentration that result from decreased intravascular volume and may lead to decreased renal perfusion.

Diagnosis 4

Altered urinary elimination related to renal disorder.

Interventions and Rationale

1. Check urine output daily at specified times.

2. Instruct clients with renal disorders to monitor their fluid intake and urine output. A decreased output may signify decreased function. Urinary output should be at a minimum of 30 mL/h. The health care provider must be notified if the urine output drops.

Diagnosis 5

Risk for infection related to dialysis and the care of the vascular access site.

Interventions and Rationale

1. Monitor temperature and white blood cell (WBC) count for elevations, which can indicate an infection.

2. Use aseptic technique in caring for the access site to reduce risk of infection.

3. Check for swelling, redness, and drainage at the access site, which can indicate an infection. Note any discharge from the access sites or wounds. Culture potentially infected sites.

4. Check for the patency of the vascular access site used for hemodialysis. A surgically re-created vascular access should have bruits and pulsation on auscultation. Blood can be aspirated and infused through femoral and subclavian catheters.

5. Check for mechanical factors, such as kinking of the tubing, displacement of the catheter, and lying on the access site, which could cause poor blood flow.

6. Observe the peritoneal catheter site for crusting or redness.

7. Instruct the client on how to care for the access site and maintain asepsis.

8. Teach the client good hygiene, to avoid crowds, and to obtain yearly inoculation for flu viruses as indicated by the health care provider.

Diagnosis 6

Risk for injury related to mechanical equipment and central nervous system dysfunction from fluid and electrolyte imbalances.

Interventions and Rationale

1. Monitor new dialysis clients and catabolic clients in ARF for signs of central nervous system dysfunction that may lead to disequilibrium syndrome. Observe for tremors, irritability, confusion, and seizures that indicate the disequilibrium syndrome.

2. Monitor serum electrolyte values associated with renal disorders and observe for symptoms of electrolyte imbalance. Report the laboratory results that indicate hyperkalemia, hypocalcemia, and hyperphosphatemia immediately. These results can be life threatening.

3. Monitor the ECG for peaked T waves that can indicate hyper-kalemia.

4. Administer phosphate binding agents as ordered to control the serum phosphorus level. A low serum calcium level can be caused by hyperphosphatemia, restricted calcium intake in the diet, and/or alterations in vitamin D metabolism needed for intestinal absorption of calcium. Overuse of aluminum-phosphate binding drugs can cause hypophosphatemia.

5. Check the symptoms of tetany when the serum calcium level is low and acidosis is corrected. Serum calcium deficits can indicate a need for vitamin D supplements.

Diagnosis 7

Ineffective breathing patterns related to peritoneal dialysate infusion.

Interventions and Rationale

1. Monitor respiratory rate. Report signs of dyspnea.

2. Check for dyspnea when administering solutions for peritoneal dialysis. Rapid infusion of dialysate can push the diaphragm upward, thus decreasing the area for lung expansion.

Evaluation/Outcome

1. Evaluate the effects of hemodialysis or peritoneal dialysis for controlling fluid, electrolyte, and acid-base balance.

2. Monitor vital signs (particularly blood pressure and pulse rate) for stability or indications of a fluid imbalance.

3. Monitor weight gain prior to and following dialysis to determine body fluid gains or losses.

4. Evaluate intake and output for fluid balance.

5. Evaluate that laboratory test results, i.e., electrolytes, creatinine, BUN, and CBC, prior to and following dialysis are in normal or in "near" normal ranges. Serum laboratory test results may be "alarmingly" elevated prior to dialysis.

6. Monitor for peripheral and pulmonary edema as a result of ECFVE.

7. Maintain a support system for the client and family.

Increased Intracranial Pressure

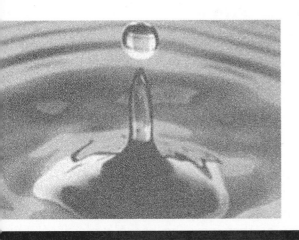

OBJECTIVES

Upon completion of this chapter, the reader should be able to:

- Explain the physiologic changes associated with fluid and electrolyte balance in clients with increased intracranial pressure.

- Describe three types of intracerebral edema.

- Describe the pathophysiologic changes that increase intracranial pressure.

- Identify complications that result from increased intracranial pressure.

- Apply principles of fluid balance in the assessment and care of a client with increased intracranial pressure.

(continued on next page)

OBJECTIVES (Continued)

● Apply principles of fluid balance in the care of a client with increased intracellular fluid (ICF).

● Describe assessment factors, diagnoses, and interventions related to increased intracranial pressure.

● Describe treatment priorities in the clinical management of increased intracranial pressure.

▶ INTRODUCTION

Intracranial pressure is that pressure within the intracranial cavity which is exerted by the volume of blood, cerebrospinal fluid, and brain parenchyma contained within the cavity. A small increase or decrease in any of these three components may have deleterious effects on brain structures and function. The health professional has a major responsibility in monitoring the neurologically impaired client for signs and symptoms of increasing intracranial pressure.

Because the brain is enclosed in the rigid cranial vault, a small increase in intracerebral fluid may result in a dramatic increase in intracranial pressure. Therefore, the health professional must closely monitor the neurologically impaired client for early signs of increasing intracranial pressure to help prevent adverse effects.

This chapter discusses the physiology of intracranial pressure, the three types of intracerebral edema, factors that increase and decrease intracranial pressure, and associated complications that may occur with intracerebral hypertension. Signs and symptoms of increasing intracranial pressure along with management priorities and principles of fluid and electrolyte balance in the management of intracerebral hypertension are discussed.

❱ PATHOPHYSIOLOGY

1

Intracranial pressure is determined by the pressure within the intracranial cavity, which is exerted by the volume of
_____ , * _____ , and * _____ .

1 blood; cerebrospinal fluid; brain parenchyma

2

A small increase in intracerebral fluid may result in a dramatic increase in intracranial pressure because * _____
_____ .

2 the brain is enclosed in a rigid cranial vault

3

In general, there are three types of cerebral edema: vasogenic, cytogenic, and interstitial. The three types of cerebral edema are
* _____ .

3 vasogenic, cytogenic, and interstitial

Vasogenic edema is the most common type of fluid accumulation within the brain. It is essentially an extracellular edema. Vasogenic edema results from damage to the cerebral blood vessels causing increased capillary permeability. This allows a transudation of proteins and an influx of water from the extracellular space into the brain parenchyma. Causes of vasogenic edema include trauma, tumors, ischemia, and infection or abscess.

4

The most common type of cerebral edema is _____ edema, which results from * _____.

4 vasogenic; damage to cerebral blood vessels causing an increase in capillary permeability

5

Increased capillary permeability results in * _____
_____ .

5 a transudation of proteins and influx of water from the extracellular space into the brain parenchyma

Cytogenic edema is intracellular. Increased capillary permeability results in an overall increase in water content within the brain and an inhibition of the sodium-potassium (Na-K) pump. This inhibition allows potassium to leave the cell and sodium chloride and water to enter the cell, causing the brain cells to swell.

Clinical causes of cytogenic edema include hypoxia from trauma or cerebral hemorrhage and hypo-osmolality.

6
Cytogenic edema is (extracellular/intracellular) _____ .
Vasogenic edema is (extracellular/intracellular) _____ .

6   intracellular; extracellular

7
Cytogenic edema inhibits the Na-K pump, resulting in _____ leaving the cell and *_____ and _____ entering the cell.

7   potassium; sodium chloride; water

8
Name three clinical conditions that may cause cytogenic edema.
*_____

8   hypoxia from trauma, cerebral hemorrhage, and hypo-osmolality

9
Interstitial edema results from obstructive conditions such as hydrocephalus, brain tumors or infections that predispose the client to an excess of fluid in the brain, and a buildup of cerebrospinal fluid in the ventricles of the brain.
    Three clinical conditions that may cause interstitial edema are
*_____

9   hydrocephalus, brain tumors, and infections

10
The three types of cerebral edema are *_____
_____ .

10   vasogenic, cytogenic, and interstitial

11
Regulators of blood flow within the central nervous system include CO_2, O_2, core body temperature, hydrogen ion concentration, and serum osmolality.
    Name five regulators of cerebral blood flow. *_____
_____

11   CO_2, O_2, core body temperature, hydrogen ion concentration, and serum osmolality

12
Hypercapnia (an increase in $PaCO_2$) causes vasodilation, which results in an increase in intracranial pressure. Hypoxemia (a decrease in PaO_2) may also cause an increase in intracranial pressure.

Hypercapnia causes a/an (increase/decrease) _____ in intracranial pressure.

12 increase; increase

Hypoxemia causes a/an (increase/decrease) _____ in intracranial pressure.

An increase in core body temperature increases metabolism and results in an increase in intracranial pressure. A decrease in core body temperature causes a decrease in body metabolism and results in a decrease in intracranial pressure.

13

What effect does an increased core body temperature have on intracranial pressure? *_____

13 It increases it.; It decreases it.

What effect does a decrease in core body temperature have on intracranial pressure? *_____

Prolonged hyperventilation causes excessive elimination of CO_2 and leads to respiratory alkalosis (increased pH and decreased $PaCO_2$). This may cause an increase in intracranial pressure.

14

Hyperventilation can cause what clinical condition? *_____

Respiratory alkalosis causes a/an (increase/decrease) _____ in intracranial pressure; prolonged hyperventilation may lead to a/an (increase/decrease) in intracranial pressure.

14 respiratory alkalosis; decrease; increase

Hypoventilation causes excessive retention of CO_2 and leads to respiratory acidosis (decreased pH and increased $PaCO_2$), which is far more dangerous than hyperventilation. Carbon dioxide is the most potent vasodilator known. As vasodilation increases, so does intracranial pressure.

15

Hypoventilation causes what clinical condition? *_____ The most potent vasodilator known is *_____. Respiratory acidosis causes a/an (increase/decrease) _____ in vasodilation and results in (increased/decreased) _____ intracranial pressure.

15 respiratory acidosis; carbon dioxide or CO_2; increase; increased

Serum osmolality is the number of formed particles in the serum and is an indication of serum concentration. Decreased serum osmolality indicates a fluid overload and may result in an increase in intracranial pressure.

16 increase; an increase in $PaCO_2$, a decrease in PaO_2, an increase in body temperature, a change in hydrogen ion concentration, and decreased serum osmolality

16

A decrease in serum osmolality may cause a/an (increase/decrease) _____ in intracranial pressure.

Five regulators that increase intracranial pressure are
*_____

_____ .

Hypo-osmolar fluids such as dextrose and water are generally avoided in the neurologically compromised client suspected of having an increase in intracranial pressure. Using intravenous fluids such as 5% dextrose in water (D_5W) results in the dextrose being metabolized, releasing free water which is absorbed by the brain cells, leading to cerebral edema.

17

Hypo-osmolar fluids may cause a/an (increase/decrease) _____ in intracranial pressure.

17 increase

▶ CLINICAL MANIFESTATIONS

Table 24-1 lists the early, progressive, and advanced clinical manifestations of increasing intracranial pressure.

18

Name at least four early signs and symptoms of increased intracranial pressure. _____

_____

18 headache, irritability, restlessness, and confusion (others: diplopia, and other visual changes)

If early signs and symptoms of intracranial pressure are missed or unable to be controlled, progressive clinical manifestations occur.

19

Name the changes that occur with the following parameters related to an increase in intracranial pressure:

Table 24-1

Clinical Manifestations of Increasing Intracranial Pressure

Early signs and symptoms	Headache
	Irritability
	Restlessness
	Confusion
	Diplopia
	Other visual changes
Progressive signs and symptoms	Nausea
	Projectile vomiting
	Bradycardia
	Decreased and/or irregular respirations
	Increased systolic pressure
	Decreased diastolic pressure
	Widened pulse pressure (difference between systolic and diastolic pressures)
	Decreased level of consciousness
	Pupillary changes
Advanced signs and symptoms	Rhinorrhea
	Otorrhea
	Changes in motor/sensory function
	Posturing, apnea, coma, death

19 a. irritability, restlessness and confusion, decreased level of consciousness; b. diplopia and/or visual changes; c. decreases; d. decreases and/or irregular; e. increases; f. decreases; g. increases, widens

a. Mental status *_____
b. Vision *_____
c. Pulse _____
d. Respiration *_____
e. Systolic blood pressure _____
f. Diastolic blood pressure _____
g. Pulse pressure _____

If the progressive clinical manifestations of increasing intracranial pressure are not controlled, more deleterious effects are likely. The symptoms are those of decompensation. Once decompensation occurs, autoregulation (the compensatory alteration in the diameter of the intracranial blood vessels designed to maintain a constant blood flow during changes in cerebral perfusion pressure) is lost with progressively increased intracranial pressure.

20 changes in motor sensory function, otorrhea, rhinorrhea, posturing, apnea, and coma (which may result in death); the compensatory alteration in the diameter of the intracranial blood vessels designed to maintain a constant blood flow during changes in cerebral perfusion pressure

20

Name six advanced clinical manifestations of increased intracranial pressure. *_____

_____

What is meant by autoregulation of cerebral blood flow?
*_____

In addition to the effects on brain metabolism and function, intracerebral hypertension has implications in the dysfunction of other major organ systems. Changes in the cardiopulmonary system include pulmonary rales (crackles), adventitious sounds, S_3, atrial fibrillation, and hypotension. Hypotension drastically worsens cerebral edema because of a resultant decrease in cerebral perfusion pressure and compensatory fluid retention.

21

In addition to changes in brain function and metabolism resulting from intracerebral hypertension, name two other body systems affected. *_____ and _____

Name at least five cardiopulmonary complications resulting from intracerebral hypertension. *_____

_____

The development of stress ulcers and gastrointestinal bleeding may occur as a result of medical treatment. Identify two changes in the gastrointestinal system that can occur as a result of the medical treatment of intracerebral hypertension.
*_____

21 cardiopulmonary; gastrointestinal; pulmonary rales, adventitious sounds, S_3, atrial fibrillation, and hypotension stress ulcers and bleeding

22

Systemic hypotension (increases/decreases) _____ cerebral perfusion pressure and results in a/an (increase/decrease) _____ in intracerebral hypertension.

22 decreases; increase

▶ CLINICAL MANAGEMENT

Clinical management of intracerebral hypertension includes careful administration of fluids and electrolytes, maintaining an airway and adequate ventilation, medication administration, temperature control, and prevention of the Valsalva maneuver, which increases intracranial pressure.

23 fluid management, ventilation, medication administration, and prevention of Valsalva maneuver (also temperature control)

24 dextrose in water (hypo-osmolar) solutions; physiological saline; Ringer's lactate (iso-osmolar solutions).

25 sodium and potassium; hypo-osmolality; for maintenance of an appropriate ratio of Na and K ions to maintain a normal serum osmolality level

23

Name four major areas for managing increasing intracranial pressure. *_____

_____

Careful fluid management in the neurologically impaired client is essential. Hypo-osmolar fluids such as dextrose and water are generally avoided. Dextrose metabolizes and free water is absorbed by brain cells, leading to cerebral edema. Physiological normal saline (0.09% NSS) or Ringer's solution are the preferred iso-osmolar intravenous fluids.

24

Intravenous fluids that should be avoided in the treatment of increased intracranial pressure include *_____

_____ .

Preferred intravenous fluids for treatment of the neurologically impaired client include *_____ and *_____ .

Extracellular fluid volume is directly dependent upon total body sodium. The principal osmotic electrolyte of extracellular fluid is sodium (Na). Most clients with hyponatremia are hypo-osmolar. The other major cation for fluid balance maintenance is potassium (K). It is essential to maintain normal Na and K levels in order to maintain normal serum osmolality. If the Na and K levels are not maintained within normal limits, the Na-K pump becomes defective. Potassium leaves the cell and Na, Cl, and water enter the cells.

25

The two major cations that regulate serum osmolality and total body water are *_____ .

Clients with hyponatremia generally have serum (hypo-osmolality/hyper-osmolality) _____ .

Explain the role of the Na-K pump in the regulation of intracerebral pressure. *_____

_____

Mannitol and urea are osmotic diuretics capable of relieving elevated intracranial pressure when given intravenously. Mannitol intravenous dosage is 1 mg/kg of body weight administered over 10–30 minutes and can be repeated once or twice every 4–6 hours. Mannitol pulls intracellular fluid into the extracellular plasma and decreases intracranial pressure. Care must be taken to monitor for possible complications of pulmonary edema and water intoxication. An additional complication that can occur with the administration of osmotic diuretics to clients with intracranial hemorrhage is rebleeding. As the brain tissue shrinks from osmotic diuretics, rebleeding may occur.

26

Two osmotic diuretics given intravenously to decrease intracranial pressure are *_____ .

The dosage and frequency of use for the administration of mannitol in increased cerebral pressure is _____ mg/kg of body weight and may be repeated *_____ every _____ hours.

Explain the mechanism of how mannitol works to decrease intracranial pressure. It is an _____ diuretic and pulls fluid from *_____ to *_____.

Two possible complications with osmotic diuretics are *_____ .

Loop diuretics such as furosemide (Lasix) may be administered in conjunction with osmotic diuretics to help eliminate excess fluid from the extracellular space.

27

Furosemide may be given in conjunction with osmotic diuretics to *_____ .

Steroids, primarily dexamethasone (Decadron), may be used to treat both acute and chronic cerebral edema. The effects of Decadron are slower in onset than osmotic diuretics and peak in 24 hours. Dexamethasone, additionally, is a potent anti-inflammatory agent and protects cell wall stability. It is especially useful in cytotoxic edema.

26 mannitol and urea; 1; once or twice; 4–6; osmotic; intracellular tissue; extracellular spaces; pulmonary edema and water intoxication

27 increase diuresis of extracellular fluid

28

The steroid used to treat both acute and chronic cerebral edema is _____.

The disadvantage of dexamethasone on acute intracranial pressure is *_____
_____ .

Dexamethasone is especially helpful in which type of cerebral edema? _____

Like all steroids, dexamethasone has the long-term complications of decreasing wound healing, electrolyte imbalance, and gastrointestinal bleeding.

29

Name three long-term complications from using dexamethasone in controlling cerebral pressure. *_____

Hyperventilation with a resultant decrease in $PaCO_2$ acts immediately to decrease cerebral blood flow and thus reduces intracranial pressure. It is preferable to give rapid ventilation of low volume to help reduce the effects of respiratory alkalosis over an extended period of time. This intervention increases the rate and decreases the volume of each breath. Clients may need long-term mechanical ventilation to prevent respiratory acidosis, which is far more serious than respiratory alkalosis. Increased concentration of $PaCO_2$ in respiratory acidosis is a more potent vasodilator than is an increase in PaO_2 resulting from respiratory alkalosis.

30

How does hyperventilation work to help reduce intracranial pressure? *_____
_____

Which clinical condition is more serious for the client with increasing intracranial pressure, respiratory acidosis or respiratory alkalosis? *_____ Why? *_____
_____

Further measures to control or decrease intracranial pressure are aimed at preventing the Valsalva maneuver and permitting gravity to help reduce intracranial pressure. Alert and cooperative clients should be encouraged not to cough, bend, stoop, lift, hold

---

28 dexamethasone (Decadron); it is slower acting and does not peak for 24 hours; cytotoxic

29 decreased wound healing, electrolyte imbalance, and gastrointestinal bleeding

30 hyperventilation reduces $PaCO_2$ concentration (a power vasodilator); respiratory acidosis; an increase in $PaCO_2$ is a more powerful vasodilator than an increase in PaO_2

their breath, sneeze, or strain at bowel elimination. To prevent a transient increase in intracranial pressure, stool softeners are administered to help prevent straining with bowel movements. The head of the bed should be elevated 30°–45° to let gravity have its effect on reducing intracranial pressure. The head and neck should be midline with no flexion, extension, or rotation. These maneuvers may result in an increase in intracranial pressure.

31

List six measures that clients should be instructed to avoid in order to prevent a transient increase in intracranial pressure.
*_____

_____ In what position should the client's bed be placed to help prevent intracranial pressure? *_____ What may occur if the client flexes, extends, or rotates the neck?
*_____ What is the purpose of administering stool softeners to the client with increased intracranial pressure? *_____

Clients with increased intracranial pressure are prone to seizures. Seizures may cause a transient increase in intracranial pressure, create safety issues for the client, or cause further hypoxia and hypercapnia. Preventive measures for seizure control include the administration and careful monitoring of anticonvulsant medications.

32

What are two deleterious effects of seizure activity in the client with increased intracranial pressure? *_____

31 cough, bend, stoop, lift, hold their breath, and sneeze (also strain at bowel movement); 30°–45° angle; transient increase in intracranial pressure; to help prevent straining with bowel movements

32 transient increase in intracranial pressure and safety issues

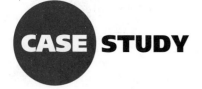

REVIEW

Mrs. Foote, age 46, was involved in a multiple vehicle accident. She suffered head trauma of unknown dimension. She was unconscious at the scene of the accident but is now alert and oriented and is admitted to an inpatient unit for observation. She is presently reporting a headache and blurred vision. Vital signs upon admission are blood pressure, 134/74; pulse, 88 and regular; respirations, 20 per minute and regular and unlabored; temperature, 98.4°F orally. You are to monitor Mrs. Foote for signs and symptoms of increasing intracranial pressure.

1. Vasogenic; cytogenic; Trauma may cause damage to cerebral blood vessels (vasogenic edema). Trauma may also cause hypoxia and/or hemorrhage (cytogenic edema).

1. If Mrs. Foote does develop signs and symptoms of increasing intracranial edema, what type(s) of edema would she have? _____ and _____
Why? *_____

2. headache, blurred vision

2. What symptoms does Mrs. Foote currently have to indicate that she might have increasing cerebral edema? *_____

3. level of consciousness

3. The most significant observation of changes in Mrs. Foote's behavior that indicates an increase in intracranial pressure is a change in her *_____ .

The health care provider places Mrs. Foote on NPO status and initiates an intravenous line. Intravenous orders include normal saline, 1000 mL at 75 mL/h, and oxygen per nasal canal at 4 L/min.

4. Hypo-osmolar fluids such as dextrose and water are metabolized into dextrose free water, which may cause the brain to swell.

4. Why did the health care provider order an IV of normal saline solution instead of a dextrose solution? *_____
_____

5. Oxygen was ordered to prevent CO_2 buildup, which is a potent vasodilator that can increase cerebral edema.

5. Mrs. Foote had no difficulty with respiration. Why was oxygen ordered? *_____ .

6. decrease

6. If Mrs. Foote develops an increase in intracranial pressure her respirations will (increase/decrease) _____ .

7. decrease

7. Her pulse rate will (increase/decrease) _____ .

8. increase

8. Her systolic blood pressure will (increase/decrease) _____ .

9. decrease

9. Her diastolic blood pressure will (increase/decrease) _____ .

10. pulse pressure

10. If Mrs. Foote's blood pressure changes from 134/74 to 145/60, this would indicate an increase in *_____ .

11. As an antipyretic to reduce core body temperature. An increase in core body temperature increases cerebral metabolism and increases brain edema.

Two hours after admission, Mrs. Foote's temperature became elevated to 99.8°F. Even though she was NPO, she was ordered and received acetaminophen (Tylenol) grains 10 by mouth with a sip of water.

11. Why was the Tylenol prescribed? *_____ .

The head of Mrs. Foote's bed is elevated to 45 degrees, and her side rails are padded.

12. cerebral edema; safety measures in case Mrs. Foote developed seizures

12. The head of the bed was elevated to 45° to help prevent *_____ . The side rails were padded for *_____ .

Mrs. Foote continued to become more restless and could not remember where she was. Vital signs were taken with the following results: blood pressure, 160/60; pulse, 66; and respirations, 16. Dexamethasone 4 mg IV push and Lasix 40 mg IV push were ordered. The IV fluid rate was decreased to 50 mL/h.

13. increasing intracranial pressure
14. restlessness and confusion, systolic blood pressure increasing, diastolic blood pressure decreasing, pulse rate decreasing, respiration decreasing, pulse pressure widening
15. decrease overall fluid intake and thereby decrease intracerebral edema
16. cause a diuresis of extracellular fluid
17. decrease intracranial pressure over a prolonged period of time
18. stabilize cell wall capillary permeability

13. Mrs. Foote is experiencing what phenomena? *_____

14. What data in question 13 indicate increased intracranial pressure? *_____

15. Mrs. Foote's IV rate was decreased in order to *_____
_____

16. Lasix was ordered to *_____

17. Dexamethasone was ordered to *_____

18. A secondary benefit of dexamethasone for Mrs. Foote is
*_____
_____

An endotracheal intubation tray and ventilator were placed on standby at the bedside. ABGs were drawn with the following results: pH 7.48, $PaCO_2$ 34, HCO_3 28, and PaO_2 96.

19. respiratory alkalosis
20. If Mrs. Foote's $PaCO_2$ increases, intubation would be considered to improve oxygenation and decrease the $PaCO_2$ level.

19. The blood gas results suggest *_____ .

20. Why was the ventilator placed on standby? *_____
_____

Mrs. Foote's confusion eased. She remained on dexamethasone with stable vital signs. She was permitted out of bed to a chair.

21. no stooping, bending, lifting, coughing, or straining at stool
22. dexamethasone increases the potential for gastrointestinal bleeding and cimetadine and Maalox may help prevent GI distress

21. What instructions should be given to Mrs. Foote to help prevent transient intracerebral edema? *_____
_____

Additional health care provider orders include cimetadine, 300 mg IV every 8 hours, and Maalox, 30 mL PO four times a day.

22. Cimetadine and Maalox are ordered because *_____
_____

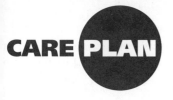
CARE PLAN

Client Management

Assessment Factors

▶ The most significant change that may indicate an increase in intracranial pressure is a change in the level of consciousness. Subtle changes initially include irritability, restlessness, and visual changes.

▶ Assess vital signs every 15–30 minutes for bradycardia, slowed and/or irregular respirations, hyperthermia, systolic hypertension, diastolic hypotension, and a widening pulse pressure. Careful monitoring of fluid balance is essential to help prevent cerebral hypertension. Hourly intake and output, careful monitoring of intravenous fluid rate, and daily weights are important assessment factors.

▶ Additional parameters to monitor include serum osmolality, arterial blood gases, and electrolytes. Decreased serum osmolality, increased $PaCO_2$, increased serum potassium, and decreased serum sodium may indicate an impending increase in intracranial pressure.

▶ Assess pulmonary sounds for rales, heart sounds for an S_3, and an increase in skin turgor as indications for fluid retention.

▶ Clients with increased intracranial pressure may develop seizures. Assess for seizure activities and additional complications of cerebral hypertension such as rhinorrhea, otorrhea, and brain stem herniation.

▶ Administration and assessment of therapeutic effects of the following medications are essential: loop diuretics, osmotic diuretics, steroids, and anticonvulsants.

Diagnosis 1

Ineffective breathing pattern related to cerebral edema and occluded/obstructed venous drainage.

Interventions and Rationale

1. Maintain head of bed elevated 30°–45° and keep body in good alignment in order for gravity to help reduce intracranial pressure.

2. Suction prn for no longer than 15 seconds to maintain clear airway and adequate oxygenation. Suction applied for longer than 15 seconds may cause a transient rise in CO_2 levels, resulting in increased intracranial pressure.

3. Administer oxygen per nasal cannula or face mask to maintain PaO_2 levels and help prevent excessive buildup of CO_2, resulting in vasodilation and increased intracranial pressure.

4. Assess rate, depth, and pattern of respirations, which indicates patency of airway.

5. Assess skin, lips, and nail beds for cyanosis as an indicator for adequate central oxygenation.

6. Monitor arterial blood gases every 4–8 hours and prn. Hypercapnia and acidosis are to be prevented. The most potent vasodilator known is an increase in $PaCO_2$ levels.

7. Maintain an ambu bag at the bedside to be used to provide controlled hyperventilation if necessary.

Diagnosis 2

Altered tissue perfusion (cerebral) related to increased intracranial pressure associated with trauma and cerebral edema.

Interventions and Rationale

1. Assess for changes in level of consciousness, arousability, irritability, agitation, memory loss, and inability to follow commands. A change in level of consciousness is the earliest and most sensitive clinical evidence of an alteration in cerebral perfusion pressure. Arousability is a reflection of the functioning of the reticular activating system (RAS).

2. Assess for headache, nausea, and vomiting. These may be early, nonspecific signs and symptoms of increasing intracranial pressure.

3. Monitor vital signs every 15–30 minutes to assess for signs and symptoms of increased intracranial pressure. Client responses to increasing intracranial pressure can change rapidly. Observe for widening of pulse pressure.

4. Assess for sensory function: visual changes, hearing changes, touch, and proprioception. this affords an evaluation of the sensory pathways in the parietal lobes.

5. Assess for motor function changes: decerebrate and decorticate posturing, muscle strength and tone, and deep-tendor reflexes. Appropriate motor function reflects total or partial intact motor pathways at the neuromuscular junction.

6. Assess pupillary reaction and ocular movements. Increasing pressure in the midbrain and pons may cause changes in cranial nerve functioning.

7. Implement proper positioning for intracranial pressure reduction: Elevate head of bed 30°–45°, avoid use of pillows, maintain body in midline, maintain head-neck alignment, avoid neck rotation, extension, and flexion, and prevent hip flexion. Head elevation allows for optimal venous drainage. Proper body alignment prevents vein compression or obstruction. Hip flexion may increase intra-abdominal pressure and impede jugular venous cerebral drainage.

8. Instruct client on measures to prevent a transient rise in intracranial pressure: no coughing, sneezing, bending, lifting, or straining with bowel movements. These physical maneuvers cause a transient rise in intracranial pressure.

9. Palpate for bladder distention, auscultate for the presence of bowel sounds, and check for constipation. These conditions may cause abdominal distension resulting in an increase in intra- abdominal pressure.

10. Maintain normal body temperature and prevent shivering. Hyperthermia and shivering may increase cerebral metabolism and result in increased intracranial pressure.

Diagnosis 3

Risk for fluid-electrolyte imbalance, related to osmotic diuresis and/or fluid retention.

Interventions and Rationale

1. Measure intake and output hourly along with fluid restriction to help decrease extracellular fluid volume that may contribute to cerebral edema. A mild dehydration status is usually maintained.

2. Auscultate for rales, rhonchi, and an S_3 to detect early signs of volume overload.

3. Monitor serum and urine osmolality every 8 hours. Increased serum osmolality helps draw fluid from brain interstitium and reduce cerebral edema.

4. Monitor urine specific gravity every 8 hours. Cerebral trauma predisposes the client to diabetes insipidus.

5. Monitor serum electrolytes, BUN, creatinine, serum proteins, hemoglobin, and hematocrit every 8 hours and prn to detect fluid volume overload or degree of dehydration.

6. Administer corticosteroids (dexamethasone or methylprednisolone) per health care provider's order. These pharmacologic agents ameliorate cerebral edema.

7. Monitor arterial blood gases every 8 hours and prn. Increased $PaCO_2$ and decreased PaO_2 may cause vasodilation and result in an increase in cerebral pressure.

8. Administer osmotic diuretics (mannitol/urea) ordered by health care provider cautiously and assess for therapeutic effect. Osmotic diuretics may have a rebound effect.

9. Monitor for rhinorrhea and otorrhea. These symptoms may indicate brain stem herniation resulting from increased cerebral pressure.

Evaluation/Outcome

1. Evaluate that the source of the health problem has been eliminated or controlled.

2. Evaluate the effectiveness of interventions in reducing symptoms (disturbed LOC, arousability, irritability, agitation, memory loss, inability to follow simple commands) and other nonspecific early signs (headache, nausea, vomiting) of cerebral edema.

3. Evaluate vital signs frequently for return to normal range and stability (observe for widening pulse pressure).

4. Evaluate fluid balance (intake and output, daily weight, and intravenous fluid rate) and electrolyte levels (Na Cl, K, Ca) for return to normal range.

5. Evaluate effectiveness of medications (loop diuretics, osmotis diuretics, steroids, anticonvulsants, etc.) in reducing edema and promoting a fluid balance.

6. Monitor blood gases for normal/stable range to ensure adequate oxygenation.

7. Monitor oxygenation of skin, lips, and nail beds for moist pink coloring.

8. Monitor pupillary reaction and ocular movements for return to normal functions of cranial nerves.

Clinical Oncology

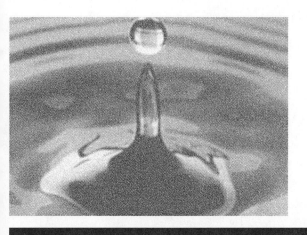

Julie Waterhouse, RN, MS

OBJECTIVES

Upon completion of this chapter, the reader should be able to:

- Describe fluid and electrolyte disturbances commonly seen in individuals with uncontrolled cancer cell growth.
- Differentiate the metabolic effects of cachexia associated with cancer.
- Give two examples of fluid and electrolyte disturbances caused by ectopic hormone secretion.
- Explain the effect of tumor lysis syndrome on fluid and electrolyte balance.
- Assess fluid and electrolyte changes in individuals with cancer.
- Describe appropriate interventions for fluid and electrolyte disturbances related to cancer.

▶ INTRODUCTION

Cancer is usually the cause of altered and uncontrolled cell growth. Cancer cells no longer look or function like normal cells and tissue. Cancer may occur in the form of a solid tumor (carcinoma or sarcoma) or may be present in the blood-forming cells of bone marrow or lymph nodes (leukemia or lymphoma). As the cancer cells move from their original location to other areas of body tissues, fluid, electrolyte, and acid-base imbalances frequently occur because of the effects of the cancer on body organs and cells. This chapter discusses various fluid, electrolyte, and acid-base changes associated with cancer.

ANSWER COLUMN

▶ PATHOPHYSIOLOGY

1

Cancer is a group of diseases characterized by abnormal and uncontrolled cell growth. Cancer cells are malignant (capable of invading normal tissues and spreading to distant sites).

Cancer is characterized by *_____

_____ .

Cancer cells are considered to be (malignant/benign)

_____ .

1   abnormal and uncontrolled cell growth; malignant

2

Fluid and electrolyte disturbances occur frequently in individuals with cancer because of the nature of the malignant cell growth and the effects of therapies used to control it.

Give two reasons why fluid and electrolyte disturbances occur frequently in individuals with cancer. *_____

_____

2   the nature of the malignant cell growth and effects of therapies used to control this cell growth

3

Cancer may begin as an individual solid tumor (carcinoma or sarcoma) or may arise throughout the body in the blood-forming cells of bone marrow or lymph nodes (leukemia and lymphoma).

Match the following types of cancer with their tissues of origin:
   a. Lymphoma
   b. Leukemia
   c. Carcinoma
   d. Sarcoma

_____ , _____   1. Epithelium or supporting tissue
            _____   2. Bone marrow
            _____   3. Lymphoid tissue

4

Malignant cells are more primitive (anaplastic) than normal cells. They may be undifferentiated or may differentiate in abnormal and bizarre ways.

This lack of normal differentiation causes malignant cells to produce unusual proteins, antigens, hormones, enzymes, and other chemicals. Because the chemicals produced by malignant cells are abnormal, they do not respond to normal regulatory mechanisms such as hormonal and metabolic controls.

Cancer of the colon may produce carcinoembryonic antigen (CEA), a fetal antigen.
Why? * _____

_____

▶ CLINICAL MANIFESTATIONS

5

One major consequence of these biochemical abnormalities is cachexia, a complex process manifested by anorexia, weight loss, wasting, weakness, anemia, fluid and electrolyte disturbances, and altered protein, lipid, and carbohydrate metabolism.

A major problem associated with cancer is _____. This serious problem is manifested by:
   a. _____
   b. _____
   c. * _____
   d. * _____

3 1. c, d; 2. b; 3. a

4 malignant cells lack normal differentiation and thus a more primitive embryonic protein may be produced

5 cachexia; a. anorexia; b. weakness; c. weight loss; d. fluid and electrolyte disturbances (others are wasting, anemia, and increased basal metabolic rate)

6

Cachexia involves changes in the metabolism of all the major nutrients. Glucose utilization is impaired and anaerobic metabolic pathways are used more often than the aerobic. This produces higher than usual concentrations of lactic acid and may result in lactic acidosis.

Glucose utilization is abnormal in cancer. What specific acid-base imbalance is caused by anaerobic metabolism? *_____

6 lactic acidosis

7

Nitrogen transferred from body tissues to the tumor often leaves the client in negative nitrogen balance. Similarly, cancer clients retain sodium, with a total of 120% that of healthy individuals. Sodium, however, is concentrated in the tumor and the serum sodium may be low (hyponatremia).

Often in clients with cancer the nitrogen balance is (positive/negative) _____ . Why? *_____

_____

7 negative; nitrogen is transferred from the body tissues to the tumor, thus causing a negative nitrogen balance

8

Does the cancer client (retain/excrete) _____ sodium? Concentration of sodium is in the _____. Because the sodium is not in the vascular fluid, (hyponatremia/ hypernatremia) _____ results.

8 retain; tumor; hyponatremia

9

The client with cancer may also experience malabsorption syndrome, which involves inflammation, ulceration, decreased patency, and decreased secretions of the GI tract. The problems that result in protein and fat absorption may compound fluid and electrolyte disturbances of cachexia.

Malabsorption syndrome may occur in cancer clients. It can involve _____, _____, and *_____.

9 inflammation, ulceration, and decreased patency OR decreased secretions of the GI tract

10

A second major consequence/problem of the primitive biochemical function of malignant cells is the secretion of abnormal hormones (ectopic hormone secretion).

An example is bronchiogenic cancer, which may secrete antidiuretic hormone (ADH), parathyroid hormone (PTH), or adrenocorticotropic hormone (ACTH). The resulting hormonal abnormalities may lead to fluid and electrolyte problems such as water intoxication (ICFVE), hyponatremia, hypokalemia, and hypophosphatemia.

The first major consequence of biochemical abnormalities in progressive cancer is _____ . The second major consequence is *_____ .

11

Abnormal hormonal secretions may occur in bronchiogenic cancer. Examples are (use abbreviations) _____ , _____ , and _____ .

What four fluid and electrolyte problems can result from these abnormal hormonal secretions? *_____

_____

12

A third problem which commonly occurs in cancer clients in whom large numbers of malignant and normal cells are destroyed by radiation or chemotherapy is catabolism (breakdown) of purine nucleic acids in cells. The result is an increase in serum uric acid.

Three problems that may result in fluid and electrolyte disturbances in cancer clients are *_____

_____ .

13

Uric acid is poorly soluble in body fluids and is excreted primarily through the kidneys. Small increases above normal serum concentrations can cause uric acid precipitation in the renal tubules and collecting ducts.

Do you know what could happen if uric acid precipitated in the renal tubules? *_____

▶ FLUID AND ELECTROLYTE DISTURBANCES

Table 25-1 lists the fluid and electrolyte disturbances commonly associated with cancer and cancer therapy. Also given are abnormal serum levels and the rationale for their occurrence.

10 cachexia; secretion of abnormal hormones OR ectopic hormone secretion

11 ADH; PTH; ACTH; water intoxication, hyponatremia, hypokalemia, and hypophosphatemia

12 cachexia, secretion of abnormal hormones (i.e., ADH, PTH, ACTH), and catabolism of purine nucleic acids

13 renal disorders and possible renal failure

Table 25-1

Fluid and Electrolyte Disturbance in Cancer and Cancer Therapy

Fluid/Electrolyte Disturbance	Commonly Associated Cancer and Cancer Therapy	Defining Characteristics	Rationale/Comments
Hypercalcemia	Breast cancer, multiple myeloma, ovarian cancer, pancreatic cancer, leukemia, lymphoma, lung cancer, bladder cancer, kidney cancer, head and neck cancer, and prostate cancer	Serum calcium >11 mg/dL	Hypercalcemia occurs in 10–20% of all cancer clients and in 40–50% of those with metastatic breast cancer or multiple myeloma. It is caused by bone destruction by metastatic tumors, elevated parathyroid hormone (PTH) levels related to some tumors, and elevated prostaglandin and osteoclast activating factor (OAF). Prolonged immobility is also a causative factor.
Hyponatremia (usually associated with dehydration)	Lung cancer, pancreatic cancer, multiple myeloma, head and neck cancer, stomach cancer, brain cancer, colon cancer, ovarian cancer, and prostate cancer; aggressive diuretic therapy. High-dose cyclophosphamide/Cytoxan therapy; daunorubicin or cytosine chemotherapy (decreases blast cell count)	Serum sodium <135 mEq/L	Hyponatremia is caused by liver, thyroid, and adrenal insufficiencies, renal failure, and congestive heart failure. A condition known as cerebral salt wasting is caused by some intracranial neoplasms. In this condition the brain releases a postulated natriuretic factor or the neural innervation to the brain is altered. The result is the kidneys' inability to conserve sodium.
Syndrome of inappropriate antidiuretic hormone (SIADH)	Lung cancer, pancreatic cancer, brain cancer, ovarian cancer, colon cancer, sarcoma, leukemia, prostate cancer, Hodgkin's disease, and other lymphomas; vincristine, cyclophosphamide chemotherapy	Serum sodium <130 mEq/L, serum osmolality <280 mOsm/kg	SIADH occurs because of increased release of ADH from posterior pituitary or ectopically from neoplastic tumors. The posterior pituitary then becomes impervious to the usual feedback control mechanism.
Hyperuricemia	Leukemias, lymphomas, multiple myeloma, any cancer treated aggressively with chemotherapy or radiation	Serum uric acid >8.0 mg/dL, uric acid crystals in urine	Breakdown of large numbers of cells causes release of uric acid into the bloodstream (tumor lysis syndrome). Precipitation of uric acid in the kidneys results in gouty nephropathy, acute hyperuricemic nephropathy, and eventual renal failure. First signs of hyperuricemic renal failure may be nausea, vomiting, and lethargy. This type of renal failure may or may not be reversible. Symptoms of hyperuricemia include hematuria, flank pain, nausea, vomiting, and symptoms of renal failure.

(continues on the following page)

Table 25-1

(Continued)

Fluid/Electrolyte Disturbance	Commonly Associated Cancer and Cancer Therapy	Defining Characteristics	Rationale/Comments
Hypokalemia	Colon cancer, multiple myeloma, Hodgkin's disease, pancreatic cancer, stomach cancer, thyroid cancer, adrenal adenoma, adrenal hyperplasia tumors, and cancers that secrete adrenocorticotropic hormone (ACTH) ectopically	Serum potassium <3.5 mEq/L	Dietary intake of potassium is deficient when the client is anorexic, vomiting, or NPO. Excessive diarrhea that leads to rapid potassium depletion occurs with many GI tumors, chemotherapy, radiation therapy to the lower abdomen, and antibiotic therapy. Excessive urinary excretion may be caused by diuretics, hypercalcemia, hypomagnesemia, antibiotic therapy, ectopic ACTH secretion, nephrotoxicity due to chemotherapy or radiation, and renal tubular necrosis due to Hodgkin's disease, multiple myeloma, and acute blast crisis. Ileostomy, colostomy, fistulas, and the diuretic phase of renal failure also contribute to hypokalemia.
Hypomagnesemia	Lung cancer, especially oat cell, ovarian cancer, and testicular cancer; total parenteral nutrition (TPN), *cis*-platinum chemotherapy	Serum magnesium <1.5 mEq/L	Low magnesium level occurs most often in clients with severe diarrhea, vomiting, malabsorption syndrome, cachexia, ADH secretion, or renal disease. The *cis*-platinum and nephrotoxic antibiotics also contribute to hypomagnesemia.
Lactic acidosis	Hodgkin's disease, lymphoma, leukemia, lymphosarcoma, and lung cancer (especially oat cell with liver metastasis)	Arterial blood pH <7.35, HCO_3 <24 mEq/L, serum CO_2 <22 mEq/L	Lactic acidosis (metabolic acidosis) occurs because rapidly growing malignant cells utilize large amounts of glucose. When the glucose is metabolized by the anaerobic pathway (glycolysis), pyruvic acid is the end product. When hypoxia exists, pyruvate is converted to lactic acid. Elevated serum lactic acid concentrations may exceed the liver's ability to metabolize and the kidneys' to excrete.

(continues on the following page)

Table 25-1

Fluid and Electrolyte Disturbance in Cancer and Cancer Therapy *(Continued)*

Fluid/Electrolyte Disturbance	Commonly Associated Cancer and Cancer Therapy	Defining Characteristics	Rationale/Comments
Hyperkalemia	Hodgkins' disease, lymphoma, leukemia, lung cancer (especially oat cell), and liver metastasis; aggressive chemotherapy	Serum potassium >5.3 mEq/L	Intracellular-extracellular redistribution occurs during respiratory and metabolic acidosis (including lactic acidosis). Extracellular hydrogen ions shift into the cell in an attempt to raise serum pH. Intracellular potassium ions then shift out of the cell to compensate. Lysis of large numbers of malignant and normal cells during radiation and chemotherapy causes the release of massive amounts of potassium from destroyed cells (tumor lysis syndrome). Renal failure and hypoaldosteronism can cause renal retention of potassium.
Hypophosphatemia	Leukemia, multiple myeloma, PTH-secreting tumors; total parenteral nutrition (TPN) (hyperalimentation)	Serum phosphorus <2.5 mg/dL	Hypophosphatemia occurs with cancers that contain and secrete PTH (PTH normally regulates the rate of phosphorus reabsorption by the kidneys). Aggressive hyperalimentation/parenteral nutrition often induces hypophosphatemia because the phosphorus influx into cells is accelerated during carbohydrate metabolism. Malabsorption, sepsis, diuretics, corticosteroids, and thrombocytopenia are other contributing factors. Symptoms of hypophosphatemia are fatigue, weakness, anorexia, irritability, paresthesia, seizures, and coma.

(continues on the following page)

Table 25-1

(Continued)

Fluid/Electrolyte Disturbance	Commonly Associated Cancer and Cancer Therapy	Defining Characteristics	Rationale/Comments
Decreased vascular volume (shift to the third space)	Liver cancer, including liver metastasis, stomach cancer, pancreatic cancer, colon cancer, and head and neck cancer	Serum albumin <3.2 g/dL, decreased BP, increased H & H, increased BUN	Decreased vascular volume occurs when serum protein is decreased, when tumor cells exude fluids, or when vascular permeability is increased by infection. Protein depletion occurs with anorexia/cachexia, nausea, and vomiting due to disease or therapy or to decreased protein synthesis in cancer clients. Some individuals with cancer have increased loss of protein via the GI tract; elevated basal metabolic rate due to disease or infection results in accelerated protein loss. Decreased serum protein leads to decreased blood volume and a drop in blood pressure. The client may have ample or excess extracellular fluid but is unable to retain it within the vascular space. Without treatment, cardiovascular failure and death result.
Hypocalcemia/hyper-phosphatemia	Leukemia, lymphoma, and multiple myeloma; aggressive chemotherapy and radiation	Serum calcium <9 mg/dL, serum phosphorus >4.5 mg/dL	Rapid cell lysis causes the release of large amounts of phosphate. Immature blast cells contain up to four times more phosphate than mature lymphocytes. The rise in serum phosphorus then causes a drop in serum calcium. Renal failure may result from precipitation of calcium phosphate in the kidneys. Symptoms include oliguria, anuria, azotemia, and tetany.

14 hypercalcemia or calcium excess; >11

14

Bone destruction that results from metastatic tumors causes what type of calcium imbalance? _____ . The serum level would be _____ mg/dL.

15 Yes; Liver, thyroid, and adrenal insufficiencies are followed by a loss of sodium. Also intracranial neoplasms could result in cerebral salt wasting and the inability of the kidneys to conserve sodium.; Not usually.

16 reabsorbed; vincristine and cyclophosphamide

17 chemotherapy; radiation; It could cause renal failure by precipitation of uric acid crystals in the kidneys.

18 hematuria, flank pain, and nausea and vomiting (also symptoms of renal failure)

19 Yes.; poor dietary intake of potassium, excessive diarrhea, and excessive urinary secretion (also vomiting, colostomy, and excess adrenal gland secretion from tumor); <3.5

20 Yes.; The breakdown of malignant and normal cells causes potassium to shift from cells to vascular fluid.; >5.3

21 because of vomiting, malabsorption syndrome, severe diarrhea, cachexia, and total parenteral nutrition (TPN)

15

Can hyponatremia be associated with cancer? _____
    Explain how? * _____
_____
    Can hypernatremia be associated with cancer? _____

16

The syndrome of inappropriate antidiuretic hormone (SIADH) can be associated with cancer. As a result, more water is (reabsorbed/excreted) _____ by the kidneys.
    The two drug therapies that contribute to SIADH are
* _____ .

17

Hyperuricemia can occur in any cancer treated aggressively with _____ or _____ .
    Explain the effect of a high-serum uric acid on kidney function. * _____
_____

18

Name three symptoms of hyperuricemia. * _____
_____

19

Can hypokalemia occur as the result of cancer? _____
    Give three reasons why there may be a low potassium level.
* _____
    The serum potassium level is _____ mEq/L.

20

Can hyperkalemia be induced by cancer? _____
    Explain why? * _____
_____
    The serum potassium level is _____ mEq/L.

21

Why does hypomagnesemia develop? * _____
_____

22 PTH secreting tumors; total parenteral nutrition (TPN)

22
Hypophosphatemia is usually associated with cancer in *_____ and *_____ .

23
A large amount of glucose is utilized by rapidly growing malignant cells. Pyruvic acid is the end product of anaerobic metabolism of glucose. When hypoxia exists, pyruvate is converted to lactic acid. The specific acid-base imbalance is *_____ .
The arterial blood pH is _____ .
The arterial bicarbonate is _____ mEq/L.

23 lactic acidosis; <7.35; <24

24
Calcium and phosphorus imbalance may be present in leukemia, lymphoma, multiple myeloma, and aggressive chemotherapy and radiation.
Identify the imbalances that occur together:
( ) a. Hypocalcemia
( ) b. Hypercalcemia
( ) c. Hypophosphatemia
( ) d. Hyperphosphatemia

24 a, d

25 decreased vascular volume of ECFV deficit (vascular); Protein loss decreases osmotic pressure and less fluid is held in the vascular space. When protein shifts to an injured or damaged site and permeability is increased, fluid shifts to the third space (to the injured or damaged site).

25
When protein depletion occurs because of anorexia/cachexia and nausea/vomiting, what type of fluid imbalance may result?
*_____
Explain why. *_____
_____
_____

26
Indicate which of the following electrolyte imbalances are frequently associated with cancer and cancer therapy:
( ) a. Hypercalcemia
( ) b. Hypernatremia
( ) c. Hypokalemia
( ) d. Hyperkalemia
( ) e. Hypomagnesemia
( ) f. Hypermagnesemia
( ) g. Hypophosphatemia
( ) h. Hypocalcemia/hyperphosphatemia

26 a, c, d, e, g, h

A less common form of cancer therapy involves lymphokine-activated killer (LAK) cell therapy and often results in vascular leak syndrome. Increased vascular permeability in this syndrome causes severe edema and cardiovascular hypotension.

27

LAK cell therapy often results in what syndrome? *_____

Two clinical findings in vascular leak syndrome are _____ and *_____ . These findings are both caused by *_____ .

27 vascular leak syndrome; edema; cardiovascular hypotension; increased vascular permeability

▶ CLINICAL APPLICATIONS

The fluid and electrolyte disturbances listed in Table 25-1 can develop in almost any individual with cancer at any time during diagnosis, treatment, recovery, or terminal stages of the disease.

Fluid and electrolyte problems are *most common,* however, with the following clinical conditions:

1. *Cachexia.* Severe anorexia, nausea, vomiting, and/or diarrhea are present.
2. *Tumor lysis syndrome.* Large numbers of cells are destroyed by chemotherapy radiation.
3. *Uncontrolled cell growth.* Rapid, widespread cell growth with multiple metastasis or multiple organ infiltration.
4. *Ectopic hormone production.* Ectopic hormones are secreted by the tumor(s).

Cachexia

Cachexia may occur because of the effects of the malignancy itself and/or be caused by radiation, immunotherapy, and chemotherapy. Contributing problems include anorexia, nausea, vomiting, diarrhea, draining wounds, and fistulas. The most frequently encountered fluid and electrolyte disturbances are hypomagnesemia, hypokalemia, and decreased vascular volume.

28

Name the two electrolytes that are most commonly lost due to cachexia. *_____

_____

Do you recall the methods/routes for replacing potassium and magnesium? See Chapters 6 and 9 on potassium and magnesium replacement.

Potassium: _____ and _____ .

Magnesium: _____ , _____ , and _____

28 potassium and magnesium; intravenously; orally; intravenously; intramuscularly; orally

29

Anorexia, nausea, and vomiting decrease protein intake; diarrhea, malabsorption syndrome, and wound drainage increase protein loss in the cancer client.

Decreased vascular volume occurs in cachexic clients because of *_____ (see Table 25-1).

Protein synthesis is (increased/decreased) _____ in many cancer clients. Metabolic changes and infections accelerate *_____ .

29 protein depletion or loss; decreased; protein loss

30

The basic goal of therapy in cancer clients with decreased vascular volume is to maintain blood pressure. Whole blood, packed red blood cells (RBCs), or albumin may be given to increase plasma oncotic pressure (colloid osmotic pressure) to restore fluid balance in the vascular space. Whole blood, packed RBCs, and albumin restore the fluid balance in the vessels by *_____ .

30 increasing plasma oncotic pressure OR increasing colloid osmotic pressure in vascular space

31

Carefully prescribed and monitored hyperalimentation (TPN) can correct hypokalemia and hypomagnesemia and improve vascular volume.

What happens to the serum phosphorus level when TPN is aggressively administered? *_____

_____ (Refer to Table 25-1.)

Prolonged parenteral nutrition without magnesium supplement can cause _____ .

31 Hypophosphatemia occurs because of phosphorus influx into cells during carbohydrate metabolism.; hypomagnesemia

Tumor Lysis Syndrome

Following the destruction of large numbers of cells by chemotherapy, usually in leukemia or lymphoma, vast numbers of intracellular electrolytes enter the bloodstream. The cancer client can develop hyperuricemia, hyperkalemia, hyperphosphatemia, and/or hypocalcemia. Renal failure or cardiac arrest may result.

32

When a large number of cells in the body is destroyed by chemotherapy what two life-threatening situations can result?
* _____

Identify the imbalances that occur during massive cell destruction:
( ) a. Hypokalemia
( ) b. Hyperkalemia
( ) c. Hypocalcemia
( ) d. Hypercalcemia
( ) e. Hyperphosphatemia
( ) f. Hyperuricemia

33

The purpose of therapy for cancer clients who are undergoing the destruction of large numbers of cells is the prevention of renal failure and *_____ .

Management includes aggressive hydration (3000 mL/day) to increase urinary volume and excretion of *_____ ,
_____ , and _____ .

34

Drugs used for the management of fluid and electrolytes include
Potent diuretics such as furosemide/Lasix when there is fluid retention;
Allopurinol to decrease uric acid;
Calcium gluconate IV infusion if hypocalcemia develops;
Sodium bicarbonate to alkalinize the urine if hyperuricemia occurs (uric acid is less soluble in acid urine).

Four imbalances found with massive cell destruction are
* _____

_____ .

---

32 renal failure and cardiac arrest; b, c, e, f

33 electrolyte imbalance. (If your answer was cardiac arrest, true, but that usually results from severe electrolyte imbalance.); uric acid; potassium; phosphorus (phosphate)

34 hyperkalemia, hyperphosphatemia, hyperuricemia, and hypocalcemia

Uncontrolled Cell Growth

Individuals with cancer may experience severe electrolyte disturbances whenever rapid and widespread malignant cell growth occurs. This uncontrolled cell growth is marked by multiple metastatic lesions (metastatic carcinoma or sarcoma) or by multiple organ infiltration (leukemias and lymphomas).

35
Hypercalcemia is usually present when *_____
_____ . (Refer to Table 25-1.)

Hypercalcemia in individuals with cancer develops more rapidly and becomes more severe than hypercalcemia from other causes. When acute hypercalcemia crisis occurs, the mortality rate is extremely high (up to 50%).

36
Management of mild and moderate hypercalcemia involves IV normal saline (NaCl 0.9%) to achieve adequate hydration and promote calcium excretion.

For severe hypercalcemia the following drugs are indicated:
Furosemide/Lasix to decrease tubular reabsorption of calcium.
Steroids to increase calcium excretion.
Calcitonin to inhibit bone resorption.
Mithramycin to inhibit bone resorption.
Biphosphonates to inhibit calcium release from bone.
Gallium nitrate to make calcium dissolution more difficult.
IV inorganic phosphates (severe side effects could be calcium precipitation in lung, kidney, or heart tissues).

With mild and moderate hypercalcemia effective management includes *_____ .

Two drugs frequently prescribed for severe hypercalcemia are *_____ . A diuretic that promotes kidney excretion of calcium is _____ .

37
Lactic acidosis and hyperkalemia may occur during periods of uncontrolled malignant cell growth.

Lactic acidosis is the result of *_____
_____ . (Refer to Table 25-1.)

What is the cause of hyperkalemia? *_____
_____ (Refer to Table 25-1.)

35 metastatic tumors cause bone destruction OR metastatic cell growth or infiltration destroys bone

36 IV normal saline; mithramycin and calcitonin; furosemide

37 rapidly growing malignant cells that utilize excess glucose with anaerobic metabolism and cause lactic acid as a by-product; Acidosis causes a compensatory shift of extracellular hydrogen ions and intracellular potassium.

Ectopic Hormone Production

Abnormal hormones may be secreted by any malignant cells. The most commonly involved cancers and hormones are those listed in Table 25-2. Study the contents in the table and refer back to it as needed.

38 ADH or antidiuretic hormone, PTH or parathyroid hormone, and ACTH or adrenocortico-tropic hormone; lung

38

Name three ectopic hormones that can be secreted by malignant cells. *_____

Ectopic hormone secretions occur most commonly with what type of cancer? _____ .

39

Acute complications caused by ectopic hormone secretions in cancer clients include fluid and electrolyte imbalances. If the imbalances are severe, cardiac arrest may occur.

Table 25-2

Hormones Commonly Secreted Ectopically by Malignant Cells

Hormones	Type of Cancer	Common Associated Problems
Antidiuretic hormone (ADH)	Lung (oat cell) Pancreas Hodgkin's disease Prostate gland Sarcoma	SIADH Hyponatremia Hypomagnesemia
Parathyroid hormone (PTH)	Lung Leukemia Multiple myeloma Breast	Hypercalcemia Hypophosphatemia Hypomagnesemia
Adrenocorticotropic hormone (ACTH)	Lung (oat cell and non-oat cell)	Hypokalemia
Osteoclast activating factor (OAF)	Multiple myeloma Lymphoma	Hypercalcemia
Prostaglandins (E series)	Breast Kidney Pancreas	Hypercalcemia

39 hypercalcemia, hypomagnesemia, hyponatremia,
and hyperphosphatemia
(also hypokalemia)

According to Table 25-2, four common electrolyte imbalances
that result from ectopic hormone secretions are *_____
_____ .

40
The primary goal of therapy in cancer clients with ectopic
hormone secretion is the eradication or reduction of the
hormone-secreting tumor. If surgery, radiation, and/or
chemotherapy do not eliminate the tumor and control the
symptoms, long-term pharmacologic therapy may be ordered.

40 surgery, radiation, and
chemotherapy

What are the three methods that can be used to reduce or
eradicate the hormone-secreting tumor? *_____
_____

41
Treatment of SIADH varies with the severity of the symptoms.
Mild SIADH: Restriction of water and fluid intake to
                       500–1000 mL/day.
Severe SIADH: 3–5% saline infusion to restore serum sodium;
                       furosemide (Lasix) to increase water excretion;
                       demeclocycline or lithium carbonate to interfere
                       with the action of ADH on renal tubules.
    Extreme care should be taken when hyperosmolar saline is
administered (3–5% saline solution) because it could raise the
serum sodium level too rapidly and cause shrinkage of CNS
neurons and neurologic dysfunction.

41 secretion (syndrome) of
inappropriate antidiuretic
hormone; restriction of
fluid to 500-1000 mL daily.

    SIADH is the abbreviation for *_____ .
    Treatment for mild SIADH is *_____ .

42
Indicate which of the following treatments may be used for
managing severe SIADH:
    ( ) a. 0.9% saline (normal saline solution)
    ( ) b. 3–5% saline infusion
    ( ) c. Radiation to tumor
    ( ) d. Chemotherapy to tumor
    ( ) e. Surgical removal of ADH-secreting tumor
    ( ) f. Lithium carbonate
    ( ) g. Ampicillin
    ( ) h. Demeclocycline

42 b, c, d, e, f, h

43 An elevated serum sodium level (hypernatremia) causes shrinkage of CNS neurons and neurologic dysfunction.

44 cachexia, tumor lysis syndrome, uncontrolled cell growth, and ectopic hormone production

43
What can happen if excessive amounts of 3–5% saline are administered to correct SIADH? * _____

_____

44
Name the four major problems found in cancer clients that are commonly associated with fluid and electrolyte disorders.
* _____

_____

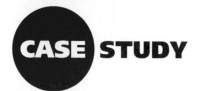

REVIEW A

Ralph Peterson, a 53-year-old auto mechanic, complained to his doctor of progressive dyspnea, a persistent, productive cough, fatigue, anorexia, and weight loss.

A chest x-ray, magnetic resonance imaging (MRI), sputum cytology, and bronchoscopy were performed and Mr. Peterson was diagnosed as having stage II squamous-cell lung cancer. The primary tumor was removed by lobectomy and radiation therapy was given a month later to reduce the risk of metastasis.

Fourteen months after his surgery Mr. Peterson was readmitted because of severe weight loss (30 pounds in 3 months), fatigue, and dyspnea. CT scans revealed that Mr. Peterson had a large metastatic lesion in the liver and two smaller tumors in the right lung.

Laboratory studies were ordered for Mr. Peterson on admission, on day 3, on day 10, on day 11, and a month later. The results of his laboratory tests are given in Table 25-3. Complete the questions related to his laboratory studies by following the table.

45
On admission, Mr. Peterson's lab tests suggested that he had decreased vascular volume, also called ECFV deficit or dehydration. (Refer to Chapter 2 on ECFV deficit if needed.)

Which of his following laboratory results are indicative of decreased vascular volume?

Table 25-3

Laboratory Studies: Mr. Peterson

Laboratory Tests	On Admission	Day 3	Day 10	Day 11	One Month
Hematology					
Hemoglobin (Hgb) (Male: 13.5–18 g)	18.5	14			
Hematocrit (Hct) (Male: 40–54%)	54	46			
Biochemistry					
BUN (10–25 mg/dL)	34	21			
Creatinine (Cr) (0.6–1.2 mg/dL)	2.1	1.5			
Uric acid (Male: 3.5–7 mg/dL)	7.8				
Lactate (serum) (6–16 mg/dL)	17				
Albumin (serum) (3.5–5.0 g/dL)	2.8	4.3			
Potassium (K) (3.5–5.3 mEq/L)	3.1	4.2	3.0		
Sodium (Na) (135–146 mEq/L)	118	135			
Chloride (Cl) (95–108 mEq/L)	103	102			
Calcium (Ca) (9–11 mg/dL)	8.8	8.8	14.4	13.4	16.6
Phosphorus (P) (2.5–4.5 mg/dL)	3.1		2.2		
Magnesium (Mg) (1.5–2.5 mEq/L)			1.3		

( ) a. Hemoglobin 18.5 g
( ) b. Hematocrit 54%
( ) c. BUN 34 mg/dL
( ) d. Serum albumin 2.8 g/dL
( ) e. Serum potassium 3.1 mEq/L (hypokalemia)
( ) f. Serum sodium 118 mEq/L (hyponatremia)
( ) g. Serum chloride 103 mEq/L
( ) h. Serum calcium 8.8 mg/dL
( ) i. Serum phosphorus 3.1 mg/dL
( ) j. Serum lactate 17 mg/dL
( ) k. Serum uric acid 7.8 mg/dL

45 a, b (very high normal), c d, e (possible), f (possible)

46

Hemoglobin and BUN may be elevated because of (hemodilution/hemoconcentration) _____ .
    Protein, sodium, and potassium are shifted to the tumor site, thus (increasing/decreasing) _____ oncotic pressure/colloid osmotic pressure. Will this have an effect on vascular fluid balance? _____ Explain *_____
_____

46 hemoconcentration; decreasing; Yes.; Decreased oncotic pressure in the vascular space causes fluid loss or dehydration.

47

On admission, Mr. Peterson's vital signs were temperature (T) 100°F, pulse rate (P) 124, respiration (R) 28, and blood pressure (BP) 96/60.
    Which of his vital signs are indicative of fluid volume deficit (vascular fluid):
    ( ) a. T 100°F
    ( ) b. P 124
    ( ) c. R 28
    ( ) d. BP 96/60

47 a, b, c (possible), d

48

IV albumin and packed RBCs were given to raise the serum oncotic pressure and to maintain vascular fluid and adequate blood pressure. He was started on hyperalimentation (TPN) to improve his overall nutritional status prior to chemotherapy. His anorexia, nausea, and fatigue gradually lessened and his BP stabilized at 116/74–110/70.
    The purpose of IV albumin and packed RBC administration is to *_____ , *_____ , and *_____ .

48 raise the serum oncotic pressure; maintain vascular fluid; maintain adequate blood pressure

49 Yes. Creatinine is slightly elevated and serum sodium is low normal.

50 hypokalemia, hypercalcemia, hypomagnesemia, and hypophosphatemia

51 to decrease the high serum calcium level; The serum calcium level was still high and both hypocalcemic agents decreased the serum level.

52 that hypercalcemia was not due to bone destruction; hypercalcemia and hypophosphatemia (also hypomagnesemia)

49

Were Mr. Peterson's laboratory results 3 days after admission of normal values? _____ Please explain. *_____

_____

50

Mr. Peterson was discharged and then readmitted 10 days after his first admission. Mr. Peterson's condition had greatly improved and chemotherapy was scheduled to begin the next day. However, he became restless and irritable and by evening was disoriented and combative. He also became increasingly weak and vomited several times.

On day ten his serum electrolytes were not within normal values. Name four electrolyte imbalances present. *_____

_____

51

His immediate treatment consisted of the following:

1. Calcitonin 100 MRC units subcutaneously every 12 hours
2. Furosemide 20 mg IV push every 6 hours
3. Sodium phosphate ($Na_2 HPO_4$) 15 mL PO three times daily
4. Potassium and magnesium increased in TPN
5. IV rate increased to 150 mL/h

On day eleven the calcitonin dose was changed:

1. Calcitonin 300 MRC units subcutaneously every 12 hours
2. Mithramycin 1 mg IV push

Why was calcitonin administered? *_____
Why were mithramycin and calcitonin given on the eleventh day? *_____

_____

52

To determine the cause of Mr. Peterson's hypercalcemia, a bone scan and PTH level was done. The bone scan was negative. This indicates *_____ .

His PTH level of 455 pg Eq/mL (norm: 163–375 pg Eq/mL) indicated that the metastatic tumors in his lung were secreting PTH ectopically. This increased PTH secretion causes the two electrolyte imbalances *_____ .

53 yes, on the lower normal side

54 hypercalcemia

53

Mr. Peterson was started on a combination of chemotherapeutics (incristine, cyclophosphamide/Cytoxan, and Doxorubicin HCI) to shrink the tumors and decrease the PTH secretion.

After 5 days of chemotherapy his serum calcium was 9 mg/dL. Is this in normal range? Explain *_____ . He was alert, oriented, and eating and drinking well; soon he was discharged.

54

A month later he was readmitted with a serum calcium level of 16.6 mg/dL. The type of imbalance present is _____ .

A similar drug regime was followed, and after his serum calcium level returned to normal, he was discharged on daily calcitonin injections.

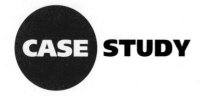
CASE STUDY

REVIEW B

Steven Blackman, 15 years old, was rushed to the local emergency room by his parents when he awakened feeling weak and short of breath. His parents told the health care provider that he had complained of feeling tired for 2 or 3 weeks and had a sore throat and swollen glands and two nosebleeds the week before. Steven's lungs were not congested, but the health care provider noted moderate lymphadenopathy and an enlarged liver and spleen. He was admitted to the adolescent unit with a suspected diagnosis of acute leukemia.

Vital signs were as follows:

T 101°F, P 124, R 30, BP 100/66

Steven Blackman's laboratory results on admission, day 1, and day 6 are given in Table 25-4. Refer to the table as needed as you proceed with this clinical example.

55

On admission, Steven's hemoglobin and hematocrit were decreased because his bone marrow had been infiltrated by

Table 25-4

Laboratory Studies: Steven Blackman

Laboratory Tests	On Admission	Day 1	Day 6
Hematology			
Hemoglobin (Hgb) (12.5–18 g/dL)	7		
Hematocrit (Hct) (40–54%)	18		
Platelets (150,000–400,000 mm^3)	56,000		
White blood cells (WBC) (5000–10,000 mm^3)	31,000		
Differential			
Blasts (0–5%)	46%		
Biochemistry			
BUN (10–25 mg/dL)	30	28	41
Creatinine (Cr) (0.6–1.2 mg/dL)	1.8	1.7	2.6
Uric acid (3.5–7 mg/dL)	8.6		19
Lactate (serum) (6–16 mg/dL)	17		
Potassium (serum) (3.5–5.3 mEq/L)	5.7	4.1	5.9
Sodium (serum) 135–146 mEq/L)	140		
Calcium (serum) (9–11 mg/dL)	9.0		7.6
Magnesium (serum) (1.5–2.5 mEq/L)	2.0		
Chloride (Cl) (95–108 mEq/L)	103		
Phosphorus (serum) (2.5–4.5 mEq/L)	3.8		8.0
Arterial Blood Gases (ABGs)			
pH (7.35–7.45)	7.28	7.38	
PaO$_2$ (70–90%)	90	92	
PaCO$_2$ (35–45 mm Hg)	34	38	
HCO$_3$ (24–28 mEq/L)	22	26	

55 weakness or fatigue; low; nosebleeds.

56 metabolic acidosis (his pH and HCO₃ are low); lactic acidosis. This is the result of an abnormal carbohydrate metabolism in the blast cells (immature WBCs).

57 renal insufficiency. Remember, if the BUN were slightly elevated and the creatinine in normal range, this insufficiency could be due to ECFV deficit or dehydration. Renal insufficiency reduces the body's ability to excrete the excess lactic acid.

58 hyperkalemia

59 As the pH rises, potassium will shift back into the cells and too much NaHCO₃ could cause alkalosis and hypokalemia.

60 tumor lysis syndrome

leukemic cells which led to decreased RBC production. This could be the reason for his _____ .

His platelet count was (high/low) _____ , a possible reason for his _____ .

His elevated WBCs are indicative of a serious problem.

56

His ABGs indicate what acid-base disorder? *_____ (Refer to Chapter 13 if needed.)

At his elevated serum lactate level the specific acid-base imbalance would be *_____ .

57

Steven's elevated BUN and creatinine could be caused by *_____ because his uric acid, in particular, is elevated.

58

His potassium level indicated _____ . This could be cellular breakdown and acidotic state.

59

Steven received NaHCO₃ in D₅W to correct acidosis. His serum potassium had to be carefully monitored while the acidotic state was being corrected. Why? *_____

_____

60

A bone marrow biopsy showed that the marrow had been almost entirely replaced by immature myeloblasts. This confirmed Steven's diagnosis of acute myelogenous leukemia (AML).

Steven was started on a chemotherapeutic regimen of doxorubicin, cytarabine, and thioquanine in an attempt to induce remission (absence of all leukemic cells).

High doses of chemotherapy result in the lysis of large numbers of malignant cells; therefore Steven was monitored for signs and symptoms of *_____ .

61

On day 6 he complained of flank pain and his urinary output decreased sharply. Laboratory values were indicative of tumor lysis syndrome.

61 hyperuricemia, hyperkalemia, hypocalcemia, and hyperphosphatemia

Name four imbalances that are significant of this disorder.

*_____

_____

62

Two other laboratory values that were indicative of his decreased urine output were *_____ .

62 elevated BUN and elevated creatinine

63

His uric acid was corrected with increased IV fluids and allopurinol (to promote uric acid excretion).

His health professional monitored his intake and output carefully and checked for edema, chest rales, and level of consciousness (LOC). Explain why? *_____

_____

63 Decreased urinary output and increased IV fluids could result in fluid overload or ECFV excess.

64

Which of the following laboratory tests should be monitored?

( ) a. Hemoglobin
( ) b. Hematocrit
( ) c. Electrolytes
( ) d. Hormones, e.g., PTH
( ) e. Phenylketonuria
( ) f. Protein and albumin

( ) g. Lactate
( ) h. Uric acid
( ) i. Lipoproteins
( ) j. BUN
( ) k. Creatinine
( ) l. ABGs

64 a, b, c, d, f, g, h, j, k, l

CASE STUDY REVIEW

ANSWER COLUMN

1. cachexia, abnormal (ectopic) hormone secretion, and increased uric acid or breakdown of purine nucleic acids

1. The three problems associated with primitive biochemical function of malignant cells are *_____ .

2. Give the names of electrolyte imbalances associated with cancer and cancer therapy:

2. a. hypercalcemia
   b. hypocalcemia;
   hyperphosphatemia
   c. hyponatremia
   d. hypokalemia;
   hyperkalemia
   e. hypophosphatemia

3. uric acid precipitates in the
   renal tubules and
   collecting ducts; a small
   increased level can cause
   renal disorder and possible
   renal failure

4. hematuria, flank pain, and
   nausea and vomiting (also
   symptoms of renal failure)

5. bone destruction which
   results from metastasis;
   elevated PTH; confusion;
   disorientation; and cardiac
   arrest (also brittle bones)

6. ADH may be secreted
   ectopically from neoplastic
   tumors, e.g., lung tumor.
   SIADH can cause severe
   water intoxication,
   hyponatremia, headaches,
   and behavioral changes.

7. decreased dietary intake,
   vomiting/diarrhea, and
   excessive urinary output
   due to diuretics (also
   ileostomy, colostomy, and
   fistulas)

8. Lactic acidosis (metabolic
   acidosis).; Anaerobic
   metabolism of glucose
   produces pyruvic acid,
   which is converted during
   hypoxia to lactic acid.

9. cachexia, tumor lysis
   syndrome, uncontrolled
   cell growth, and ectopic
   hormone production

10. dehydration, fluid loss, or
   hemoconcentration

11. dehydration; renal
   insufficiency (If the BUN
   returns to normal after
   hydration the problem is
   dehydration.)

a. Calcium _____
b. Calcium _____
   and phosphorus _____
c. Sodium _____
d. Potassium _____
e. Phosphorus _____

3. Hyperuricemia is a serious condition that results from massive cell destruction by radiation or chemotherapy. What is its effect on the renal tubules? *_____ What could happen to the body? *_____
   _____

4. Three symptoms of hyperuricemia are *_____
   _____

5. Hypercalcemia is a serious condition. It is generally caused by
   *_____
   or *_____
   A very high calcium level can cause _____, _____,
   and *_____ .

6. SIADH is another serious condition. Why? *_____
   _____

7. Give three reasons why hypokalemia may occur. *_____
   _____

8. What type of acid-base imbalance is caused by anaerobic metabolism of glucose? *_____

   Explain how. *_____
   _____

9. Name the four most common causes of fluid and electrolyte imbalance in cancer clients. *_____
   _____

   Mr. Peterson had been diagnosed 14 months before as having lung cancer. He was readmitted to the hospital because of severe weight loss, fatigue, and dyspnea.

10. Mr. Peterson's hemoglobin and hematocrit were elevated. This may be the result of _____ .

11. His BUN and creatinine were slightly elevated. This may be caused by _____ or _____ .

12. Decreased vascular volume.; Protein shifts to tumor site, thus decreasing oncotic pressure.

12. What effects do low serum protein and albumin levels have on the vascular fluid?* _____ Why?* _____
_____

On day 10 after admission Mr. Peterson's calcium level was high. He was restless, irritable, disoriented, combative, weak, and vomiting.

13. Calcitonin and mithramycin

13. Two drugs Mr. Peterson received to decrease his serum calcium level were * _____ .

Steven Blackman, 15 years old, was diagnosed as having acute leukemia. The results of his hematology on admission indicated a low hemoglobin, hematocrit, and platelet count and an elevated WBC.

14. lactic acidosis (if the results were based on ABGs, metabolic acidosis)

14. Steven's pH and HCO_3 were low and his serum lactate was slightly elevated. What acid-base disorder do you suspect? * _____

15. hyperkalemia; cellular breakdown and acidotic state

15. His serum potassium level was 5.7 mEq/L. What potassium imbalance is present? _____ Why?* _____
_____

16. hypokalemic alkalosis (potassium shifts back into cells)

16. When correcting acidosis with $NaHCO_3$, name the imbalance that may occur.* _____

17. tumor lysis syndrome; hyperuricemia

17. Steven was given chemotherapy in massive doses to destroy the large numbers of malignant cells. His uric acid was 19 mg/dL. What disorder frequently results from elevated uric acid?* _____
What imbalance did he have? _____

18. high uric acid or hyperuricemia

18. Steven was given increased amounts of IV fluids, allopurinol, and $NaHCO_3$ (which alkalinizes the urine) to correct what imbalance?* _____

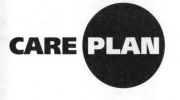

CARE PLAN

Client Management

Assessment Factors

▶ Fluid and electrolyte balance must be monitored carefully in clients with any type of cancer and at all stages of diagnosis and treatment. Assessment is particularly important in clients during and after treatment with chemotherapy, radiation, surgery, biologic response modifiers, and/or bone marrow transplantation. In addition, fluid and electrolyte problems are particularly common in clients dying from cancer.

▶ Assess for anorexia, nausea, vomiting, diarrhea, edema, weight loss or gain, neurologic status, fatigue, and activity levels. Laboratory values of sodium, calcium, potassium, magnesium, and phosphorus should be checked and reported frequently. Arterial blood pH, serum albumin, and serum uric acid should also be assessed as indicated.

▶ Assessment of fluid and electrolyte disturbances is particularly difficult in individuals with cancer because symptoms of these disturbances mimic symptoms often related to other causes, such as chemotherapy, systemic effects of tumor growth, and psychological responses to cancer.

Assessment for and recognition of fluid and electrolyte imbalance in clients with cancer are especially difficult because the symptoms (e.g., anorexia, vomiting, fatigue, diarrhea, and muscle weakness) mimic those of chemotherapy, radiation, or general deterioration in advanced cancer.

Many fluid and electrolyte conditions in cancer clients can be reversed or controlled. It is essential that health professionals assess them. Table 25-5 provides the assessment guideline for fluid and electrolyte imbalance in cancer clients. This table can be used in hospitals and clinics or at home. To use it as an assessment tool, check the blanks in the assessment column. For additional information or clarification use the comment column.

Diagnosis 1

Fluid volume deficit related to decreased serum protein, excessive sodium excretion, and/or decreased concentrating ability of renal tubules.

Interventions and Rationale

1. Check frequently for signs and symptoms of dehydration. Signs such as rapid pulse and dry mucous membranes may be the first indication of fluid volume deficit.

2. Check BP in supine and standing positions. Report a fall of more than 15 mm Hg systolic or more than 10 mm Hg diastolic. A drop of this extent may signal marked dehydration.

3. Monitor intake and output, weight, pulse rate, serum electrolytes, and serum protein. These signs may be early indicators of fluid volume deficit.

Table 25-5

Assessment of Fluid and Electrolyte Imbalance

Type of Primary Cancer: _____

Stage: _____ **Liver metastasis:** _____ **Bone metastasis:** _____

Observation	Assessment		Comments
Vital signs	Temperature	_____	
	Pulse	_____	
	Respiration	_____	
	Blood pressure	_____	
		_____	
	Heart sounds	_____	
	Peripheral pulses	_____	
Intake	PO	_____	
	IV infusions	_____	
	Amounts	_____	
Output	Amounts	_____	
	Specific gravity	_____	
	Urine osmolality	_____	
	Polyuria	_____	
	Oliguria	_____	
	Anuria	_____	
Weight and skin changes	Daily weight	_____	
	Skin turgor	_____	
	Skin temperature	_____	
	Edema	_____	
	Ascites	_____	
GI changes	Anorexia	_____	
	Nausea	_____	
	Vomiting	_____	
	Diarrhea	_____	
	Constipation	_____	
	Bowel sounds	_____	
	Abdominal distention	_____	
	Abdominal cramps	_____	
	Fistula	_____	
	GI suction	_____	
	Draining tube	_____	
Respiratory changes	Dyspnea	_____	
	Hyperpnea	_____	
	Chest crackles	_____	
	Sputum	_____	

(continues on the following page)

Table 25-5

Assessment of Fluid and Electrolyte Imbalance *(Continued)*

Type of Primary Cancer: _____

Stage: _____ **Liver metastasis:** _____ **Bone metastasis:** _____

Observation	Assessment		Comments
Neurologic changes	Headache	_____	
	LOC changes	_____	
	Irritability	_____	
	Disorientation	_____	
	Confusion	_____	
	Paresthesia	_____	
	Altered perception	_____	
	Seizures	_____	
	Coma	_____	
State of being	Alert	_____	
	Fatigue		
	Lethargic	_____	
Muscular changes	Muscle weakness	_____	
	Hyporeflexia	_____	
	Hyperreflexia	_____	
	Muscle cramps	_____	
	Twitching	_____	
	Tetany signs	_____	
Body chemistry and hematology changes	Hemoglobin	_____	
	Hematocrit	_____	
	Platelets	_____	
	WBCs	_____	
	Differential	_____	
	Electrolytes:		
	Potassium	_____	
	Sodium	_____	
	Calcium	_____	
	Magnesium	_____	
	Chloride	_____	
	Phosphorus	_____	
	Serum osmolality	_____	
	Protein	_____	
	Albumin	_____	
	BUN	_____	
	Creatinine	_____	
	Uric acid	_____	
	Lactate	_____	

(continues on the following page)

Table 25-5

(Continued)

Type of Primary Cancer: _____

Stage: _____ **Liver metastasis:** _____ **Bone metastasis:** _____

Observation	Assessment		Comments
	ABGs:		
	pH	_____	
	PaO_2	_____	
	$PaCO_2$	_____	
	HCO_3	_____	
Chemotherapy	Drug	_____	
	Dose, route	_____	
	Side effects	_____	
Radiation therapy	Dose	_____	
	Times	_____	
	Target area	_____	

4. Maintain adequate hydration, with oral fluids if appropriate or with IV fluids as ordered. Fluids are necessary to replace or maintain the serum volume.

5. Administer albumin, packed cells, whole blood, or other blood products as ordered. Albumin helps to maintain the colloid osmotic pressure of the blood and increase plasma volume. Administration of blood products helps to raise blood pressure and improve renal flow.

6. Maintain optimal nutritional status, especially protein intake. An adequate protein intake is essential to maintain normal colloidal pressure and retain fluid in the vascular space.

Diagnosis 2

Altered nutrition: less than body requirements, related to anorexia, vomiting, diarrhea, wound drainage, and/or malabsorption.

Interventions and Rationale

1. Assess current and normal height and weight, diet history, caloric intake, anthropometric measurements, and physiologic factors such as difficulty swallowing or anorexia. This

assessment facilitates identification of individuals with existing nutritional abnormalities or at high risk for nutritional problems. These data are also required to plan and monitor nutritional interventions.

2. Monitor serum albumin, creatinine, lymphocyte count, and nitrogen balance. These values are the most likely to be affected in malnutrition related to cancer.

3. Enhance oral nutrition by encouraging a high-protein, high-calorie diet fortified with commercial supplements. If adequate nutrition can be obtained orally, this route is safer and easier for the client.

4. Encourage small, frequent feedings of calorie-dense and nonacidic foods. Cancer patients often experience an early sensation of fullness, so feedings should be small and spaced apart and should avoid empty calories.

5. Administer medications to control or reduce nausea, vomiting, mouth pain, and diarrhea as needed. Medications that reduce these symptoms increase the client's potential intake and absorption of nutrients.

6. Ease swallowing by implementing measures to relieve dryness of mucous membranes and/or reduce severity of stomatitis, such as oral hygiene, mouth rinses, and lubricants.

7. Compensate for taste alterations by substituting fish, chicken, eggs, and cheese for meats; adding extra sweetness or flavorings; etc.

8. If oral nutrition is inadequate, administer tube feedings through nasogastric, gastrostomy, or jejunostomy tube. The enteral route for provision of nutrition is preferable to the parenteral route.

9. Assist in administration and monitoring of total parenteral nutrition if needed. The parenteral route for administering nutritional support is the least preferable due to the risk of complications, expense, and potential difficulties.

Diagnosis 3

Fluid volume excess related to dilutional hyponatremia and increased levels of ADH.

Interventions and Rationale

1. Monitor intake and output, urine specific gravity, breath sounds, heart sounds, peripheral pulses, edema, nausea, vomiting, anorexia, weakness, and fatigue. Congestive heart failure, weakness, nausea, and vomiting can occur due to hyponatremia and water toxicity.

2. Monitor serum electrolytes and notify physician of Na <120 mEq/L, K <3.5 mEq/L, Ca <8.5 mg/dL, or serum osmolality <280 mOsm/kg. Symptoms of hyponatremia and water toxicity begin near these levels.

3. Monitor and report changes in LOC. Irritability, restlessness, confusion, convulsions, and unresponsiveness can occur.

4. Report weight gain of greater than 2 kg/day. Sudden weight gain may indicate fluid retention.

5. Restrict fluid intake as ordered. Mild cases of SIADH may be controlled simply by restricting fluid intake.

6. Administer 3% saline IV and drugs (furosemide, demeclocycline, or lithium carbonate) as ordered. IV saline raises serum sodium, and diuretics prevent circulatory overload.

7. Decrease or discontinue the dosage of vincristine and cyclophosphamide chemotherapy, which can induce SIADH per order.

Diagnosis 4

Risk for injury related to bone demineralization or alterations in potassium balance.

Interventions and Rationale

1. Check for fatigue, apathy, depression, confusion, and weakness. These are neuromuscular symptoms of hypercalcemia and hypokalemia.

2. Institute safety precautions to prevent accidental falls. Fractures are more likely because of bone demineralization and mental changes.

3. Report new or worsening metastasis, especially bone metastasis. Hypercalcemia is more likely in the presence of bony metastasis. Hypokalemia can be caused by vomiting, diarrhea, nephrotoxicity, and hypercalcemia.

4. Monitor serum calcium levels and notify the health care provider of calcium levels above 11 mg/dL. Elevated serum calcium can lead to pathologic fractures and cardiac arrest.

Diagnosis 5

Decreased cardiac output related to increased serum potassium.

Interventions and Rationale

1. Monitor potassium levels frequently, especially during and after aggressive radiation or chemotherapy. Hyperkalemia is particularly likely following the destruction of large numbers of cells.

2. Report potassium levels above 5.3 mEq/L. Cardiac dysrhythmias become more common as serum potassium increases above this level.

3. Carefully monitor cardiac rhythm and EKG pattern and report abnormalities. Peaked T waves are an early sign of hyperkalemia. Tachycardia, bradycardia, heart block, and cardiac arrest may follow.

4. Administer Kayexalate in sorbitol PO or by enema to correct hyperkalemia. These agents cause a sodium-potassium ion exchange resulting in the excretion of excess potassium.

Diagnosis 6

Altered thought processes related to altered electrolyte balance.

Interventions and Rationale

1. Assess fluid and electrolyte balance frequently, particularly during periods of uncontrolled cell growth, tumor lysis, cachexia, ectopic hormone secretion, chemotherapy, and radiation. Fluid and electrolyte disturbances are most likely in cancer patients at these times, and many of these abnormalities (hypercalcemia, hypokalemia, hyponatremia, hypomagnesemia, etc.) can influence neuromuscular function.

2. Administer agents to correct acidosis and/or electrolyte imbalance. Medicate for nausea, vomiting, diarrhea, or cardiac dysrhythmias as ordered. Control of these processes is necessary to prevent progression of neurological problems.

3. Monitor serum potassium levels frequently. Administer potassium in IV solution as ordered. If potassium is excreted by the kidneys or shifts back into the cells hypokalemia may occur.

4. Reorient to time, place, and person if confusion or disorientation is apparent. Impairment of thought processes can cause increased anxiety for the client and family.

5. Check LOC, respiratory status, cardiac rhythm, renal function, and blood gases and report changes. Changes in these parameters may signal worsening of the fluid and electrolyte disturbance.

Diagnosis 7

Altered urinary elimination related to cell lysis and buildup of uric acid in the nephron.

Interventions and Rationale

1. Monitor urinary output and urine color, clarity, hematuria, and specific gravity. It is particularly important to monitor these factors during and after chemotherapy, particularly in leukemia and lymphoma.

2. Check for flank pain and medicate appropriately. Uric acid renal stones may cause acute, severe pain.

3. Report signs of renal failure. Obstruction of urine flow by renal calculi can cause kidney damage and eventual renal failure.

4. Report serum uric acid >8.0 mg/dL, urinary output <30 mL per hour, BUN >25 mg/dL, creatinine >1.2 mg/dL, or sudden weight gain with elevated BP, lung congestion, or edema.

5. Administer allopurinol and increase IV fluid rate as ordered before chemotherapy or radiation. Allopurinol reduces uric acid concentration, and increased IV fluids help to maintain hydration and adequate renal function.

6. Teach the client and family dietary modifications to increase the alkalinity of the urine. Uric acid is more likely to precipitate in acidic urine.

Evaluation/Outcome

1. Maintain fluid balance through intake and output measures.

2. Evaluate electrolyte balance through serum electrolyte tests while client is receiving chemotherapeutic agents and/or other anticancer therapy.

3. Remain free of signs and symptoms of fluid and electrolyte imbalances during anticancer therapy.

4. Monitor weight frequently (losses can be common in client with cancer).

5. Evaluate effectiveness of interventions through laboratory test findings and client's physical and mental status.

6. Evaluate that a support system is available for the client and family.

Chronic Diseases with Fluid and Electrolyte Imbalances

CHAPTER

26

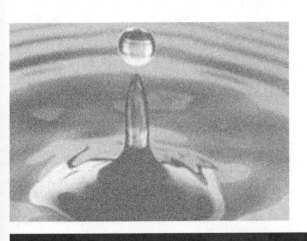

OBJECTIVES

Upon completion of this chapter, the reader should be able to:

- Identify the physiologic changes in fluid and electrolytes associated with chronic diseases such as congestive heart failure (CHF), diabetes mellitus (DM), and chronic obstructive pulmonary disease (COPD).
- Explain the clinical manifestations related to CHF, DM, and COPD.
- Identify abnormal laboratory results associated with CHF, DM, and COPD.
- Discuss the major treatment modalities for correcting fluid and electrolyte imbalances associated with CHF, DM, and COPD.
- Identify selected diagnoses and interventions with rationales for CHF, DM, and COPD.

▶ INTRODUCTION

A chronic disease, defined by the U.S. National Center for Health Statistics, is a chronic condition that has a duration of 3 months or longer. Chronic conditions usually progress slowly over a long period of time. Chronic illnesses frequently do not occur as a single health problem but are associated with multiple chronic health problems, e.g., a person with uncontrolled diabetes mellitus or chronic obstructive pulmonary disease (COPD) often develop heart failure. This chapter addresses three common chronic diseases; congestive heart failure (CHF), diabetes mellitus, and COPD.

Congestive heart failure (CHF) is a chronic disease process secondary to major disease entities, i.e., long-time diabetes mellitus, coronary heart disease, hypertension, pulmonary diseases, kidney diseases, and hyperthyroidism. CHF is a type of heart failure characterized by an inability of the heart to pump an adequate supply of blood (pump failure) to meet the needs for tissue perfusion. CHF is circulatory congestion related to pump failure. It develops slowly, begins with milder symptoms, and usually does not become severe until compensatory mechanisms fail.

Diabetes mellitus (DM) results from a malfunction of the beta cells of the pancreas. Thus, the body is unable to utilize sugar due to a lack of insulin secretion from the beta cells. Approximately 11 million people in the United States are affected by some form of DM. There are two common types of DM: insulin-dependent diabetes mellitus (IDDM), Type I, and non-insulin-dependent diabetes mellitus (NIDDM), Type II. With NIDDM, usually some insulin secretion occurs. The old term for Type I is juvenile-onset diabetes and for Type II is maturity-onset diabetes. These are misleading terms because either type of diabetes can occur in the very young or very old.

Diabetic ketoacidosis (DKA) is associated with IDDM, Type I, and results from a severe or complete deficit of insulin secretion. DKA is characterized by a blood sugar exceeding 300 mg/dL, ketosis, a blood pH < 7.30, and a bicarbonate level < 14 mEq/L. *Hyperglycemic hyperosmolar nonketotic (HHNK)* is characterized by a blood sugar > 500 mg/dL, dehydration, and a serum osmolality > 300 mOsm/kg.

Chronic obstructive pulmonary disease (COPD) is a chronic pulmonary disease associated with airway obstruction. The narrowing of the bronchioles increases the resistance to air flow. It is the second most common cause of hospital admissions. This chronic condition can result in disabilities. Examples of COPD are emphysema, chronic bronchitis, bronchiectasis, and asthma. Smoking is the leading cause of emphysema and chronic bronchitis. Other causes for COPD include alpha$_1$-antitrypsin deficiency (hereditary trait), chronic bacterial infection, air pollution, and inhalation of chemical irritants.

In this chapter, the three chronic diseases are presented in sections: Congestive Heart Failure, Diabetes Mellitus, and Chronic Obstructive Pulmonary Disease. The pathophysiology, clinical manifestations, clinical applications, and clinical management associated with specific diagnoses and clinical interventions are included in each section.

ANSWER COLUMN

▶ CONGESTIVE HEART FAILURE (CHF)

Pathophysiology

1

With CHF, there is circulatory congestion related to the heart's inability to pump *_____ . (Refer to introduction as needed).

CHF is referred to as pump _____ .

1 an adequate supply of blood; failure

2

Congestive heart failure is frequently (primary/secondary) _____ to other major disease entities.

2 secondary

Table 26-1 lists the pathophysiologic factors associated with CHF and the compensatory mechanisms to prevent heart failure. Left-sided and right-sided heart failure present different symptoms. Each type is included as a part of the pathophysiologic factors. Study the table and refer to it as necessary.

Table 26-1

Physiologic Changes Associated With CHF

Physiologic Changes	Rationale
Cardiac reserve (decreased) ↓	Decreased cardiac reserve is the inability of heart to respond to increased burden, e.g., fever, exercise, or excitement.
Cardiac compensation	The heart, in early heart failure, compensates for loss of cardiac reserve. Over an extended period of time the heart increases its cardiac output through ventricular dilatation, ventricular hypertrophy, and tachycardia.
Ventricular dilatation	Muscle fibers of myocardium increase in length and the ventricle enlarges to augment its output. Heart muscle stretches to a certain point and then ceases to increase heart contractility. A dilated heart needs more oxygen than a "normal" heart; however, the decreased coronary blood flow limits the O_2 supply to the heart muscle.
Ventricular hypertrophy	There is increased thickening of ventricular wall, which increases the weight of the heart. Ventricular hypertrophy mostly follows dilatation, and hypertrophy aids in heart contractility. A hypertrophied heart works harder than a normal heart and has a greater O_2 need.
Tachycardia	The increased heart rate is the least effective of the three compensatory mechanisms. The heart rate increases to a point that the ventricles are unable to fill adequately. As the heart rate increases, diastole time is reduced. The stroke volume first decreases, causing the cardiac output to increase, and later decreases as the heart rate greatly increases and diastole time shortens.
Cardiac decompensation	Occurs when the three compensatory mechanisms fail to maintain heart function and adequate circulation. Symptoms begin to develop with normal activity.
Left-sided heart failure	Generally results from left ventricular damage to the myocardium. The heart at first is unable to eject the full blood volume from the ventricle. Three compensatory mechanisms come into play. With compensatory mechanism failure, residual blood remains in the dilated ventricle. The left atrium dilates and atrial hypertrophy results. When the atrium is unable to receive blood from pulmonary veins, pulmonary congestion or pulmonary edema occurs. Etiologic factors include hypertension, myocardial infarction (heart attack), rheumatic fever affecting aortic valve, or syphilis. Symptoms of left-sided heart failure are similar to symptoms of overhydration, i.e., irritated cough, dizziness, engorged neck veins, moist rales.
Right-sided heart failure	Generally results from increased pressure in the pulmonary vascular system. The right ventricle tries to pump blood into the congested lungs, thus meeting resistance. Blood and fluids "back up" into the venous circulation, causing congestion in the GI tract, liver, and kidneys. Peripheral edema also occurs. Right-sided heart failure generally follows left-sided heart failure; however, occasionally, it is independent of left-sided failure. Symptoms of right-sided heart failure include liver congestion and enlargement, fullness in abdomen, and peripheral edema of lower extremities, mostly refractory and pitting.

3 decrease; ability of the heart to respond to increased burden

3

With CHF, there is a(n) (increase/decrease) _____ in cardiac reserve.

What is cardiac reserve? *_____

4 ventricular dilatation, ventricular hypertrophy, and tachycardia

4

In early heart failure, the heart compensates in order to meet oxygen and circulatory needs. The three methods by which the heart compensates are *_____

_____

5 the muscle fibers of the myocardium increase in length, thus the ventricle enlarges to increase output and circulation; more

5

Physiologically, how does ventricular dilatation occur? *_____

_____

With ventricular dilatation the heart needs (more/less) _____ oxygen.

6 An increased thickening of the ventricle wall increases heart contractility

6

Explain the rationale for ventricular hypertrophy in CHF. *_____

_____

7 a fast heart rate or pulse rate over 100; unable to fill adequately

7

Tachycardia is *_____ .

Tachycardia increases in rate until the ventricles are *_____ .

8 failure of the three compensatory mechanisms to maintain heart function

8

What is cardiac decompensation? *_____

_____

9 left ventricle damage; The ventricle remains dilated with residual blood. The atrium dilates and atrial hypertrophy results.

9

Left-sided heart failure generally results from *_____ .

When the compensatory mechanisms fail with left-sided failure, what happens to the ventricle and atrium? *_____

_____

10 pulmonary; constant, irritating cough, dyspnea, engorged veins, and moist rales

10

What type of edema occurs from left-sided heart failure?

_____

Name four symptoms of left-sided heart failure (overhydration). *_____

_____

11 increased pressure in the pulmonary vascular system; Blood and fluids "back up" in the venous circulation, increasing venous pressure and causing GI, liver, and kidney congestion. Peripheral edema in the lower extremities also results.

12 Right-sided heart failure generally follows left-sided heart failure.; Refractory or nondependent edema, also pitting edema; in the morning

11

Right-sided heart failure generally results from *_____

_____

What occurs when the right ventricle fails to adequately pump blood to the lungs? *_____

_____

_____

12

Explain the occurrence of right-sided heart failure in relation to left-sided heart failure. *_____

What type of peripheral edema occurs? *_____ Should it be assessed in the morning or in the evening? *_____

Clinical Manifestations

The heart compensates for inadequate blood flow by increasing the heart rate. Table 26-2 lists the common clinical manifestations and rationale associated with CHF. Study the table carefully, noting the reasons for the signs and symptoms related to CHF.

13 a. increased; b. increased; c. increased

13

Vital sign changes associated with CHF are:
   a. Pulse rate is _____ .
   b. Respiratory rate is _____ .
   c. Blood pressure may be _____ .

14 tachypnea; gas exchange; oxygen

14

A rapid increase in respiration is known as _____ .
The reason for an increased respiratory rate is to improve the *_____ . More (oxygen/carbon dioxide) _____ intake occurs.

15 pulmonary and peripheral; pulmonary; peripheral

15

The two types of edema associated with CHF are *_____

_____

Initially, left-sided heart failure causes _____ edema.
Right-sided heart failure is associated with _____ edema.

Table 26-2

Clinical Manifestations Associated with CHF

Clinical Manifestations	Rationale
Vital Signs (VSs)	
Increased pulse rate (tachycardia)	Increased heart rate is a compensatory mechanism to improve circulation of the blood.
Increased respiration (tachypnea)	Respirations increase to increase oxygen intake for tissue oxygenation.
Increased blood pressure (hypertension)	When hypertension occurs, it is usually because of atherosclerosis. Noncirculating vascular fluid can also increase blood pressure.
Edema	
Pulmonary	Caused by left-sided heart failure. (Because of pump failure, fluid "back up" in the pulmonary system, causing fluid congestion in the lung tissues.) Fluid inhibits adequate gas exchange (O_2 and CO_2). Signs and symptoms of pulmonary edema are similar to the signs and symptoms of overhydration.
Peripheral	May result from right-sided heart failure. Fluids accumulate in the extremities due to the fluid back-up in the venous circulation.
Cyanosis	Cyanosis is a sign of hypoxia due to inadequate blood flow to body tissues.
Laboratory Results	
Plasma/serum sodium: increased (hypernatremia) or normal	Sodium retention in the extracellular fluid (ECF) usually occurs even when the serum sodium is within normal range or lower. Hemodilution can cause a normal or slightly lower serum sodium level.
Plasma/serum potassium: normal or decreased (hypokalemia)	The serum potassium level can be decreased with the use of potassium-wasting diuretics and due to hemodilution from fluid volume excess.
Plasma/serum magnesium: normal or decreased (hypomagnesemia)	Long-term use of potassium-wasting diuretics can cause both hypomagnesemia and hypokalemia.
Serum osmolality: < 280 mOsm/kg	Due to hemodilution. If the serum sodium level is increased, the serum osmolality increases.

16

Indicate which serum electrolyte results are related to CHF.

( ) a. Hypernatremia

( ) b. Hyperkalemia

( ) c. Hypermagnesemia

( ) d. Normal serum sodium level

( ) e. Hypokalemia

( ) f. Hypomagnesemia

16 a, d, e, f

Clinical Applications

Mrs. Allen, age 68, was admitted to the hospital with CHF. She has shortness of breath when walking up a flight of stairs. The health professional assessed Mrs. Allen's physiologic status and noted an irritating cough, dyspnea on exertion, moist rales in the lungs, hand vein engorgement in upward position after 30 seconds, and swelling in the ankles and feet. Her blood pressure is 154/96 and pulse was 110. Her ECG showed ventricular hypertrophy.

17

Mrs. Allen presents two compensatory physiologic changes essential for maintaining cardiac function, these compensatory mechanisms are *_____ .

Are these compensatory mechanisms effective?_____

Explain why. *_____

_____

17 tachycardia and ventricular hypertrophy; No. Most likely, ventricular dilatation is present and limiting the effectiveness of the increased heart rate and ventricular hypertrophy.

18

According to Mrs. Allen's symptoms, which type(s) of heart failure is (are) present?

( ) a. Left-sided heart failure

( ) b. Right-sided heart failure

18 a, b

19

The assessment of Mrs. Allen identifies four symptoms of pulmonary congestion, which are: *_____

_____

19 irritating cough, dyspnea, moist rales, and hand vein engorgement

20 right

20

Swelling in the feet and ankles is indicative of _____-sided heart failure.

Table 26-3 gives the laboratory results for Mrs. Allen on the day of admission and the second and fourth days after admission. Be able to identify laboratory results that are normal and which are not. Explain the abnormal laboratory findings.

21 elevated or increased; rise; edema or ECFVE

21

Mrs. Allen's serum sodium is _____ . Sodium retention can cause Mrs. Allen's extracellular fluid volume to (rise/decrease) _____ .

What type of fluid imbalance was present? _____

22 increase; Potassium may be diluted due to the increase of ECF or hemodilution.; A lack of adequate food intake containing potassium.; If she were receiving diuretics, this might cause a low serum K.

22

Mrs. Allen's low-average serum potassium may be due to a(n) (increase/decrease) _____ in ECF. Explain why. *_____

_____

Another reason why Mrs. Allen's serum potassium may be low-average is *_____ .

Table 26-3

Laboratory Studies of Mrs. Allen

Laboratory Tests	On Admission	Day 1	Day 4
Hematology			
Hemoglobin (12.9–17.0 g)	12.5		
Hematocrit (40–46%)	40		
WBC (white blood count)	8200		
Biochemistry			
BUN (blood urea nitrogen) (10–25 mg/dL)*	28	24	18
Plasma/serum CO_2[†] (22–32 mEq/L)	22	24	24
Plasma/serum chloride (95–108 mEq/L)	107	106	107
Plasma/serum sodium (135–146 mEq/L)	151	148	143
Plasma/serum potassium (3.5–5.3 mEq/L)	3.6	3.8	4.0

*mg/100 mL = mg/dL.

[†]*Plasma* and *serum* are used interchangeably.

Clinical Management

The "three D's" frequently employed in the management of congestive heart failure are:

1. Diet

2. Digitalization

3. Diuretics

The clinical management for CHF in Mrs. Allen's case incorporates the "three D's."

Diet

23

Mrs. Allen was placed on a low-sodium diet and her fluid intake was limited to 1200 mL (300 mL below daily requirement).

Salt and water intake is limited for which of the following reasons:

( ) a. Increase edema

( ) b. Prohibit further increase of edema

( ) c. Decrease water intoxication

23 b

Digitalization or Loading Doses

Digitalization is the process of increasing the serum level of digitalis to achieve the desired physiologic effect. It is also referred to as a loading dose or doses.

Digitalis preparations are classified as cardiac glycosides (cardiotonic). The action of digitalis is to slow the ventricular contractions and increase the forcefulness of the contractions. Examples of digitalis preparations are digoxin, digitoxin, gitaligin, deslanoside (Cedilanid), and digitalis leaf. Digoxin is the choice cardiac glycoside for prolonged use in the treatment of CHF.

24

Digitalis is classified as a *_____ .

This drug slows the *_____ and makes the heart beat *_____ .

24 cardiac glycoside; ventricular contractions (heart rate); more forcefully (stronger)

25

Mrs. Allen was digitalized with digoxin and then placed on a daily maintenance dose of digoxin, 0.25 mg. This

25 increases; improved or increased; increased

(increases/decreases) _____ cardiac output. Blood circulation is then _____ . The urinary output is _____ .

It is important that you remember the toxic effects of digitalis preparations, which include pulse below 60, nausea, vomiting, and anorexia.

Diuretics

26

Diuretics are used for the excretion of sodium and water. Many diuretics increase the excretion of sodium, water, and chloride, and the valuable electrolyte _____ .

26 potassium

27

Frequently, a potassium-sparing diuretic is prescribed with a potassium-wasting diuretic to prevent excessive loss of what ion? _____

27 Potassium

28

Identify diuretics that are potassium-wasting and potassium-sparing by placing K-W for potassium-wasting diuretics and K-S for potassium-sparing diuretics.

_____ a. Hydrochlorothiazide (HydroDIURIL)
_____ b. Triameterene (Dyrenium)
_____ c. Furosemide (Lasix)
_____ d. Mannitol
_____ e. Spironolactone (Aldactone)

28 a. K-W; b. K-S; c. K-W; d. K-W; e. K-S

29 muscular weakness; dizziness, arrhythmia, silent ileus (decrease peristalsis), and abdominal distention

29

Identify at least five symptoms of hypokalemia (potassium deficit). (Refer to Chapter 6 if necessary.) *_____
_____

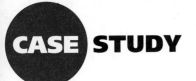

REVIEW

Mrs. Allen, age 68, is in congestive heart failure on admission. The clinical assessment of her symptoms and findings are stated under clinical applications.

ANSWER COLUMN

1. ventricular dilatation, ventricular hypertrophy, and tachycardia
2. decompensation; The compensatory mechanisms failed to maintain cardiac output, since symptoms were present.

3. more

4. increased; The blood is backed up in the venous system, causing increased pressure.

5. a. irritating cough; b. dyspnea on exertion; c. moist rales; d. hand vein engorgement; e. pulse 110 (tachycardia); f. ventricular hypertrophy

6. overhydration

7. swelling in the ankles and feet

8. diet, digitalization, and diuretics

9. potassium-wasting; hypokalemia

---

1. In early heart failure, name the three compensatory mechanisms that assisted Mrs. Allen to maintain her cardiac output to maintain circulation. *_____

   _____

2. Is Mrs. Allen in cardiac (compensation/decompensation)? _____ Explain your answer. *_____

   _____

3. Does the heart need (more/less) _____ blood when there is ventricular dilatation and hypertrophy?

4. With right-sided heart failure, the venous (hydrostatic) pressure is (increased/decreased) _____ . Explain why.
   *
   _____

   _____

   The health professional assessed Mrs. Allen's physiologic status and identified symptoms of left-and right-sided heart failure.

5. Mrs. Allen's signs and symptoms of left-sided heart failure include:
   a. *_____
   b. *_____
   c. *_____
   d. *_____
   e. *_____
   f. *_____

6. The symptoms of left-sided heart failure are similar to symptoms of _____ .

7. Mrs. Allen's symptom of right-sided heart failure is *_____

   _____ .

8. Clinical management for Mrs. Allen consisted of the "three D's," which are *_____ .

9. Mrs. Allen is receiving HydroDIURIL. Is this a (potassium-wasting/potassium-sparing) _____ diuretic? The potassium imbalance that can occur is (hypokalemia/hyperkalemia) _____ .

10. Hypokalemia enhances the action of any digitalis preparation, making the digoxin stronger (cumulative action can occur).

11. a. bradycardia—pulse ↓ 60 or arrhythmia, or both; b.anorexia; c. nausea and vomiting

10. If Mrs. Allen's serum potassium was below average, what effect does this have on digoxin. (Review Chapter 6 if necessary.) * _____

_____

11. Give three symptoms of digitalis toxicity.
    a. * _____
    b. * _____
    c. * _____

CARE PLAN

Client Management

Assessment Factors

▶ Obtain baseline vital signs to determine abnormal changes and for comparison with future vital signs.

▶ Assess for signs and symptoms of left-sided heart failure (overhydration or pulmonary edema), i.e., constant, irritating cough, dyspnea, neck and/or hand vein engorgement, chest rales.

▶ Assess for signs and symptoms of right-sided heart failure, i.e., pitting peripheral edema, liver enlargement, fullness of abdomen.

▶ Check serum electrolyte levels, especially potassium and sodium. Report abnormal findings. Use baseline electrolyte results for comparison with future serum electrolytes.

Diagnosis 1

Fluid volume excess related to cardiac decompensation secondary to left-sided and right-sided heart failure.

Interventions and Rationale

1. Auscultate lung areas to detect abnormal breath sounds, such as moist rales due to lung congestion (pulmonary edema).

2. Monitor vein engorgement by checking hand veins for fluid overload. Lower the hand below the heart level until the hand veins are engorged; then raise the hand above the heart level. If the hand veins remain engorged above heart level after 15 seconds, fluid volume excess is most likely present.

3. Check the feet and ankles daily in the early morning before client rises. If edema is present, the reason is probably due to cardiac and/or renal dysfunction.

4. Instruct client not to use table salt to season foods. Salt contains sodium, which can cause water retention. Suggest other ways to enhance flavor of foods.

5. Instruct the client to eat foods rich in potassium (fruits, vegetables) if he or she is taking a potassium-wasting diuretic and digoxin. Hypokalemia can enhance the action of digoxin and can cause digitalis toxicity (slow, irregular pulse, nausea/ vomiting).

6. Assess for signs and symptoms of hypokalemia (serum potassium deficit), i.e., dizziness, muscular weakness, abdominal distention, diminished peristalsis, and dysrhythmia, if client has been receiving potassium-wasting diuretics for several months.

Diagnosis 2

Ineffective breathing patterns related to fluid in the lung tissues.

Interventions and Rationale

1. Monitor breathing patterns. Report the presence of dyspnea, shortness of breath, rapid breathing, and wheezing.

2. Elevate the head of the bed 30°–75° to lower the diaphragm and increase aveoli spaces for gas exchange. Client may sit upright in a chair or in an orthopneic position to increase available air space.

Diagnosis 3

Impaired tissue integrity related to fluid accumulation in the extremities and buttocks.

Interventions and Rationale

1. Encourage the client to change positions frequently. Edematous tissue can break down due to hypoxia and constant pressure on skin surface.

2. Provide skin care, especially to edematous areas, at least twice daily.

Diagnosis 4

Self-care deficit: feeding, bathing, and hygiene, related to fatigue and breathlessness secondary to CHF.

Interventions and Rationale

1. Assist client with activities of daily living such as feeding and bathing. CHF increases body fatigue and the inability to perform small tasks without extreme exhaustion.

2. Encourage family member(s) to participate in meeting client's needs as necessary.

3. Encourage the client to be self-sufficient if he or she is able to perform basic tasks and meet his or her needs, such as dressing, bathing, and hygiene care (brushing teeth).

Other Diagnoses to Consider

Altered tissue perfusion related to cardiopulmonary insufficiency.

Evaluation/Outcome

1. Evaluate the therapeutic effect of interventions to correct the underlying cause of CHF.

2. Remain free of signs and symptoms of left-sided heart failure and right-sided heart failure.

3. Evaluate the effectiveness of medications in reducing pulmonary and/or peripheral edema and cardiac symptoms.

4. Evaluate the dietary intake and fluid intake and output.

5. Evaluate that a support system for the client is available.

▶ DIABETES MELLITUS (DM) AND DIABETIC KETOACIDOSIS (DKA)

Pathophysiology

With an insulin deficit, glucose utilization is reduced and the cells are starved of important nutrients. Fat and protein catabolism (breakdown) occurs to provide the body with needed energy. Fatty acids are released from the breakdown of adipose (fat) tissue. Acids are further broken down into ketonic acids (ketones) and acetoacetate (acetone). Since the liver cannot oxidize the excess ketones, these ketone bodies accumulate in the blood. The acetone is excreted by the lungs.

30
A cessation or deficit of insulin secretions (increases/decreases) _____ the body's utilization of glucose.

30 decreases

31
Diabetic ketoacidosis (DKA) is more likely to occur with which type of diabetes mellitus? (IDDM/NIDDM) _____

31 IDDM

32
Failure to metabolize glucose leads to a(n) (increase/decrease) _____ in fat catabolism. Ketosis occurs, which results in a(n) (deficit/excess) _____ of ketone bodies (ketonic acids) in the blood.

32 increase; excess

33
With an increase in bicarbonate ion excreted by the kidneys due to osmotic diuresis, more hydrogen ions are reabsorbed into the circulation. Cellular breakdown causes lactic acid to be released from the cells. The increase in ketone bodies, hydrogen ions, and lactic acid increases the (acidotic/alkalotic) _____ state of the body.

33 acidotic

34
Failure of glucose metabolism can cause which of the following:
( ) a. Glucose utilization for energy
( ) b. fat catabolism which releases excessive amounts of ketone bodies
An excessive number of ketone bodies in the body is known as

_____ .

Ketosis leads to diabetic _____ .

34 b; ketosis; ketoacidosis

35
An elevation of the blood sugar level, >180 mg/dL, increases the glucose concentration in the glomeruli of the kidneys. When

the concentration of glucose in the glomeruli exceeds the renal threshold for tubular reabsorption, glycosuria results. Increased glucose concentration acts as an osmotic diuretic which causes diuresis.

What does *glycosuria* mean? *_____

What does *diuresis* mean? *_____

35 sugar in the urine; excess urine excretion

36

An elevated blood sugar also increases the hyperosmolality of the extracellular fluid.

The hyperosmolality of the extracellular fluid leads to a withdrawal of fluid from the cells. Thus the ECF space is increased.

The fluid from the cells dilutes the extracellular sodium concentration, producing (hypernatremia/hyponatremia)

_____ .

The migration of intracellular fluid into the extracellular fluid results in which of the following:

( ) a. Cellular dehydration

( ) b. Cellular hydration

36 hyponatremia; a

37

In renal excretion, the ketones (strong acids) combine with the cation sodium, causing sodium depletion. Ketone bodies (ketones) are excreted as ketonuria. The additional solute load of ketones in the glomeruli results in which of the following:

( ) a. A decreased loss of water in the formation of ketonuria

( ) b. An increased loss of water in the formation of ketonuria

37 b

38

Polyuria can result from which of the following:

( ) a. Glycosuria

( ) b. Anuria

( ) c. Ketonuria

With the loss of water, the solute concentration of the blood (increases/decreases) _____ and the blood volume (increases/decreases) _____ .

38 a, c; increases; decreases

39

As a result of DKA, nausea and vomiting occur, causing a severe fluid and electrolyte imbalance.

There is an increase in water loss by way of the lungs due to Kussmaul breathing (rapid vigorous breathing).

Dehydration occurs from which of the following:

( ) a. Nausea and vomiting

( ) b. Kussmaul breathing

( ) c. Oliguria

( ) d. Polyuria

39 a, b, d

40

The failure of cellular utilization of glucose causes potassium to leave the cells. The serum potassium level may therefore reflect normal or high serum values.

When serum potassium loss is the result of vomiting and renal excretion, the hemoconcentration can cause the serum potassium level to appear *_____ .

40 normal or high

Etiology

Between 20% and 25% of DKA clients are those who are newly diagnosed with DM, Type I. Table 26-4 lists the causes of DKA.

Table 26-4

Causes of DKA

Categories	Causes
Insulin deficiency	Undiagnosed DM, Type I Omission of prescribed insulin
Acute incidence	Infection Trauma Pancreatitis Major surgical interventions Gastroenteritis
Miscellaneous	Hyperthyroidism Steroids Adrenergic agonists

41 undiagnosed DM and omission of a prescribed insulin dose	**41** Two common causes of DKA due to insulin deficiency are * _____ .
42 infection, trauma, and pancreatitis (others: major surgery, gastroenteritis)	**42** Name three causes of an acute incidence of DKA. * _____ _____

Clinical Manifestations

The most common symptoms of DKA are extreme thirst, polyuria, weakness, and fatigue. Hyperglycemia induces osmotic diuresis. Table 26-5 describes the signs and symptoms and laboratory results related to DKA. This table should be used as a guide for the assessment of clients with probable DKA.

Table 26-5

Clinical Manifestations of DKA

Signs and Symptoms	Rationale
Extreme Thirst *Polyuria*	Elevated blood sugar and ketones increase the serum osmolality, causing thirst and osmotic diuresis.
Weakness, Fatigue	Reduced cellular metabolism results in low energy levels.
Nausea, Vomiting	Continuous vomiting causes a loss of body fluids and electrolytes. Dehydration results.
Vital Signs Temperature elevated or N	Infection causes an elevated temperature; dehydration can cause a slightly elevated temperature.
Pulse rapid	With a loss of body fluid, the heart beats faster to compensate in order to maintain circulation. Tachycardia of greater than 140 bpm denotes a severe fluid loss.
Blood pressure slightly to severely decreased	With early fluid loss from diuresis, the blood pressure decreases by 10–15 mm Hg.
Respiration rapid, vigorous breathing	Kussmaul breathing is a compensatory mechanism to decrease H_2CO_2 (acid) by blowing off CO_2
Poor Skin Turgor; Dry, Parched Lips; Disorientation, Confusion	Dehydration frequently results in these symptoms; poor skin turgor; dry, parched lips; and confusion.
Abdominal Pain with Tenderness	Abdominal pain usually indicates severe ketoacidosis.

Note: N = normal; ↑ = elevated; ↓ = decreased; bpm = beats per minute.   *(continues on the following page)*

Table 26-5

Clinical Manifestations of DKA *(Continued)*

Signs and Symptoms	Rationale
Laboratory Test Results Blood sugar 300–800 mg/dL	Blood sugar level is high; at times, it is not as high as HHNK. Sugar is not metabolized and utilized by the cells.
Electrolytes Potassium N, ↓, ↑	Potassium in the cells is low, but the serum potassium level may be high due to a hemoconcentration. Normal or low levels can also occur.
Sodium N, ↓, ↑	Sodium is lost because of diuresis. Serum levels can be elevated due to dehydration.
Magnesium N, ↓, ↑ Chloride N, ↓ Phosphorus low N or ↓	Magnesium and phosphorus react the same as potassium. Chloride is excreted with sodium and water.
CO_2 ↓	The serum CO_2 is a bicarbonate determinant. With the loss of bicarbonate, the serum CO_2 is greatly decreased (<14 mEq/L).
Serum osmolality 300–350 mOsm/kg	Fluid loss (dehydration) increases the serum osmolality.
Hematology Hemoglobin, hematocrit ↑ WBC ↑	Because of fluid loss, hemoconcentration results, increasing the hemoglobin and hematocrit levels. Elevated white blood cells can indicate an infection.
Arterial Blood Gases (ABGs) pH ↓ $PaCO_2$ ↓ HCO_3 ↓	The pH is low in the acidotic state. The $PaCO_2$ may be decreased as the lungs are expelling CO_2 (compensatory mechanism). The bicarbonate is lost through diuresis with an increase in hydrogen and ketone (acid) levels.
Urine Glycosuria Ketonuria	Glucose and ketones spill into the urine.

Note: N = normal; ↑ = elevated; ↓ = decreased; bpm = beats per minute.

---

43 extreme thirst, polyuria, fatigue, and weakness

43

The four early clinical manifestations related to DKA are
* _____

44

Indicate which of the following vital signs are related to DKA:

( ) a. Elevated temperature
( ) b. Tachycardia
( ) c. Bradycardia
( ) d. Decreased blood pressure of 10–15 mm Hg
( ) e. High blood pressure
( ) f. Vigorous, rapid breathing
( ) g. apnea

44 a, b, d, f

45

Identify the changes that result in (a) the skin, (b) the lips and (c) the sensorium from dehydration associated with fluid loss and diuresis:

a. *_____
b. *_____
c. *_____

45 a. poor skin turgor; b. dry and/or parched lips; c. disorientation or confusion

46

The five electrolytes that frequently result in an imbalance due to DKA are *_____

_____

_____ .

46 potassium, sodium, magnesium, phosphorus (phosphate), and bicarbonate or serum CO_2 (also chloride)

47

With cellular breakdown, potassium is (lost/reabsorbed) _____ (from/into) _____ the cells.
    When the acidotic state is corrected, potassium re-enters the cells and (hypokalemia/hyperkalemia) _____ may result.

47 lost; from; hypokalemia

48

With early fluid loss, the sodium level may be elevated because of increased aldosterone secretion (sodium-retaining hormone) response.
    With continuous diuresis, the serum sodium level is

_____ .

48 decreased

49

What causes the hemoglobin and hematocrit to be elevated?
*_____

An elevated white blood cell (WBC) count is often due to an

_____ .

49 hemoconcentration (due to fluid volume deficit); infection

50 acidosis; it is a respiratory compensatory mechanism where the lungs blow off CO_2 to decrease the acidity in the blood

50

A decrease in the pH and the arterial bicarbonate (HCO_3) indicates metabolic (acidosis/alkalosis) _____ resulting from DKA.

Why is the $PaCO_2$ (arterial partial pressure carbon dioxide) decreased in DKA? * _____

_____

Clinical Applications

51

Dehydration is one of the major symptoms and concerns for persons in DKA.

When there is a marked intracellular and extracellular fluid depletion, the end result is which of the following:

( ) a. Decreased hemoconcentration
( ) b. Increased hemoconcentration
( ) c. Decreased blood volume
( ) d. Increased blood volume

51 b, c

52

While the client is receiving IV fluids and insulin, observe for symptoms of hypoglycemia, also known as an insulin reaction, or a hypoglycemic reaction. These symptoms include cold, clammy skin; nervousness; weakness; dizziness; tachycardia; low blood pressure; and slurred speech. The blood sugar is frequently 50 mg/dL or lower.

How can the insulin reaction be corrected quickly? * _____

_____

52 You may need to consult a medical text; however, a glass or two of orange juice can raise the blood sugar rapidly.

53

When persons are treated for DKA with large doses of insulin, the health professional should observe for what type of reaction? * _____

Too much insulin will cause symptoms similar to shock. Name three symptoms. _____

53 insulin reaction; tachycardia, nervousness, and weakness (also low blood pressure, dizziness, and slurred speech)

54

Clients with diabetes who are ill are advised to go to bed because rest reduces metabolism. This decreases fat and protein catabolism.

These persons should also be protected from overheating and chilling. If they are in a state of vascular collapse, extra heat should *not* be applied since it can increase vasodilatation and intensify the failure of the circulation.

Rest reduces metabolism in an ill diabetic person; therefore, rest decreases the chance of _____ and _____ catabolism.

In the state of vascular collapse, extra heat may cause further (vasoconstriction/vasodilatation) _____ .

54 fat; protein; vasodilatation

55

Jill Thompson arrived in the emergency room in a semicomatose state. Prior to admission, she had been vomiting and had complained of "feeling weak." The family stated she had a severe cold with a fever for weeks. They felt the vomiting was due to a viral infection.

The mucosa in her mouth was dry. Vomiting and dry mucosa would indicate _____ .

Her respirations were rapid and deep, this can be an indication of which of the following:

( ) a. Kussmaul breathing
( ) b. Dyspnea

Her heart sinus rhythm was sinus tachycardia (pulse rate 120). Her breath had a very sweet smell. The family stated she did not have diabetes mellitus, but there was a familial history of it.

In the emergency room, a stat blood chemistry was done and a retention catheter was inserted. The blood sugar was 476 mg/dL, the normal range being 70–110 mg/dL. This indicates a (hypoglycemic/hyperglycemic) _____ state. The serum CO_2 combining power was very low, which indicates an _____ state.

55 dehydration; a; hyperglycemic; acidotic

Table 26-6 identifies the laboratory studies of Jill Thompson, which show how her results deviated from the normal values at the time of her illness.

56

Her urinalysis was as follows:
Color, dark yellow
Specific gravity, 1.024
Reaction, acid

Table 26-6

Laboratory Studies for Jill Thompson

Laboratory Tests	On Admission	Day 1			Day 2	Day 3
Hematology						
Hemoglobin (12.9–17.0 g)	17.8					
Hematocrit (40–46%)	52					
Biochemistry						
BUN (blood urea nitrogen) (10–25 mg/dL)*	15					
Sugar feasting—postprandial (under 150 mg/dL)	476	825	458	382	60	144
Acetone	+1 / 1:10	+1 / 1:10	Trace / 1:8			
Plasma/serum CO_2† 50–70 vol %	7	10	14	18	34	44
22–32 mEq/L	3	4	6	8	15	20
Plasma/serum chloride (95–108 mEq/L)	104		130	132	133	110
Plasma/serum sodium (135–146 mEq/L)	137		151	159	164	145
Plasma/serum potassium (3.5–5.3 mEq/L)	4.8		2.7	3.2	4.2	4.5

*mg/100 mL = mg/dL
†*Plasma* and *serum* are used interchangeably.

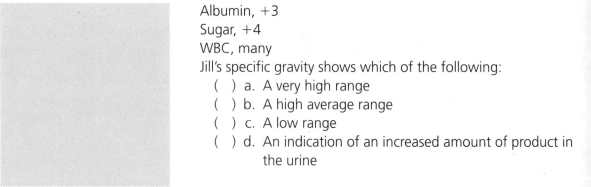

Albumin, +3
Sugar, +4
WBC, many
Jill's specific gravity shows which of the following:
( ) a. A very high range
( ) b. A high average range
( ) c. A low range
( ) d. An indication of an increased amount of product in the urine

The +4 sugar in the urine indicates (hypoglycemia/ hyperglycemia) _____ .

The +3 albumin in the urine indicates which of the following:

( ) a. Normal range
( ) b. Pathologic involvement

57

Jill's hemoglobin and hematocrit counts were which of the following:

( ) a. Normal
( ) b. Below normal
( ) c. Above normal
( ) d. An indication of mild edema
( ) e. An indication of mild dehydration

58

The feasting blood sugars (blood drawn after eating) on admission and the first day were which of the following:

( ) a. Normal
( ) b. Below normal
( ) c. Above normal
( ) d. An indication of hyperglycemia
( ) e. An indication of hypoglycemia

The second day her blood sugar was 60 mg/dL, which indicates a _____ reaction.

59

Jill Thompson's CO_2 combining power would indicate which of the following:

( ) a. Metabolic acidosis
( ) b. Metabolic alkalosis
( ) c. A bicarbonate loss
( ) d. A bicarbonate increase

60

On admission, Jill Thompson's serum chloride, sodium, and potassium were in the (high/low/normal) _____ range.

On the first day, the laboratory studies indicated which of the following:

56 b, d; hyperglycemia; b

57 c, e

58 c, d; hypoglycemic or insulin

59 a, c

( ) a. Hyperchloremia
( ) b. Hypochloremia
( ) c. Hypernatremia
( ) d. Hyponatremia
( ) e. Hyperkalemia
( ) f. Hypokalemia

60 normal; a, c, f

61
In DKA there is frequently a serum sodium decrease before treatment due to which of the following:
( ) a. Fluid intake
( ) b. Vomiting
( ) c. Urine excretion

61 b, c

Clinical Management

Treatment modalities for DKA include (1) vigorous fluid replacement, (2) insulin replacement, and (3) electrolyte correction Osmotic diuresis can cause a fluid volume deficit of 4–8 liters of body fluid. In such a case immediate restoration of fluid loss is essential.

Fluid Replacement
62
In the first 24 hours, 80% of the total water and salt deficit should be replaced. There is less urgency for the other electrolytes since the rate of assimilation of the intracellular electrolytes is limited. Administration of potassium must be included, but *not in early treatment* (unless indicated) since an elevated serum potassium can be toxic.

With DKA, 80% of (salt and water/potassium and magnesium) *_____ should be replaced in the first 24 hours.

Cellular assimilation of electrolytes is (faster/slower) _____ than extracellular assimilation of electrolytes.

62 salt and water; slower

63
For the first hour, 1–2 liters of a crystalloid [normal saline solution (0.9% NaCl)] or lactated Ringer's solution may be rapidly infused to reestablish the fluid volume balance. This may be followed by 1 liter every hour for the next 2 hours as indicated.

63 hemodilution

Rapid fluid replacement decreases the hyperglycemic state by causing a (hemoconcentration/hemodilution) _____ .

64

Alternating normal saline solution with lactated Ringer's solution may be the IV therapy of choice for improving fluid balance, renal perfusion, and blood pressure. ECF is restored directly from IV therapy. ICF replacement occurs in approximately 2 days.

When reestablishing fluid balance in the ECF space, the suggested amount of IV fluids for the first hour is *_____ . The purpose of rapid infusion of IV fluids is to improve
*_____ , *_____ , and *_____ .

64 1–2 liters; fluid balance; renal perfusion; blood pressure

65

Restoration of ICF balance is somewhat (slower/faster) _____ than restoration of the ECF balance.

Indicate which solutions are used initially to correct the fluid imbalance:

( ) a. Dextrose in water (D₅W)
( ) b. Lactated Ringer's solution
( ) c. Normal saline solution (0.9% NaCl)

65 slower; b, c

66

A fluid overload in the ECF space should be avoided. What are four of the symptoms of overhydration or hypervolemia?
*_____

_____

66 constant, irritating cough, difficulty breathing (dyspnea), neck and hand vein engorgement, and chest rales

Insulin Replacement

Ten to 15 years ago, massive doses of insulin were administered for the treatment of DKA. Today, less insulin is used when correcting DKA. Regular or crystalline insulin is given either intravenously and/or intramuscularly.

67

The parenteral routes used for correcting DKA include which of the following:

( ) a. Intravenous
( ) b. Subcutaneous
( ) c. Intramuscular

67 a, c

68

An initial bolus of 20–50 units of regular insulin is a practice of many health care providers. The somewhat standard guideline for IV insulin replacement is an insulin bolus of 0.1–0.4 U/kg, followed by 0.1 U/kg per hour in IV fluids until the blood sugar level reaches 200–250 mg/dL.

Sample Problem: A client weighs 154 pounds or 70 kg. The order reads regular insulin bolus of 0.4 U/kg and 0.1 U/kg per hour in normal saline solution. The amount of regular insulin to be administered as a bolus is _____ units, and the amount of regular insulin to be administered per hour in intravenous normal saline solution is _____ units. How much regular insulin is added to a 500-mL normal saline solution bag to run for 5 hours? _____ units

68 28; 7; 35

69

The blood sugar must be closely monitored during insulin replacement.

When the blood sugar level reaches _____ mg/dL, the IV fluids are usually switched to 5% dextrose in water. This prevents the possible occurrence of a (hypoglycemic/ hyperglycemic) _____ reaction.

69 200–250; hypoglycemic

70

The longer the acidosis persists, the more resistant the person is likely to be to insulin.

If acidosis persists, the person may require (more/less) _____ insulin.

Which of the following types of insulin can be administered intravenously?
( ) a. NPH
( ) b. Regular
( ) c. Protamine zinc insulin (PZI)
( ) d. Crystalline

70 more; b, d

Electrolyte Correction

71

Potassium (K) replacement should start approximately 6–8 hours after the first dose of insulin has been administered (intravenously or intramuscularly) and as the acidotic state is being corrected. Serum potassium levels should be taken frequently. Potassium moves back into cells as fluid balance and the acidotic state are corrected.

If potassium is *not* given as acidosis is corrected, the serum potassium level may be (high/low) _____ . State the rationale for the reaction. *_____

_____

72

While fluid and insulin replacements are occurring, the serum potassium levels should be constantly monitored.

The serum potassium level (increases/decreases) _____ as fluids and insulin are being administered.

73

As acidosis is corrected, insulin is utilized more rapidly by the body for metabolizing sugar (glucose).

(Hypoglycemia/hyperglycemia) _____ is most likely to result. Can you explain why? *_____

_____

_____

74

Magnesium, phosphate, and bicarbonate serum levels should be closely monitored. If the serum magnesium level is low, correcting hypokalemia does not fully result until the magnesium level is corrected.

There is controversy related to phosphate replacement when treating DKA. Phosphates are needed for neuromuscular function; thus serum phosphorus should be monitored along with the other electrolytes.

Another controversial issue is the use of bicarbonate therapy in the treatment of DKA. Usually, fluids and insulin replacement correct the acidotic state. If the pH falls below 7.1, bicarbonate replacement is usually prescribed.

The three electrolytes other than potassium and sodium that should be closely monitored are *_____

_____ .

75

Indicate when a bicarbonate infusion may be ordered:

Margin answers:

71 low; Potassium moves back into the cells leaving a serum potassium (K) deficit.

72 decreases

73 hypoglycemia.; When acidosis is corrected, there is less resistance to insulin. The insulin that had been previously administered (nonfunctional insulin due to acidosis) metabolizes the sugars for cellular use, causing a low blood sugar (hypoglycemia).

74 magnesium, phosphate (phosphorus), and bicarbonate

( ) a. pH 7.15
( ) b. pH 7.05
( ) c. pH 6.95
( ) d. pH 7.21

75 b, c

CASE STUDY REVIEW

Jill Thompson, age 22, unknown diabetic, was admitted to the emergency room in a semicomatose state. Her respirations were deep and rapid, and her breath had a sweet smell. She had been urinating frequently. She had been vomiting for several days. Her laboratory results were Hgb 17.8 g, Hct 52, sugar feasting or post-prandial 476 mg/dL, serum CO_2 3 mEq/L, serum sodium 137 mEq/L, serum chloride 104 mEq/L, and serum potassium 4.8 mEq/L.

ANSWER COLUMN

1. deep, rapid respirations (Kussmaul breathing), sweet smelling breath, and frequent urination

2. frequent urination and prolonged vomiting; hemoglobin and hematocrit

3. 476; 70–110; 150 or lower

4. hyperosmolar

5. glycosuria

6. decreased; metabolic acidosis

1. According to Jill Thompson's history, identify three clinical symptoms of hyperglycemia. *_____
_____

2. Two clinical symptoms that indicated dehydration were
*_____.
What two laboratory results also indicated dehydration?
*_____

3. Her feasting sugar or postprandial blood sugar was _____ mg/dL. The normal range for a fasting blood sugar is _____ mg/dL and for feasting sugar is _____ mg/dL.

4. Jill Thompson's increased blood sugar causes the body fluids to be (hypo-osmolar/hyperosmolar) _____ ; thus, os-motic diuresis results.

5. Polyuria can occur from ketonuria and _____ .

6. Her serum CO_2 was markedly _____ . What type of acid-base imbalance is present? *_____
_____

7. ketone bodies or ketosis (strong acid); diabetic ketoacidosis

8. The 2 liters of normal saline solutions. One liter of normal saline (0.9% NaCl) supplies 154 mEq/L of Na^+ and 154 mEq/L of Cl^-.

9. Rehydration causing dilution of potassium. Also, some of the potassium may be returning to the cells with the correction of DKA.

10. 6–8

11. 200–250 mg/dL or lower

12. nervousness, cold and clammy skin, tachycardia, and slurred speech (others: hunger, dizziness, low blood pressure)

13. 2 liters of normal saline solutions administered the first day

---

7. Her acidosis is the result of fat catabolism, producing
   * _____ . This type of acidosis is referred to as
   * _____ .

In the emergency room, Jill Thompson received 2 liters of normal saline (0.9% NaCl), $NaHCO_3$, and insulin. The health professional checked her laboratory results and noted that her blood sugar remained high and her serum CO_2 remained low. Her electrolytes were Na 151 mEq/L, Cl 130 mEq/L, and K 2.7 mEq/L.

8. Her elevated serum sodium and chloride may be due to
   * _____
   _____ .

9. The low serum potassium level may be due to * _____
   _____ .

10. Potassium should be administered * _____ hours after correction of acidosis.

In the emergency room, Jill Thompson received 35 units of regular insulin. The first day of admission she received a total of 275 units of regular insulin and 2 liters of normal saline solution (1 liter contained 5% dextrose). Also, the first day she received KCl—100 mEq/L in 2 liters of IV fluids.

Her laboratory results the second day were blood sugar 60 mg/dL, serum CO_2 15 mEq/L and 20 mEq/L, serum Na 164 mEq/L, Cl 133 mEq/L, and K 4.2 mEq/L.

11. Blood sugars need to be monitored frequently. When the blood sugar level drops to * _____ , 5% dextrose in water should be given.

12. The health professional should observe for symptoms of hypoglycemia. Four of the symptoms are * _____
   _____ .

13. Her serum sodium and serum chloride levels were still elevated the second day. This may be due to * _____
   _____ .

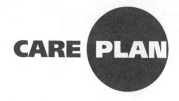

Client Management

Assessment Factors

▶ Obtain a client's history of signs and symptoms related to fluid loss and incidences leading to the health problem. Record the vital signs and note abnormal findings such as tachycardia, slightly decreased blood pressure, vigorous-rapid breathing, and slightly elevated or high temperature. These can indicate dehydration and a possible acidotic state.

▶ Check for abnormal laboratory results that indicate DKA, such as elevated blood sugar (>300 mg/dL); elevated hemoglobin and hematocrit; decreased serum CO_2, normal or low serum potassium, sodium, magnesium, chloride, and/or phosphorus levels; decreased pH; decreased arterial HCO_3; and decreased $PaCO_2$.

▶ Check urine for glycosuria and ketonuria. These are additional indicators of DKA.

▶ Assess urine output. Polyuria is an indicator of osmotic diuresis.

Diagnosis 1

Fluid volume deficit related to hyperglycemia and osmotic diuresis (polyuria).

Interventions and Rationale

1. Monitor vital signs (VS). Vital signs that are indicative of fluid loss or dehydration include rapid, thready pulse rate; slightly decreased systolic blood pressure; rapid, vigorous breathing (Kussmaul breathing); and slightly elevated temperature.

2. Check for other signs and symptoms of fluid loss such as poor skin turgor; dry, parched lips; dry, warm skin; and dry mucous membranes.

3. Check the serum osmolality from laboratory results or from assessment of physical changes. Normal serum osmolality is 280–295 mOsm/kg. The serum osmolality level may also be obtained by doubling the serum sodium level or by using the formula given in Chapter 1.

4. Monitor blood sugar level. Levels greater than 200 mg/dL indicate hyperglycemia. Increased blood sugar levels can cause osmotic diuresis.

5. Observe for signs and symptoms of hypokalemia and hyperkalemia. Symptoms of hypokalemia are malaise, dizziness,

arrhythmias, hypotension, muscular weakness, abdominal distention, and diminished peristalsis. Hypokalemia can occur as the acidotic state is corrected. Symptoms of hyperkalemia are tachycardia and then bradycardia, abdominal cramps, oliguria, numbness, and tingling in extremities.

6. Instruct the client to monitor blood sugar levels and/or urine to denote glycosuria. Clients can test their blood sugars with the use of a glucometer or some other approved testing device.

7. Administer normal saline solution and/or lactated Ringer's solution as prescribed to reestablish ECF. IV fluids for the first hour are usually given rapidly.

Diagnosis 2

Altered nutrition: less than body requirements, related to insufficient utilization of glucose and nutrients.

Interventions and Rationale

1. Administer regular (crystalline) insulin intravenously as prescribed in a bolus and in IV fluids to correct insulin deficiency. Recognize that 20–50 units or 0.1–0.4 U/kg of regular insulin may be given as a bolus. It is usually followed by administering 0.1 U/kg per hour in IV fluids.

2. Observe for signs and symptoms of a hypoglycemic reaction (insulin reaction) from possible overcorrection of hyperglycemia. The symptoms include cold, clammy skin, nervousness, weakness, dizziness, tachycardia, low blood pressure, and slurred speech.

3. Monitor IV fluids and adjust flow rate according to orders. If IV fluids are to run fast, observe for symptoms of overhydration.

Diagnosis 3

Altered tissue perfusion: renal, cardiopulmonary, and peripheral, related to fluid volume deficit and lack of glucose utilization.

Interventions and Rationale

1. Monitor urine output, heart rate, blood pressure, and chest sounds for abnormalities. Fluid deficit limits tissue perfusion and decreases circulatory volume and nutrients available to the vital organs. Report abnormal findings.

2. Monitor arterial blood gases (ABGs), particularly the pH, $PaCO_2$, PaO_2, and HCO_3. A decrease in pH and arterial HCO_3 determines the severity of the acidotic state. Tissue perfusion is decreased during acidosis.

Other Diagnoses to Consider

Risk for injury: cells and tissues, related to glucose intolerance and infection secondary to DKA. Fluid volume excess, related to excess administration of IV fluids.

Evaluation/Outcome

1. Evaluate the therapeutic effect of interventions to correct the underlying cause of diabetic ketoacidosis.
2. Remain free of signs and symptoms of diabetic ketoacidosis.
3. Monitor the laboratory tests, serum electrolytes and glucose, and ABGs, that these tests remain within normal ranges.
4. Evaluate the dietary intake and fluid intake and output.
5. Evaluate that a support system for the client is available.

▶ CHRONIC OBSTRUCTIVE PULMONARY DISEASE (COPD)

Pathophysiology

Morphologic changes in emphysema are (1) thickening of bronchial walls caused by submucosal edema and excess mucous secretion; (2) loss of elastic recoil of lung tissue; and (3) destruction of the alveolar septa that promote overdistention and dead air space.

ANSWER COLUMN

76 a. thickening of bronchial walls, b. loss of elastic recoil of lung tissue, c. destruction to alveolar septa or overdistended alveoli

76

Name three morphologic changes in COPD.

a. * _____

b. * _____

c. * _____

Bronchitis and emphysema generally coexist. Table 26-7 lists the pathophysiologic changes associated with COPD conditions. The rationale for pathophysiologic changes is included.

77
Airway obstruction is greatest on (inspiration/expiration) _____ .

77 expiration

78
The normal value of $PaCO_2$ is _____ mm Hg.
The term for CO_2 retention is _____ and the $PaCO_2$ is _____ mm Hg.

78 35–45; hypercapnia; >45

79
A serious acid-base imbalance that occurs in advanced COPD is
* _____ .
   Explain how this acid-base imbalance occurs. * _____
_____
   The pH is _____ and the $PaCO_2$ is _____ .

79 respiratory acidosis; CO_2 combines with water to produce carbonic acid, thus causing acidosis; <7.35; >45 mm Hg

80
The name for reduced oxygen (O_2) concentration in the blood is
_____ .
Decreased arterial O_2 causes the number of red blood cells to (increase/decrease) _____ .
The hemoglobin and hematocrit is (increased/decreased)
_____ .
Why? * _____

80 hypoxemia; increase; increased. More RBCs and hemoglobin are needed to carry oxygen.

81
Could a nonsmoker with an alpha$_1$-antitrypsin deficiency develop emphysema? _____ .
   Explain the rationale for your answer. * _____
_____

81 Yes. Antitrypsin deficiency permits the proteolytic enzymes in the lungs to damage lung tissue.

82
Cor pulmonale is right-sided heart failure caused by * _____
_____ .
It can result in COPD when alveolar tissue destruction leads to
* _____ .

82 pulmonary hypertension; a reduction in the size of the pulmonary capillary bed

Table 26-7

Pathophysiologic Changes in Chronic Obstructive Pulmonary Disease (COPD)

Pathophysiologic Changes	Rationale
Decreased elasticity of bronchiolar walls (loss of elastic recoil)	Loss of elastic recoil causes a premature collapse of airways with expiration. Alveoli become overdistended when air is trapped in the affected lung tissue and dead air space is increased. Overdistention leads to rupture and coalescence of several alveoli.
Alveolar damage	Chronic air trapping and airway inflammation lead to weakened bronchiolar walls and alveolar disruption. Coalescence of adjacent alveoli results in bullae (parenchymal air-filled spaces > 1 cm in diameter). The total area of gas exchange is greatly reduced and pulmonary hypertension may develop.
Mucous gland hyperplasia and increased mucous production	Oversecretion of mucous is commonly found in bronchitis and advanced emphysema. Increased mucous production can cause mucous plugs which lead to airway obstruction.
Inflammation of bronchial mucosa	Inflammatory infiltration and edema of the bronchial mucosa commonly occur in bronchitis but are also found in advanced emphysema. Edema and infiltration cause thickening of bronchiolar walls.
Airway obstruction	This condition is caused primarily by narrowed bronchioles, edema and mucous plugs. Obstruction is greatest on expiration. During inspiration bronchial lumina widen to admit air; the lumina collapse during expiration.
CO_2 retention Increased $PaCO_2$ >45 mm Hg (hypercapnia) Norms: 35–45 mm Hg	Accumulation of carbon dioxide (CO_2) concentration in the arterial blood from inadequate gas exchange is the result of hypoventilation. CO_2 excess, >60 mm Hg, can lead to ventricular fibrillation.
Respiratory acidosis	CO_2 retention results from hypoventilation. Water combines with CO_2 to produce carbonic acid, and with increased CO_2 retention respiratory acidosis occurs (H_2O) + CO_2 = H_2CO_3). The arterial blood gases reflect pH < 7.35; $PaCO_2$ > 45 mm Hg.
Hypoxemia	Hypoxemia, or reduced oxygen (O_2) in the blood, is frequently caused by airway obstruction and alveolar hypoventilation. The thickened alveolar capillary membrane reduces O_2 diffusion.
Cor pulmonale (right-sided heart failure due to pulmonary hypertension)	Destruction of alveolar tissue leads to a reduction of the size of the pulmonary capillary bed. Pulmonary hypertension occurs when $\frac{2}{3}$ to $\frac{3}{4}$ of the vascular bed is destroyed. The workload of the right ventricle is then increased, thus causing right ventricular hypertrophy and eventually CHF.
Increased red blood cell (RBC) count	Secondary polycythemia occurs as a compensatory mechanism with prolonged hypoxemia. Hemoglobin and hematocrit are increased to enhance O_2 transport.
Alpha$_1$-antitrypsin deficiency	A genetic predisposition to alpha$_1$-antitrypsin deficiency is present. An antitrypsin or trypsin inhibitor is produced in the liver. A deficit of antitrypsin allows proteolytic enzymes (released in the lungs from bacteria or phagocytic cells) to damage lung tissue. The result is emphysema.

Clinical Manifestations

Early signs and symptoms of bronchitis and/or emphysema are fatigue and dyspnea after exertion. Table 26-8 lists the signs and symptoms of early to advanced COPD (chronic bronchitis and emphysema). Study the table carefully and refer to it as needed.

Table 26-8

Clinical Manifestations of COPD

Signs and Symptoms	Rationale
Chronic Fatigue	Fatigue, an early sign of COPD, is caused by hypoxia and the increased effort required to move air into and out of the lungs.
Dyspnea	Difficulty in breathing and shortness of breath following exertion are early signs of COPD. In advanced COPD dyspnea occurs with little or no exertion.
Vital Signs BP increased	Increased blood pressure is due to increased sympathetic stimulation from stress.
Pulse rate increased	Increased pulse rate results from poor oxygenation. The body's attempts to compensate for hypoxemia (decreased oxygen in the blood) by increasing the heart rate to carry more oxygen.
Respirations labored and increased	Loss of elasticity of lung tissue causes the bronchioles to collapse during normal expiration, thus prolonging the expiratory phase of respiration. Accessory respiratory muscles are used to improve alveolar ventilation and gas exchange.
Barrel-Shaped Chest (AP diameter > lateral diameter)	This is the result of loss of lung elasticity, chronic air trapping, and chest wall expansion with chest rigidity. It may also be compounded by dorsal kyphosis which results from a bent-forward position used to facilitate breathing. Shoulders are elevated and the neck appears to shorten. Accessory muscles of respiration are used for breathing.
Cough (productive)	A cough is usually associated with bronchitis because of the excessive secretion of the mucous glands. In emphysema a cough is associated with respiratory infection or cardiac failure. Bacterial growth in retained mucous secretions leads to repeated infections and a chronic cough.
Cyanosis	In advanced COPD, marked cyanosis is due to poor tissue perfusion, which results from hypoxemia. Signs of cyanosis may also appear when the hemoglobin is below 5 g.
Clubbing of Nails	Clubbing of nails is commonly seen in association with hypoxemia and polycythemia. It may be due to capillary dilation in an attempt to draw more oxygen to the fingertips.

(continues on the following page)

Table 26-8

Clinical Manifestations of COPD (Continued)

Signs and Symptoms	Rationale
Laboratory Results Arterial blood gases (ABGs) pH < 7.35 PaCO$_2$ > 45 mm Hg HCO$_3$ > 28 mEq/L PaO$_2$ < 70 mm Hg BE >+ 2 (respiratory acidosis with metabolic compensation)	Increased CO$_2$ retention and water cause an excessive amount of carbonic acid. As a result of too much carbonic acid in the blood, acidosis develops and the pH is decreased. The PaCO$_2$ is the respiratory component of the ABGs. A decreased pH and an increased PaCO$_2$ indicate respiratory acidosis. The PaO$_2$ may be normal or greatly reduced, depending on the degree of distortion of ventilation/perfusion ratio. An increased bicarbonate (HCO$_3$) level indicates metabolic compensation to neutralize or decrease the acidotic state. A normal HCO$_3$ (24–28 mEq/L) indicates no compensation.
Hemoglobin (Hgb) and Hematocrit (Hct) Increased (hemoglobin may increase to 20 g)	Increased Hgb and Hct are due to hypoxemia. More hemoglobin can carry more oxygen. An elevated hemoglobin is a sign that cyanosis is more likely.
Electrolytes: Potassium, low to low normal Sodium, normal to slightly elevated	The serum potassium level may be 3.0–3.7 mEq/L and can be the result of poor dietary intake related to breathlessness, potassium-wasting diuretics, or chronic use of steroid (e.g., cortisone). Usually the sodium level is normal but it can be elevated due to cardiac failure, excess IV saline infusions, or chronic use of steroids.

---

83 fatigue and dyspnea on exertion.

84 increased; increased; labored; prolonged

85 loss of lung elasticity and chest wall expansion with chest rigidity or dorsal kyphosis from a bent position and using accessory respiratory muscles

83

Two early signs and symptoms of COPD are * _____

_____ .

84

Changes in VS may include the following:

    1. Blood pressure: _____

    2. Pulse rate: _____

    3. Respiration: _____

The expiratory phase of respiration is _____ .

85

A common characteristic of COPD is a barrel-shaped chest. Explain. * _____

_____

86

A cough is more common with what COPD problem? _____
Respiratory infection is a complication of COPD. Explain why?
*_____

_____

87

What major type of acid-base imbalance occurs in COPD?
*_____ .
Indicate the arterial blood gases that occur with this acid-base
imbalance:
    ( ) a. pH 7.46
    ( ) b. pH 7.32
    ( ) c. PaCO$_2$ 55 mm Hg
    ( ) d. PaCO$_2$ 32 mm Hg

88

Explain the significance of an elevated bicarbonate (HCO$_3$) level
in respiratory acidosis. *_____

_____

89

Which of the following laboratory results frequently occur in
chronic COPD? Correct the incorrect responses.
    ( ) a. Hemoglobin decreased
    ( ) b. Hematocrit decreased
    ( ) c. Potassium low or low normal
    ( ) d. Sodium loss

Clinical Applications

    Joseph Hall, age 54, has smoked two packs of cigarettes for the last 35 years. He has repeatedly been admitted to the hospital over the last 7 years for COPD or emphysema. The health professional assessed Mr. Hall's physiologic status and noted dyspnea following exertion (breathlessness), barrel-shaped chest, and mild cyanosis. Joseph complained of constant fatigue. When checking his breath sounds, the health professional noted a prolonged expiration rate. Vital signs were BP 150/86, pulse rate 94, and respiration 26 and labored.

---

86 bronchitis; Bacteria grows in retained mucous secretions and respiratory infection results.

87 respiratory acidosis; b, c
88 Elevated HCO$_3$ level indicates metabolic compensation. Conservation of bicarbonate helps to decrease the acidotic state.

89 a.—, increased to carry more oxygen; b.—, increased; c. X; d.—; sodium normal or slightly elevated

90 a, b, c, d, e

91 smoking

92 poor oxygenation or hypoxemia

93 poor nutritional intake. He can be given a potassium-wasting diuretic for heart failure as a result of prolonged respiratory distress.

94 normal

95 metabolic (renal) compensation

96 respiratory acidosis; without; The pH is low, $PaCO_2$ is high, and HCO_3 and BE are normal values and thus there is no compensation.

90

Which of Mr. Hall's clinical signs and symptoms taken on admission indicate COPD?
( ) a. Breathlessness
( ) b. Barrel-shaped chest
( ) c. Mild cyanosis
( ) d. Fatigue
( ) e. Prolonged expiration

91

A risk factor of COPD which can be linked to Mr. Hall's problem is _____ .

The results of the laboratory studies ordered for Mr. Hall are given in Table 26-9

92

Mr. Hall's RBC, hemoglobin, and hematocrit were elevated because of *_____ .

93

His potassium is low average. This can be the result of *_____
_____ .

94

Sodium level may be normal or slightly elevated. His serum sodium value is in the (high/normal/low) _____ range.

95

The serum CO_2 is a bicarbonate determinant. An increased value (alkalosis) may be due to base excess from bicarbonate intake or to metabolic (renal) compensation.
    In Mr. Hall's situation the cause is most likely *_____ .

96

On admission, his arterial blood gases (ABGs) indicate (respiratory alkalosis/respiratory acidosis) *_____ (with/without) _____ metabolic compensation.
    Explain his ABGs in response to your previous answer.
*_____
_____

Table 26-9

Laboratory Studies: Joseph Hall

Laboratory Tests	On Admission	Day 1	Day 2
Hematology			
Red blood cells (4.5–6 million)	6.6	6.5	6.2
Hemoglobin (Male: 13.5–18 g)	16.8	16.6	16.2
Hematocrit (Male: 40–54%)	57.8	57.2	55.6
White blood cells (5–10 mm^3)	12.8	13.0	10.5
Biochemistry			
Potassium (K) (3.5–5.3 mEq/L)	3.5	3.6	3.7
Sodium (Na) (135–146 mEq/L)	140	138	139
Chloride (Cl) (95–108 mEq/L)	107	106	106
Carbon dioxide (CO_2) (22–32 mEq/L)	30	36	38
Arterial Blood Gases (ABGs)			
pH (7.35–7.45)	7.24	7.32	7.34
$PaCO_2$ (35–45 mm Hg)	73	68	60
PaO_2 (70–100 mm Hg)	45	70 (with O_2)	76 (with O_2)
HCO_3 (24–28 mEq/L)	28	34	37
BE (−2 to +2)	+2	+6	+9

97 respiratory acidosis; Yes.; The HCO_3 and BE are elevated. This is a compensatory mechanism that brings the pH close to normal value.

97

On day 1 and day 2 his acid-base imbalance reflects
* _____ .

Is there metabolic compensation? _____ Explain. *_____

_____

98 It delivers a high concentration of O_2, >90%. This decreases the hypoxic respiratory drive and can cause CO_2 narcosis.; 2 L/min

99 low; hypoxemia or low oxygen content in the blood

100 respiratory infection. This is the result of trapped mucous secretions and the presence of bacteria.

101 1–2 L/min; A high concentration of O_2 decreases hypoxic respiratory drive.

102 to liquify secretions and ease in expectoration; cor pulmonale; CHF

98
Oxygen was administered to Mr. Hall at 2 L/min with a nasal O_2 cannula (nasal prongs). A ventimask delivered 24, 28, 35, and 40% of oxygen. A nonbreathing oxygen mask should *not* be used. Explain. *_____

_____

The rate of O_2 flow with a nasal cannula should be no greater than _____ .

99
Mr. Hall's PaO_2 is (high/low) _____ . His PaO_2 indicates *_____

_____

100
The health professional rechecked his breath sounds and noted rhonchi in the lower base of both lungs.
    Mr. Hall's WBCs are elevated. Rhonchi and elevated WBCs could be indicative of *_____

_____

Clinical Management

    Mr. Hall received bronchodilators and 2 L/min of oxygen. Breathing exercises were explained to him.
    Table 26-10 lists methods of managing COPD.

101
Low-flow oxygen is frequently needed to decrease hypoxemia. When a nasal O_2 cannula is used, the flow should be

_____

    If a high concentration of oxygen is delivered, what might happen to the respiratory drive? *_____

102
Why is hydration important in the management of COPD? *_____

_____

Increased fluid intake should be contraindicated when _____ and/or _____ are present.

Table 26-10

Clinical Management of COPD

Management Methods	Rationale
Oxygen (O_2)	Low-flow oxygen: 1–2 L/min with a nasal O_2 cannula or ventimask with 24 or 28% is suggested. Mechanical ventilators may be needed to decrease CO_2 retention and to aid in ventilation. Care should be taken to avoid CO_2 narcosis; O_2 that is too high decreases the hypoxic respiratory drive.
Hydration	Fluid intake should be increased to 3–4 L/day to liquify secretions and ease in expectoration *unless* cor pulmonale and/or CHF is present.
Bronchodilators: Isoproterenol (Isuprel) Metaproterenol (Alupent) Terbutaline (Brethine) Aminophylline Theophylline products	The purpose of these agents is to dilate bronchial tubes (bronchioles), to expectorate mucus, and to improve ventilation. Following use of a bronchodilator the client should deep breathe and cough. Bronchodilators can be administered through nebulizers (pressurized aerosols or IPPB with low-flow O_2 or compressed air), intravenously in IV fluids (aminophylline), or orally (theophylline products). Side effects of these drugs are tachycardia, cardiac dysrhythmias, and nausea/vomiting.
Antibiotics	When a respiratory infection is present, antibiotics are given intravenously (diluted in 50–100 mL of solution) or orally.
Chest Physiotherapy	Chest clapping loosens the thick, tenacious mucous secretions that must be "coughed up." Deep breathing and coughing should follow. Diaphragmatic breathing improves tidal volume and increases alveolar ventilation. Pursed-lip breathing prevents airway collapse so that trapped air in the alveoli can be expelled.
Exercise	Walking and stationary bicycling improve respiratory status and state of well being.
Relaxation Techniques	Practicing relaxation techniques decreases anxiety, fear, and panic. Decreased dyspnea can result from relaxation.

103 a. to dilate the bronchial tubes/bronchioles; b. to expectorate mucous; c. to improve ventilation

103

Bronchodilators are used for the following purposes:

a. * _____

b. * _____

c. * _____

104

Indicate which of the following side effects may result from constant use or overuse of bronchodilators:

( ) a. Bradycardia
( ) b. Tachycardia
( ) c. Nausea, vomiting
( ) d. Cardiac dysrhythmias
( ) e. Hypotension
( ) f. Skin rash

104 b, c, d

105

Identify three examples of chest physiotherapy and explain their purposes:

   a. *_____
     Purpose *_____
   b. *_____
     Purpose *_____
   c. *_____
     Purpose *_____

105 a. chest clapping; to loosen thick, tenacious mucous secretions;
b. diaphragmatic breathing; to increase alveolar ventilation;
c. pursed-lip breathing; to prevent airway collapse

106

Use of a relaxation technique performed daily can improve ventilation. Explain how. *_____

106 It decreases anxiety, fear, and panic related to breathlessness.

CASE STUDY

REVIEW

Mr. Joseph Hall, age 54, has had numerous admissions for severe dyspnea related to emphysema. His clinical signs, symptoms, and findings are stated under clinical applications.

ANSWER COLUMN

1. chronic obstructive lung disease (COPD); bronchitis and asthma
2. decreased elasticity of lung tissue or loss of elastic recoil, alveoli overdistention and damage, and excess mucous production (others: edema of the bronchial mucosa, hypoxemia)
3. smoking

1. Emphysema is classified as a *_____
Two other lung disorders under this classification are
  *_____ .

2. Name three physiologic changes that occur in COPD. *_____
_____
_____

3. What is the major risk factor in COPD? _____

4. antitrypsin; damage to lung tissue; emphysema or COPD

5. fatigue, dyspnea, barrel-shaped chest, and coughing (others: cyanosis, abnormal ABGs)

6. poor oxygenation or hypoxemia

7. respiratory acidosis; no

8. respiratory acidosis; Yes; HCO_3 and BE are elevated to decrease acidotic state.

9. Delivery of a high concentration of oxygen decreases hypoxic respiratory drive.

0. His WBC is elevated, indicating a possible infection (respiratory).

1. chest clapping, teaching diaphragmatic breathing, and teaching pursed-lip breathing [others: explaining relaxation technique, mild exercise, increase fluids (hydration)]

4. Name the protein produced in the liver that inhibits proteolytic enzymes in the lung. _____ A deficit of this protein causes *_____ and the disease _____ .

5. Four signs and symptoms of COPD are *_____

_____ .

6. Mr. Hall's RBC, hemoglobin, and hematocrit values are elevated. Identify the reason.

*_____

Mr. Hall's ABG on admission are pH 7.35, $PaCO_2$ 73 mm Hg, and HCO_3 28 mEq/L. On day 2 his ABG were pH 7.34, $PaCO_2$ 60 mm Hg, HCO_3 37 mEq/L, BE +9.

7. Mr. Hall's acid-base imbalance on admission is *_____

_____ . Is there metabolic compensation? _____

8. On day 2 his ABGs indicate *_____ .
Is there metabolic compensation? _____ Explain.

*_____

Mr. Hall received 2 liters per minute of oxygen and ampicillin in IV fluids.

9. Clients with emphysema should not be given a high concentration of oxygen.
Why? *_____

10. Why was Mr. Hall given ampicillin? *_____

_____ .

11. Name three actions to assist Mr. Hall with his breathing.
*_____
*_____
*_____ .

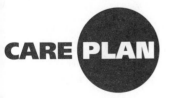

Client Management

Assessment Factors

▶ Obtain a client history of respiratory-related problems such as dyspnea at rest and on exertion, increasing shortness of breath, wheezing, fatigue, and activity intolerance.

▶ Auscultate and percuss the lung areas noting diminishe[d] breath sounds, decreased lung expansion, wheezing, crackle[s] and hyperresonance (hollow sound).

▶ Check vital signs (VS) for baseline reading to compare with fu[-] ture VS readings.

▶ Check the arterial blood gas (ABGs) report. Compare result[s] with the norms: pH 7.35–7.45, PaCO$_2$ 35–45 mm Hg, HCO$_3$ 24–2[6] mEq/L, BE −2 to +2.

Diagnosis 1

Impaired gas exchange related to alveoli damage and the collaps[e] of the bronchial tubes (bronchioles).

Interventions and Rationale

1. Monitor ABGs. Report abnormal changes as noted. A marke[d] decrease in pH and a marked increase in PaCO$_2$ (respirator[y] acidosis) should be reported immediately.

2. Check the electrolytes and hematology findings when re[-] turned and report abnormal results. Elevated hemoglobi[n] and hematocrit indicate hypoxemia.

3. Monitor breath sounds and lung expansion by ausculatin[g] and percussing lung area.

4. Assist with the use of aerosol bronchodilators. Check breat[h] sounds after use of aerosol treatments. If breath sounds ar[e] not clear or improved, the health care provider should be no[-] tified.

Diagnosis 2

Ineffective airway clearance related to excess mucous secretion[s] and the collapse of the bronchial tubes secondary to COPD.

Interventions and Rationale

1. Check breath sounds for rhonchi and rales. Provide ches[t] physiotherapy (chest clapping) for rhonchi and have clien[t] deep breathe and cough to clear bronchial secretions.

2. Instruct the client how to do breathing exercises; i.e., pursed[-] lip breathing (to prevent airway collapse) and diaphragmati[c] breathing (to increase alveolar ventilation).

3. Instruct the client not to get overfatigued and to avoid smoking, carefully use chemical irritants (bleaches, paints, and aerosol hair spray), avoid people with respiratory infections, air pollution, excess dust, pollen, and extreme heat or cold weather, all of which increase breathlessness.

4. Instruct the client to use bronchodilators as directed. Overuse of pressurized bronchodilator aerosol can cause a rebound effect.

5. Monitor fluid and food intake. Hydration is important to liquify tenacious mucous secretions. Frequent small feedings may be necessary.

6. Instruct the client to recognize early signs of respiratory infections, i.e., change in sputum color, elevated temperature, and coughing.

Diagnosis 3

Decreased cardiac output related to breathlessness and hypoxemia secondary to COPD.

Interventions and Rationale

1. Monitor vital signs. Report increase in pulse rate and changes in the rate of respiration. Labored breathing is a common sign of a respiratory problem.

2. Encourage the client to limit activities that increase the body's need for oxygen.

Diagnosis 4

Anxiety related to breathlessness, dependence on others, and the treatment regime.

Interventions and Rationale

1. Encourage the client to select and engage in a relaxation technique; help in the selection. Relaxation helps to decrease oxygen need by body tissues.

2. Explain the treatment and care to the client and family members and answer questions or refer them to the health care provider.

3. Be supportive of client and family members.

4. Refer to support groups, community agencies, and/or assistance programs.

Diagnosis 5

Activity intolerance related to breathlessness and fatigue.

Interventions and Rationale

1. Assist the client with the activities of daily living (ADLs) as needed.

2. Encourage the client to try mild exercises in the afternoon or when breathlessness is not severe. Avoid early mornings when mucous secretions are increased and after meals when energy is needed for digestion.

3. Observe for signs and symptoms for COPD, i.e., changes in vital signs, dyspnea, fatigue, barrel-shaped chest and cyanosis. Barrel-shaped chest results from dilated alveoli, inability to expel trapped air in the alveoli, and long-term effect of COPD.

Other Diagnoses to Consider

1. Ineffective breathing patterns related to CO_2 retention and poor gas exchange secondary to COPD.

2. Altered tissue perfusion related to hypoxemia.

3. Altered nutrition: less than body requirements, related to breathlessness.

4. Altered comfort related to breathlessness and muscle pain (diaphragm, intercostal).

5. Ineffective coping related to breathlessness and life style changes.

6. Risk for injury: lungs, related to smoking and respiratory infections.

7. Impaired physical mobility related to breathlessness.

8. Self-care deficit related to the inability to take part in ADLs because of dyspnea or breathlessness.

Evaluation/Outcome

1. Evaluate the therapeutic effect of interventions to correct the underlying cause of COPD.

2. Remain free of signs and symptoms of respiratory acidosis.

3. Determine that ABGs have returned to normal or within client's ABG normal range.

4. Evaluate the effectiveness of medications in reducing acute phases of COPD.

5. Evaluate that a support system for the client is available.

Appendix A

Clinical Pathways

Clinical pathways are designed to be used when providing ca[re] for clients with specific health problems. The form for clinical pat[h]ways can vary among institutions. Clinical pathways frequently a[re] accompanied with guidelines related to the health problem.

Two examples of a clinical pathway form are:

1. Congestive heart failure (CHF), in the acute phase, eme[r]gency department and the first day, in the improving phas[e] and in the discharge phase.

2. Home care pathway for newborn hyperbilirubinemia for vi[sit] 1 and visit 2.

These two pathways are from two different settings; the fir[st] is from an institution such as a hospital, the second in a home ca[re] environment.

Clinical Pathway - | DRAFT | CONGESTIVE HEART FAILURE

ACUTE PHASE - EMERGENCY DEPARTMENT   DATE ____/____/____

Disclaimer for Pathways and Guidelines: Clinical Pathways and Guidelines are developed by a multidisciplinary team. They are guidelines for care. They are not compulsory or mandatory plans of treatment or standards of care. When considering individual patient needs, alternative independent clinical assessments and judgements may be necessary.

BELOW: SELECT SHIFT & INITIAL

		0700-1500	1500-2300	2300-0700
Assessment	H&P per ED Protocol...............	☐ ____	☐ ____	☐ ____
	Vital signs & multisystem assessment per ED protocol.............................	☐ ____	☐ ____	☐ ____
	Advanced directives addressed..........	☐ ____	☐ ____	☐ ____
	Guideline I: S&S Diagnosis of CHF......	☐ ____	☐ ____	☐ ____
	Guideline II: CHF Pathway/Risk Stratification.....................	☐ ____	☐ ____	☐ ____
	Guideline VI: Level of Care for CHF Patients...........................	☐ ____	☐ ____	☐ ____
Treatments	Continuous cardiac monitoring..........	☐ ____	☐ ____	☐ ____
	Weight prior to diuresis (if appropriate)....	☐ ____	☐ ____	☐ ____
	Foley catheter as indicated..............	☐ ____	☐ ____	☐ ____
Tests/Labs	**Guideline III / IV: Diagnostic Procedures in New Onset/Established CHF** (EKG,CXR,CBC, complete chemistry profile, Mg, thyroid function, other as indicated).........................	☐ ____	☐ ____	☐ ____
	Pulse Oximetry per protocol..............	☐ ____	☐ ____	☐ ____
Medications/IVs	IV access............................	☐ ____	☐ ____	☐ ____
	Oxygen therapy per protocol.............	☐ ____	☐ ____	☐ ____
	Guideline IX: Diuresis.................	☐ ____	☐ ____	☐ ____
	Evaluate patient's routine medications.....	☐ ____	☐ ____	☐ ____
Consults	Cardiology consult as indicated..........	☐ ____	☐ ____	☐ ____
Nutrition	NPO except for medications.............	☐ ____	☐ ____	☐ ____
Activity/Safety	Bedrest.............................	☐ ____	☐ ____	☐ ____
	High Fowlers position...................	☐ ____	☐ ____	☐ ____
Discharge Planning	Responsible support person identified......	☐ ____	☐ ____	☐ ____
	Residence prior to admission identified.....	☐ ____	☐ ____	☐ ____
Patient/Family Teaching Outcomes	Verbalizes understanding of: Treatment plan and need for admission...	☐ ____	☐ ____	☐ ____
	Importance of notifying the staff when experiencing SOB or chest pain........	☐ ____	☐ ____	☐ ____
	Need for limited activity................	☐ ____	☐ ____	☐ ____
Clinical Processes/ Outcomes	If patient meets criteria, meds given in ED: • Furosemide....................	☐ ____	☐ ____	☐ ____
	• Bumetanide.....................	☐ ____	☐ ____	☐ ____
	• Morphine......................	☐ ____	☐ ____	☐ ____
	• Nitrates.......................	☐ ____	☐ ____	☐ ____
	• Heparin.......................	☐ ____	☐ ____	☐ ____
	Documentation of support person on record. Residence and telephone documented on record..............................	☐ ____	☐ ____	☐ ____

INITIAL	SIGNATURE	TITLE	INITIAL	SIGNATURE	TITLE

PHYSICIAN SIGNATURE: _____

Clinical Pathway -   DRAFT   CONGESTIVE HEART FAILURE

ACUTE PHASE - DAY 1	(ICU/TELEMETRY/MS UNIT)	DATE ____/____/____

(ADMISSION DAY or OBSERVATION DAY (0-24 hrs))

Disclaimer for Pathways and Guidelines: Clinical Pathways and Guidelines are developed by a multidisciplinary team. They are guidelines for care. They are not compulsory or mandatory plans of treatment or standards of care. When considering individual patient needs, alternative independent clinical assessments and judgements may be necessary.

		BELOW: SELECT SHIFT & INITIAL		
		0700-1500	1500-2300	2300-0700
Assessment	Vital signs & systems assessment per unit protocol	☐ ___	☐ ___	☐ ___
	Advanced directives addressed	☐ ___	☐ ___	☐ ___
	Monitor for signs & symptoms of SOB, JVD, rales, peripheral edema, S3,S4, murmur, arrthymias .	☐ ___	☐ ___	☐ ___
	Guideline VI: Level of Care for CHF Patients ...	☐ ___	☐ ___	☐ ___
Treatments	Continuous cardiac monitoring as indicated	☐ ___	☐ ___	☐ ___
	Weight q AM	☐ ___	☐ ___	☐ ___
	Intake & output	☐ ___	☐ ___	☐ ___
Tests/Labs	Pulse Oximetry per protocol	☐ ___	☐ ___	☐ ___
	Guideline III: Diagnostic Procedures in New Onset CHF.	☐ ___	☐ ___	☐ ___
	Guideline IV: Diagnostic Procedures in Established CHF.	☐ ___	☐ ___	☐ ___
	GuidelineV: Assessment of LV Function in CHF	☐ ___	☐ ___	☐ ___
Medications/IVs	IV access	☐ ___	☐ ___	☐ ___
	Oxygen therapy per protocol	☐ ___	☐ ___	☐ ___
	Guideline IX: Diuresis	☐ ___	☐ ___	☐ ___
	Guideline X: ACE Inhibitors	☐ ___	☐ ___	☐ ___
	Guideline XII: Digoxin	☐ ___	☐ ___	☐ ___
	Guideline XIII: Indications for Anticoagulation .	☐ ___	☐ ___	☐ ___
	Guideline XIV, XV, XVI and XVII.	☐ ___	☐ ___	☐ ___
	Patient's routine medications as indicated	☐ ___	☐ ___	☐ ___
Consults	Cardiology consult as indicated	☐ ___	☐ ___	☐ ___
Nutrition	Cardiac diet as tolerated, (additional Na and fluid restrictions as indicated)	☐ ___	☐ ___	☐ ___
	Nutrition screen, Diet Teaching Needs Assessment	☐ ___	☐ ___	☐ ___
Activity/Safety	Bedrest with BRP/bedside commode	☐ ___	☐ ___	☐ ___
	Fall risk assessment completed	☐ ___	☐ ___	☐ ___
	Maintain semi-Fowlers position	☐ ___	☐ ___	☐ ___
Discharge Planning	• Care management assessment:			
	• Evaluation of support system and discharge needs	☐ ___	☐ ___	☐ ___
	• Preadmission compliance with diet and medication evaluated	☐ ___	☐ ___	☐ ___
	• Initial discharge plan addressed, with patient and care giver.	☐ ___	☐ ___	☐ ___
	• Need for DME and home weight scale identified.	☐ ___	☐ ___	☐ ___
Patient/Family Teaching Outcomes	• Verbalizes basic understanding of disease process, (reason for SOB and decreased activity level etc.)	☐ ___	☐ ___	☐ ___
Clinical Processes/ Outcomes	• Decreasing SOB	☐ ___	☐ ___	☐ ___
	• JVD decreasing	☐ ___	☐ ___	☐ ___
	• Improved breath sounds	☐ ___	☐ ___	☐ ___
	• Negative fluid balance >500(8hr), 750(12hr) ...	☐ ___	☐ ___	☐ ___
	• LV Function ordered or documented in record (ås appropriate).	☐ ___	☐ ___	☐ ___
	• O₂ Sat maintained > 92%			

INITIAL SIGNATURE		TITLE	INITIAL SIGNATURE	TITLE

PHYSICIAN SIGNATURE: _____

Clinical Pathway - | DRAFT | CONGESTIVE HEART FAILURE

IMPROVING PHASE - DAY 2 ICU/Telemetry/MS Unit   DATE ____/____/____

Disclaimer for Pathways and Guidelines: Clinical Pathways and Guidelines are developed by a multidisciplinary team. They are guidelines for care. They are not compulsory or mandatory plans of treatment or standards of care. When considering individual patient needs, alternative independent clinical assessments and judgements may be necessary.

		BELOW: Select Shift & Initial		
		0700-1500	1500-2300	2300-0700
Assessment	Vital signs & multisystem assessment per unit protocol	☐ ____	☐ ____	☐ ____
	Monitor for signs & symptoms SOB, JVD, rales, peripheral edema	☐ ____	☐ ____	☐ ____
	Guideline VI: Level of Care for CHF Patients ...	☐ ____	☐ ____	☐ ____
Treatments	Continuous cardiac monitoring as indicated	☐ ____	☐ ____	☐ ____
	Weight AM	☐ ____	☐ ____	☐ ____
	Intake & output q 8 hours	☐ ____	☐ ____	☐ ____
	D/C foley if indicated	☐ ____	☐ ____	☐ ____
Tests/Labs	**Guideline III: Diagnostic Procedures in New Onset CHF ....**	☐ ____	☐ ____	☐ ____
	Guideline IV: Diagnostic Procedure in Established CHF	☐ ____	☐ ____	☐ ____
	Guideline V: Assessment of LV Function in CHF	☐ ____	☐ ____	☐ ____
	Pulse Oximetry per protocol	☐ ____	☐ ____	☐ ____
Medications/IVs	Oxygen therapy per protocol	☐ ____	☐ ____	☐ ____
	Guideline IX: Diuresis	☐ ____	☐ ____	☐ ____
	Guideline X: ACE Inhibitors	☐ ____	☐ ____	☐ ____
	Guideline XII: Digoxin	☐ ____	☐ ____	☐ ____
	Guideline XIII: Anticoagulation in CHF	☐ ____	☐ ____	☐ ____
	Guideline XIV, XV, XVI and XVII.	☐ ____	☐ ____	☐ ____
	Patient's routine medications as indicated	☐ ____	☐ ____	☐ ____
Consults	Nutrition for Level 4 Malnutrition Risk and diet teaching..	☐ ____	☐ ____	☐ ____
Nutrition	Cardiac diet (additional Na and fluid restrictions as indicated)	☐ ____	☐ ____	☐ ____
Activity/Safety	OOB X 3 with assistance, (meals in chair, remain up for 30 minutes)	☐ ____	☐ ____	☐ ____
	Encourage high to semi-Fowlers position when in bed and during meals	☐ ____	☐ ____	☐ ____
Discharge Planning	• Care manager reassessment of discharge plan, assess needs for Home O_2 and refer as indicated..	☐ ____	☐ ____	☐ ____
	• Assess need for Home Health, Telemanagement, Cardiac Rehab referral.	☐ ____	☐ ____	☐ ____
Patient/Family Teaching Outcomes	• Demonstrates understanding of activity level....	☐ ____	☐ ____	☐ ____
	• Medication instructions initiated.	☐ ____	☐ ____	☐ ____
	• Verbalizes understanding of relationship of increased Na and fluid intake with SOB, weight gain and peripheral edema.	☐ ____	☐ ____	☐ ____
	• Verbalizes rationale for daily weight monitoring. .	☐ ____	☐ ____	☐ ____
Clinical Processes/ Outcomes	• Decreased weight	☐ ____	☐ ____	☐ ____
	• Increased activity without increased SOB.	☐ ____	☐ ____	☐ ____
	• Negative fluid balance.	☐ ____	☐ ____	☐ ____
	• ECHO completed.	☐ ____	☐ ____	☐ ____
	• Receiving Ace inhibitors.	☐ ____	☐ ____	☐ ____
	• Receiving Digoxin.	☐ ____	☐ ____	☐ ____
	• Receiving diuretics.	☐ ____	☐ ____	☐ ____

Initial	Signature	Title	Initial	Signature	Title

PHYSICIAN SIGNATURE: _____

Clinical Pathway - | DRAFT | CONGESTIVE HEART FAILURE

DISCHARGE PHASE - DAY 3, 4, ___ (TELEMETRY/MS UNIT)   DATE ___/___/___

Disclaimer for Pathways and Guidelines: Clinical Pathways and Guidelines are developed by a multidisciplinary team. They are guidelines for care. They are not compulsory or mandatory plans of treatment or standards of care. When considering individual patient needs, alternative independent clinical assessments and judgements may be necessary.

		BELOW: SELECT SHIFT & INITIAL		
		0700-1500	1500-2300	2300-0700
Assessment	Vital signs & system assessment per unit protocol	. . .☐ _____	☐ _____	☐ _____
	Advanced directives addressed	. . .☐ _____	☐ _____	☐ _____
	Guideline VI: Level of Care for CHF Patients	. . .☐ _____	☐ _____	☐ _____
	Guideline VIII: NYHA Classification Circle - I , II , III , IV)	. . .☐ _____	☐ _____	☐ _____
Treatments	Continuous cardiac monitoring as indicated . . .	. . .☐ _____	☐ _____	☐ _____
	Weight q AM	. . .☐ _____	☐ _____	☐ _____
	Intake and output q 8 hours	. . .☐ _____	☐ _____	☐ _____
Tests/Labs	Pulse Oximetry per protocol	. . .☐ _____	☐ _____	☐ _____
Medications/IVs	Oxygen Therapy per protocol	. . .☐ _____	☐ _____	☐ _____
	Guideline IX: Diureses	. . .☐ _____	☐ _____	☐ _____
	Guideline X: Ace Inhibitors	. . .☐ _____	☐ _____	☐ _____
	Guideline XII: Digoxin	. . .☐ _____	☐ _____	☐ _____
	Guideline XIII: Anticoagulation in CHF	. . .☐ _____	☐ _____	☐ _____
	Guideline XIV, XV, XVI and XVII.	. . .☐ _____	☐ _____	☐ _____
	Patient's routine medications as indicated	. . .☐ _____	☐ _____	☐ _____
Consults	High risk patients meeting nutrition needs.	. . .☐ _____	☐ _____	☐ _____
	Diet education completed.	. . .☐ _____	☐ _____	☐ _____
Nutrition	Cardiac diet (additional Na and fluid restrictions as indicated)	. . .☐ _____	☐ _____	☐ _____
Activity/Safety	OOB and ambulating as tolerated	. . .☐ _____	☐ _____	☐ _____
	Meals in chair, remain up for 30 minutes	. . .☐ _____	☐ _____	☐ _____
	Encourage self care	. . .☐ _____	☐ _____	☐ _____
Discharge Planning	Discharge resources identified and referrals made as indicated:			
	• Smoking cessation program	. . .☐ _____	☐ _____	☐ _____
	• Home Health referral.	. . .☐ _____	☐ _____	☐ _____
	• Cardiac Rehabilitation.	. . .☐ _____	☐ _____	☐ _____
Patient/Family Teaching Outcomes	Verbalizes understanding of:			
	• Discharge medication regimen, action, side effects, drug and food interaction.	. . .☐ _____	☐ _____	☐ _____
	• Importance of monitoring daily wt - notify MD with increase of 3lbs in weight and or increasing SOB.	. . .☐ _____	☐ _____	☐ _____
	• Cardiac diet as indicated.	. . .☐ _____	☐ _____	☐ _____
Clinical Processes/ Outcomes	Resp. rate at baseline with increased activity. . .	. . .☐ _____	☐ _____	☐ _____
	Stable rate, rhythm, &BP with increased activity.	. . .☐ _____	☐ _____	☐ _____
	• Receiving ACE Inhibitors.	. . .☐ _____	☐ _____	☐ _____
	• Receiving digoxin	. . .☐ _____	☐ _____	☐ _____
	• Receiving diuretics.	. . .☐ _____	☐ _____	☐ _____
	• **Guideline VII: Discharge Criteria met :** (Y = D/C) (N= reapply next day).	. . .☐ _____	☐ _____	☐ _____

INITIAL	SIGNATURE	TITLE	INITIAL	SIGNATURE	TITLE

PHYSICIAN SIGNATURE: _____

Christiana Care
Visiting Nurse Association

Page 1 of 5   Client Name:_____
Newborn Hyperbilirubinemia   Admission #:_____
Home Care Pathway   ID #:_____

Outcomes: 1. Newborn's weight stabilizes and begins to rise.
             2. Bilirubin level decreases.
             3. Newborn has normal skin reactions to phototherapy.

KEY

✓ = Done   ∅ = None   NA = Not Applicable   I = Instructed   R = Reinstructed V = Variance A= Achieved

Admission	Discharge
1. OASIS	Outcomes Met: 1. Y___ N___ V___ 2. Y___ N___ V___ 3. Y___ N___ V___
2. Client / Family Data	
3. HCFA Certification	Discharged to : Family _____ Other ____ ED_____
4. Consent to Treat	Rehospitalized ___ Reason:_____
5. Client payment responsibilities	Plans for discharge (include MD follow - up):_____
6. Medication List	_____
7. DME used & company name:_____	_____
8. Bilirubin level on hospital discharge (or most recent level):_____	_____
9. DAT=_____	_____
10. Additional Comments:_____	_____
_____	Physician notified of discharge:_____
_____	
_____	Spoke to:_____ Date/Time:_____
_____	
	Nurse's Signature:_____ Date:_____

Assessment Visit # 1 Date:	**Assessment Visit # 2 Date:**
1. Vital signs: Temperature_____	1. Vital signs: Temperature_____
Apical pulse_____	Apical pulse_____
Regular_____	Regular_____
Irregular_____	Irregular_____
Murmur_____ (S1/S2?)	Murmur_____ (S1/S2?)
Respirations_____	Respirations_____
2. STATE: Deep Sleep____ Light Sleep____ Drowsy____	2. STATE: Deep Sleep____ Light Sleep____ Drowsy____
Alert, Eyes Bright____ Eyes Open, Motor Activity ____	Alert, Eyes Bright____ Eyes Open, Motor Activity____
Crying (consolable)____ Crying (not consolable)____	Crying (consolable)____ Crying (not consolable)____
3. Presence of NB reflexes: Moro_____ TN_____	3. Presence of NB reflexes: Moro_____ TN_____
Root_____ Suck_____	Root_____ Suck____
Grasp_____ Plantar____	Grasp_____ Plantar_____
4. Fontanels:	4. Fontanels:
Flat_____ Depressed_____ Bulging_____	Flat_____ Depressed_____ Bulging_____
5. Skin color, including which areas of the skin area jaundiced:	5. Skin color, including which areas of the skin area jaundiced:
_____	_____
_____	_____
Skin turgor:_____	Skin turgor:_____
Areas of pressure/ skin breakdown:_____	Areas of pressure/ skin breakdown:_____
_____	_____
Signs of birth trauma (describe and measure):_____	Signs of birth trauma (describe and measure):_____
6. Current weight (Calibrate scale using known weight measure prior to weighing newborn):_____	6. Current weight (Calibrate scale using known weight measure prior to weighing newborn):_____
_____ weight loss over_____ (hours, days)	_____ weight loss over_____ (hours, days)
_____ weight gain over_____ (hours, days)	_____ weight gain over_____ (hours, days)
Nurse's Signature:_____	**Nurse's Signature:_____**
Print Name:_____ Initial:_____	**Print Name:_____ Initial:_____**

Christiana Care
Visiting Nurse Association

Newborn Hyperbilirubinemia
Home Care Pathway

Client Name:_____
ID #:_____

Assessment Visit # 1 Date:	Assessment Vist #2 Date:

6. Feeding
  Breastfeeding:_____minutes, q._____hour(s)
  Do breast(s) feel lighter after feeding? Yes____No__
  Is suck strong and coordinated? Yes____No_____
  Formula Type:_____
    Amount and frequency:_____
	6. Feeding
	  Breastfeeding:_____minutes, q._____hour(s)
	  Do breast(s) feel lighter after feeding? Yes____No__
	  Is suck strong and coordinated? Yes____No_____
	  Formula Type:_____
	    Amount and frequency:_____

7. Elimination
  Diapers wet:_____(over_____hours)
    Soiled:_____(over_____hours)
	7. Elimination
	  Diapers wet:_____(over_____hours)
	    Soiled:_____(over_____hours)

8. Circumcision? Yes_____No_____N/A_____	8. Circumcision? Yes_____No_____N/A_____
Goals: ☐ Newborn is normothermic. ☐ Adequate # wet/soiled diapers (If BF: 2 wet,2 soiled on day 2). ☐ Vital signs wnl. ☐ Newborn is alert and responsive. ☐ Skin is intact. ☐ No S/Sx of dehydration. ☐ Newborn is feeding well.	**Goals:** ☐ Newborn is normothermic. ☐ Adequate # wet/soiled diapers (If BF: 2 wet,2 soiled on day 2). ☐ Vital signs wnl. ☐ Newborn is alert and responsive. ☐ Skin is intact. ☐ No S/Sx of dehydration. ☐ Newborn is feeding well.
Comments:_____ _____ _____ _____ _____	Comments:_____ _____ _____ _____ _____
Treatment Visit	**Treatment Visit**

1. Heelstick for serum bilirubin level=_____
    Area: L heel_____R heel_____
      Medial____Lateral_____
2. Laboratory should call physician with results.
3. Home care nurse should communicate with physician for further orders (Record communication with MD office here: Name of person spoken to, date/time):_____
4. Phototherapy unit placed in accordance with manufacturer's guidelines. Intensity selected is HIGH.
    Single_____ or Double____Phototherapy
Goals:
☐ Bilirubin level is decreasing.
☐ Skin is intact at heelstick site(s).
☐ Phototherapy unit is correctly placed.
 	
Comments:_____
_____
_____
_____
_____
	1. Heelstick for serum bilirubin level=_____
	    Area: L heel_____R heel_____
	      Medial____Lateral_____
	2. Laboratory should call physician with results.
	3. Home care nurse should communicate with physician for further orders (Record communication with MD office here: Name of person spoken to, date/time):_____
	4. Phototherapy unit placed in accordance with manufacturer's guidelines. Intensity selected is HIGH.
	    Single_____ or Double____Phototherapy
	Goals:
	☐ Bilirubin level is decreasing.
	☐ Skin is intact at heelstick site(s).
	☐ Phototherapy unit is correctly placed.
	
	Comments:_____
	_____
	_____
	_____
	_____

Medications	**Medications**
Record on Medication List. Untoward side effects of medications:_____ _____ _____	Document changes on Medication List. Untoward side effects of medications:_____ _____ _____
Goal: ❏ Medications given by caregiver as directed.	**Goal:** ❏ Medications given by caregiver as directed.
Nurse's Signature:	**Nurse's Signature:**
Print Name: **Initial:**	**Print Name:** **Initial:**

Courtesy of Christiana Care Visiting Nurse Association, New Castle, DE

Christiana Care
Visiting Nurse Association

Page 3 of 5

Client Name:_____

Newborn Hyperbilirubinemia

ID#:_____

Home Care Pathway

Instruction Visit 1 Date:	Instruction Visit 2 Date:

1. Instruct caregiver in the following:
  • Cause of newborn hyperbilirubinemia
  • Normal breakdown mechanism of hemoglobin and excretion (urobilinogen in urine: dark urine; sterobilingen in stool: brown stool)
  • Record-keeping: Axillary temperature
                        Oral intake
                        Elimination
 	
2. Instruct on use of phototherapy unit(s)
  • Keep newborn on phototherapy 23 out of 24 hours
  • Phototherapy unit should be on highest intensity
  • Changing light bulb
  • Unit should be placed so ventilation is not obstructed
 	
3. Instruct caregiver on skin care:
  • Avoidance of skin lotion
  • Appearance of maculopapular rash is common and disappears spontaneously
  • Reporting extreme skin erythema, dryness, and blistering
 	
4. Instruct caregiver to do the following:
  • Check axillary temperature qid
  • Report 97.4 <T>99.4F to VNA nurse
  • Offer frequent feedings
  • If breastfeeding, encourage at least 8 feedings daily
  • Positioning
  • Report decreased intake or urine output or projectile vomiting to VNA nurse
 	
Patient education materials provided/used:_____
_____
_____
_____
_____
 	
Goals:
❑ **Newborn is properly placed on phototherapy unit(s).**
❑ **Caregiver demonstrates ability to assemble and use phototherapy unit(s).**
❑ **Caregiver verbalizes knowledge of disease, purpose, and phototherapy procedure.**
 	
Comments:_____
_____
_____
_____
_____
_____
_____
_____
_____
_____
 	
Nurse's Signarture:
 	
Print Name: **Initial**
	1. Instruct caregiver in the following:
	  • Cause of newborn hyperbilirubinemia
	  • Normal breakdown mechanism of hemoglobin and Excretion (urobilinogen in urine: dark urine; sterobilingen in stool: brown stool)
	  • Record-keeping: Axillary temperature
	                        Oral intake
	                        Elimination
	
	2. Instruct on use of phototherapy unit(s)
	  • Keep newborn on phototherapy 23 out of 24 hours
	  • Phototherapy unit should be on highest intensity
	  • Changing light bulb
	  • Unit should be placed so ventilation is not obstructed
	
	3. Instruct caregiver on skin care:
	  • Avoidance of skin lotion
	  • Appearance of maculopapular rash is common and disappears spontaneously
	  • Reporting extreme skin erythema, dryness, and blistering
	
	4. Instruct caregiver to do the following:
	  • Check axillary temperature qid
	  • Report 97.4 <T>99.4F to VNA nurse
	  • Offer frequent feedings
	  • If breastfeeding, encourage at least 8 feedings daily
	  • Positioning
	  • Report if decreased intake or urine output or projectile vomiting to VNA nurse
	
	Patient education materials provided/used:_____
	_____
	_____
	_____
	_____
	
	Goals:
	❑ **Newborn is properly placed on phototherapy unit(s).**
	❑ **Caregiver demonstrates ability to assemble and use phototherapy unit(s).**
	❑ **Caregiver verbalizes knowledge of disease, purpose, and phototherapy procedure.**
	
	Comments:_____
	_____
	_____
	_____
	_____
	_____
	_____
	_____
	_____
	_____
	
	Nurse's Signature:
	
	Print Name: **Initial:**

Christiana Care
Visiting Nurse Association

Page 4 of 5
Newborn Hyperbilirubinemia
Home Care Pathway

Client Name:_____
ID#:_____

Psychosocial Visit 1 Date:	**Psychosocial Visit 2 Date:**
1. Comprehension (Ability to grasp concepts and respond to?) Exhibits: High _____ Medium _____ Low _____ 2. Motivation Level (Code: F=Family/Caregiver C=Client) _____Asks questions _____Eager to learn _____Extremely anxious _____Uncooperative _____Seems uninterested _____Denies educational need 3. Language barrier:____Yes ____No 4. Literate:____Yes ____No Comments:_____	1. Family Relationships: _____ _____ _____ _____ _____ _____ 2. Family Stressors: _____ _____ _____ 3. Financial Problems: _____ _____
Goal: ❏ Caregiver is comfortable using phototherapy unit(s) **Referrals / Interdisciplinary Services** 1. Smoking cessation for caregiver/ family 2. MSW 3. Lactation Consultant 4. La Leche League International: 1(800)La Leche(525-3243) 5. Nursing Mother's, Inc.: (302)733-0973 6. The Warm Line: (302)762-8938 7. Other:_____ **Goal:** ❏ **Client / Family can list resources available.** Comments:_____	4. Other: _____ _____ **Goal:** ❏ Caregiver / Family gaining increasing sense of control over treatment of hyperbilirubinemia. **Referrals / Interdisciplinary Services** 1. Smoking cessation for caregiver/ family 2. MSW 3. Lactation Consultant 4. La Leche League International: 1(800)La Leche(525-3243) 5. Nursing Mother's, Inc.: (302)733-0973 6. The Warm Line (302)762-8938 7. Other:_____ **Goal:** ❏ **Client / Family can list resources available.** Comments:_____
Nurse's Signature_____	**Nurses's Signature:**_____
Print Name: **Initial:**	**Print Name:** **Initial:**

Christiana Care
Visiting Nurse Association

Page 5 of 5
Clinical Pathway for Home Care: Hyperbilirubinemia
Outcome Record

Client Name:_____
Admission #:_____
ID #:_____

ICD9 Code:_____

Pathway Start Date:_____   Pathway Stop Date:_____
# of Home Visits:_____

Client Variance

❑ A1 Readmitted to hospital   ❑ A5 Other_____
❑ A2 Death
❑ A3 Caregiver noncompliance
❑ A4 Continues home care r/t_____

System Variance
   Internal   ❑ B1 Equipment not available
                     ❑ B2 Visit delay impending progress or treatment

System Variance
   External   ❑ B3 Insurance Problem
                     ❑ B4 Transportation problem

Nurse's Initial	Date	Visit Day	Variance Code	Variance/Explanation/Comments	Variance Caused Delay (Y/N)	Action Taken

Note: Y= Yes, N= No

Nurse's Signature:	Initials:	Nurse's Signature:	Initials:
Print Name:		Print Name:	
Nurse's Signature:	Initials:	Nurse's Signature:	Intials:
Print Name:		Print Name:	
Nurse's Signature:	Initials:	Nurse's Signature:	Initials:
Print Name:		Print Name:	

Hyperout 698 Gale

Courtesy of Christiana Care Visiting Nurse Association, New Castle, DE

Appendix B

Summary of Acid-Base Imbalances

Metabolic Acidosis	Metabolic Alkalosis
	Clinical Manifestations
Kussmaul breathing (rapid and vigorous)	Shallow breathing
Flushing of the skin (capillary dilation)	Tetanylike symptoms
Decrease in heart rate and cardiac output	Irritability, confusion
Nausea, vomiting, abdominal pain	Vomiting
Dehydration	
	Laboratory Findings
Bicarbonate deficit	*Bicarbonate excess*
pH<7.35, HCO_3<24 mEq/L,	pH>7.45, HCO_3>28 mEq/L, BE>+2,
BE<−2, plasma CO_2<22 mEq/L	plasma CO_2 >32 mEq/L
	Causes
Diabetic acidosis, severe diarrhea or starvation, tissue trauma, renal and heart failure, shock, severe infection	Peptic ulcer, vomiting, gastric suction

Respiratory Acidosis	Respiratory Alkalosis
	Clinical Manifestations
Dyspnea, inadequate gas exchange	Rapid shallow breathing
Flushing and warm skin	Tetanylike symptoms (numbness, tingling of fingers)
Tachycardia	Palpitations
Weakness	Vertigo
	Laboratory Findings
Carbonic acid excess (CO_2 retention)	*Carbonic acid deficit*
pH<7.35, $PaCO_2$ >45mm Hg	pH>7.45, $PaCO_2$ <35 mm Hg
	Causes
COPD (emphysema, chronic bronchitis, severe asthma), narcotics, anesthetics, barbiturates, pneumonia, chest injuries	Anxiety, hysteria, drug toxicity, fever, pain, brain tumors, early salicylate poisoning, excessive exercise

Appendix C

Clinical Problems Associated with Fluid Imbalances

Clinical Problems	ECFVD	ECFVE	ECFV Shift	ICFVE
Gastrointestinal				
Vomiting and diarrhea	+			
GI fistula	+			
GI suctioning	+			
Increased salt intake	+			
Intestinal obstruction	+		+	
Perforated ulcer	+		+	
Excessive hypotonic fluids oral and intravenous				+
Renal				
Renal failure		+		
Renal disease		+		
Cardiac				
Congestive heart failure		+		
Miscellaneous				
Brain tumor/injury				+
Fever	+			
Profused diaphoresis	+			
SIADH (syndrome of inappropriate antidiuretic hormone)		Initially +		+
Burns	+	+	+	
Diabetic ketoacidosis	+			
Ascites (cirrhosis)		+	+	
Venous obstruction		+		
Sprain			+	
Massive trauma	+		+	
Drugs				
Cortisone group of drugs		+		

Appendix D

Clinical Problems Associated with Electrolyte Imbalances

Clinical Problems	Potassium	Sodium	Calcium	Magnesium	Phosphorus
Gastrointestinal					
Vomiting and diarrhea	K↓	Na↓	Ca↓	Mg↓	P↓
Malnutrition	K↓	Na↓	Ca↓	Mg↓	P↓
Anorexia nervosa	K↓	Na↓	Ca↓	Mg↓	P↓
Intestinal fistula	K↓	Na↓		Mg↓	P↓
GI surgery	K↓	Na↓		Mg↓	P↓
Chronic alcoholism	K↓	Na↓	Ca↓	Mg↓	P↓
Lack of vitamin D			Ca↓		
Hyperphosphatemia			Ca↓		
Transfusion of citrated blood			Ca↓		
Cardiac					
Myocardial infarction	K↓	Na↓		Mg↓	
		Hypervolemia			
Congestive heart failure (CHF)	K↓/N	Na↑		Mg↓/N	
Endocrine					
Cushing's syndrome	K↓	Na↑		Mg↓	
Addison's disease	K↑	Na↓		Mg↑	
Diabetic ketoacidosis	K↑	Na↑/↓	Ca↓	Mg↑	P↓/N
	Diuresis K↓		(ionized)	Diuresis Mg↓	
Parathyroidism					
Hypo:			Ca↓		P↑
Hyper:			Ca↑		P↓

(continues on the following page)

Continued)

Clinical Problems	Potassium	Sodium	Calcium	Magnesium	Phosphorus
Renal					
Acute renal failure	Oliguria K↑	Na↑		Mg↑	P↑
	Diuresis K↓				
Chronic renal failure	K↑	Na↑	Ca↑/↓	Mg↑	P↑
Miscellaneous					
Cancer	K↓/↑	Na↓	Ca↑	Mg↓	P↓
Bone destruction			Ca↑		
Burns	K↓/↑	Na↓	Ca↓	Mg↓	P↓
Acute pancreatitis			Ca↓		
SIADH (syndrome of inappropriate antidiuretic hormone)		Na↓			
Metabolic acidosis	K↑		Ca↓		
Metabolic alkalosis	K↓				
Drugs					
Diuretics					
Potassium wasting	K↓	Na↓	Ca↑/↓	Mg↓	
Potassium sparing	K↑/N	Na↓		Mg↓	
ACE inhibitors	K↑	Na↓/N			

Appendix E

Clinical Assessment Tool: Fluid, Electrolyte, and Acid-Base

This assessment tool can be used for assessing fluid, electrolyte, and acid-base imbalances in all clinical settings.

A. Health history of the clinical problem
   1. Chief complaint
   2. History of the present illness
      a. Date of onset
      b. Duration
      c. Effects of bodily function
      d. Treatment and medications—effective or noneffective
   3. Past history of clinical condition
B. Fluid balance assessment
   1. Skin turgor
   2. Mucous membrane
   3. Vital signs—P↑, BP↓, T sl↑
   4. Insensible fluid loss
      a. Diaphoresis
      b. Hyperventilation
   5. Body weight loss—2.2 pounds = 1 liter of water
   6. Intake and output
      a. Intake: oral; IV fluids
      b. Output: urine; stool; GI fluids; blood; wound
   7. Edema

8. Behavioral changes—confusion and irritability (ECFV↓ and ICFV↑)
9. Neck and/or hand vein engorgement
10. Chest sounds—rales
11. Laboratory results
    a. Serum osmolality   <280 mOsm/kg, overhydration
       >295 mOsm/kg, dehydration
    b. Hemoglobin   <12 g/dL, anemia
       >17 g/dL, dehydration
    c. Hematocrit   >52%, possible dehydration
    d. BUN (10–25 mg/dL range)   >25–35 mg/dL, possible dehydration
    e. Creatinine (0.7–1.4 mg/dL range)   >1.5 mg/dL, possible dehydration

C. Electrolyte balance assessment
   1. Serum electrolytes
      a. Potassium: 3.5–5.3 mEq/L
      b. Sodium: 135–146 mEq/L
      c. Calcium: 4.5–5.5 mEq/L; 9–11 mg/dL; 2.3–2.8 mmol/L (SI units)
         Ionized calcium: 2.2–2.5 mEq/L; 4.4–5.0 mg/dL; 1.1–1.24 mmol/L
      d. Magnesium: 1.8–2.4 mEq/L
      e. Chloride: 95–108 mEq/L
      f. Phosphorus: 1.7–2.6 mEq/L; 2.5–4.5 mg/dL
   2. Signs and symptoms of hypo-hyperkalemia, hypo-hypernatremia, hypo-hypercalcemia
   3. Urine osmolality 50–1400 mOsm/L (range); 500–800 mOsm/L (average)
      Urine specific gravity: 1.010–1.030
   4. Urine electrolytes
      a. Potassium: 25–120 mEq/24 h
      b. Sodium: 40–220 mEq/24 h
      c. Calcium: 50–150 mg/24 h
      d. Chloride: 110–250 mEq/24 h
      Example: Urine sodium 20 mOsm/L 24 hr: body retaining sodium even if serum sodium is low. Commonly seen with CHF and cirrhosis of the liver.

5. Vital signs (VS): pulse irregular
6. ECG: changes with potassium, sodium, calcium, and magnesium imbalances
7. Behavioral changes: potassium imbalance
8. Drug therapy: diuretics, steroids, digitalis preparations, antibiotics
9. Continuous GI suctioning: loss of major electrolytes

D. Acid-base balance assessment
1. Arterial blood gases (ABGs)
   a. pH: <7.35, acidosis; >7.45, alkalosis
   b. $PaCO_2$: <35 mmHg, respiratory alkalosis; >45 mmHg, respiratory acidosis
   c. HCO_3: <24 mEq/L, metabolic acidosis; >28 mEq/L, metabolic alkalosis
      Base excess (BE): <-2, metabolic acidosis; $>+2$, metabolic alkalosis
2. Serum CO_2: 22–32 mEq/L
3. Overbreathing or underbreathing
4. Chest sounds: rales, rhonchi
5. Assisted ventilator
6. Behavioral changes: acid-base imbalance present
7. Intubations
8. Electrolyte imbalance: loss of potassium (K) and hydrochloric acid (HCl): hypokalemic alkalosis

Foods Rich in Potassium, Sodium, Calcium, Magnesium, Chloride, and Phosphorus

Classes	Potassium	Sodium	Calcium	Magnesium	Chloride	Phosphorus
Daily requirements	3–4 g	2–4 g	800 mg	300–350 mg	3–9 g	800–1200 mg
Beverages	Cocoa, Coca Cola, coffee, wines	Pepsi-Cola, tea, decaffeinated coffee		Cocoa		
Fruit and fruit juices	Citrus fruits: oranges, grapefruit Juices: grapefruit (canned), orange (canned), prune (canned), tomato (canned)					
	Fruits: apricots (dry), bananas, cantaloupe, dates, raisins (dry), watermelon, prunes			Average	High only in dates and bananas	
Bread products and cereal	Average to low amount	White bread, soda crackers, and wheat flakes		Cereals with oats		Whole grain cereal
Dairy products	Average to low—milk, buttermilk	Butter, cheese, and margarine	Milk, cheese	Milk (average)	Cheese, milk	Cheese, milk, eggs
Nuts	Almonds, Brazil nuts, cashews, and peanuts	Low, except if salted	Brazil nuts (moderate)	Almonds, Brazil nuts, peanuts, and walnuts		Peanuts

(continues on the following page)

(Continued)

Classes	Potassium	Sodium	Calcium	Magnesium	Chloride	Phosphorus
Vegetables	Baked beans, carrots (raw), celery (raw), dandelion greens, lima beans (canned), mustard greens, tomatoes, spinach *Note:* Nearly all vegetables are rich in potassium when raw, but K will be lost if water used in cooking is discarded.	Average to low Celery (high average)	Baked beans, kale, mustard and turnip greens, broccoli	Green, leafy	Spinach, celery	Dry beans
Meat, fish, and poultry	Average—meats High average—sardines, codfish, scallops	Corned beef, bacon, ham, crab, tuna fish, sausage (pork) Low in poultry	Salmon, meats	Fish, shrimp Low in poultry Low in meats Egg, average	Eggs, crabs, fish (average), turkey	Beef, pork, fish, chicken, turkey
Miscellaneous	Catsup (average), spices, potato chips, and peanut butter	Catsup, mayonnaise, potato chips, pretzels, pickles, dill, olives, mustard, Worcestershire sauce, celery salt, salad dressing—French and Italian	Molasses	Chocolate and chocolate bars, chocolate syrup Molasses Table salt		

Glossary

abdomen the portion of the body lying between the chest and the pelvis.

acid any substance that is sour in taste and that neutralizes a basic substance.

acid metabolites see metabolites.

ACTH abbreviation for adrenocorticotropic hormone. A hormone secreted by the hypophysis or pituitary gland. It stimulates the adrenal cortex to secrete cortisone.

afterload resistance in the vessels against which the ventricle ejects blood during systole.

aged age of 65 years or older.

albumin simple protein. It is the main protein from the blood.

serum primary function to maintain the colloid osmotic pressure of the blood.

alimentary pertaining to nutrition; the alimentary tract is a digestive tube from the mouth to the anus.

alkaline any substance that can neutralize an acid and that, when combined with an acid, forms a salt.

alveolus air sac or cell of the lung.

amphoteric ability to bind or release excess H^+.

anesthetic an agent causing an insensibility to pain or touch.

anion a negatively charged ion.

anorexia a loss of appetite.

anoxia oxygen deficiency.

antipyretic a medication that reduces body core temperature.

anuria a complete urinary suppression.

aortic arch the arch of the aorta soon after it leaves the heart.

aphasia a loss of the power of speech.

arrhythmia irregular heart rhythm.

arterioles minute arteries leading into a capillary.

arteriosclerosis pertaining to thickening, hardening, and loss of elasticity of the walls of the blood vessels.

artery a vessel carrying blood from the heart to the tissue.

ascites an accumulation of serous fluid in the peritoneal cavity.

atrium a chamber. In the heart it is the upper chamber of each half of the heart.

atrophy decrease in size of structure.

autoregulation control of blood flow to tissue by a change in the tissue.

azotemia an excessive quantity of nitrogenous waste products in the blood increased BUN and creatinine.

BE abbreviation for base excess.

biliary pertaining to or conveying bile.

blood intravascular fluid composed of red and white blood cells and platelets.

bradycardia pulse rate less than 50 beats per minute.

brain interstitium spaces between the brain tissues.

brain parenchyma functional tissue of the brain.

brain stem herniation protrusion of the medulla, pons, and midbrain into the spinal canal.

bronchiectasis dilatation of a bronchus.

BUN abbreviation for blood urea nitrogen. Urea is a by-product of protein metabolism.

butterfly (winged tip) an infusion device designed for short-term parenteral therapy. Each set consists of a wing-tip needle with a metal cannula, plastic or rubber wings, and plastic catheter or hub. The needle is $\frac{1}{2}$–$1\frac{1}{2}$ inches long with needle gauges of 15–26. The infusion needle and clear tubing are bonded into a single unit. It is commonly used for children and elderly who may have small or fragile veins.

capillary a minute blood vessel connecting the smallest arteries (arterioles) with the smallest veins (venules).

capillary permeability diffusion of substances from capillary walls into tissue spaces.

carbonic anhydrase inhibitor an agent used as a diuretic that inhibits the enzyme carbonic anhydrase.

cardiac output amount of blood ejected by the heart each minute.

cardiac reserve capacity of the heart to respond to increased burden.

carotid sinus a dilated area at the bifurcation of the carotid artery that is richly supplied with sensory nerve endings of the sinus branch of the vagus nerve.

cation a positively charged ion.

cerebral hemorrhage bleeding into brain tissue from rupture in a blood vessel.

cerebral spinal fluid fluid contained within the ventricles of the brain and spinal cord.

cerebrospinal fluid fluid found and circulating through the brain and spinal cord.

cirrhosis a chronic disease of the liver characterized by degenerative changes in the liver cells.

colloid gelatinlike substance, e.g., protein.

colloid osmotic pressure pressure exerted by non-diffusible substances.

congestive heart failure (CHF) circulatory congestion related to pump failure.

contraindication nonindicated form of therapy.

conversion table:
1 kilogram (kg) = 2.2 pounds (lb)
1 gram = 1000 milligrams (mg) or 15 grains (gr)
1 liter (L) = 1 quart or 1000 milliliters (mL)
1 cubic centimeter (cc) = 1 milliliter (mL); 100 mL = 1dL
1 deciliter (dL) = 100 mL
1 drop (gtt) = 1 minim (m)
qh = every hour
x = times

cortisone a hormone secreted by the adrenal cortex

creatinine end product of creatine (amino acid).

crystalloids diffusible substances dissolved in solut that pass through a selectively permeable membran

CVP abbreviation for central venous pressure. It is the nous pressure in the vena cava or the heart's rig atrium.

cyanosis a bluish or grayish discoloration of the skin d to a lack of oxygen in the hemoglobin of the bloo

cytogenic originating within the cell.

decerebrate condition wherein the brain cells are a fected, causing the extremities to be in rigid exte sion.

decompensation failure to compensate.

decorticate condition wherein the cortex of the bra is affected, causing the extremities to be in rig flexion.

deficit lack of.

dependent edema see edema.

dermis the true skin layer.

dextran colloid hyperosmolar solution.

dextrose a simple sugar, also known as glucose.

diabetes mellitus a disorder of carbohydrate metabo lism due to an inadequate production or utilizatior of insulin.

diabetic acidosis an excessive production of ketone bodies (acid) due to a lack of insulin and inability tc utilize carbohydrates, also called diabetic keto-acidosis.

dialysate an isotonic solution used in dialysis that has similar electrolyte content to plasma or Ringer's solu-tion, with the exception of potassium.

diaphoresis excessive perspiration.

diffusion the movement of each molecule along its own pathway irrespective of all other molecules; go-ing in various directions, mostly from greater to lesser concentration.

diplopia double vision.

disequilibrium syndrome rapid shift of fluids and electrolytes during hemodialysis which causes CNS disturbances.

dissociation a separation.

diuresis an abnormal increase in urine excretion.

diuretic a drug used to increase the secretion of urine.
  potassium-sparing diuretic retains potassium and excretes other electrolytes.
  potassium-wasting diuretic excretes potassium and other electrolytes.

verticulum a sac or pouch in the wall of an organ.

y weight normal body weight without excess water.

odenal pertaining to the duodenum, which is the first part of the small intestine.

spnea a labored or difficult breathing.

dema an abnormal retention of fluid in the interstitial spaces.

dependent edema fluid present in the interstitial spaces due to gravity (frequency found in extremities after being in standing or sitting position).

nondependent edema fluid present in the interstitial spaces, but not necessarily due to gravity alone, e.g., cardiac, liver, or kidney dysfunction.

pitting edema depression in the edematous tissue.

pulmonary edema fluid throughout the lung tissue.

refractory edema fluid in the interstitial spaces that does not respond to diuretics.

e.g. for example.

electrolyte a substance that, when in solution, conducts an electric current.

endothelium flat cells that line the blood and lymphatic vessels.

enzyme a catalyst, capable of inducting chemical changes in other substances.

epidermis an outer layer of the skin.

erythrocytes red blood cells.

erythropoietin factor secreted by the kidneys that stimulates bone marrow to produce red blood cells.

excess too much.

excretion an elimination of waste products from the body.

excretory pertaining to excretion.

extracellular fluid volume shift (ECF shift) shift of fluid within the ECF compartment from intravascular to interstitial spaces or from interstitial to intravascular spaces.

extract outside of.

extravasation the accumulation of vesicant or an irritant in the subcutaneous tissue.

febrile pertaining to a fever.

flatus gas in the alimentary tract.

generic name reflects the chemical family to which a drug belongs. The name never changes.

globulin a group of simple proteins.

glomerulus a capillary loop enclosed within the Bowman's capsule of the kidney.

glucose formed from carbohydrates during digestion and frequently called dextrose.

glycogen a stored form of sugar in the liver or muscle that can be converted to glucose.

glycosuria sugar in the urine.

gt abbreviation for drop.

gtt abbreviation for drops.

hematocrit the volume of red blood cells or erythrocytes in a given volume of blood.

hemoconcentration increase in number of red blood cells and solutes and a decrease in plasma volume.

hemodilution an increase in the volume of blood plasma due to a lack of red blood cells and solutes or an excess of intravascular fluid.

hemoglobin conjugated protein consisting of iron-containing pigment in the erythrocyte.

hemolysis destruction of red blood cells and causing release of hemoglobin into the serum.

heparin anticoagulant.

hepatic coma liver failure.

hernia a protrusion of an organ through the wall of a cavity.

inguinal protrusion of the intestine at the inguinal opening.

homeostasis uniformity or stability. State of equilibrium of the internal environment.

hormone a chemical substance originating in an organ or gland, which travels through the blood and is capable of increasing body activity or secretion.

ADH abbreviation for antidiuretic hormone; a hormone to lessen urine secretion.

hydrocephalus increased fluid retention in the ventricles of the brain.

hydrostatic pressure pressure of fluids at equilibrium.

hyperalimentation intravenous administration of a hyperosmolar solution of glucose, protein, vitamins, and electrolytes to promote tissue synthesis.

hyperbaric oxygenation oxygen under pressure carried in the plasma.

hypercalcemia a high serum calcium.

hypercapnia increased carbon dioxide in the blood.

hyperchloremia a high serum chloride.

hyperglycemia condition where blood glucose levels are elevated above normal.

hyperkalemia a high serum potassium.

hypernatremia a high serum sodium.

hyperosmolar increased number of osmols per solution. Increased solute concentration as compared to plasma.

hypertension high blood pressure.

essential a high blood pressure that develops in the absence of kidney disease. It is also called primary hypertension.

hypertonic a higher solute concentration than plasma.

hypertrophy increased thickening of a structure.

hyperventilation breathing at a rate greater than needed for body requirements.

hypervolemia an increase in blood volume.

hypocalcemia a low-serum calcium.

hypochloremia a low-serum chloride.

hypoglycemia low blood sugar.

hypokalemia a low-serum potassium.

hyponatremia a low-serum sodium.

hypo-osmolality condition where number for formed particles in the serum is decreased.

hypo-osmolar decreased number of osmols per solution. Decreased solute concentration as compared to plasma.

hypophysis the pituitary gland.

hypotension a low blood pressure.

hypotonic a lower solute concentration than plasma.

hypoventilation breathing at a rate lower than required to meet metabolic demands.

hypovolemia a decrease in blood volume.

hypoxemia reduced oxygen content in the blood.

hypoxia decreased oxygen content in body tissue.

i.e. that is.

incarcerated constricted, as an irreducible hernia.

infusion an injection of a solution directly into a vein.

insensible perspiration water loss by diffusion through the skin.

inside-needle catheter (INC) an infusion device designed for short-term parenteral therapy (opposite of the over-needle catheter—ONC) that is constructed exactly opposite the ONC. Needle length is $1\frac{1}{2}$–3 inches with a catheter length of 8–36 inches. The catheter is available in gauges of 8–22. The INC set comes with a catheter sleeve guard that must be secured over the needle bevel to prevent severing the catheter. It is commonly used for more prolonged infusions. Catheters used in INCs and ONCs are constructed of silicone, Teflon, polyvinyl chloride, or polyethylene.

insulin a hormone secreted by the beta cells of the islets of Langerhans found in the pancreas. It is important in the oxidation and utilization of blood sugar (glucose).

inter between.

interstitial edema accumulation of excess fluid tween cells; this is extracellular fluid.

intervention action.

intra within.

intracerebral edema accumulation of excess fl within the brain tissue and structures.

intracerebral hypertension increased press within the brain structures.

intracranial pressure pressure exerted by fluid with the brain structures.

ion a particle carrying either a positive or negati charge.

ionization separation into ions.

ionizing separating into ions.

iso-osmolar same number of osmols per solution compared to plasma.

isotonic same solute concentration as plasma.

ketone bodies oxidation of fatty acids.

ketonuria excess ketones in urine.

Kussmaul breathing hyperactive, abnormally vigor ous breathing.

lassitude weariness.

lidocaine also known as xylocaine. A drug used as a sur face anesthetic. It also can be used to treat ventricu lar arrhythmias.

lymph an alkaline fluid. It is similar to plasma except that its protein content is lower.

lymphatic system the conveyance of lymph from the tissues to the blood.

malaise uneasiness, ill feeling.

medulla the central portion of an organ, e.g., adrenal gland.

membrane a layer of tissue that covers a surface or organ or separates a space.

mercurial diuretic a drug that affects the proximal tubules of the kidneys by inhibiting reabsorption of sodium.

metabolism the physical and chemical changes involved in the utilization of particular substances.

metabolites the by-products of cellular metabolism or catabolism.

midbrain connects the pons and cerebellum with the cerebral hemispheres.

milliequivalent the chemical activity of elements.

milligram measures the weight of ions.

milliosmol 1/1000th of an osmol. It involves the osmotic activity of a solution.

olar 1 gram molecular weight of a substance.

yocardium the muscle of the heart.

arcotic a drug that depresses the central nervous system, relieves pain, and can induce sleep.

ecrosis destroyed tissue.

ephritis inflammation of the kidney.

ephrosis degenerative changes in the kidney.

euromuscular pertaining to the nerve and muscle.

euromuscular junction the innervation of the nerve with a muscle.

ondependent edema see edema.

nonvolatile acid fixed acid resulting from metabolic processes, excreted by the kidneys.

oliguria a diminished amount of urine.

oral rehydration fluid oral fluids designed to replace fluid and electrolyte losses in clients (usually children) who are able to tolerate liquids. These fluids are made up of similar concentrations of glucose, sodium, potassium, chloride, and bicarbonate of soda. Examples include WHO, Hydra-lyte, Rehydra-lyte, Lytren, ReSol, and Infalyte.

osmol a unit of osmotic pressure.

osmolality osmols or milliosmols per kilogram of water. Osmolality is the concentration of body fluids, i.e., electrolytes, BUN, glucose, etc.

osmolarity osmols or milliosmols per liter of solution.

osmosis the passage of a solvent through a partition from a solution of lesser solute concentration to one of greater solute concentration.

osmotic pressure the pressure or force that develops when two solutions are of different concentrations and are separated by a selectively permeable membrane.

otorrhea drainage from the ear.

over-needle catheter an infusion device designed for short-term parenteral therapy (opposite of the INC). The bevel of the needle extends beyond the catheter, which is $1\frac{1}{4}$–8 inches in length. The needle is available in gauges of 8–22. It is more comfortable for the client. See also inside-needle catheter.

oxygenation the combination of oxygen in tissues and blood.

oxyhemoglobin hemoglobin carrying oxygen.

packed cells red blood cells (RBCs).

pallor or pallid pale.

PAP abbreviation for pulmonary artery pressure. It measures the pressure in the pulmonary artery.

paracentesis the surgical puncture of a cavity, e.g., abdomen.

parathyroid an endocrine gland secreting the hormone parathormone, which regulates calcium and phosphorus metabolism.

parenteral therapy introduction of fluids into the body by means other than the alimentary tract.

parietal lobe lobe on the side of the brain lying under the parietal bone.

patency the state of being opened.

PCWP abbreviation for pulmonary capillary wedge pressure. Its reading indicates the pumping ability of the left ventricle. Left ventricular end-diastolic pressure (LVEDP) is the best indicator of ventricular function. PCWP reflects LVEDP.

perfusion passing of fluid through body space.

pericardial sac fibroserous sac enclosing the heart.

pericarditis inflammation of the pericardium or the membrane that encloses the heart.

peristalsis wavelike movement occurring with hollow tubes such as the intestine for the movement of contents.

peritoneal cavity a lining covering the abdominal organs with the exclusion of the kidneys.

permeability capability of fluids and/or other substances, e.g., ions, to diffuse through a human membrane.

   selectively permeable membrane refers to the human membrane.

   semipermeable membrane refers to artificial membranes.

phlebitis inflammation of the vein.

physiologic pertaining to body function.

pitting edema see edema.

plasma intravascular fluid composed of water, ions, and colloid. Plasma is frequently referred to as serum.

plasmanate commercially prepared protein product used in place of plasma.

pleural cavity the space between the two pleuras.

pleurisy inflammation of the pleura or the membranes that enclose the lung.

polyionic many ions or ionic changes.

polyuria an excessive amount or discharge of urine.

pons that part of the brain that connects the cerebral hemispheres.

porosity the state of being porous.

portal circulation circulation of the blood through the liver.

postoperative following an operation.

potassium-sparing diuretics see diuretics.

potassium-wasting diuretics see diuretics.

prednisone synthetic hormonal drug resembling cortisone.

preload pressure of the blood that fills the left ventricle during diastole.

pressoreceptor sensory nerve ending in the aorta and carotid sinus, which when stimulated causes a change in the blood pressure.

pressure gradient the difference in pressure that makes the fluid flow.

proprioception awareness of one's movement and position in space.

protein nitrogenous compounds essential to all living organisms.

    plasma relates to albumin, globulin, and fibrinogen.
    serum relates to albumin and globulin.

pruritis itching

psychogenic polydipsia psychologic effect of drinking excessive amounts of water.

pulmonary artery pressure see PAP.

pulmonary capillary wedge pressure see PCWP.

pulmonary edema see edema.

pulse pressure the arithmetic difference between the systolic and diastolic blood pressure.

rales pertaining to rattle. It is the sound heard in the chest due to the passage of air through the bronchi, which contain secretions or fluid.

rationale the reason.

reabsorption the act of absorbing again an excreted substance.

refractory edema see edema.

retention retaining or holding back in the body.

reticular activating system alert awareness system of the brain formed from the thalamus, hypothalamus, and cortex.

rhinorrhea drainage from the nose.

sclerosis hardening of an organ or tissue.

selectively permeable membrane see permeability.

semi-Fowler's position 45° elevation.

semipermeable membrane see permeability.

sensible perspiration the loss of water on the skin due to sweat gland activity.

serous cavity a cavity lined by a serous membrane.

serum consists of plasma minus the fibrinogen. It is the same as plasma except that after coagulation of blood, the fibrinogen is removed. Serum is frequently referred to as plasma.

sign an objective indication of disease.

solute a substance dissolved in a solution.

solvent a liquid with a substance in solution.

specific gravity a weight of a substance, e.g., urin Water has a specific gravity of 1.000. The specif gravity of urine is higher.

steroid an organic compound. It is frequently referred t as an adrenal cortex hormone.

stress effect of a harmful condition or disease(s) affec ing the body.

stroke volume amount of blood ejected by the le ventricle with each contraction.

sympathetic nervous system a part of the auto nomic nervous system. It can act in an emergency.

symptom subjective indication.

tachycardia a fast heart beat.

TBSA abbreviation for total body surface area

tetany a nervous affection characterized by tonic spasms of muscles.

thrombophlebitis inflammation of a vein with a thrombus or a blood clot.

tonicity effect of fluid on cellular volume, i.e., electrolytes, BUN, glucose.

total parenteral nutrition (TPN) also known as hyperalimentation.

trade name the name given to a drug by its manufacturer.

transudation the passage of fluid through the pores of a membrane.

trauma an injury.

urea the final product of protein metabolism that is normally excreted by the kidneys.

uremia a toxic condition due to the retention of nitrogenous substances (protein by-products), such as urea, which cannot be excreted by the kidneys.

Valsalva maneuver procedure in which individual takes deep breath and bears down to increase intrathoracic pressure for prevention of air injection. Forced exhalation closes the glottis.

vasoconstriction decrease in size of a blood vessel.

vasodilation increase in size of a blood vessel.

vasogenic originating within the blood vessels.

vasomotor pertaining to the nerves having a muscular contraction or relaxation control of the blood vessel walls.

pressors drugs given to contract muscles of the blood vessel walls to increase the blood pressure.

a vessel carrying unoxygenated blood to the heart.

tilation the circulation of air.

lmonary the inspiration and expiration of air from the lungs.

ventricles the lower chambers of the heart.

venules minute veins moving from capillaries.

vertigo dizziness.

volatile acid acid excreted as a gas by the lungs.

winged-tip infusion device see butterfly.

References/Bibliography

Abraham, W. T., & Schriert, R. W. (1994). Body fluid volume regulation in health and disease. *Advances in Internal Medicine, 39,* 23–43.

American Burn Association. (1984). Guidelines for service standards and severity classification in the treatment burn injury. *Bulletin of the American College of Surgeons, 69*(10), 24–28.

American Nurses Association. (1991). *Standards of clinical nursing practice.* Kansas City: American Nurses Association.

Andrews, B. T. (1994). Fluid and electrolyte disorders in neurosurgical intensive care. *Neurosurgical Clinics of North America, 5*(4), 707–723.

Baird, S. B., McConkle, R., & Grant, M. (1996). *Cancer nursing: A comprehensive textbook.* Philadelphia: Saunders.

Barone, M. A. (Ed.). (1996). *The Harriet Lane handbook* (14th ed.). St. Louis: Mosby.

Baxter, C. R., & Waeckerle, J. F. (1988). Emergency treatment of burn trauma. *Journal of Trauma, 17,* 1305–131

Beckwith, N. (1987). Fundamentals of fluid resuscitation. *Nursing Life, 2*(3), 51–55.

Bezerra, J. A., Stathos, T. H., Duncan, B., Gaines, J. A., & Udall, J. N. (1992). Treatment of infants with acute diarrhea: What's recommended and what's practiced. *Pediatrics, 90,* 1–4.

Birney, M. H., & Penney, D. G. (1990). Atrial natriuretic peptide: A hormone with implications for clinical practice *Heart and Lung, 19*(2), 174–182.

Bloch, A. S. (1990). *Nutrition management of the cancer patient.* Rockville, MD: Aspen.

Bove, L. A. (1994). How fluids and electrolytes shift after surgery. *Nursing 1994, 24*(8), 34–39.

Brensilver, J. M., & Goldberger, E. (1996). *A primer of water, electrolyte, and acid-base syndromes* (8th ed.). Philadelphia: Davis.

Brown, R. G. (1993). Disorders of water *and* sodium balance. *Postgraduate Medicine, 93*(4), 227, 228, 231–234, 239–244.

Bryant, K. K. (1991). Burn trauma: The emergent phase of care. *Contemporary perspectives in trauma nursing.* An independent home study course for individual continuing education. Chicago: Forum Medicum.

Burgess, M. (1991). Initial management of a patient with extensive burn injury. *Critical Care Nursing Clinics of North America, 3*(2), 165–179.

Butts, E. E. (1987). Fluid and electrolyte disorders associated with diabetic ketoacidosis and hyperglycemic hyperosmolar nonketotic coma. *Nursing Clinics of North America, 22*(4), 827–836.

Cannon, P. J. (1989). Sodium retention in heart failure. *Cardiology Clinics, 7*(1), 49–59.

Carleton, S. C. (1995). Cardiac problems associated with burns. *Cardiology Clinics, 13*(2), 257–262.

Carpentito, L. J. (1997). *Nursing diagnosis application to clinical practice* (7th ed.). Philadelphia: Lippincott.

Cefalu, W. T. (1991). Diabetic ketoacidosis. *Critical Care Clinics, 7*(1), 89–107.

Chambers, J. K. (1987). Fluid and electrolyte problems in renal and urologic disorders. *Nursing Clinics of North America, 22*(4), 815–825.

Chernow, B., Bamberger, E., & Stoiko, M. (1989). Hypomagnesemia in patients in postoperative intensive care. *Chest, 95*(2), 391–396.

Christopher, K. L. (1980). The use of a model for hemodynamic balance to describe burn shock. *Nursing Clinics of North America, 15*(3), 617–627.

Clark, B. A., & Brown, R. S. (1995). Potassium homeostasis and hyperkalemic syndromes. *Endocrinology and Metabolism Clinics of North America, 24*(3), 573–591.

Clark, J. C., & McGee, R. N. (1992). *Core curriculum for oncology nursing.* Philadelphia: Saunders.

Cornell, S. (1997). Maintaining a fluid balance. *Advance for Nurse Practitioners, 5*(12), 43–44.

Coroenwald, S., Frogge, M. H., Goodman, M., & Yarbro, C. H. (1992). *Comprehensive cancer nursing review.* Boston: Jones & Bartlett.

Cunningham, S. G. (1982). Fluid and electrolyte disturbances associated with cancer and its treatment. *Nursing Clinics of North America, 17*(4), 579–591.

Davis, K. D., & Attie, M. F. (1991). Management of severe hypercalcemia. *Critical Care Clinics, 7*(1), 175–189.

Doran, A. (1992). S.I.A.D.D.: Is your patient at risk? *Nursing 92, 22*(6), 60–63.

Ebersole, P., & Hess, P. (1998). *Toward healthy aging: human needs and nursing response* (5th ed.). Baltimore: Mosby.

Faldo, L., & Kravitz, M. (1993). Management of acute burns and burn shock resuscitation. *AACN Clinical Issues in Critical Care Nursing, 4*(2), 351–366.

Felver, L., & Pendarvis, J. H. (1989). Electrolyte imbalances. *AORN Journal, 49*(4), 992–1005.

Foster, E. E., & Lefor, A. T. (1996). General management of gastrointestinal fistulas. *Surgical Clinics of North America, 76*(5), 1019–1033.

Freeman, B. I., & Burkart, J. M. (1991). Hypokalemia. *Critical Care Clinics, 7*(1), 143–153.

Fundamentals of fluid and electrolyte imbalances. (1982). Travenol Laboratories, Parenteral Products, Deerfield, IL.

German, K. (1987). Fluid and electrolyte problems associated with diabetes insipidus and syndrome of inappropriate antidiuretic hormone. *Nursing Clinics of North America, 22*(4), 785–795.

Gershan, J. A., Freeman, C. M., Ross, M. C., & members of the Research committee, Greater Milwaukee area chapter of the American Association of Critical Care Nurses. (1990). *Heart and Lung, 19*(2), 152–156.

Giesecke, A. H., Grande, C. M., & Whitten, C. W. (1990). Fluid therapy and the resuscitation of traumatic shock. *Critical Care Clinics, 6*(1), 61–71.

Guyton, A. C. (1989). *Textbook of medical physiology* (7th ed.). Philadelphia: Saunders.

Hecker, J. (1988). Improve techniques in IV therapy. *Nursing Times, 84*(34), 28–33.

Heitkemper, M. M., & Bond, E. (1988). Fluid and electrolytes: Assessment and interventions. *Journal of Enterostomal Therapy, 15*(1), 18–23.

Held, J. L. (1995). Correcting fluid and electrolyte imbalance. *Nursing 1995, 25*(4), 71.

Hollifield, J. W. (1989). Electrolyte disarray and cardiovascular disease. *American Journal of Cardiology, 63,* 21B–26B.

Innerarity, S., & Stark, J. (1997). *Fluid and electrolytes.* Springhouse, PA.: Springhouse.

Intravenous Nurses's Society. (1990). *Intravenous nursing standards of practice.* Belmont, ME: Intravenous Nurses's Society.

Jones, A. M., Moseley, M. J., Halfmann, S. J., Heath, A. H., & Henkelman, N. J. (1991). Fluid volume dynamics *Critical Care Nurse, 11*(4), 74–76.

Jones, D. H. (1991). Fluid therapy in the PACU. *Critical Care Nursing Clinics of North America, 3*(1), 109–130.

Kamel, K. S., Ethier, J. H., & Richardson, M. A. (1990). Urine electrolytes and osmolality: When and how to us them. *American Journal of Nephrology, 10*(2), 89–102.

Kamel, K. S., Magner, P. O. C., Ethier, J. H., & Halperin, M. L. (1989). Urine electrolytes in the assessment of extracellular fluid volume contraction. *American Journal of Nephrology, 9*(4), 344–347.

Karb, V. B. (1989). Electrolyte abnormalities and drugs which commonly cause them. *Journal of Neuroscience Nursing, 21*(2), 125–128.

Karch, A. (1998). *Nursing Drug Guide.* Philadelphia: Lippincott.

Kee, J. L. (1987). Potassium imbalance. *Nursing 1987, 17*(9), 32 K, M, P.

Kee, J. L. (1998). *Laboratory and diagnostic tests with nursing implications* (5th ed.). Stamford, CT: Appleton a Lange.

Kee, J. L., & Boyda, E. K. (1998). Knowledge base for patients with fluid, electrolyte, and acid-base imbalances F. D. Monahan & M. Neighbors (Eds.), *Medical-surgical nursing* (2nd ed., pp. 75–112). Philadelphia; Saunders.

Kehoe, C. (1991). Malignant ascites: Etiology, diagnosis, and treatment. *Oncology Nursing Forum, 18,* 523–530

Keyes, J. L. (1974). Blood-gas and blood-gas transport. *Heart and Lung, 3*(6), 945–954.

Keyes, J. L. (1976). Blood-gas analysis and the assessment of acid-base status. *Heart and Lung, 5*(2), 247–255.

King, C. R., Hoffart, N., & Murray, M. E. (1992). Acute renal failure in bone marrow transplantation. *Oncology Nursing Forum, 19,* 1327–1335.

Kleihenz, T. J. (1985). Preload and afterload. *Nursing 1985, 15*(5), 50–55.

Klemm, P. (1992). *Total nutritional admixture (TNA): Programmed instruction.* Baltimore: Johns Hopkins Hospital Department of Nursing.

Kokko, J. P., & Tanner, R. L. (1996). *Fluids and electrolytes* (3rd. ed.). Philadelphia: Saunders.

Kositzke, J. A. (1990). A question of balance, dehydration in the elderly. *Journal of Gerontologic Nursing, 16*(5), 4–11, 40–41.

Kravitz, M. (1993). Immune consequences of burn injury. *AACN Clinical Issues in Critical Care Nursing, 4*(2), 399–413.

Lancaster, L. E. (1987a). *Core curriculum for nephrology nursing.* Pitman, NJ: Jannetti, Anthony J.

Lancaster, L. E. (1987b). Renal and endocrine regulation of water and electrolyte balance. *Nursing Clinics of North America, 22*(4), 761–772.

Lancour, J. (1978). ADH and aldosterone: How to recognize their effects. *Nursing 1978, 8*(9), 36–41.

Leaf, A., & Cotran, R. (1985). *Renal pathophysiology* (3rd ed.). New York: Oxford University Press.

Levy, D. B., & Peppers, M. P. (1991). IV fluids used in shock. *Emergency, 23*(4), 22–26.

Lorenz, J. M. (1997). Assessing fluid and electrolyte status in the newborn. *Clinical Chemistry, 43*(1), 205–210.

Lueckenotte, A. G. (1996). *Gerontologic nursing.* St. Louis: Mosby.

Martin, R. Y., & Schrier, R. W. (1995). Renal sodium excretion and edematous disorders. *Endocrinology and Metabolism Clinics of North America, 24*(3), 459–475.

Mathenson, M. (1989). Intravenous therapy. *Critical Care Nurse, 9*(2), 21–34.

Matz, R. (1994). Parallels between treated uncontrolled diabetes and the refeeding syndrome with emphasis on fluid and electrolyte abnormalities. *Diabetes Care, 17*(10), 1209–1213.

McCance, K., & Huether, S. (1990). *Pathophysiology: The biologic basis for disease in adults and children.* St. Louis: Mosby.

McConnell, E. A. (1987). Fluid and electrolyte concerns in intestinal surgical procedures. *Nursing Clinics of North America, 22*(4), 853–859.

McDermott, K. C., Almadrones, L. A., & Bajorunas, D. R. (1991). The diagnosis and management of hypomagnesemia: A unique treatment approach and case report. *Oncology Nursing Forum, 18,* 1145–1152.

McFadden, M. E., & Gatoricos, S. E. (1992). Multiple systems organ failure in the patient with cancer, Part I: Pathophysiologic perspectives. *Oncology Nursing Forum, 19,* 719–727.

Meador, B. (1982). Cardiogenic shock. *RN, 45*(4), 38–42.

Medical Center of Delaware. (1992). *Calculating infusion rate.* Newark, DE: Medical Center Orientation Materials.

Metheny, N. (1996). *Fluid and electrolyte balance* (3rd ed.). Philadelphia: Lippincott.

Meyers, K. A., & Hickey, M. K. (1988). Nursing management of hypovolemic shock. *Critical Care Nursing Quarterly, 11*(1), 57–67.

Millam, D. (1991). Myths and facts . . . About IV therapy. *Nursing 91, 21*(6), 75–76.

Miller, C. A. (1990). *Nursing care of older adults: Theory and practice.* Glenview, IL: Scott Foresman/Little, Brown.

Moiser, L. C. (1991). Anaphylaxis: A preventable complication of home infusion therapy. *Journal of Intravenous Nursing, 14*(2), 108–112.

Mueller, K. D., & Boisen, A. M. (1989). Keeping your patient's water level up. *RN, 52*(7), 65–68.

Nanji, A. (1983). Drug-induced electrolyte disorder. *Drug Intelligence and Clinical Pharmacy, 17,* 175–185.

Narins, R. G. (1982). Diagnostic strategies in disorders of fluid, electrolyte and acid-base homeostasis. *American Journal of Medicine, 72,* 496–518.

Norris, M. K. (1989). Dialysis disequilibrium syndrome. Action stat! *Nursing 1989, 19*(4), 33.

O'Donnell, M. E. (1995). Assessing fluid and electrolyte balance in elders. *American Journal of Nursing, 95*(11), 40–45.

Olinger, M. L. (1989). Disorders of calcium and magnesium metabolism. *Emergency Medicine Clinics of North America, 7*(4), 795–819.

Oster, J. R., Reston, R. A., & Materson, B. J. (1994). Fluid and electrolyte disorders in congestive heart failure. *Seminar Nephrology, 14*(5), 485–505.

Otto, S. (1991). *Oncology nursing.* St. Louis: Mosby.

Peppers, M. P., Geheb, M., & Desai, T. (1991). Hypophosphatemia and hyperphosphatemia. *Critical Care Clinics, 7*(1), 201–213.

Perkin, R., & Levin, D. L. (1980). Common fluid and electrolyte problems in the pediatric intensive care unit. *Pediatric Clinics of North America, 27*(3), 567–586.

Poe, C. M., & Radford, A. L. (1985). The challenge of hypercalcemia in cancer. *Oncology Nursing Forum, 12*(6), 29–34.

Porth, C. M. (1998). *Pathophysiology* (4th ed.). Philadelphia: Lippincott.

Practice parameter: The management of acute gastroenteritis in young children. (1996). *Pediatrics, 97,* 424–436.

Price, C. (1989). Continuous renal replacement therapy, from a professional nursing perspective. *Nephrology News and Issues, 3*(7), 31–34.

Ragland, G. (1990). Electrolyte abnormalities in the alcoholic patient. *Emergency Medicine Clinics of North America, 8*(4), 761–771.

Robson, A. (1997). Parenteral fluid therapy. In R. Behrman (Ed.), *Nelson textbook of pediatrics* (14th ed. pp. 171–211). Philadelphia: Saunders.

Rose, B. D. (1997). *Clinical physiology of acid-base and electrolyte disorders* (5th ed.). New York: McGraw-Hill.

Ross Roundtable Report, 12th. (1992). Enteral nutrition support for the 1990's: Innovations in nutrition, technology and techniques. Columbus, OH: Ross Laboratories (Division of Abbott Laboratories).

Rutherford, C. (1989). Fluid and electrolyte therapy: Considerations for patient care. *Journal of Intravenous Nursing, 12*(3), 175–183.

Salem, M., Munoz, R., & Chernow, B. (1991). Hypomagnesemia in critical illness. *Critical Care Clinics, 7*(1), 225–247.

Samson, L. F., & Ouzts, K. M. (1996). Fluid and electrolyte regulation. In M. Curley, J. Smith, & P. Moloney-Harmon (Eds.), *Critical care nursing of infants and children* (pp. 385–409). Philadelphia: Saunders.

Schrier, R. W. (1997). *Renal and electrolyte disorders* (5th ed.). Boston: Little, Brown.

Shakir, K. M., & Amin, R. M. (1991). Hypoglycemia. *Critical Care Clinics, 7*(1), 75–87.

Smith, Z. H., & VanGeilick, A. J. (1992). Management of neutropenic enterocolitis in the patient with cancer. *Oncology Nursing Forum, 19,* 1337–1342.

Sommers, M. (1990). Rapid fluid resuscitation: How to correct dangerous deficits. *Nursing 1990, 20*(1), 52–6

Stein, J. H. (1988). Hypokalemia: Common and uncommon causes. *Hospital Practice,* March 30.

Sterns, R. H. (1991). The management of hyponatremic emergencies. *Critical Care Clinics, 7*(1), 127–141.

Szerlip, H., & Goldfarb, S. (1993). *Fluid and electrolyte disorders.* New York: Churchill Livingstone.

Terry, J. (1994). The major electrolytes. *Journal of Intravenous Nursing, 17*(5), 240–247.

Twombly, M. (1983). Shift to third space. *Monitoring fluid and electrolytes precisely: Nursing skillbook.* Horsha PA: Intermed Communications.

Valle, G. A., & Lemberg, L. (1988). Electrolyte imbalances in cardiovascular disease: The forgotten factor. *Heart and Lung, 17*(3), 324–329.

VanHook, J. W. (1991). Hypermagnesemia. *Critical Care Clinics, 7*(1), 215–223.

Votey, S. R., Peters, A. L., & Hoffman, J. R. (1989). Disorders of water metabolism: Hyponatremia and hypernatremia. *Emergency Medicine Clinics of North America, 7*(4), 749–765.

Waltman, N. L., Bergstrom, N., Armstrong, N., Norrell, K., & Braden, B. (1991). Nutritional status, pressure sore and mortality in elderly patients with cancer. *Oncology Nursing Forum, 18,* 867–873.

Watkins, S. L. (1995). The basics of fluid and electrolyte therapy. *Pediatric Annuals, 24*(1), 16–22.

Watson, J. E. (1987). Fluid and electrolyte disorders in cardiovascular patients. *Nursing Clinics of North America 22*(4), 797–803.

Wittaker, A. (1985). Acute renal dysfunction. *Focus on Critical Care, 12*(3), 12–17.

Wong, D. (1998). *Essentials of pediatric nursing* (4th ed.). Philadelphia: Mosby.

Wong, D. L. (1995). *Whaley & Wong's nursing care of infants and children* (5th ed.). St. Louis: Mosby.

Young, M. E., & Flynn, K. T. (1988). Third-spacing. When the body conceals fluid loss. *RN, 51*(8), 46–48.

Zalaga, G. P. (1991). Hypocalcemic crisis. *Critical Care Clinics, 7*(1), 191–199.

Zull, D. N. (1989). Disorders of potassium metabolism. *Emergency Medicine Clinics of North America, 7*(1), 771–793.

Index